Cerebrospinal Fluid Disorders

David D. Limbrick Jr. • Jeffrey R. Leonard
Editors

Cerebrospinal Fluid Disorders

Lifelong Implications

Springer

Editors
David D. Limbrick Jr.
Department of Neurological Surgery
Washington University School of Medicine
St. Louis Children's Hospital
St. Louis, MO
USA

Jeffrey R. Leonard
Nationwide Children's Hospital
Department of Neurosurgery
The Ohio State University College of Medicine
Columbus, OH
USA

ISBN 978-3-319-97927-4 ISBN 978-3-319-97928-1 (eBook)
https://doi.org/10.1007/978-3-319-97928-1

Library of Congress Control Number: 2018959740

This Springer imprint is published by the registered company Springer Nature Switzerland AG
The registered company address is: Gewerbestrasse 11, 6330 Cham, Switzerland

Preface

Disturbances in cerebrospinal fluid (CSF) physiology can occur at any stage across the lifespan, with clinical presentation, natural history, and neurological implications of pathology dependent upon patient age and etiology. While the result is often hydrocephalus, risk factors and biological mechanisms are myriad. In 2018 at least, treatment, however, remains relatively uniform: diversion of cerebrospinal fluid (CSF). While there have been advances in the gold standard treatment for hydrocephalus, the CSF shunt, technical advances in endoscopic third ventriculostomy (ETV) with or without adjuvant choroid plexus cauterization (CPC) have resulted in increased interest in and investigation of these procedures. As neurosurgical methods advance, it is best to view hydrocephalus—regardless of the age of onset—as a lifelong chronic problem. Even with optimal treatment, there remains neurological morbidity and mortality and a significant cost to the evolving healthcare system. Because of this, patients and their families demand rapid improvements in treatment methods for this challenging disease.

This text is designed to provide the current "state of the field" for CSF disorders that occur across the lifespan. The authors of the following chapters are true content experts and provide their accumulated knowledge, experience, and wisdom in addition to a thoughtful view forward. We begin with a discussion of the ventricles themselves, with changes in the ependyma that occur throughout development and as the brain matures and then ages. Pathophysiological changes and their role in hydrocephalus of various etiologies are considered. Alterations in CSF composition, physiology, and flow are also discussed in the context of neurodevelopment and neurodegeneration.

In recent years, we have come to a detailed understanding of the etiologies of hydrocephalus—congenital, acquired, and those observed in the aging brain. This book contains chapters that chronicle the rapidly evolving discoveries that identify the genetic basis of hydrocephalus. Considerable advances have been made in genetic etiologies, and, in many cases, these findings have provided insight into mechanisms underlying the pathogenesis of hydrocephalus. Novel methods in neuroimaging and biochemical biomarkers have also provided novel insights both into the disease itself and into its effects on the nervous system, from infancy through adulthood.

The most common cause of pediatric hydrocephalus in high-income countries is posthemorrhagic hydrocephalus, while globally, in low- and middle-income countries, postinfectious hydrocephalus predominates. Because of the relevance to public health, both of these disorders are considered in detail in the ensuing chapters. Likewise, full consideration is also given to hydrocephalus-associated spina bifida, which has taken on new significance in the era of fetal myelomeningocele repair and the emerging role of ETV in this setting.

While the causes of hydrocephalus in adults may differ from those that affect children, there is certainly overlap. For example, trauma and brain tumors may cause hydrocephalus in individuals of any age. Other etiologies may converge as well; though often noted in preterm infants (e.g., from hemorrhage in the immature germinal matrix), posthemorrhagic hydrocephalus occurs frequently in adults after subarachnoid hemorrhage or other common forms of intracranial hemorrhage. Perhaps the most vexing form of adult-onset hydrocephalus is idiopathic normal pressure hydrocephalus (iNPH). iNPH deserves special consideration, as its pathophysiology, diagnosis, and treatment remain controversial.

Though simple in principle, the management of hydrocephalus can be exceedingly difficult. Multiloculated hydrocephalus is notoriously challenging, often requiring multiple fenestration procedures and complex shunt configurations. Intracranial hypotension presents a different sort of challenge; the diagnosis and definition of a CSF leak may be more difficult than its treatment.

Over the past decade, there has been increasing emphasis on improving the quality and safety of neurosurgical care for hydrocephalus patients of all ages. Committed experts have built consortia to study hydrocephalus and conduct sophisticated clinical trials to help determine best practices. Others have worked to improve existing shunt designs and catheter components or to develop the next generation of devices to help neurosurgeons treat this chronic disease.

We would like to conclude by thanking each of the contributing authors for their commitment and their efforts in compiling this book. We hope that you find this collection valuable as you build your expertise in this complex disease and its treatment!

Sincerely,

St. Louis, MO, USA
Columbus, OH, USA

David D. Limbrick Jr.
Jeffrey R. Leonard

Contents

Contributors

Prince Antwi, BA Department of Neurosurgery, Yale School of Medicine, New Haven, CT, USA

Samuel R. Browd, MD, PhD Seattle Children's Hospital, University of Washington, Department of Neurological Surgery, Seattle, WA, USA

Shlomi Constantini, MD, MSc Dana Children's Hospital, Tel-Aviv Medical Center, Pediatric Neurosurgery, Tel Aviv, Israel

Michael C. Dewan, MD, MSCI Vanderbilt University Medical Center, Monroe Carell Jr. Children's Hospital at Vanderbilt, Department of Neurological Surgery, Nashville, TN, USA

William Dobyns, MD Department of Genetics, University of Washington, Center for Integrative Brain Research, Seattle Children's Research Institute, Seattle, WA, USA

Dan Doherty, MD, PhD Department of Pediatrics, University of Washington and Seattle Children's Hospital, Center for Integrative Brain Research, Seattle Children's Research Institute, Seattle, WA, USA

David L. Dornbos III, MD Department of Neurological Surgery, The Ohio State University Wexner Medical Center, Columbus, OH, USA

Per Kristian Eide, MD, PhD Oslo University Hospital – Rikshospitalet, Department of Neurosurgery, Oslo, Norway

Johannes Marthinus Nicolaas Enslin, BPhysT, MBChB, MMed, FCNeurosurg Red Cross Children's Hospital, Department of Neurosurgery, Cape Town, South Africa

Anthony Graham Fieggen, MBChB, MSc, MD, FCS(SA) Division of Neurosurgery, University of Cape Town, Department of Surgery, Cape Town, South Africa

Charuta Gavankar Furey, MD Department of Neurosurgery, Yale School of Medicine, New Haven, CT, USA

Thomas Garton, BS University of Michigan, Department of Neurosurgery, Ann Arbor, MI, USA

Maria Montserrat Guerra, PhD Instituto de Anatomía, Histología y Patología, Facultad de Medicina, Universidad Austral de Chile, Valdivia, Chile

Mark Halverson, MD Department of Radiology, Nationwide Children's Hospital, Columbus, OH, USA

Mark G. Hamilton, MDCM, FRCSC, FAANS Division of Neurosurgery, Department of Clinical Neuroscience, University of Calgary, Calgary, AB, Canada

Brian W. Hanak, MD University of Washington, Neurological Surgery, Seattle, WA, USA

Prashant Hariharan, MS, MEng Department of Chemical Engineering and Materials Science, Department of Biomedical Engineering, Wayne State University, Detroit, MI, USA

Carolyn A. Harris, PhD Department of Chemical Engineering and Materials Science, Department of Biomedical Engineering, Department of Neurosurgery, Wayne State University Medical School, Detroit, MI, USA

Jason S. Hauptman, MD, PhD Seattle Children's Hospital, University of Washington, Department of Neurosurgery, Seattle, WA, USA

Albert M. Isaacs, MD Division of Biology and Biomedical Sciences, Washington University in St. Louis, St. Louis, MO, USA

Division of Neurosurgery, Department of Clinical Neuroscience, University of Calgary, Calgary, AB, Canada

Evan J. Joyce, MD, MS University of Utah, Department of Neurological Surgery, Salt Lake City, UT, USA

Kristopher Thomas Kahle, MD, PhD Departments of Neurosurgery, Pediatrics, and Cellular and Molecular Physiology, Yale School of Medicine, New Haven, CT, USA

John R. W. Kestle, MD Primary Children's Hospital, University of Utah, Department of Neurosurgery, Salt Lake City, UT, USA

Abhaya V. Kulkarni, MD, PhD Division of Neurosurgery, Hospital for Sick Children, University of Toronto, Toronto, ON, Canada

Annie Laquerriere, MD, PhD Pathology Laboratory, Rouen University Hospital and Inserm Unit 1245, Team Genetics and Pathophysiology of Neurodevelopmental Disorders, IRIB, Rouen, France

Jeffrey R. Leonard, MD Nationwide Children's Hospital, Department of Neurosurgery, The Ohio State University College of Medicine, Columbus, OH, USA

David D. Limbrick Jr., MD, PhD Department of Neurological Surgery, Washington University School of Medicine, St. Louis Children's Hospital, St. Louis, MO, USA

William B. Lo, MBBChir, FRCS(SN), FEBNS Division of Neurosurgery, Hospital for Sick Children, University of Toronto, Toronto, ON, Canada

Barry R. Lutz, PhD Department of Bioengineering, University of Washington, Seattle, WA, USA

Francesco T. Mangano, DO Division of Pediatric Neurosurgery, Cincinnati Children's Hospital Medical Center, Department of Neurological Surgery, University of Cincinnati College of Medicine, Cincinnati, OH, USA

John M. McGregor, MD Department of Neurological Surgery, The Ohio State University Wexner Medical Center, Columbus, OH, USA

Jason Milton, DO, PharmD, MBA Department of Neurosurgery, OhioHealth, Columbus, OH, USA

Nicholas Musgrave, BS The Ohio State University Medical Center, Columbus, OH, USA

Robert P. Naftel, MD Monroe Carell Jr. Children's Hospital at Vanderbilt, Neurological Surgery, Division of Pediatric Neurosurgery, Nashville, TN, USA

Shahid M. Nimjee, MD, PhD Department of Neurological Surgery, The Ohio State University Wexner Medical Center, Columbus, OH, USA

Eduardo Ortega, MD Hospital Regional de Valdivia, Unidad de Neurocirugía, Instituto de Neurociencias Clínicas, Medical School, Valdivia, Chile

Smruti K. Patel, MD Division of Pediatric Neurosurgery, Cincinnati Children's Hospital Medical Center, Department of Neurological Surgery, University of Cincinnati College of Medicine, Cincinnati, OH, USA

Jonathan A. Pindrik, MD Division of Pediatric Neurosurgery, Department of Neurological Surgery, Nationwide Children's Hospital, The Ohio State University College of Medicine, Columbus, OH, USA

Ciarán J. Powers, MD, PhD Department of Neurological Surgery, The Ohio State University Wexner Medical Center, Columbus, OH, USA

Geir Ringstad, MD Oslo University Hospital – Rikshospitalet, Department of Radiology, Oslo, Norway

Jay Riva-Cambrin, MD, MSc, FRCS(C) Alberta Children's Hospital, Department of Clinical Neurosciences, Calgary, AB, Canada

Esteban M. Rodríguez, MD, PhD Instituto de Anatomía, Histología y Patología, Facultad de Medicina, Universidad Austral de Chile, Valdivia, Chile

Jonathan Roth, MD Dana Children's Hospital, Tel-Aviv Medical Center, Pediatric Neurosurgery, Tel Aviv, Israel

Varun Shah, BS The Ohio State University Medical Center, Columbus, OH, USA

Ammar Shaikhouni, MD, PhD Department of Neurological Surgery, The Ohio State University Wexner Medical Center, Columbus, OH, USA

H. Wayne Slone, MD Department of Radiology, The Ohio State University Wexner Medical Center, Columbus, OH, USA

Luke G. F. Smith, MD Department of Neurological Surgery, The Ohio State University Wexner Medical Center, Columbus, OH, USA

Eric Anthony Sribnick, MD, PhD Division of Neurosurgery, Nationwide Children's Hospital, Department of Neurosurgery, The Ohio State University College of Medicine, Columbus, OH, USA

Jennifer M. Strahle, MD Washington Univeristy in St. Louis, Department of Neurosurgery, St. Louis, MO, USA

Nathaniel Toop, MD Department of Neurological Surgery, The Ohio State University Wexner Medical Center, Columbus, OH, USA

Hannah Tully, MD, MSc Department of Neurology, University of Washington and Seattle Children's Hospital, Center for Integrative Brain Research, Seattle Children's Research Institute, Seattle, WA, USA

Shawn M. Vuong, MD Division of Pediatric Neurosurgery, Cincinnati Children's Hospital Medical Center, Department of Neurological Surgery, University of Cincinnati College of Medicine, Cincinnati, OH, USA

John C. Wellons III, MD, MSPH Monroe Carell Jr. Children's Hospital at Vanderbilt, Neurological Surgery, Division of Pediatric Neurosurgery, Nashville, TN, USA

William E. Whitehead, MD Texas Children's Hospital, Department of Neurosurgery, Houston, TX, USA

Michael A. Williams, MD Departments of Neurology and Neurological Surgery, University of Washington School of Medicine, Seattle, WA, USA

Patrick P. Youssef, MD Department of Neurological Surgery, The Ohio State University Wexner Medical Center, Columbus, OH, USA

Weihong Yuan, PhD Department of Radiology, University of Cincinnati, Cincinnati Children's Hospital Medical Center, Cincinnati, OH, USA

Part I

Normal and Abnormal CSF Physiology

Physiopathology of Foetal Onset Hydrocephalus

1

Esteban M. Rodríguez, Maria Montserrat Guerra, and Eduardo Ortega

Abbreviations

AQP4	Aquaporin 4
CSF	Cerebrospinal fluid
GW	Gestational week
NPC	Neural progenitor cell
NSC	Neural stem cells
SA	Sylvius aqueduct
SVZ	Subventricular zone
VZ	Ventricular zone

Balanced View of CSF Physiology

Aiming to a Balanced View of CSF Physiology

Several functions have been ascribed to the cerebrospinal fluid (CSF), including protection to the brain, excretion of metabolites, homeostasis of the brain chemical environment, and as a transport pathway between different brain areas [18, 80, 98, 108]. These various functions, coupled with its rapid turnover, perpetual formation,

E. M. Rodríguez (✉) · M. M. Guerra
Instituto de Anatomía, Histología y Patología, Facultad de Medicina,
Universidad Austral de Chile, Valdivia, Chile
e-mail: erodrigu@uach.cl

E. Ortega
Hospital Regional de Valdivia, Unidad de Neurocirugía, Instituto de Neurociencias Clínicas,
Medical School, Valdivia, Chile

D. D. Limbrick, J. R. Leonard (eds.), *Cerebrospinal Fluid Disorders*,
https://doi.org/10.1007/978-3-319-97928-1_1

and continuous circulation and absorption have led to consider the CSF as the "third circulation," as first referred to by Cushing [16].

For decades, the CSF was regarded as a water solution of ions and few other components, such as glucose and vitamins. The concept of waste drainage was also associated to the "physiology" of CSF. Furthermore, the functional significance of the complex structure of the ventricular and subarachnoid compartments and the multiple populations of cell types lining discrete areas of the ventricular walls were, and still are, overlooked or neglected.

When the cerebrospinal fluid-contacting neurons were discovered, the concept that the CSF could be a pathway for signal molecules started to develop. This idea was strongly substantiated by the demonstration that the choroid plexus is a true gland that, in addition to transport water and ions, it also has the capacity to transport peptides and proteins from blood to CSF and to synthesize and secrete into the CSF a series of biologically active molecules [14, 78, 98]. Although the series of peptides, proteins, and neurotransmitters detected in the CSF using different methods increased throughout three decades, it was the analysis by mass spectrometry that suddenly revealed the enormous complexity of the molecular composition of the CSF.

In recent years, the discovery of aquaporins and other water transporters, all highly selective for water molecules, has again moved the balance to the oversimplified view that CSF physiology refers almost exclusively to water exchange between brain compartments. The glymphatic concept emphasizes the transport of water and waste molecules from the brain parenchyma into subarachnoid space along perivascular pathways of the Virchow Robin spaces, overlooking the fact that this "brain parenchyma" refers to the most superficial region of the brain cortex. It is really disturbing when the physiology of CSF is only associated with the movement of water through the different brain compartment, what leads several authors to talk about CSF secretion when in actuality they are only referring to water transport, completely disregarding the rich heterogeneity of the ventricular walls (circumventricular organs included) and the wealth of signal molecules that use the CSF as a pathway.

The CSF as a Pathway for a Cross Talk Between Different Periventricular Regions

CSF proteomics is showing a wealth of over 200 proteins [113]. A long series of peptides and neurotransmitters are also present in the CSF. Some of these compounds move by bulk flow from the interstitial fluid of brain parenchyma, many are secreted by neurons, glia, and ependyma into the CSF, others are transported by specific transport systems from blood to ventricular CSF (choroid plexus) while a few of them originate from cells present in the CSF. For many of these compounds, CSF levels bear hardly any relationship to peripheral levels in the blood [98].

The long series of biologically active proteins, peptides, and neurotransmitters present in the CSF reach this fluid through different mechanisms: (1)

Neurotransmitters and their metabolites reach the CSF via the bulk flow of parenchymal fluid. (2) Regulated secretion into the CSF of biologically active compounds by the circumventricular organs (subcommissural organ, pineal gland, choroid plexuses, and median eminence), such as SCO-spondin, basic fibroblast growth factor, melatonin, transthyretin, transthyretin-T4 complex, transthyretin-T3 complex, nerve growth factor (NGF), transforming growth factor-β (TGFβ), vascular endothelial growth factor (VEGF), transferrin and vasopressin [28, 42, 43, 81]. (3) Selective and circadian regulated secretion by CSF-contacting neurons of serotonin and neuropeptides such vasopressin, oxytocin, and somatostatin [80, 99, 100]. (4) Transport of peripheral hormones through the choroid plexus. Most of the transported hormones, such as leptin, prolactin, and thyroxin, have specific targets, mostly the hypothalamus [14, 81]. The concentrations of these neuroactive compounds vary between locations, suggesting they are important for the changes in brain activity that underlie different brain states [98].

Furthermore, a series of findings indicate that cells forming the ventricular walls release into the CSF microvesicles containing signalling and intracellular proteins [13, 22, 32, 55, 96]. Harrington et al. [32] suggested that this bulk flow of nanostructures generates a dispersed signal delivery, of longer duration.

Thus, the early view that the CSF is a medium carrying brain-borne and blood-borne signals to distant targets within the brain [80] has largely been supported by numerous investigations [42, 45, 81, 108]. Worth mentioning here is the much neglected system of CSF-contacting neurons most likely playing receptive functions sensing CSF composition. Most of these neurons are bipolar with the dendritic process reaching the CSF and endowed with a 9 + 0 single cilium [100].

In brief, a good body of evidence is revealing that the dynamic and molecular composition of the CSF and, consequently, the CSF physiology is much more complex and fascinating than the simplistic view held for decades. Signal molecules, either specifically transported from blood to CSF or secreted into the CSF by a series of periventricular structures, use the CSF to reach their targets in the brain. This allows a cross talk between brain regions located beyond the blood-brain-barrier, thus keeping the brain milieu private [29, 98].

Changing of CSF Composition as It Moves Through the Ventricular System

The ventricular CSF changes its molecular composition as it unidirectionally moves through the various ventricular and subarachnoid compartments (Fig. 1.1a). The choroid plexus of the lateral ventricles, the interstitial fluid of the parenchyma surrounding these ventricles, and axon endings secreting into these cavities are the source of molecules forming this "first" fluid. At the third ventricle, new compounds are added to the CSF by hypothalamic neurons, the pineal gland, and the local choroid plexus [42, 69, 80]. When entering the Sylvius aqueduct (SA), the CSF is enriched by the secretion of the subcommissural organ [101] (Fig. 1.1a). Consequently, the CSF of the fourth ventricle is different as compared to that of the

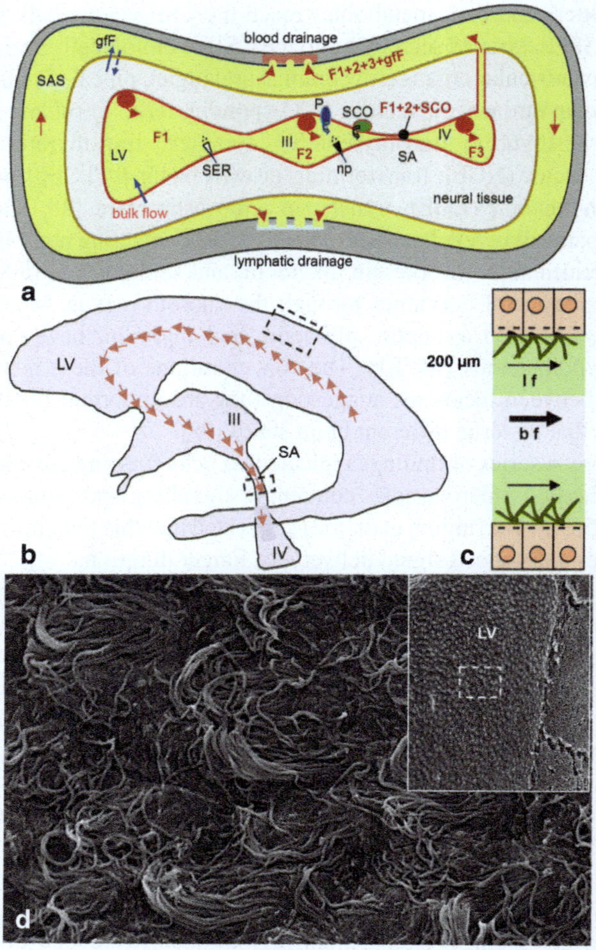

Fig. 1.1 (**a**) Line drawing depicting the changes in the CSF compositions as it moves throughout the lateral (LV), third (III) and fourth (IV) ventricles. F1 = CSF of the lateral ventricles contains molecules from the bulk flow of the parenchyma and compounds secreted by the choroid plexus and CSF-contacting neurons, such as serotonin (SER). F2 = CSF of the third ventricle contains F1 plus compounds secreted by the choroid plexus and hypothalamic CSF-contacting neurons (np, neuropeptides) and the pineal (P). SA = the Sylvius aqueduct contains F1 + F2 plus the secretion of the subcommissural organ (SCO). F3 = CSF of the fourth ventricle contains F1 + F2 + SA fluid plus compounds secreted by the choroid plexus and CSF-contacting neurons. The CSF of the subarachnoid space contains F1 + F2 + F3 plus molecules from the glymphatic flow (gfF) draining the most superficial region of the brain cortex. (**b**) Line drawing representing the laminar CSF flow (arrows) generated by the cilia beating. (**c**) Scheme representing the laminar (lf) and bulk (bf) of CSF though the Sylvius aqueduct (for orientation see rectangle in **b**). The broken line on top of ependymal cells depicts the negative charges from sialoglycoproteins of the glycocalix. (**d**) Scanning electron microscopy of the lateral wall of a normal rat showing the bundles of cilia of each cells beating in the same direction. *Inset.* Low SEM magnification of a lateral wall of a lateral ventricle (LV). Rectangle frames an area similar to that shown in **d**

lateral ventricles [113]. This partially explains the different protein composition between the CSF collected from the lateral ventricles and that obtained from a subarachnoid compartment [101].

Furthermore, at the interphase brain cortex/subarachnoid space there is a bidirectional flow of CSF and interstitial fluid along the large paravascular spaces that surround the penetrating arteries and the draining veins (Fig. 1.1a). Since water movement along this pathway is mediated by astroglial aquaporin-4 (AQP4) water channels, this paravascular pathway has been termed "glymphatic system" [35, 36]. This pathway facilitates efficient clearance of interstitial solutes, and its failure may lead to neurodegeneration [37].

Multiciliated Ependyma and CSF Flow

The mechanisms responsible for the CSF circulation are not fully understood. The following factors do play a role: (1) the hydrostatic difference between the production and drainage sites; (2) the pulsations of the cerebral arterial tree; (3) the directional beating of ependymal cilia [18, 106, 107]. The relative contribution of each of these forces is still controversial.

The flow of the CSF throughout the ventricular system involves two different mechanisms, the bulk flow and the laminar flow. Bulk flow is driven by arteriovenous pressure gradients and arterial pulsations. The laminar flow occurs in a thin layer along the walls in a variety of directions [98]. It has been shown that cilia beating is responsible for the laminar flow of CSF, whereas its role in the bulk of CSF taking place in the core of the ventricular cavities is probably insignificant [15, 59, 66, 106]. The cilia beating of the ependyma of the lateral ventricles generate currents as far as 200 μm away from the surface [66] (Fig. 1.1b–d). In the frog brain, about 75% of the CSF within the ventricles is mixed as a result of ciliary activity [66]. Ciliary currents adjacent to the ependyma have been observed in rats, dogs, and humans [109].

The ciliary beating is supported by a sialic acid-induced hydration mantle on the ependymal surface [98]. The frequency of cilia beating is stimulated by the activation of serotonin receptors [68]. Serotonin is released by axon terminals of the suprapendymal serotonergic plexus originated in raphe nuclei [12, 68, 102].

Using computational fluid dynamics, the relative impact of macroscale (choroid plexus pulsation and ventricular wall motion) and microscale (beating of cilia) effects on near-wall CSF dynamics has been investigated [95]. This study revealed a marked effect of the cilia on the near-wall dynamics and directionality but not on the bulk flow. Conversely, the bulk flow alone does not produce any notable directionality of the flow near or on the surface of the lateral ventricles. The authors concluded that in the lateral ventricles, near-wall CSF dynamics is dominated by ependymal cilia action [95]. This confirms early observations that the ciliary movement plays a key role in the maintenance of an adequate CSF flow [31, 109, 111]. The role of the multiciliated ependyma in CSF dynamics is strongly supported by the demonstration that primary cilia dyskinesia, a syndrome that impairs ciliary activity, leads to the development of hydrocephalus [2, 17, 27, 34, 50, 51, 97]. Shimizu and Koto [93] have suggested that immotility of cilia is of particular importance in narrow canals, such as the Sylvius aqueduct, for the development of hydrocephalus.

Human Ependymogenesis

The Wall of the Lateral Ventricles of the Human Developing Brain Is a Complex and Dynamic Mosaic

Very little, if any, attention has been paid to the complexity of the cell organization of different domains of the ventricular walls. To make it even more complex, such a mosaic undergoes changes during foetal development. This dynamic complexity of the ventricular walls partially resembles that of the ventricular walls of the rodent developing brain. During the last few day of foetal life, the medial wall of the lateral ventricles of the rat is already lined by multiciliated ependyma while the lateral and dorsal walls continue formed by neural stem cells (NSC) [29]. In human embryos, there is also an early division of labour between the medial and the latero-dorsal walls of the lateral ventricles [57]. Such a partition of labour seems an efficient design; while the latter is permanently involved in neurogenesis, the medial wall is progressively engaged in the flow of CSF. Indeed, coupled multiciliated ependymal cells generate the laminar flow of CSF [59, 66] that is essential for the CSF flow along the ventricular system (see above).

In the human developing telencephalon, ependymogenesis starts about the 18th gestational week (GW) (Fig. 1.2a) in the medial wall of the lateral ventricles and progressively continues through the lateral and then to the dorsal walls [57, 83]. Thus, in young foetuses, the lateral wall of the ventricle is fully involved in neurogenesis while the medial wall starts to change its role, from neurogenesis to ependymogenesis. In pre-term foetuses, while the medial wall is fully lined by multiciliated mature ependyma, the lateral wall has mixed populations of cells suggestive of neurogenesis and ependymogenesis.

Fig. 1.2 (**a**) Panel summarizing the timetable of key events in the developing human brain. The bulk of neural proliferation and neural migration occurs between 12 and 22 GW; then both processes decrease progressively. The process of ependymogenesis starts at about 18th GW and is completed after birth. Gliogenesis starts at about the 15th GW and continues for several months after birth. In the hydrocephalic, human brain disruption of the ventricular zone starts at about 17 GW (*red arrow*). (**b**, **c**) Photomicrographs of a hydrocephalic foetus (23 GW) illustrating the VZ formed by two types of cells: radial GFAP-positive cells (NSC) and radial GFAP/βIV-tubulin positive cells. The subventricular zone (SVZ) contains βIII-tubulin+ progenitor cells. (**d**) The VZ of a 31 GW hydrocephalic foetus appears formed by multiciliated βIV-tubulin+ ependyma (Ep). (**e**) Hydrocephalic HTx rat, PN7. Scanning electron microscopy of the dorsal wall of a lateral ventricle showing the disruption wave, leaving the subventricular zone nude. *Inset.* Similar region with double immunofluorescence for βIV-tubulin (multiciliated ependyma) and connexin 43 (gap junctions). (Source: **a**–**d** from [83])

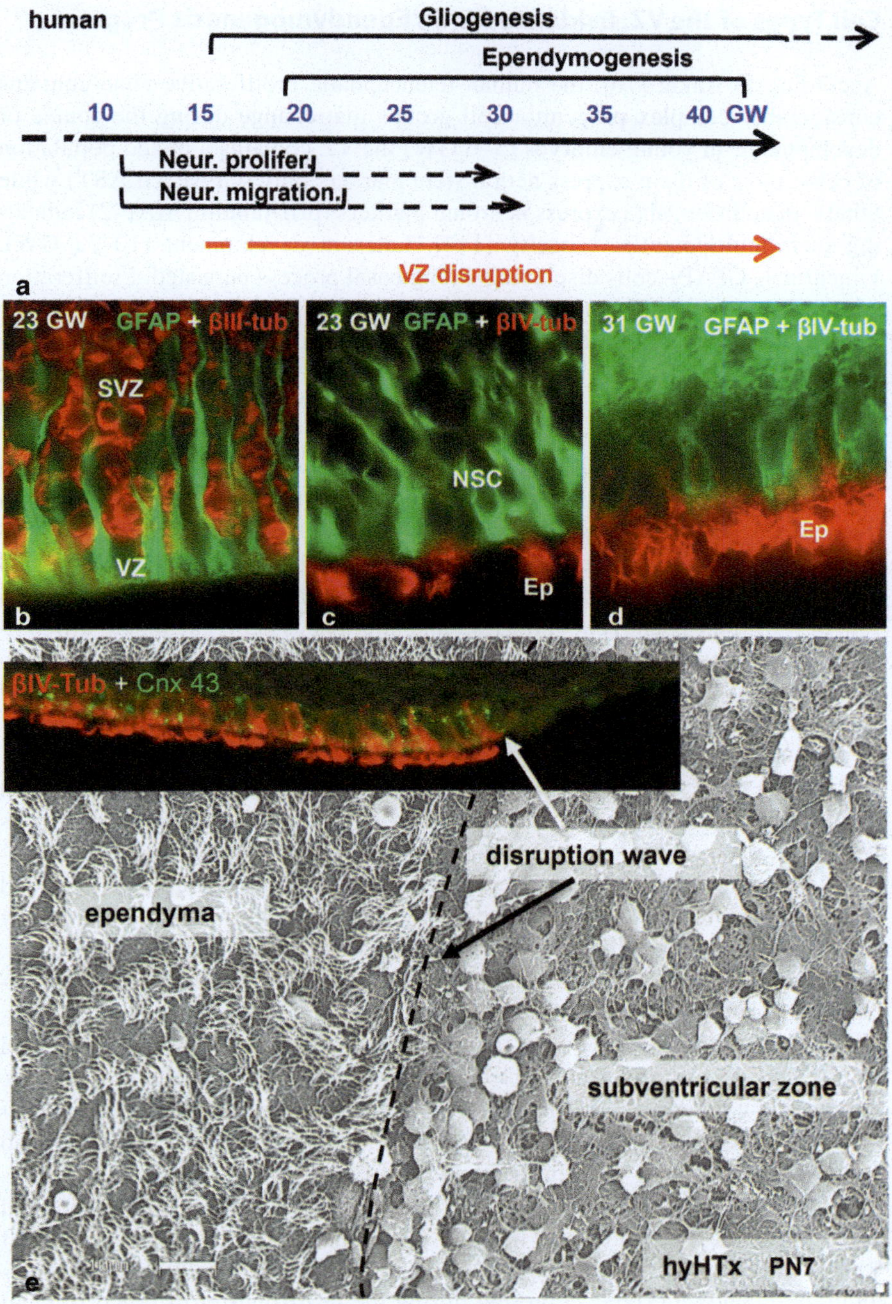

human
Gliogenesis
Ependymogenesis
10
15
20
25
30
35
40 GW
Neur. prolifer.
Neur. migration.
VZ disruption
a
23 GW GFAP + βIII-tub
SVZ
VZ
b
23 GW GFAP + βIV-tub
NSC
Ep
c
31 GW GFAP + βIV-tub
Ep
d
βIV-Tub + Cnx 43
disruption wave
ependyma
subventricular zone
hyHTx PN7
e

Cell Types of the VZ. Evidence for an Ependymogenesis Program

According to Rakic [76], the human telencephalic proliferative zone contains considerably complex progenitor cell groups that change during the course of development. In young embryos (5–6 GW) the VZ contains a mixed population of cells; most of them express neural stem markers only (GFAP, GLAST) while others, in addition, also express neuronal markers (βIII-tubulin, MAP-2) indicating their multipotential capacity [114]. Later in development (10–22 GW), vimentin +, GFAP+ cells displaying a long basal process persisted. Proliferation of GFAP+ cells of the ventricular zone (VZ) occurs until the 23rd GW, coinciding with the formation of the ependyma [114]. According to Gould et al. [26], in early pregnancy, the VZ is formed by GFAP+ radial glia/neural stem cells, whereas in late pregnancy, the VZ is formed by GFAP+ ependymal cells with a short basal process,

By use of several markers, Sarnat [85, 86, 88] has followed in human foetuses the temporal and spatial differentiation of cells lining the ventricular walls. In these studies, Sarnat has regarded as ependyma all cells lining the foetal ventricular system. Using this criterion, he concluded that the expression of GFAP and vimentin in foetal ependymal cells follows a regional and temporal distribution [85, 86], with the ependyma of the roof and floor plates being the first to differentiate. During several gestational weeks, GFAP is co-expressed with vimentin in most foetal ependymal cells. At birth, only scattered ependymal cells of the lateral ventricles still express GFAP, and it disappears entirely within the first few weeks of postnatal life [88].

The true process of ependymogenesis in the human remains largely unknown due, to a great extent, to limitations to obtain samples of the ventricular walls from systematically selected regions and selected gestational ages, and to process these samples for different methods. A recent investigation has provided some new evidence on ependymogenesis [57]. Based on the immunoreactivity to GFAP, AQP4, βIV-tubulin, and βIII-tubulin, their morphology (basal process, one or multiple cilia) and their spatial and temporal distribution, we have distinguished seven cell types in the VZ of the lateral ventricles of human foetuses [57, 83]. Type 1 cells with a long radial process, expressing AQP4 in the plasma membrane domain and GFAP throughout the cytoplasm, displaying a single cilium, is the main cell type in the VZ of young foetuses and most likely correspond to NSC (Fig. 1.2b). Type 2 cells are identical to type 1 cells but also express βIV-tubulin, a well-known marker of multiciliated ependyma, suggesting they correspond to NSC that have started to differentiate into ependymal cells (Fig. 1.2c). Cells type 3 through 6 would reflect progressive stages of ependymal differentiation ending in the differentiated multiciliated, βIV-tubulin+, ependyma (type 7) present during the last trimester of foetal life and throughout adulthood (Fig. 1.2d).

Hydrocephalus

A Concept

Foetal-onset hydrocephalus is a heterogeneous disease. Genetic and environmental factors, such as vitamin B or folic acid deficiency [40], viral infection of ependyma [44], and prematurity-related germinal matrix and intraventricular haemorrhage [7], contribute to its occurrence.

Numerous investigations in humans and mutant animals have substantiated the view that hydrocephalus is not only a disorder of CSF dynamics but also a brain disorder, and that derivative surgery does not resolve most aspects of the disease [46]. Actually, 80–90% of the neurological impairment of neonates with foetal onset hydrocephalus is not reversed by derivative surgery. *How can we explain the inborn and, so far, irreparable neurological impairment of children born with hydrocephalus?* In 2001, Miyan and his co-workers asked a key question [60]: "Humanity lost: the cost of cortical maldevelopment in hydrocephalus. Is there light ahead?" Although this appealing question has not been responded, there is some light in the horizon. A strong body of evidence indicates that the common past of hydrocephalus and brain maldevelopment starts early in the embryonic life with the disruption of the ventricular (VZ) and subventricular (SVZ) zone. However, the nature, mechanisms, and extent of the brain impairment linked to hydrocephalus are far from been fully unfolded. Certainly, a better treatment of hydrocephalus and the associated neurological impairment will come from a better understanding of the biological basis of the brain abnormalities in hydrocephalus [19, 105]. This view may represent one of the "lost highways" in hydrocephalus research, as described by Jones and Klinge [46].

To have clarity of the timetable of neurogenesis and ependymogenesis in normal rodents and humans seems essential for a better understanding of the early events occurring in foetal onset hydrocephalus.

Prenatal Neurogenesis. Timetable of Neural Proliferation and Migration, Gliogenesis, and Ependymogenesis

Virtually, all cells of the developing mammalian brain are produced in two germinal zones that form the ventricular walls, the VZ and the SVZ [6, 8, 25, 58, 39, 53]. The VZ is a pseudostratified neuroepithelium that contains multipotent radial glia/stem cells, hereafter called neural stem cells (NSC). NSC line the ventricular lumen and through a long basal process reach the pial surface. A landmark of NSC is their primary cilia that project to the ventricle and are bathed by the foetal CSF [47, 64]. During a fixed period of brain development, NSC divide asymmetrically, with one daughter cell remaining as a NSC and the other becoming a neural progenitor cell (NPC). NPC proliferate and cluster underneath the VZ, forming the so-called

SVZ. NPC differentiate into neuroblasts that start migration using the basal process of NSC as scaffold. In the human, the bulk of neural proliferation and neuroblast migration occurs at a rather short period, between GW 12 and 18 (Fig. 1.2a).

Gliogenesis starts at about the 15th GW and continues for several months after birth. Ependymal cell differentiation starts at about the 18th GW and is completed after birth (Fig. 1.2a) [83, 85, 86].

Over the years, based on our own and other investigators' evidence, we have progressively come to the view that a *disruption of the VZ and SVZ*, in most cases due to genetic defects, triggers onset of congenital hydrocephalus *and* abnormal neurogenesis (Fig. 1.2a, c). We will discuss this evidence below.

Brain Damage Versus Brain Defects

A distinction must be made between (1) brain *maldevelopment* due to a primary pathology of the VZ that precedes or accompanies onset of hydrocephalus and (2) brain *damage* caused by hydrocephalus. The former occurs during development, and consequently neonates *are born* with a neurological deficit. Brain *damage* is mainly a postnatal acquired defect, essentially caused by ventricular hypertension and abnormal CSF flow and composition.

Brain damage may be associated to regional ischemia, disruption of white matter pathways, and alteration of microenvironment of neural cells [19, 20]. Derivative surgery, the almost exclusive treatment of hydrocephalus today, is aimed to prevent or diminish brain *damage*. It is clear that hydrocephalic patients improve clinically after surgery due to correction of intracranial pressure, improvement in white matter blood flow [19], and probably to resumption of the clearance role of CSF. However, *derivative surgery does not reverse the inborn brain defects*. This has led a study group on hydrocephalus to conclude that "Fifty years after the introduction of shunts for the treatment of hydrocephalus, we must acknowledge that the shunt is not a cure for hydrocephalus" [5].

Ventricular Zone Disruption

A Concept and Definitions

For clarity purposes, we shall define the terms used in the present chapter to refer to the ventricular zone. At stages of development when the VZ is mostly formed by neural stem cells (NSC), the acronym VZ will be used. When the VZ is mostly or exclusively formed by multiciliated ependymal cells, the term "ependyma" will be used. The terms "denudation," "disruption," or "loss" will be alternatively used to refer to the disassembling, disorganization, or loss of the VZ cells [81]. A solid body of evidence indicates that radial glial cells are neural stem cells. Throughout the present text, we shall use the term neural stem cells, and its acronym NSC, to refer to the cells forming the embryonic ventricular zone, characterized by a long basal process, a single 9 + 0 cilium projecting to the ventricle and by expressing certain markers such a nestin [57].

In mutant animals, the disruption of the VZ follows a program that has temporal and spatial patterns, progressing as a "tsunami" wave running from caudal to rostral regions of the developing ventricular system, leaving behind a severe damage (Fig. 1.2e) [29, 41, 74, 81, 103]. A similar process of VZ disruption occurs in human hydrocephalic foetuses [21, 29, 82, 83, 94]. Since the VZ disruption is a continuous process, starting during the embryonic life and continuing during the first postnatal week, the pathology first affects NSC, then the NSC differentiating into ependymal cells and finally the differentiated multiciliated ependyma. These three cell types have distinct phenotypes and certainly play quite different roles. What do they have in common so that the denudation wave will hit them all? Junction proteins appear to be the key to understanding this devastating phenomenon [29].

A Stormy Intracellular Traffic of Junction Proteins in NSC and Ependymal Cells Leads to Ventricular Zone Disruption

What is the molecular mechanism underlying the VZ disruption occurring in human hydrocephalic foetuses, the HTx rat and in various mutant mice developing hydrocephalus? Overall, a series of findings indicates that disruption of VZ arises from a final common pathway involving alterations of vesicle trafficking, abnormal cell junctions, and loss of VZ integrity [23, 38, 48, 52, 77]. The abnormal localization of N-cadherin and connexin 43 in NSC and ependymal cells and the formation of subependymal rosettes suggest that VZ disruption results from a defect in cell polarity and in cell–cell adhesion of VZ cells. The accumulation of N-cadherin and connexin 43 in the soon-to-detach VZ cells and their virtual absence from the plasma membrane indicate that they are synthesized by the disrupting cells but are not properly transported to the plasma membrane (Fig. 1.3a–d) [29]. The mechanism actually involved in this abnormal expression and translocation of N-cadherin is unknown. The specific disruption of N-cadherin-based junctions is enough to induce ependymal disruption. Indeed, antibodies against chicken N-cadherin injected into the CSF of chick embryos disrupt the VZ, lead to denudation of the SVZ and formation of periventricular rosettes [24]. Similarly, the use of N-cadherin antibodies or synthetic peptides harbouring a cadherin-recognition sequence triggers the detachment of ependymal cells from explants of the dorsal wall of the bovine Sylvius aqueduct [71]. The abnormal localization of connexin 43 in the NSC and ependymal cells could be associated to the faulty localization of N-cadherin. Indeed, it has been reported that gap junction proteins are delivered to the plasma membrane at adherent junction sites [90].

In mutant mice, several gene mutations leading to abnormal trafficking of junction proteins and resulting in VZ disruption have been reported [11, 38, 41, 48, 52, 54, 91]. The nature of the genetic defect in hydrocephalic patients [21, 72, 94] is unknown. It may be postulated that they all carry a defect at one or another point of the pathways assembling adherent and gap junctions.

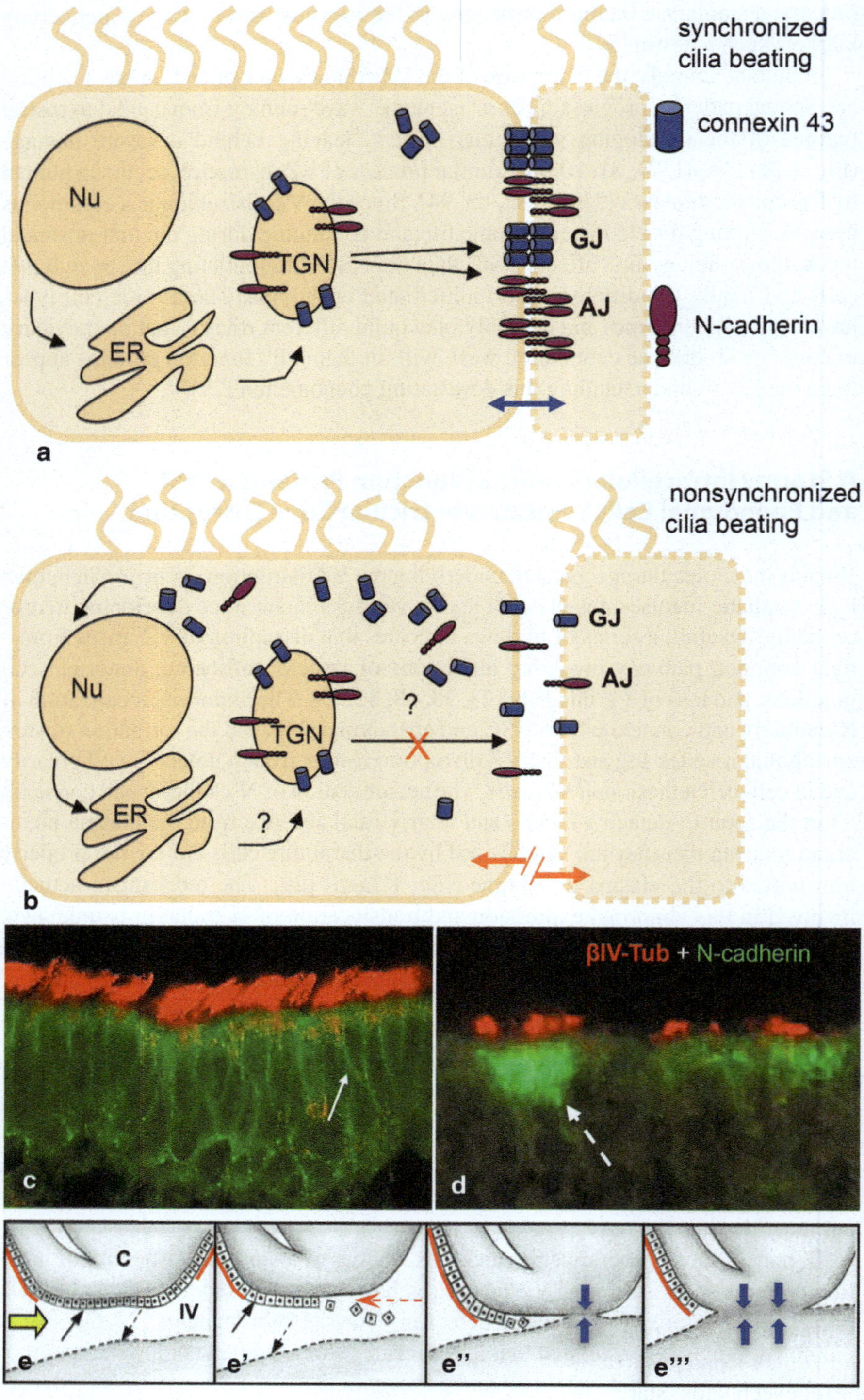
synchronized
cilia beating
connexin 43
Nu
TGN
ER
GJ
AJ
N-cadherin
a
nonsynchronized
cilia beating
Nu
TGN
ER
GJ
AJ
?
?
b
βIV-Tub + N-cadherin
c
d
C
IV
e
e'
e''
e'''

Fig. 1.3 Proposed mechanisms underlying ependymal denudation and abnormal CSF flow in the Sylvius aqueduct of spina bifida aperta (SBA) patients. The ependyma of the Sylvius aqueduct (SA) of control foetuses display a normal expression and a normal transport to the plasma membrane of the junction proteins N-cadherin and connexin 43 (**a**). This results in normal gap (GJ) and adherent (AJ) junctions. In the SA of SBA patients, N-cadherin and connexin 43 are expressed but their transport to the plasma membrane is impaired. N-cadherin and connexin 43 are abnormally accumulated in the cytoplasm, whereas functional adherent and gap junctions fail (**b**). All together, this may induce: (i) ependymal denudation, aqueduct stenosis, and CSF obstruction; (ii) nonsynchronized cilia beating, abnormal CSF flow, and may finally contribute to (iii) hydrocephalus. ER, rough endoplasmic reticulum; Nu, cell nucleus; TGN, trans-Golgi network. (**c, d**) Pallium of a human hydrocephalic foetus showing zones lined by normal (**c**) or abnormal (**d**) ependyma. In areas of intact ependyma, N-cadherin is localized at the plasma membrane (**c**, full arrow). Close to the disruption front, ependymal cells displayed abnormal expression of N-cadherin (**d**, broken arrows). (**e–e‴**). In *hyh* mice, disruption of the VZ lining the ventral wall of the aqueduct occurs during early foetal life (**e**, broken line). Disruption of the dorsal wall of aqueduct occurs shortly after birth (**e′**, red arrow). Then the ventral and dorsal denuded walls fuse, leading to aqueduct obliteration (**e″**, **e‴**, arrows) and hydrocephalus. (Source: **a, b** from [94]; **c, d** from [29]; **e–e″** modified after [103])

Nongenetic mechanisms leading to VZ disruption have to be considered also [92, 112]. In fact, lysophosphatidic acid, a blood-borne factor found in intraventricular haemorrhages, binds to receptors expressed by the VZ cells resulting in abnormal N-cadherin trafficking, VZ disruption, and hydrocephalus [112]. The vascular endothelial growth factor is elevated in the CSF of patients with hydrocephalus, and when administered into the CSF of normal rats, it causes alterations of adherent junctions, ependyma disruption, and hydrocephalus [92]. Thus, the possibility that signals from the hydrocephalic CSF may contribute, or even trigger VZ disruption, has to be kept in mind. Furthermore, it should be kept in mind that foetal CSF is the internal milieu of NSC [42]. Interestingly, the CSF of hydrocephalic HTx rats has an abnormal protein composition that contribute to the abnormal neurogenesis occurring in this mutant [56, 61, 62, 101].

Temporal and Spatial Programs of VZ Disruption

The process of VZ disruption has temporal and spatial patterns. The temporal program implies that disruption starts when the VZ is formed by NSC and finishes when the VZ is formed by multiciliated ependyma. In the mean time, a progressive transition from NSC to multiciliated ependyma occurs. The spatial program discloses that disruption begins in caudal regions of the ventricular system and progresses rostrally to reach the lateral ventricles [41, 74, 103]. Each of the two programs has its own outcomes.

In the temporal program, the early VZ disruption implies the loss of NSC and abnormal neurogenesis, while the late VZ disruption results in the loss of multiciliated ependyma and alterations in the laminar flow of CSF and hydrocephalus [29, 94]. In the *hyh* mutant mouse, the program is turned on at E12 and turned off by the end of the second postnatal week [41, 74, 103]. In the HTx mutant rat, disruption in the telencephalon starts at E19 and finishes at the first postnatal week [29].

In hydrocephalic foetuses, disruption of the VZ in the telencephalon has been shown as early as 16 GW [21, 29].

In the spatial program, the disruption of the VZ of the SA implies aqueduct stenosis/obliteration, alteration of the laminar, and bulk flow of CSF and hydrocephalus. At variance, the disruption of the VZ of the telencephalon leads to abnormal neurogenesis [29, 83].

With the years and based on solid evidence, we have progressively come to the conclusion that *foetal onset hydrocephalus and abnormal neurogenesis are two inseparable phenomena, because they are linked at the etiological level.*

In the pathophysiologic programs of VZ disruption, the loss of NSC and ependyma occurs in *specific regions* of the SA and ventricular walls, and also at *specific stages* of brain development. This explains why only certain brain structures have an abnormal development, which in turn results in a specific neurological impairment.

Pathophysiology of Foetal Onset Hydrocephalus

The Complex Cell Organization of the Walls of the Sylvius Aqueduct

The walls of the Sylvius aqueduct of wild-type *hyh* mice are formed by several populations of ependymal cells [103]. Interestingly, in mutant hydrocephalic *hyh* mice, some of these ependymal populations undergo proliferation, others are resistant to denudation whereas others denude [4, 74, 103]. In full-term human foetuses, the dorsal, lateral, and ventral walls of the SA three populations of ependymal cells have been described [94]. The functional significance of three ependymal populations is unclear. However, in spina bifida aperta foetuses, there seems to be an association between ependymal lineages of SA and the observed SA pathology. The ependymal cells lining the ventral wall display a normal subcellular distribution of N-cadherin and connexin 43; these cells do not detach. At variance, the ependymal cells of the lateral SA walls display an abnormal intracellular location of junction proteins and are likely to undergo denudation. The formation of large rosettes is mostly associated to this ependyma [94].

Ventricular Zone Disruption in the Sylvius Aqueduct, Aqueduct Stenosis/Obliteration, and Noncommunicating Hydrocephalus

In the *hyh* mouse, a programmed disruption of the VZ of the ventral wall of the SA starts early in foetal life (E12.5) and *precedes* the onset of a moderate communicating hydrocephalus. The loss of the ependyma of the dorsal wall of the SA occurring shortly after birth leads to fusion of the denuded ventral and dorsal walls of SA, resulting in aqueduct obliteration and severe hydrocephalus (Fig. 1.3e–e′′′) [41, 74, 103]. The phenomenon of VZ denudation associated with the onset of hydrocephalus has also been found in other mutant mice [38, 48, 52, 65, 77].

In human hydrocephalic foetuses, ependymal denudation of SA precedes and probably triggers the onset of hydrocephalus [21, 72, 94]. It can be postulated, on solid grounds, that a primary alteration of the VZ of the aqueduct due to various genetic defects triggers the onset of congenital hydrocephalus.

Ventricular Zone Disruption in the Sylvius Aqueduct, Loss of Multiciliated Ependyma and Communicating Hydrocephalus

In full-term human foetuses and in the perinatal period of mice the SA is mostly lined by multiciliated ependymal cells [94, 103]. The disruption occurring in this period in hydrocephalic humans and mutant mice implies the loss of multiciliated ependyma. Prior to denudation, the abnormal ependymal cells display abnormalities in the amount and subcellular distribution of N-cadherin and connexin 43 (Fig. 1.3) [94]. Since connexin 43 and N-cadherin co-assemble during their traffic to the plasma membrane [104], the abnormal formation of adherent junctions would also result in abnormal gap junctions. Thus, defects of adherent junctions between ependymal cells in hydrocephalic foetuses could alter gap junction-dependent ependymal physiology prior to, or in the absence of, ependymal disruption. An alteration of the CSF laminar flow through the SA of human hydrocephalic foetuses could be envisaged, even if denudation is confined to small areas of the aqueduct wall and hydrocephalus courses with a patent aqueduct (Fig. 1.3a, b). This could be part of the mechanism resulting in a communicating hydrocephalus.

At Late Gestational Stages, the Disruption in the Ventricular Zone of the Telencephalon Leads to the Loss of Multiciliated Cells and Likely Alterations in the Laminar CSF Flow

The disruption wave starting in the fourth ventricle, after a few days, reaches the telencephalon; then it continues along the walls of the lateral ventricles following a fixed route but avoiding certain discrete regions that are disruption resistant. This phenomenon occurs in certain mutant animals [41, 103] and part or most of it also occurs in human hydrocephalic foetuses [21, 29] and in premature hydrocephalic foetuses with intraventricular haemorrhage [57].

Ciliary beating of ependymal cells is responsible, at least in part, for the laminar flow of CSF occurring on the ventricular surface (see above). Long ago, Worthington and Cathcart [109] concluded that in humans, small areas of ependymal injury and ciliary destruction may affect CSF flow far beyond the region of local damage. During the third trimester of gestation, VZ disruption occurring in hydrocephalic foetuses and in cases with posthaemorrhagic hydrocephalus leaves large areas of the ventricular walls denuded [21, 29, 57]. It seems likely that these local disturbances may impair laminar CSF flow and contribute to the development of hydrocephalus.

Abnormal Neurogenesis Linked to Foetal Onset Hydrocephalus

Disruption of the Ventricular Zone of the Telencephalon Is Associated to Abnormal Neurogenesis

In human hydrocephalic foetuses [21, 29], premature infants with posthaemorrhagic hydrocephalus [57], the HTx rat [29] and the *hyh* mouse [23], the VZ disruption results in two neuropathological events: formation of periventricular heterotopias and translocation of NSC/NPC to the CSF (Fig. 1.4a–d).

At regions of disruption where NSC have been lost, the neuroblasts generated in the SVZ no longer have the structural scaffold to migrate and consequently accumulate in periventricular areas forming periventricular heterotopias. In human hydrocephalic foetuses, periventricular heterotopias have been found in young (21 GW) and full-term (40 GW) foetuses, indicating that they were formed early in development and had remained in situ until the end of foetal life and, probably, after birth (Fig. 1.4a, b). Interestingly, a 2-month-old child with a disrupted VZ carried periventricular heterotopias [23]. Humans with disruption in the VZ of the telencephalon carry periventricular heterotopias primarily composed of later-born neurons [23]. Periventricular heterotopias behave as epileptogenic foci [30]. This may explain why 6–30% of hydrocephalic children, including the present case, develop epilepsy that is not solved by CSF drainage surgery [72, 89].

The Cerebrospinal Fluid Is the Main Fate of the Disrupting NSC/NPC

In hydrocephalic human foetuses [21, 29] and premature infants with posthaemorrhagic hydrocephalus [49], NSC/NPC reach the ventricle at sites of VZ disruption and can be collected from the CSF. Furthermore, cells collected from CSF of two SBA foetuses develop into neurospheres [83].

hydrocephalic foetus, 40 GW, with a large denuded area covered by a layer of glial fibrillary acidic protein (GFAP) positive astrocytes. Periventricular heterotopias (PH) are associated with disruption of the VZ. (**c**) In the HTx rat, disruption of the VZ results in shedding of proliferative neural progenitor cells into the CSF, as shown by injection of BrdU in living animals and tracking the BrdU+ cells in tissue sections (**c**, arrow) and CSF cell pellets (**d**). βIII-tubulin+ or nestin+ cells are present in the cell pellet (**d**). (**e**, **f**) Under proper culture conditions, cells grow forming neurospheres displaying a similar junction pathology than hydrocephalic living animals. In neurospheres from non-affected HTx rat, N-cadherin is located at the plasma membrane (**e**); in neurospheres from hydrocephalic CSF N-cadherin accumulates in the cytoplasm (**f**). (**g**) Line drawing depicting the pathology of ventricular zone (VZ). Whereas disruption in the aqueduct of Sylvius leads to hydrocephalus, VZ disruption in the telencephalon results in abnormal neurogenesis. A cell junction pathology appears to be a final common pathway of multiple genetic and environmental factors that finally result in the disruption of the VZ. (Source: **a**–**g** from [29])

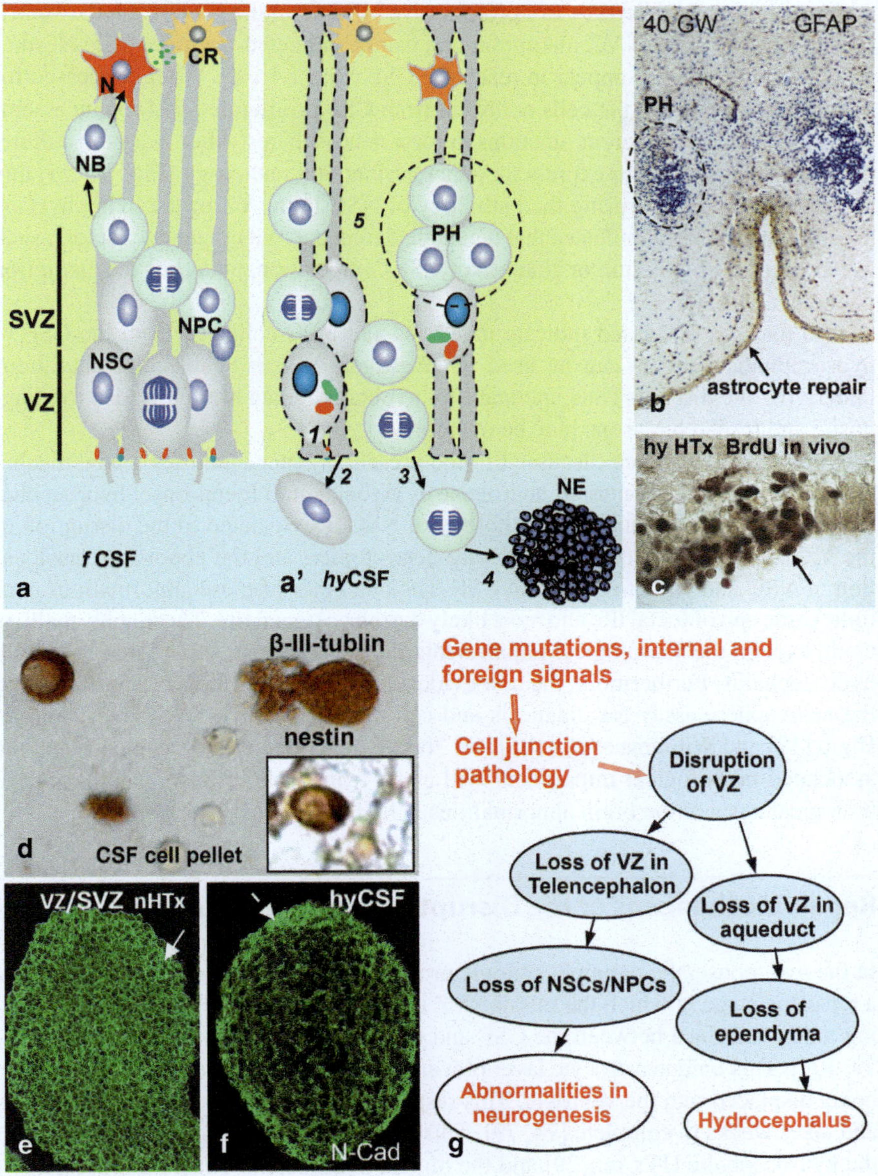

Fig. 1.4 Neuropathological events associated to the disruption of the ventricular zone in the telencephalon. (**a**, **a′**) Line drawings depicting the pathology. (**a**) Neural stem cells (NSC) in the ventricular zone (VZ) proliferate to raise proliferative neural progenitor cells (NPC), which migrate as neuroblasts (NB) along radial processes of NSC and differentiate into neurons (N). NSC are joined by adherent and gap junctions. CR, Cajal-Retzius cell; fCSF, foetal cerebrospinal fluid; SVZ, subventricular zone. (**a′**) Disruption of the VZ results in displacement of NSC [1] and NPC [2] into the CSF [3]. These cells can be collected from the CSF of hydrocephalic rats and cultured. They develop abnormal neurospheres [4]. The absence of the scaffold provided by NSC results in arrested neuroblasts that form periventricular heterotopias (PH) [5]. (**b**) Telencephalon of a human

In the hydrocephalic HTx rat, proliferative NPC from the SVZ reach the ventricle through the sites of VZ disruption and can be collected from the CSF. Nestin+ NSC from the VZ also appear to reach the CSF (Fig. 1.1c, d). When processed for the neurosphere assay, the cells collected from CSF proliferate and become assembled again through adherent junctions to form neurospheres. After 2 days in culture, the neurospheres start to express an adherent junction pathology (Fig. 1.4e, f) and become disrupted, mirroring the pathology of NSC in the VZ of the living hyHTx. This finding strongly indicates that a genetic defect and not epigenetic factors, such as increased CSF pressure or changes of CSF composition, underlies the disruption phenomenon.

The findings discussed indicate that NSC and NPC collected from the CSF of hydrocephalic patients can be used to investigate cell and molecular alterations underlying the disease. Thus, the inability to obtain human brain biopsies for diagnostic and research reasons may be overcome.

In brief, the evidence discussed in the present chapter identifies a new mechanism underlying the abnormal neurogenesis associated to foetal-onset hydrocephalus (Fig. 1.4g). A cell junction pathology of NSC is associated to the disruption of the VZ, the formation of periventricular heterotopias, and the abnormal translocation of NSC and NPC to the foetal CSF. The outcomes of these abnormalities continue to the end of foetal life and most likely during postnatal life. These abnormalities could explain the neurological impairments, such as epilepsy, of children born with hydrocephalus. Furthermore, the new evidence also provides the basis for the use of the neurosphere assay for diagnosis and cell therapy [29, 83]. We agree with Del Bigio [19] and Williams et al. [105] that "better treatment of hydrocephalus and the associated neurological impairment will come from a better understanding of the biological basis of the brain abnormalities in hydrocephalus."

Repair Mechanisms of the Disrupted Ventricular Zone

In the *hyh* mouse, the pathophysiologic program leading to hydrocephalus includes a repairing stage in which the missing VZ is replaced by a layer of astrocytes forming a new interface between the CSF and the brain parenchyma (Fig. 1.5a–c) [74, 79, 103]. This unique astrocyte layer prevents the NPC still present in the SVZ from being displaced into the ventricle. This response occurs shortly after VZ disruption and takes weeks to complete [74, 79]. This phenomenon has also been described in the hydrocephalic HTx rat [29] and the human hydrocephalic foetuses [21, 29, 57, 87, 94].

The astrocytes re-populating the denuded areas are different from astrocytes of the normal brain parenchyma and from reactive astrocytes found after brain injury. They share several cytological features with multiciliated ependyma and similar para-cellular and intra-cellular routes of transport of cargo molecules moving between CSF, the subependymal neuropile and the pericapillary space (Fig. 1.5a–c) [79]. How do astrocytes arriving at the denuded ventricular surface become arranged into a compact cell layer? In the *hyh* mice, the numerous interdigitations between the cell bodies of astrocytes and the dense network formed by their processes might explain the stability of this newly formed cell layer (Fig. 1.5b, c) [79]. What are the signals mediating this response? In *hyh* mice and human hydrocephalic foetuses, VZ disruption takes place at prenatal stages previous to a detectable hydrocephalus. Therefore, intraventricular pressure or expanding ventricles cannot be considered responsible for the denudation of the VZ or its repairing by astrocytes [79].

In *hyh* mice, the periventricular astrocyte reaction appears at stages when ventriculomegaly is starting to develop. The most robust astrocyte layer occurs in the denuded floor of the fourth ventricle, a cavity displaying a minor dilatation [79]. What are the physiopathological consequences for the brain of the assembly of a compact layer of astrocytes replacing the lost ependyma? This is an important question open to investigation. Still, there are already some clues. Astrocytes replacing the denuded ependyma have a high expression of AQP4 and a high endocytosis and transcytosis activity, suggesting they function as a new CSF–brain interphase involved in water and solute transport, contributing to re-establish some of the functions of the lost ependyma [79].

Interestingly, the disruption of the VZ that occurs in foetal life of the hydrocephalic HTx rat and the repairing astrocyte mechanisms occurring postnatally is followed by a second disruption process, this time affecting the astroglial layer. The outcome of this new disruption is the massive translocation of neurons into the ventricle [73]. This second and devastating disruption process observed in 1-month-old rats could be part of the mechanism leading to death.

Cell Therapy in the Horizon

Once establishing that foetal-onset hydrocephalus and abnormal neurogenesis are two inseparable phenomena turned on by a cell junction pathology first affecting NSC/NPC and later the multiciliated ependyma; the grafting of stem cells into hydrocephalic foetuses appears as a valid therapeutic task to repair the VZ disruption and its outcomes.

Growing evidence has shown that stem cell transplantation represents a great opportunity for the treatment of many neurological diseases. Stem cells used for transplantation into the central nervous system (CNS) include mesenchymal stem cells (MSC) [84], NSC [3, 9], and NPC [70, 110]. In most of the early investigations, the stem cells were grafted in the vicinity of the injured or altered neural tissue. However, delivery of stem cells into the CSF is emerging as an alternative, particularly for those diseases with a broad distribution in the central nervous system [3, 67, 75, 110]. A key question whether the hydrocephalic CSF would be a friendly medium to host grafted NSC has been recently solved. When neurospheres obtained from non-affected HTx rats are further cultured in the presence of CSF from hydrocephalic HTx rats, neural stem cells differentiate into neurons, astrocytes, and ependyma [33].

On-going experiments in our laboratory grafting normal neurospheres into the lateral ventricle of hydrocephalic HTx rats has shown that 48 hs after

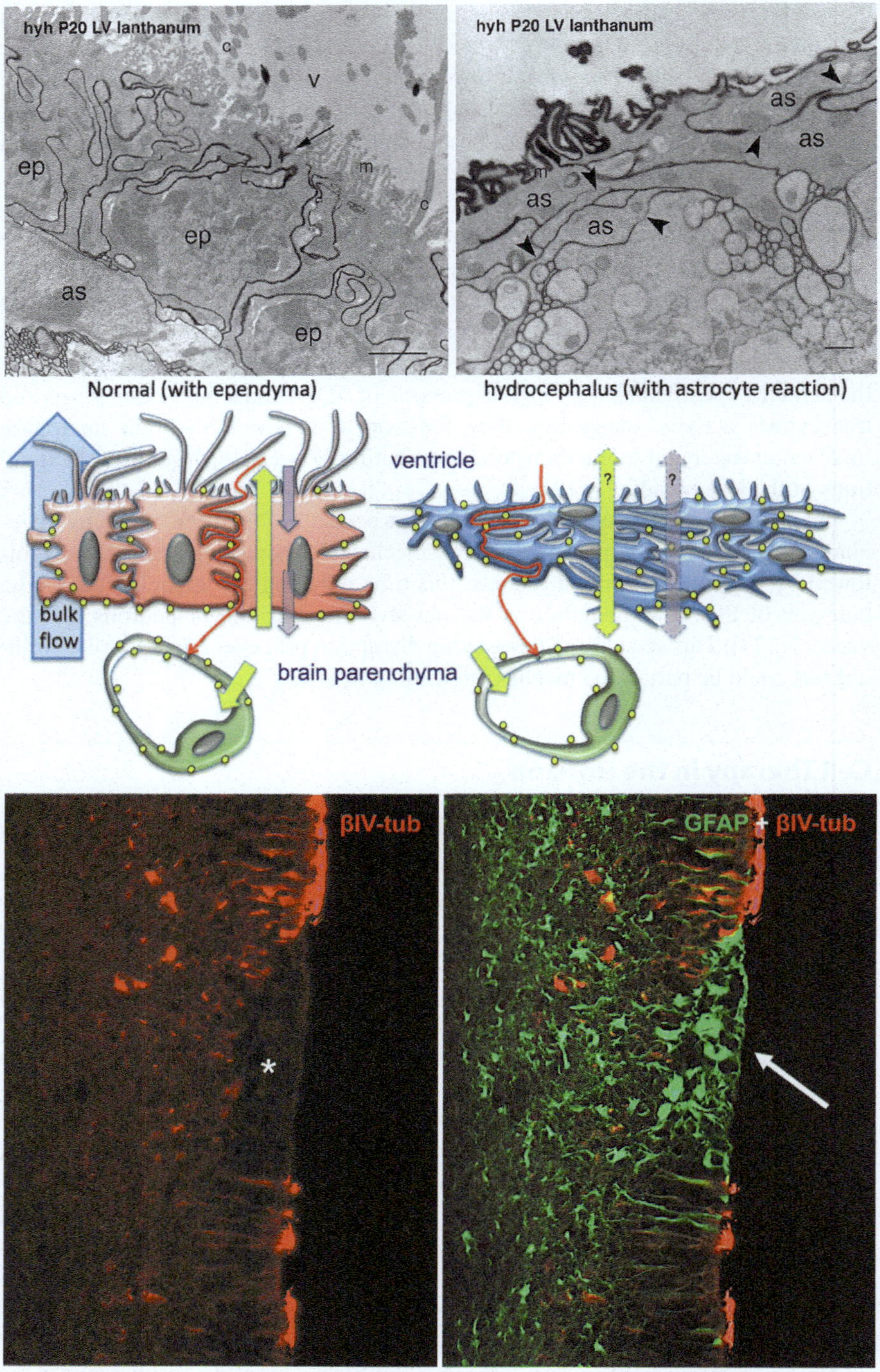
hyh P20 LV lanthanum
ep
ep
as
ep
hyh P20 LV lanthanum
as
as
as
as
Normal (with ependyma)
hydrocephalus (with astrocyte reaction)
ventricle
bulk flow
brain parenchyma
βIV-tub
GFAP + βIV-tub

Fig. 1.5 (**a**) Lanthanum nitrate applied into the lateral ventricle of a P20 *hyh* mouse penetrates from the lateral ventricle (V, arrow) toward the brain parenchyma through the winding extracellular spaces of the denudation-resistant, ciliated ependyma (ep). (**b**) In the astrocyte layer (as) lining the denuded ventricular surface of a *hyh* mouse, the tracer penetrates through the extracellular spaces and bypasses the gap junctions joining the astrocytes (arrowheads). **c**, cilia; m, microvilli. (**c**) Representation of the transcellular and paracellular transport mechanisms that would operate at the ependyma and at the layer of repairing astrocytes. In the ependymal cells of wt mice (left), most aquaporin 4 (yellow dots) is located at the basolateral domains, suggesting that the ependyma transports water from the brain parenchyma (bottom) toward the ventricular CSF (upper) (thick arrow across the ependyma). There is pinocytosis and transcytosis directed in the opposite direction through this barrier (purple arrow). In *hyh* mouse (right), a layer of astrocytes covering the denuded surface express aquaporin 4 throughout the cell body and processes (yellow dots) and could be involved in water transport from or to the CSF (double-headed yellow arrow). Pinocytosis in the astrocytes would also operate in both directions (double-head purple arrows). The ependymal and the astrocyte barriers would transport molecules from the CSF to the brain parenchyma through a paracellular route (winding red arrows). (**d**, **d′**). Disruption process affecting the VZ and SVZ of preterm neonates with intraventricular hemorrhage. The VZ formed by multiciliated cells also undergoes disruption (**d**, asterisk); the disrupted foci are sealed by a layer of GFAP+ astrocytes (**d′**, arrow). (Source: **a**–**c** from [79]; **d**, **d′** from [57])

transplantation, the grafted NSC moves *selectively* to the area devoid of VZ, proliferate, and differentiate into patches of multiciliated ependyma; a second subpopulation move into the cerebral cortex. According to our current investigations, it seems likely that the new multiciliated ependyma formed after NSC grafting would help the laminar flow of CSF and, consequently, attenuate the hydrocephalus condition. If NSC grafting results in a functional recovery of the neurological deficit of the rats born with hydrocephalus is under research.

Toward the frontier of the bed side The isolation and expansion of NSC of human origin are crucial for the successful development of cell therapy approaches in human brain diseases. A relevant step forward has been achieved by scientists of the Neuroscience Center of Lund (Sweden) who developed an immortal neural stem cell line and have standardized a protocol to obtain neurospheres from foetal striatum-derived neural stem [10, 63]. An additional key point to consider is the time and opportunity when NSC should be transplanted. It seems reasonable to suggest that NSC grafting should be performed shortly after the disruption process of the VZ had been turned on. In human hydrocephalic foetuses, VZ disruption starts at about the 16th GW and continues throughout the second and third trimester of pregnancy (see above). The opportunity for transplantation may be the foetal surgery performed to repair neural tube defects, such as spina bifida aperta, that is performed within a well-defined gestational period (19th–25th GW) [1]. It may be hoped that grafting of stem cells into the hydrocephalic brain would result in the repopulation of the disrupted areas of the VZ and/or the generation of a protective microenvironment to diminish/prevent the outcomes of VZ disruption. (Fig. 1.6).

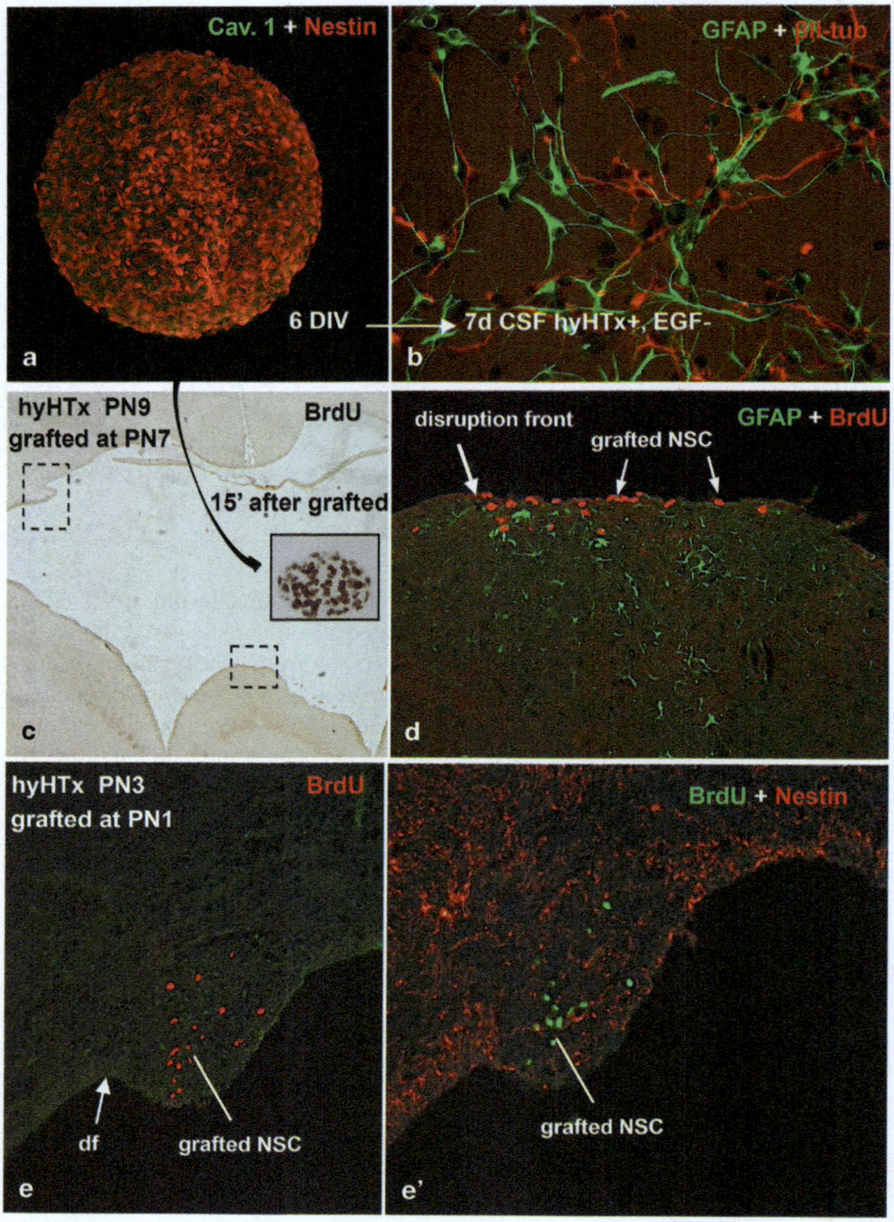

Fig. 1.6 Neural stem cells grafted into the cerebrospinal fluid (CSF) of a hydrocephalic HTx rat move selectively to the disrupted areas of the ventricular zone (VZ). (**a**) Neurosphere after 6 days in culture immunostained for nestin. (**b**) In the presence of hydrocephalic CSF and devoid of epidermal growth factor, neural stem cells differentiate into βIII-tubulin+ neurons and GFAP+ astrocytes. (**c–e′**) Grafting of neurospheres obtained from a non-affected HTx rat on postnatal day 1 (PN1) to PN1 and PN7 hydrocephalic HTx rats. Grafted neurospheres were labelled with BrdU during the last 24 h in culture. (**c**) 15 min after grafting neurospheres remain proliferative and free inside the dilated lateral ventricles *(inset)*. (**d–e′**) Two days after grafting, neurospheres disassemble and the NSC move selectively to the disrupted areas of the VZ. df, disruption front. (Source: **a–e′** from [83])

References

1. Adzick NS, Thom EA, Spong CY, Brock JW, Burrows PK, Johnson MP, Howell LJ, Farrell JA, Dabrowiak ME, Sutton LN, Gupta N, Tulipan NB, D'Alton ME, Farmer DL, Investigators MOMS. A randomized trial of prenatal versus postnatal repair of myelomeningocele. N Engl J Med. 2011;364:993–1000.
2. Afzelius BA. The immotile-cilia syndrome: a microtubule-associated defet. CRC Crit Rev Biochem. 1985;19:63–87.
3. Bai H, Suzuki Y, Noda T, Wu S, Kataoka K, Kitada K, Ohta M, Chou H, Ide C. Dissemination and proliferation of neural stem cells on injection into the fourth ventricle of the rat: a transplantation. J Neurosci Methods. 2003;124:181–7.
4. Bátiz LF, Páez P, Jiménez AJ, Rodríguez S, Wagner C, Pérez-Fígares JM, Rodríguez EM. Heterogeneous expression of hydrocephalic phenotype in the *hyh* mice carrying a point mutation in alpha-SNAP. Neurobiol Dis. 2006;23:152–68.
5. Bergsneider M, Egnor MR, Johnston M, Kranz D, Madsen JR, JP MA 2nd, Stewart C, Walker ML, Williams MA. What we don't (but should) know about hydrocephalus. J Neurosurg. 2006;104:157–9.
6. Bonfanti L, Peretto P. Radial glial origin of the adult neural stem cells in the subventricular zone. Prog Neurobiol. 2007;83:24–36.
7. Boop FA. Posthemorrhagic hydrocephalus of prematurity. In: Cinalli C, Maixner WJ, Sainte-Rose C, editors. Pediatric hydrocephalus. Milan: Springer-Verlag; 2004.
8. Brazel CY, Romanko MJ, Rothstein RP, Levison SW. Roles of the mammalian subventricular zone in brain development. Prog Neurobiol. 2003;69:49–69.
9. Buddensiek J, Dressel A, Kowalski M, Runge U, Schroeder H, Hermann A, Kirsch M, Storch A, Sabolek M. Cerebrospinal fluid promotes survival and astroglial differentiation of adult human neural progenitor cells but inhibits proliferation and neuronal differentiation. BMC Neurosci. 2010;11:48.
10. Cacci E, Villa A, Parmar M, Cavallaro M, Mandahl N, Lindvall O, Martinez-Serrano A, Kokaia Z. Generation of human cortical neurons from a new immortal fetal neural stem cell line. Exp Cell Res. 2007;313:588–601.
11. Chae TH, Kim S, Marz KE, Hanson PI, Walsh CA. The *hyh* mutation uncovers roles for Snap in apical protein localization and control of neural cell fate. Nat Genet. 2004;36:264–70.
12. Chan-Paly V. Serotonin axons in the supra- and subependymal plexuses and in the leptomeninges; their roles in local alterations of cerebrospinal fluid and vasomotor activity. Brain Res. 1976;102:103–30.
13. Chiasserini D, van Weering JR, Piersma SR, Pham TV, Malekzadeh A, Teunissen CE, de Wit H, Jiménez CR. Proteomic analysis of cerebrospinal fluid extracellular vesicles: a comprehensive dataset. J Proteome. 2014;106:191–204.
14. Chodobski A, Szmydynger-Chodobska J. Choroid plexus: target for polypeptides and site of their synthesis. Microsc Res Tech. 2001;52:865–82.
15. Cifuentes M, Rodríguez S, Pérez J, Grondona JM, Rodríguez EM, Fernández-Llebrez P. Decreased cerebrospinal fluid flow through the central canal of the spinal cord of rats immunologically deprived of Reissner's fibre. Exp Brain Res. 1994;98:431–40.
16. Cushing H. Studies in intracranial physiology and surgery: the third circulation, the hypophysis, the gliomas. Serie: Cameron-prize lecture. London: H. Milford, Oxford University Press; 1926.
17. Davis RE, Swiderski RE, Rahmouni K, Nishimura DY, Mullins RF, Agassandian K, Philp AR, Searby CC, Andrews MP, Thompson S, Berry CJ, Thedens DR, Yang B, Weiss RM, Cassell MD, Stone EM, Sheffield VC. A knockin mouse model of the Bardet-Biedl syndrome 1 M390R mutation has cilia defects, ventriculomegaly, retinopathy, and obesity. Proc Natl Acad Sci U S A. 2007;104:19422–7.
18. Davson H, Segal MB. Physiology of the CSF and blood–brain barriers. Boca Raton: CRC Press; 1995.

19. Del Bigio MR. Pathophysiologic consequences of hydrocephalus. Neurosurg Clin N Am. 2001;12:639–49.
20. Del Bigio MR. Neuropathology and structural changes in hydrocephalus. Dev Disabil Res Rev. 2010;16:16–22.
21. Domínguez-Pinos MD, Páez P, Jiménez AJ, Weil B, Arráez MA, Pérez-Fígares JM, Rodríguez EM. Ependymal denudation and alterations of the subventricular zone occur in human fetuses with a moderate communicating hydrocephalus. J Neuropathol Exp Neurol. 2005;64:595–604.
22. Feliciano DM, Zhang S, Nasrallah CM, Lisgo SN, Bordey A. Embryonic cerebrospinal fluid nanovesicles carry evolutionarily conserved molecules and promote neural stem cell amplification. PLoS One. 2014;9(2):e88810.
23. Ferland RJ, Bátiz LF, Neal J, Lian G, Bundock E, Lu J, Hsiao YC, Diamond R, Mei D, Banham AH, Brown PJ, Vanderburg CR, Joseph J, Hecht JL, Folkerth R, Guerrini R, Walsh CA, Rodríguez EM, Sheen VL. Disruption of neural progenitors along the ventricular and subventricular zones in periventricular heterotopia. Hum Mol Genet. 2009;18:497–516.
24. Ganzler-Odenthal SI, Redies C. Blocking N-cadherin function disrupts the epithelial structure of differentiating neural tissue in the embryonic chicken brain. J Neurosci. 1998;18:5415–25.
25. Götz M, Huttner WB. The cell biology of neurogenesis. Nat Rev Mol Cell Biol. 2005;6:777–88.
26. Gould SJ, Howard S, Papadaki L. The development of ependyma in the human fetal brain: an immunohistological and electron microscopic study. Dev Brain Res. 1990;55:255–67.
27. Greenstone MA, Jones RWA, Dewar A, Neville BGR, Cole PJ. Hydrocephalus and primary ciliary dyskinesia. Arch Dis Child. 1984;59:481–2.
28. Gross PM. Circumventricular organs and body fluids, Vol. I, II, and III. Boca Raton: CRC Press; 1987.
29. Guerra M, Henzi R, Ortloff A, Lichtin N, Vío K, Jimémez A, Dominguez-Pinos MD, González C, Jara MC, Hinostroza F, Rodríguez S, Jara M, Ortega E, Guerra F, Sival DA, den Dunnen WFA, Pérez-Figares JM, McAllister JP, Johanson CE, Rodríguez EM. Cell junction pathology of neural stem cells is associated with ventricular zone disruption, hydrocephalus, and abnormal neurogenesis. J Neuropathol Exp Neurol. 2015;74:653–71.
30. Guerrini R, Barba C. Malformations of cortical development and aberrant cortical networks: epileptogenesis and functional organization. J Clin Neurophysiol. 2010;27:372–9.
31. Hagenlocher C, Walentek P, M Ller C, Thumberger T, Feistel K. Ciliogenesis and cerebrospinal fluid flow in the developing Xenopus brain are regulated by foxj1. Cilia. 2013;2:12.
32. Harrington MG, Fonteh AN, Oborina E, Liao P, Cowan RP, McComb G, Chavez JN, Rush J, Biringer RG, Huhmer AF. The morphology and biochemistry of nanostructures provide evidence for synthesis and signaling functions in human cerebrospinal fluid. Cerebrospinal Fluid Res. 2009;6:10.
33. Henzi R, Guerra M, Vío K, González C, Herrera C, McAllister JP, Johanson C, Rodríguez EM. Neurospheres from neural stem/neural progenitor cells (NSPC) of non-hydrocephalic HTx rats produce neurons, astrocytes and multiciliated ependyma. The cerebrospinal fluid of normal and hydrocephalic rats supports such a differentiation. Cell Tissue Res. 2018;373:421–38.
34. Ibañez-Tallon I, Pagenstecher A, Fliegauf M, Olbrich H, Kispert A, Ketelsen UP, North A, Heintz N, Omran H. Dysfunction of axonemal dynein heavy chain Mdnah5 inhibits ependymal flow and reveals a novel mechanism for hydrocephalus formation. Hum Mol Genet. 2004;13:2133–41.
35. Iliff JJ, Wang M, Liao Y, Plogg BA, Peng W, Gundersen GA, Benveniste H, Vates GE, Deane R, Goldman SA, Nagelhus EA, Nedergaard M. A paravascular pathway facilitates CSF flow through the brain parenchyma and the clearance of interstitial solutes, including amyloid β. Sci Transl Med. 2012;4(147):147ra111.
36. Iliff JJ, Wang M, Zeppenfeld DM, Venkataraman A, Plog BA, Liao Y, Deane R, Nedergaard M. Cerebral arterial pulsation drives paravascular CSF-interstitial fluid exchange in the murine brain. J Neurosci. 2013;33:18190–9.
37. Iliff JJ, Chen MJ, Plog BA, Zeppenfeld DM, Soltero M, Yang L, Singh I, Deane R, Nedergaard M. Impairment of glymphatic pathway function promotes tau pathology after traumatic brain injury. J Neurosci. 2014;34:16180–93.

38. Imai F, Akimoto K, Koyama H, Miyata T, Ogawa M, Noguchi S, Sasaoka T, Noda T, Ohno S. Inactivation of aPKClambda results in the loss of adherens junctions in neuroepithelial cells without affecting neurogenesis in mouse neocortex. Development. 2006;133:1735–44.
39. Jacobsen M. Developmental neurobiology. New York: Plenum; 1991.
40. Jellinger G. Anatomopathology of nontumoral aqueductal stenosis. J Neurosurg Sci. 1986;30:1Y16.
41. Jiménez AJ, Tomé M, Páez P, Wagner C, Rodríguez S, Fernández-Llebrez P, Rodríguez EM, Pérez-Fígares JM. A programmed ependymal denudation precedes congenital hydrocephalus in the hyh mutant mouse. J Neuropathol Exp Neurol. 2001;60:1105–19.
42. Johanson CE, Duncan JA 3rd, Klinge PM, Brinker T, Stopa EG, Silverberg GD. Multiplicity of cerebrospinal fluid functions: new challenges in health and disease. Cerebrospinal Fluid Res. 2008;5:10.
43. Johansson PA. The choroid plexuses and their impact on developmental neurogenesis. Front Neurosci. 2014;8:340.
44. Johnson RT, Johnson KP, Edmonds CJ. Virus-induced hydrocephalus: development of aqueductal stenosis in hamsters after mumps infection. Science. 1967;157:1066Y67.
45. Johnson AK, Gross PM. Sensory circumventricular organs and brain homeostatic pathways. FASEB J. 1993;7:678–86.
46. Jones HC, Klinge PM. Hydrocephalus, 17–20th September, Hannover Germany: a conference report. Cerebrospinal Fluid Res. 2008;5:19.
47. Kazanis I, Lathia J, Moss L, ffrench-Constant C. The neural stem cell microenvironment. StemBook [Internet]. Cambridge, MA: Harvard Stem Cell Institute; 2008.
48. Klezovitch O, Fernandez TE, Tapscott SJ, Vasioukhin V. Loss of cell polarity causes severe brain dysplasia in Lgl1 knockout mice. Genes Dev. 2004;18:559–71.
49. Krueger RC, Wu H, Zandian M, Daniel-PouRM KP, Yu JS, Sun YE. Neural progenitors populate the cerebrospinal fluid of pre-term patients with hydrocephalus. J Pediatr. 2006;148: 337–40.
50. Lechtreck KF, Delmotte P, Robinson ML, Sanderson MJ, Witman GB. Mutations in Hydin impair ciliary motility in mice. J Cell Biol. 2008;180:633–43.
51. Lee L. Riding the wave of ependymal cilia: genetic susceptibility to hydrocephalus in primary ciliary dyskinesia. J Neurosci Res. 2013;91:1117–32.
52. Ma X, Bao J, Adelstein RS. Loss of cell adhesion causes hydrocephalus in nonmuscle myosin II-B-ablated and mutated mice. Mol Biol Cell. 2007;18:2305–12.
53. Malatesta P, Appolloni I, Calzolari F. Radial glia and neural stem cells. Cell Tissue Res. 2008;331:165–78.
54. Markham NO, Doll CA, Dohn MR, Miller RK, Yu H, Coffey RJ, McCrea PD, Gamse JT, Reynolds AB. DIPA-family coiled-coils bind conserved isoform-specific head domain of p120-catenin family: potential roles in hydrocephalus and heterotopia. Mol Biol Cell. 2014;25:2592–603.
55. Marzesco AM, Janich P, Wilsch-Bräuninger M, Dubreuil V, Langenfeld K, Corbeil D, Huttner WB. Release of extracellular membrane particles carrying the stem cell marker prominin-1 (CD133) from neural progenitors and other epithelial cells. J Cell Sci. 2005;118:2849–58.
56. Mashayekhi F, Draper CE, Bannister CM, Pourghasem M, Owen-Lynch PJ, Miyan JA. Deficient cortical development in the hydrocephalic Texas (H-Tx) rat: a role for CSF. Brain. 2002;125:1859–74.
57. McAllister P, Guerra M, Lc R, Jimenez AJ, Dominguez-Pinos D, Sival D, den Dunnen W, Morales DM, Schmidt RE, Rodríguez EM, Limbrick DD. Ventricular zone disruption in human neonates with intraventricular hemorrhage. J Neuropathol Exp Neurol. 2017;76(5):358–75.
58. Merkle FT, Alvarez-Buylla A. Neural stem cells in mammalian development. Curr Opin Cell Biol. 2006;18:704–9.
59. Milhorat TH. The third circulation revisited. J Neurosurg. 1975;42:628–45.
60. Miyan J, Sobkowiak C, Draper C. Humanity lost: the cost of cortical maldevelopment. Is there light ahead? Eur J Pediatr Surg. 2001;11(Suppl 1):S4–9.

61. Miyan JA, Nabiyouni M, Zendah M. Development of the brain: a vital role for cerebrospinal fluid. Can J Physiol Pharmacol. 2003;81:317–28.
62. Miyan JA, Zendah M, Mashayekhi F, Owen-Lynch PJ. Cerebrospinal fluid supports viability and proliferation of cortical cells in vitro, mirroring in vivo development. Cerebrospinal Fluid Res. 2006;3:2.
63. Monni E, Cusulin C, Cavallaro M, Lindvall O, Kokaia Z. Human fetal striatum-derived neural stem (NS) cells differentiate to mature neurons in vitro and in vivo. Curr Stem Cell Res Ther. 2014;9:338–46.
64. Mori T, Buffo A, Gotz M. The novel roles of glial cells revisited: the contribution of radial glia and astrocytes to neurogenesis. Curr Top Dev Biol. 2005;69:67–99.
65. Nechiporuk T, Fernández TE, Vasioukhin V. Failure of epithelial tube maintenance causes hydrocephalus and renal cysts in Dlg5-/- mice. Dev Cell. 2007;13:338–50.
66. Nelson DJ, Wright EM. The distribution, activity, and function of the cilia in the frog brain. J Physiol Lond. 1974;243:63–78.
67. Neuhuber B, Barshinger AL, Paul C, Shumsky JS, Mitsui T, Fischer I. Stem cell delivery by lumbar puncture as a therapeutic alternative to direct injection into injured spinal cord. J Neurosurg Spine. 2008;9:390–9.
68. Nguyen T, Chin WC, O'Brien JA, Verdugo P, Berger AJ. Intracellular pathways regulating ciliary beating of rat brain ependymal cells. J Physiol. 2001;531.(Pt 1:131–40.
69. Nicholson C. Signals that go with the flow. Trends Neurosci. 1999;22:143–5.
70. Ohta M, Suzuki Y, Noda T, Kataoka K, Chou H, Ishikawa N, Kitada M, Matsumoto N, Dezawa M, Suzuki S, Ide C. Implantation of neural stem cells via cerebrospinal fluid into the injured root. Neuroreport. 2004;15:1249–53.
71. Oliver C, González C, Alvial G, Flores CA, Rodríguez EM, Batiz LF. Disruption of CDH2/N-cadherin-based adherens junctions leads to apoptosis of ependymal cells and denudation of brain ventricular walls. J Neuropathol Exp Neurol. 2013;72:846–60.
72. Ortega E, Muñoz RI, Luza N, Guerra F, Guerra M, Vio K, Henzi R, Jaque J, Rodriguez S, McAllister JP, Rodriguez EM. The value of early and comprehensive diagnoses in a human fetus with hydrocephalus and progressive obliteration of the aqueduct of Sylvius: case report. BMC Neurol. 2016;16:45.
73. Ortloff A, Lichtin N, Guerra M, Vío K, Rodríguez EM. The disruption of the ventricular zone that occurs in foetal life of the hydrocephalic HTx rat is followed by a second disruption in the postnatal life. 57th annual meeting of Society of Research into Hydrocephalus and Spina Bifida, Cologne, Germany, 2013.
74. Páez P, Bátiz LF, Roales-Buján R, Rodríguez-Pérez LM, Rodríguez S, Jiménez AJ, Rodríguez EM, Pérez-Fígares JM. Patterned neuropathologic events occurring in *hyh* congenital hydrocephalic mutant mice. J Neuropathol Exp Neurol. 2007;66:1082–92.
75. Pluchino S, Quattrini A, Brambilla E, Gritti A, Salani G, Dina G, Galli R, Del Carro U, Amadio S, Bergami A, Furlan R, Comi G, Vescovi AL, Martino G. Injection of adult neurospheres induces recovery in a chronic model of multiple sclerosis. Nature. 2003;422:688–94.
76. Rakic P. Elusive radial glial cells: historical and evolutionary perspective. Glia. 2003;43:19–32.
77. Rasin M, Gazula V, Breunig J, Kwan KY, Johnson MB, Liu-Chen S, Li HS, Jan LY, Jan YN, Rakic P, Sestan N. Numb and Numbl are required for maintenance of cadherin-based adhesion and polarity of neural progenitors. Nat Neurosci. 2007;10:819–27.
78. Redzic ZB, Segal MB. The structure of the choroid plexus and the physiology of the choroid plexus epithelium. Adv Drug Deliv Rev. 2004;56:1695–716.
79. Roales-Buján R, Páez P, Guerra M, Rodríguez S, Vío K, Ho-Plagaro A, García-Bonilla M, Rodríguez-Pérez LM, Domínguez-Pinos MD, Rodríguez EM, Pérez-Fígares JM, Jiménez AJ. Astrocytes acquire morphological and functional characteristics of ependymal cells following disruption of ependyma in hydrocephalus. Acta Neuropathol. 2012;124:531–46.
80. Rodríguez EM. The cerebrospinal fluid as a pathway in neuroendocrine integration. J Endocrinol. 1976;71:407–43.
81. Rodríguez EM, Blázquez JL, Guerra M. The design of barriers in the hypothalamus allows the median eminence and the arcuate nucleus to enjoy private milieus: the former opens to the portal blood and the latter to the cerebrospinal fluid. Peptides. 2010;31:757–76.

82. Rodríguez EM, Guerra MM, Vío K, González C, Ortloff A, Bátiz LF, Rodríguez S, Jara MC, Muñoz RI, Ortega E, Jaque J, Guerra F, Sival DA, den Dunnen WF, Jiménez AJ, Domínguez-Pinos MD, Pérez-Fígares JM, McAllister JP, Johanson C. A cell junction pathology of neural stem cells leads to abnormal neurogenesis and hydrocephalus. Biol Res. 2012;45:231–42.
83. Rodríguez EM, Guerra M. Neural stem cells and fetal onset hydrocephalus. Pediatr Neurosurg. 2017; https://doi.org/10.1159/000453074.
84. Satake K, Lou J, Lenke LG. Migration of mesenchymal stem cells through cerebrospinal fl uid into injured spinal cord tissue. Spine. 2004;29:1971–9.
85. Sarnat HB. Role of human fetal ependyma. Pediatr Neurol. 1992a;8:163–78.
86. Sarnat HB. Regional differentiation of the human fetal ependyma: immunocytochemical markers. J Neuropathol Exp Neurol. 1992b;51:58–75.
87. Sarnat HB. Ependymal reactions to injury. A review. J Neuropathol Exp Neurol. 1995;54:1–15.
88. Sarnat HB. Histochemistry and immunocytochemistry of the developing ependyma and choroid plexus. Microsc Res Tech. 1998;41:14–28.
89. Sato O, Yamguchi T, Kittaka M, Toyama H. Hydrocephalus and epilepsy. Childs Nerv Syst. 2001;17(1–2):76–86.
90. Shaw RF, Fay AJ, Puthenveedu M, et al. Microtubule plus-end-tracking proteins target gap junctions directly from the cell interior to adherens junctions. Cell. 2007;128:547–60.
91. Shibasaki T, Tokunaga A, Sakamoto R, Sagara H, Noguchi S, Sasaoka T, Yoshida N. PTB deficiency causes the loss of adherens junctions in the dorsal telencephalon and leads to lethal hydrocephalus. Cereb Cortex. 2013;23:1824–35.
92. Shim JW, Sandlund J, Han CH, Hameed MQ, Connors S, Klagsbrun M, Madsen JR, Irwin N. VEGF, which is elevated in the CSF of patients with hydrocephalus, causes ventriculomegaly and ependymal changes in rats. Exp Neurol. 2013;247:703–9.
93. Shimizu A, Koto M. Ultrastructure and movement of the ependymal and tracheal cilia in congenitally hydrocephalic WIC-Hyd rats. Childs Nerv Syst. 1992;8:25–32.
94. Sival DA, Guerra M, den Dunnen WFA, Bátiz LF, Alvial G, Rodríguez EM. Neuroependymal denudation is in progress in full-term human foetal spina bifida aperta. Brain Pathol. 2011;21:163–79.
95. Siyahhan B, Knobloch V, de Zélicourt D, Asgari M, Schmid Daners M, Poulikakos D, Kurtcuoglu V. Flow induced by ependymal cilia dominates near-wall cerebrospinal fluid dynamics in the lateral ventricles. J R Soc Interface. 2014;11:20131189.
96. Street JM, Barran PE, Mackay CL, Weidt S, Balmforth C, Walsh TS, Chalmers RT, Webb DJ, Dear JW. Identification and proteomic profiling of exosomes in human cerebrospinal fluid. J Transl Med. 2012;5:10–5.
97. Tissir F, Qu Y, Montcouquiol M, et al. Lack of cadherins Celsr2 and Celsr3 impairs ependymal ciliogenesis, leading to fatal hydrocephalus. Nat Neurosci. 2010;13:700–7.
98. Veening JG, Barendregt HP. The regulation of brain states by neuroactive substances distributed via the cerebrospinal fluid; a review. Cerebrospinal Fluid Res. 2010;7:1.
99. Vigh-Teichmann I, Vigh B. The cerebrospinal fluid-contacting neuron: a peculiar cell type of the central nervous system. Immunocytochemical aspects. Arch Histol Cytol. 1989;52:195–207.
100. Vigh B, Manzano e Silva MJ, Frank CL, Vincze C, Czirok SJ, Szabó A, Lukáts A, Szél A. The system of cerebrospinal fluid-contacting neurons. Its supposed role in the nonsynaptic signal transmission of the brain. Histol Histopathol. 2004;19:607–28.
101. Vío K, Rodríguez S, Yulis CR, Oliver C, Rodríguez EM. The subcommissural organ of the rat secretes Reissner's fiber glycoproteins and CSF-soluble proteins reaching the internal and external CSF compartments. Cerebrospinal Fluid Res. 2008;5:3.
102. Voutsinos B, Chouaf L, Mertens P, Ruiz-Flandes P, Joubert Y, Belin MF, Didier-Bazes M. Tropism of serotonergic neurons towards glial targets in the rat ependyma. Neuroscience. 1994;59:663–72.
103. Wagner C, Bátiz LF, Rodríguez S, Jiménez AJ, Páez P, Tomé M, Pérez-Fígares JM, Rodríguez EM. Cellular mechanisms involved in the stenosis and obliteration of the cerebral aqueduct of *hyh* mutant mice developing congenital hydrocephalus. J Neuropathol Exp Neurol. 2003;62:1019–40.

104. Wei CJ, Francis R, Xu X, Lo CW. Connexin43 associated with an N-cadherin-containing multiprotein complex is required for gap junction formation in NIH3T3 cells. J Biol Chem. 2005;280:19925–36.
105. Williams MA, McAllister JP, Walker ML, Kranz DA, Bergsneider M, Del Bigio MR, Fleming L, Frim DM, Gwinn K, Kestle JR, Luciano MG, Madsen JR, Oster-Granite ML, Spinella G. Priorities for hydrocephalus research: report from a National Institutes of Health-sponsored workshop. J Neurosurg. 2007;107:345–57.
106. Wrigh EM. Transport processes in the formation of the cerebrospinal fluid. Rev Physiol Biochem Pharmacol. 1978;83:1–34.
107. Wright EM. Secretion and circulation of the cerebrospinal fluid. In: Rodriguez EM, van Wimersma Greidanus TB, editors. Front Horm Res. Basel: Karger; 1981.
108. Wood JH. Neurobiology of cerebrospinal fluid. New York: Plenum; 1983.
109. Worthington WC Jr, Cathcart RS 3rd. Ciliary currents on ependymal surfaces. Ann N Y Acad Sci. 1966;130:944–50.
110. Wu S, Suzuki Y, Noda Y, Bai H, Kitada M, Kataoka K, Nishimura Y, Ide C. Immunohistochemical and electron microscopic study of invasion and differentiation in spinal cord lesion of neural stem cells grafted through cerebrospinal fluid in rat. J Neurosci Res. 2002;69:940–5.
111. Yamadori T, Nara K. The directions of ciliary beat on the wall of the lateral ventricle and the currents of the cerebrospinal fluid in the brain ventricles. Scan Electron Microsc. 1979;3:335–40.
112. Yung YC, Mutoh T, Lin ME, Noguchi K, Rivera RR, Choi JW, Kingsbury MA, Chun J. Lysophosphatidic acid signaling may initiate fetal hydrocephalus. Sci Transl Med. 2011;3:99ra87.
113. Zappaterra MD, Lisgo SN, Lindsay S, Gygi SP, Walsh CA, Ballif BA. A comparative proteomic analysis of human and rat embryonic cerebrospinal fluid. J Proteome Res. 2007;6:3537–48.
114. Zecevic N. Specific characteristic of radial glia in the human fetal telencephalon. Glia. 2004;48:27–35.

Iron and Hydrocephalus

2

Thomas Garton and Jennifer M. Strahle

Introduction

Iron is arguably one of the most important metals in biology. It plays vital roles in everything from oxygen and electron transport to cell division and nucleotide biosynthesis to myelination and redox cycles [35]. However, iron excess can lead to a myriad of disorders such as hemochromatosis and siderosis. Cerebral-specific disorders such as Alzheimer's and Parkinson's disease are intricately linked to iron overload in the brain. The majority of iron found in the body is contained within hemoglobin (Hb), the tetrameric oxygen transport protein, which contains a ferrous (Fe^{2+}) cation within each of its four heme cores. Under normal circumstances, CSF hemoglobin levels are low within the cerebrospinal fluid compared to other proteins such as serum albumin [72]. Moreover, there is no nonprotein-bound iron normally present within cerebrospinal fluid, or CSF [53]. CSF is therefore relatively iron-free in normal conditions.

The link between iron and hydrocephalus predominantly stems from the relationship between hydrocephalus and intracranial hemorrhage (specifically, intracerebral, intraventricular, or subarachnoid hemorrhage—ICH, IVH, and SAH, respectively). Hydrocephalus is more common when blood enters the ventricles as is the case in IVH or the suabarachnoid space in the setting of SAH. In preterm infants, germinal matrix hemorrhage (GMH) may extend into the ventricles, and in the case of high grade (grade 3 or 4), GMH-IVH results in hydrocephalus in up to 28% of infants [13]. Following intraventricular or subarachnoid hemorrhage, hemoglobin enters the CSF, and as a result, large amounts of iron collect within the

T. Garton
University of Michigan, Department of Neurosurgery, Ann Arbor, MI, USA

J. M. Strahle (✉)
Washington Univeristy in St. Louis, Department of Neurosurgery, St. Louis, MO, USA
e-mail: strahlej@wustl.edu

D. D. Limbrick, J. R. Leonard (eds.), *Cerebrospinal Fluid Disorders*,
https://doi.org/10.1007/978-3-319-97928-1_2

ventricular system. Current lines of research are investigating the connection between the iron released into the CSF during such hemorrhages and the formation of hydrocephalus.

Iron Homeostasis in the Brain

In order to understand how iron contributes to the induction of hydrocephalus, it is important to understand how iron is managed in the brain under normal conditions. Because of the dangers associated with iron overload, levels are closely controlled in the brain. Some iron is bound to small organic molecules such as citrate, ATP, or ascorbic acid [6], while almost no iron is found floating in free ferrous or ferric forms. Iron can also be found as an important structural or catalytic component of many proteins and enzymes in the brain including the electron transport chain complexes I and II. However, the most significant source of iron is the heme cores of proteins such as neuroglobin and hemoglobin.

Non-heme-Bound Iron

As a cation often bound to proteins or other larger molecules, iron cannot freely diffuse across cell membranes, and thus it requires specific transport proteins. One of the most common uptake mechanisms is the transferrin-transferrin receptor system (Tf-TfR) (Fig. 2.1). Transferrin (Tf) is an 80 kDa glycoprotein with high affinity for iron [1], found to be expressed in nearly every cell type in the CNS. Tf is responsible for the majority of iron found within the CSF in physiological conditions. The primary job of Tf is to scavenge free iron in the extracellular space or CSF. Tf binds ferric iron and is subsequently endocytosed by the Tf Receptor [32]. The resulting endosome is acidified, which releases ferric iron from Tf and facilitates its reduction to the ferrous state [48]. Once in its ferrous form, iron escapes from the endosome via the Divalent Metal Transporter 1 (DMT1), a ubiquitous protein capable of transporting a large number of divalent ions including iron, zinc, manganese, cobalt, cadmium, copper, nickel, and lead [32]. Cytosolic iron is still not free but rather sequestered within lysosomes and an iron-binding protein, ferritin (Ft) [79], a highly stable spherical protein that sequesters Fe^{2+} in ferroxidase centers (Fig. 2.1). Should the available Ft become saturated, a transporter called ferroportin 1 (FP1) can transport excess iron out of the cell into the interstitial fluid. This FP1-mediated transport is paired with oxidation of the toxic Fe^{2+} to Fe^{3+} by the multicopper ferroxidase ceruloplasmin (CP). Once outside the cell, transferrin can bind to ferric iron, and thus the cycle is restarted. Ceruloplasmin may be stabilized by amyloid precursor protein (APP), but the role of APP in iron homeostasis is still unclear [74]. It has been suggested that neuronal APP lacks ferroxidase capabilities but is rather essential for FP1's association to the neuronal cell membrane [74]. The precise mechanism by which APP stabilizes FP1, however, is undetermined.

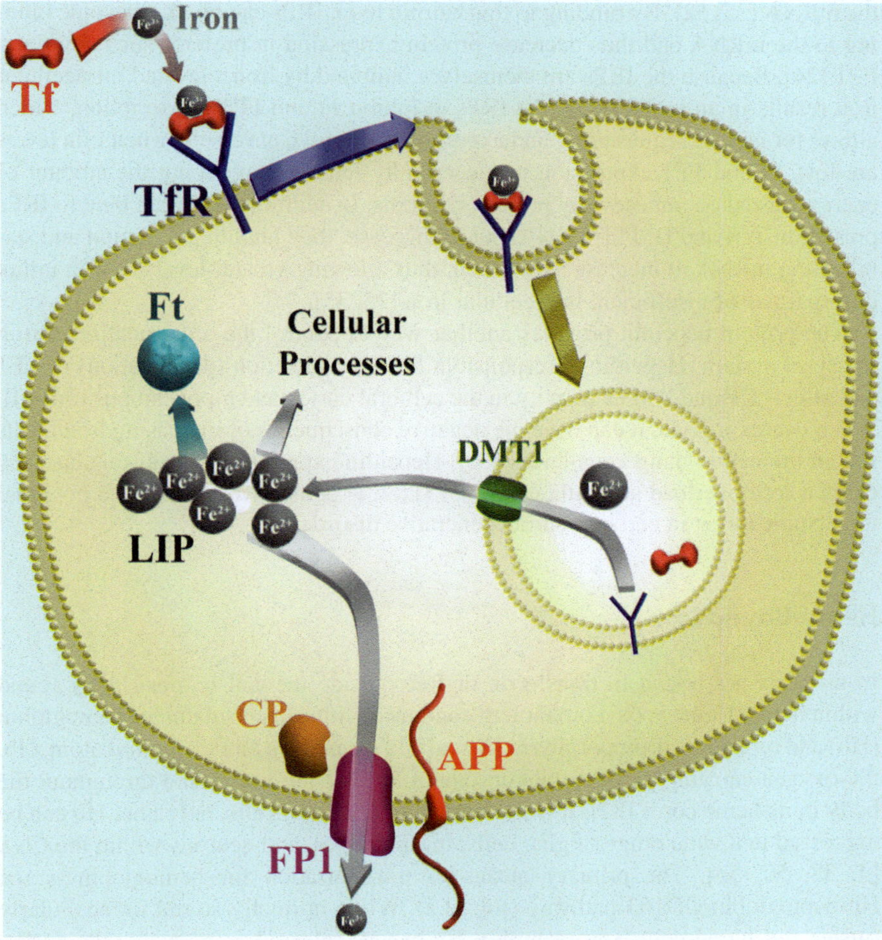

Fig. 2.1 The Non-heme-Iron Homeostatic Pathway in the Brain. Iron is captured by Transferrin (Tf), which is subsequently internalized by Transferrin Receptor (TfR) via receptor-mediated endocytosis. Once internalized into the early endosome, iron is released from TfR and leaves the endosome via Divalent Metal Transporter 1 (DMT1) where it joins the Labile Iron Pool (LIP) in the cytosol. This iron is either used for cellular processes, sequestered in Ferritin (Ft), or is pushed out of the cell via Ferroportin 1 (FP1), which is stabilized by Ceruloplasmin (CP) and Amyloid Precursor Protein (APP)

Regulation of Iron Homeostasis

The transport systems described above are fairly ubiquitous throughout the CNS. Regulation of these systems is achieved primarily via the iron regulatory proteins, IRP-1 and IRP-2. When IRPs are not bound to iron, they can bind to a region of the mRNA coding for each of these iron-related proteins called the iron-responsive element (IRE); the IRE is a relatively conserved specific hairpin loop in the 5′-UTR of the mRNA [35, 52]. By binding to this hairpin loop, IRPs can block ribosome binding to the mRNA and thus decrease protein expression in proteins such as Ft and FP1 [24]. Because the IRPs are themselves inhibited by iron, elevated intracellular iron results in an inability for the IRPs to inhibit Ft and FP1 transcription, which allows for greater sequestering and export of iron [26]. Conversely, when iron levels are low, Ft and FP1 expression is successfully inhibited, reducing the amount of energy wasted on unnecessary protein synthesis. In addition, IRPs can bind to IREs present in TfR and DMT1 mRNA, but in this case, they bind to a 3′ region and stabilize the mRNA to increase expression, thus allowing greater levels of iron influx during times of insufficient intracellular iron [25, 35].

The protein hepcidin provides another way to control the aforementioned iron transport system. Hepcidin is responsible for internalization (deactivation) of FP1 and affects CP and DMT1 activity in the cerebral cortex and hippocampus [36, 43]. When overexpressed, it can have the negative consequence of increasing iron levels within the cell to dangerous levels [66]. Hepcidin expression is itself regulated by cellular iron overload and inflammation [51]. It is being investigated as a potential therapeutic target in certain neurodegenerative disorders.

Heme-Bound Iron

Iron that is not bound to transferrin or free outside the cell is most likely found within heme. Heme is the core moiety contained within each subunit of hemoglobin (Hb) and refers to a protoporphyrin IX scaffold supporting an Fe^{2+} central atom. Hb, the oxygen carrying protein, contains about 70% of the iron found throughout the body in its heme cores [82]. It is not limited to erythroid cells, but rather Hb can be expressed in a wide range of glial cells, macrophages, and neurons within the CNS [4, 38, 50, 55]. The primary means of transportation for hemoglobin is the Hb-haptoglobin-CD163 pathway (Fig. 2.2). While normally stored intracellularly (inside red blood cells, for example), Hb can be released from such cells during hemolysis. Once extracellular, hemoglobin becomes unstable, and therefore it must be quickly scavenged by the protein haptoglobin (Hp), a plasma glycoprotein that binds to Hb with incredibly high affinity [73]. Hp is a tetrameric serine protease in which the two β subunits bind to Hb after it naturally dissociates into dimers in the extracellular fluid [67]. Importantly, this Hb–Hp complex is incapable of performing redox reactions, possibly due to Hp's ability to halt reactions between the heme core and hydrogen peroxide (see section "Mechanisms of Iron Toxicity") [2].

After associating, this Hb–Hp complex is bound with high affinity by the membrane-bound receptor CD163, a 130 kDa transmembrane member of the scavenger receptor cysteine-rich (SRCR) domain-containing protein family (Fig. 2.2). CD163 endocytoses the complex, preventing accumulation of Hb in the extracellular space [23]. Following endocytosis, the Hb–Hp complex dissociates, allowing Hb to be degraded to heme and the Hp to return to the extracellular space [18, 54]. Once released from its protein scaffold, heme is broken down by heme oxygenase (HO) proteins (namely the inducible HO-1 or the constitutively expressed HO-2). HO-1

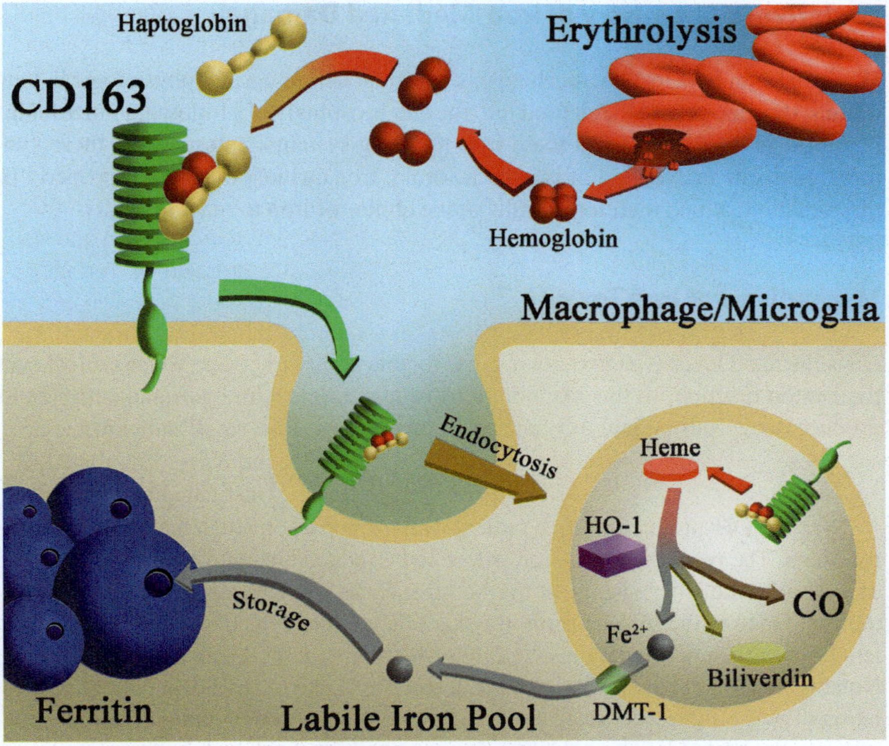

Fig. 2.2 Heme-bound Iron Transport Pathway in the Brain. Iron that is contained within heme can be released into the extracellular space via hemolysis. Hemoglobin is scavenged by haptoglobin before being endocytosed by CD163. Heme is released from hemoglobin in the early endosome due to increased acidity and is subsequently degraded by Heme Oxygenase (HO) proteins to release carbon monoxide (CO), Biliverdin, and Ferrous iron. This ferrous iron is then able to exit the endosome via DMT-1 and join the Labile Iron Pool, where it is homeostatically managed as depicted in Fig. 2.1. (Reprinted with permission from Garton et al. [22])

is upregulated by the presence of heme as well as a variety of other proinflammatory signal molecules [68]. HO proteins decompose heme into carbon monoxide, biliverdin, and Fe^{2+} [69]. The biliverdin is subsequently converted to bilirubin (an antioxidant known to be neurotoxic in preterm neonates) [44, 71], while the iron is bound by Ferritin (Ft) and sequestered according to normal iron homeostatic systems.

The regulation of the transporter CD163 in the brain is not well understood though it seems to be upregulated by inflammatory cytokines and by the presence of Hp–Hb complexes [5, 16]. CD163 contains a 9-subunit ectodomain, which can be shed from the cell membrane by ADAM17, a membrane-bound serine protease involved in Aβ formation in Alzheimer's Disease [37, 42, 49]. The cleaved ectodomain is called "soluble" CD163 (sCD163) and is used as an inflammatory biomarker. CD163 has recently been discovered to be expressed in neurons following IVH and other hemorrhagic conditions [10, 21, 22, 39]. This provides a pathway for iron bound within hemoglobin to gain access to neurons in addition to glial cells.

Underlying Chemistry of Iron-Mediated Damage

While the iron homeostatic mechanisms function well in normal physiological conditions, the amount of Hb released into the cerebrospinal fluid following intracranial hemorrhage may overwhelm these iron-handling systems. Saturation of these systems results in an overload of iron in the brain. Iron cannot be managed properly in this situation, which therefore results in the ability of iron to react toxically.

Mechanisms of Iron Toxicity

On a chemical level, iron toxicity results from its ability to generate free radicals via the Fenton reaction. In this reaction, ferrous iron reacts with hydrogen peroxide to produce dangerous radical oxygen species according to the reaction below:

$$Fe^{2+} + H_2O_2 \rightarrow Fe^{3+} + OH^{\cdot} + OH^{-}$$

Note the $OH^{\cdot}$ product is a free radical which can participate in harmful oxidizing reactions. The resulting ferric iron is free to be reduced back to Fe^{2+} by the myriad of available reducing agents in the body, such as glutathione or superoxide dismutase. Once in the ferrous form, the reaction can begin again with a new equivalent of hydrogen peroxide, thus continuously pumping out reactive oxygen species. Notably, H_2O_2 is relatively abundant in the brain. It plays significant roles in modulation of neurotransmitter release and is therefore produced by mitochondrial respiration in the brain [3]. The oxidative damage resulting from such iron overload then returns to target the mitochondrial inner membrane [7, 59]. Reactive oxygen species can react with cytochrome proteins in the mitochondrial membrane, resulting in oxidation of mitochondrial lipid molecules. This can fragment the mitochondrial membrane sufficiently to allow for escape of the caspase proteins, notoriously involved in apoptosis. Additional mitochondria-related pathways for iron damage exist, however. Iron overload in vitro has been demonstrated to induce mitochondrial fragmentation in neurons; the mechanism of this fragmentation involves the dephosphorylation of dynamin-related protein 1 (Drp1), a mitochondrial GTPase that functions in mitochondrial fission [12, 47]. This fission pathway interacts with the Calcineurin phosphatase signal pathways [8, 61], which are also influenced by iron [47]. Therefore, there exists an abundance of pathways by which iron overload can lead to cell damage and death, which has resulted in its highlighting as a key target for new hemorrhagic therapies.

How Does Iron Induce Hydrocephalus after ICH/IVH?

When it comes to exactly how iron is linked to hydrocephalus independent of cell death, the answer is less clear. For each subtype of intracranial hemorrhage, there exists a few potential mechanisms through which hydrocephalus develops. With respect to ICH, hydrocephalus is more likely to occur in the setting of ICH with clot location adjacent to the ventricle such as in the thalamus [41, 81]. Although presence of intraventricular blood is a risk factor for hydrocephalus, in the aforementioned studies, location of blood in the ventricle was not associated with need for placement of a shunt for long-term treatment of hydrocephalus or in the presence of intraventricular extension.

Traditional thoughts on the formation of hydrocephalus after ICH maintain that hemorrhage may be responsible for upregulating inflammatory responses and damaging the arachnoid granulations, which are the sites of CSF outflow from the brain [29]. However, studies investigating the arachnoid granulations after hemorrhage are scarce, partially due to the difficulty in identifying them in infant populations (which are one of the most affected demographics for posthemorrhagic hydrocephalus, or PHH) [45, 62]. There may be additional pathways for iron-mediated damage, however. Intriguingly, ICH with IVH extension seems to be linked to more severe hydrocephalus than IVH that does not contain an intraparenchymal hematoma component [9]. This is likely due to the role the hematoma plays in the development of hydrocephalus. Chen et al. demonstrated that the hematoma acts as a source of iron over extended periods of time. In rats with experimental IVH without ICH, the amount of iron in the CSF was higher than in rats with both ICH/IVH in an acute time window. However, after 3 days, the combined ICH/IVH rats had higher iron levels in the CSF, indicating the progressive release of iron from the hematoma. Moreover, it is likely that the iron is inducing hydrocephalus via its ability to damage the ependymal cells lining the ventricular wall. These cells have motile (and primary) cilia that are thought to be involved in the flow of CSF throughout the ventricular system. Chen et al. reported an association between severe ependymal cilia damage and the severity of hydrocephalus and further linked the level of damage to the amount of iron being released into the CSF [9]. This finding of iron-mediated ependymal cell loss and cilia damage was also corroborated by a study that specifically injected iron into the ventricles of rats [19]. Thus, it is clear that the acting factor in the ependymal cilia loss is the presence of high levels of iron in the CSF.

As previously mentioned, neonatal populations are particularly at risk for developing PHH. Therefore, a substantial body of work has aimed to assess the role of iron in neonatal IVH and subsequent PHH. Earlier studies demonstrated that preterm-birth infants suffering from posthemorrhagic ventricular dilation had significantly elevated levels of nonheme-bound iron in their CSF [53]. Intriguingly, Savman et al. postulated that the amount of iron present in the collected CSF was too great to be simply due to hemolysis; rather they expected that a significant contributor must be the release of iron from ferritin within brain parenchyma. However, intraventricular iron alone is sufficient to induce hydrocephalus in neonatal rat models [62]. Therefore, it is likely that initial hemolysis results in sufficient intraventricular iron levels to inflict damage on the ependymal walls and choroid plexus, resulting in the release of yet more iron from ferritin into the extracellular space.

It is important to note that ependymal loss is sufficient to produce hydrocephalus, but it is unknown whether it is necessary. In other words, nearly every study investigating the role of iron during the development of PHH has observed ependymal cilia damage, but it is possible that there exist other pathways of action for iron that have gone unnoticed but that must also be addressed in order to fully combat the formation of hydrocephalus after ICH/IVH. For example, one study by Schweizer et al. demonstrated that by deleting the Ferritin H gene from the choroid plexus, hydrocephalus can be generated 100% of the time [56]. While this study was not specifically investigating hemorrhagic conditions, it raises the possibility that should the choroid plexus become unable to handle the amount of iron present, it could result in hydrocephalus perhaps via overproduction of CSF [20].

How Does Iron Induce Hydrocephalus after SAH?

Research investigating the link between hydrocephalus and SAH has mostly focused on noncommunicating or obstructive hydrocephalus. In this form of hydrocephalus, blood products may block the CSF outflow pathways. It has also been hypothesized that SAH could result in overproduction of CSF leading to chronic communicating hydrocephalus although this has not been confirmed [31]. It is possible that the inflammatory upregulation caused by iron's production of ROS's could be related to scarring around these narrow pathways and therefore be linked indirectly to PHH. However, there exists clear evidence for acute (within 6 h) development of communicating hydrocephalus following SAH [60]. While Siler et al. noted the role of the inflammatory response in the generation of their communicating hydrocephalus model, they did not investigate whether iron was involved in the generation of the inflammatory response. However, clinical studies have identified a link between elevated levels of iron (as measured by the iron-sequestering protein Ferritin) in the CSF and severe hydrocephalus, as well as a link between the levels of CSF iron and the number of inflammatory cells in the CSF [63]. Furthermore, it has been demonstrated that accumulation of iron around the ventricles following SAH is related to hydrocephalus [46]. Therefore, it is clear that iron is linked to hydrocephalus in some way, but the manner in which it is related is still a matter for further investigation.

Animal Models

While there exist many models for evaluating the role of iron in posthemorrhagic cell death, the number of animal models devoted to analyzing the connection between iron and hydrocephalus are relatively limited. In their entirety, these models investigate this relationship in the broader context of hemorrhagic stroke (specifically SAH or IVH). With regard to SAH, the method of induction is usually endovascular perforation in rats, with subsequent experiments monitoring iron levels via Perl's staining or via iron chelators [46]. Among them is the model by Strahle et al. who directly injected $FeCl_2$ and $FeCl_3$ into the lateral ventricles to observe the effects on ventriculomegaly and the development of hydrocephalus [62]. Moreover, this model also specified that the iron within heme is the key component of hemoglobin-mediated hydrocephalus by comparing heme with protoporphyrin IX (the latter being the heme scaffold without the iron core) which demonstrated that protoporphyrin IX injection had no effect on ventricular volume compared to controls [62]. Many of the studies that have indicated iron's role in hydrocephalus do so by demonstrating the efficacy of iron chelators at ameliorating the damage.

Preclinical Treatments Focusing on Iron

The information provided by the animal models previously discussed demonstrates the clear involvement of iron in the formation of hydrocephalus and the cell death seen after IVH and SAH. Preclinical studies have targeted iron in the search for potential treatments, focusing on the iron chelators Deferoxamine (DFX) and Minocycline.

Deferoxamine

Deferoxamine (DFX) is a ferric ion chelator that is used clinically for systemic iron overload. The efficacy of DFX in treating hemorrhage-induced brain damage in preclinical models has been reviewed previously [15, 30, 57]. A stratified meta-analysis showed DFX to be effective in experimental ICH, particularly when administered 2–4 h after hemorrhage, and with a dosage of 10–50 mg/kg [15]. DFX has been repeatedly demonstrated to ameliorate iron-induced edema [76], neuronal death [28], hippocampal degeneration [21], and inflammation [14, 75, 76, 86]. During SAH, DFX treatment chelates free iron before it can form ROS, thus ameliorating vasospasm [70]. More specific to the nature of this chapter, DFX has been shown to reduce post-hemorrhagic hydrocephalus (PHH) [9, 84]. Gao et al. showed that hydrocephalus developed after intraventricular injection of lysed but not packed erythrocytes into adult rats, and that DFX co-injection reduced this ventricular enlargement by 27% [19]. Strahle et al. also demonstrated that iron injection alone could cause hydrocephalus in neonatal rats, and that DFX reduced this ventricular enlargement by 57% [62]. Iron may induce PHH through free radical production and oxidative stress, but it is possible that it also activates the Wnt signaling pathway [40]. The Wnt signaling pathway is involved in fibrosis in a variety of tissues and, therefore, it may play a role in obstructive noncommunicating hydrocephalus formation following hemorrhage. DFX reduced Wnt1/Wnt3a upregulation following IVH most likely via iron chelation [40]. Regardless of its mechanism of action, studies evaluating DFX consistently demonstrate its ability to reduce iron-mediated hydrocephalus, suggesting that it may be a viable drug for implementation into clinical trials.

Minocycline

Minocycline is another iron chelator that has received attention with respect to alleviating the effects of iron on hydrocephalus. As a tetracycline derivative, it has high lipophilicity allowing it to cross the blood-brain-barrier (BBB) and likely the blood-CSF-barrier as well [33]. In vitro, Minocycline has been shown to reduce iron-induced injury in cortical neurons with even higher activity than DFX [11]. In vivo, it reduces iron overload, neuronal death, and iron-induced brain edema and BBB disruption following hemorrhage [83]. Co-injection of minocycline + $FeCl_2$ compared to $FeCl_2$ alone decreased Ft, CP, HO-1, Tf, and TfR upregulation [85]. A study by Guo et al. demonstrated the viability of minocycline as a method of alleviating the post-hemorrhagic hydrocephalus induced by collagenase injection into the striatum of the brain [27]. Ventricular volume was decreased after minocycline treatment at both 7 days and 1 month. They identified that this decrease coincided with a reduction in the iron overload of the brain. During treatment of hydrocephalus with minocycline, another group identified a reduction of reactive gliosis that was associated with the reduced ventricular dilation [77]. However, there was not complete resolution of the ventriculomegaly compared to controls. Therefore, the potential for minocycline to be used as an iron-centered treatment for PHH remains a matter for further investigation and potential improvement.

Clinical Trials of Iron-Centered Treatments

Neither DFX nor Minocycline have been the center of a hydrocephalus-oriented clinical trial. Both have been evaluated for their effectiveness in reducing hemorrhagic injury. In 2011, a Phase-I dose-finding study assessed DFX treatment in ICH and found it to be feasible and well-tolerated [58]. That led to a Phase-II trial of DFX in human ICH patients, the High Dose Deferoxamine in Intracerebral Hemorrhage (HI-DEF) trial [78]. In the trial, there were some concerns over the occurrence of acute respiratory distress syndrome (ARDS) and currently a lower dose of DFX is being tested in the Intracerebral Hemorrhage Deferoxamine Trial (iDEF; NCT02175225). In addition, a recent 42-patient study investigating DFX treatment for ICH concluded that DFX may slow hematoma absorption and inhibit edema formation [80]. Unfortunately, there has been a lack of DFX clinical trials that investigate the effects of DFX on the development of hydrocephalus. Given the preclinical effects of DFX, advancement of DFX into large-scale clinical trials for IVH, SAH, and PHH should be considered.

In the ongoing MINOS (Minocycline to Improve Neurologic Outcome in Stroke) trial, minocycline treatment has been shown to be safe in 10 mg/kg intravenous dosages [17]. The trial has shown that minocycline decreases the expression of the potentially harmful matrix metalloproteinase-9 and the inflammatory cytokine IL-6 after stroke [64, 65]. However, it has yet to release results on the overall efficacy of minocycline. However, a pilot study conducted in 2013 involving 95 participants investigated the effects of minocycline in ischemic and hemorrhagic stroke. It found that minocycline is safe but not particularly efficacious [34]. There is, therefore, significant controversy about the efficacy of minocycline in human trials. Given the agreement of preclinical studies on the safety of the treatment, however, it seems reasonable to consider moving forward toward a larger clinical trial and specifically a clinical trial investigating hydrocephalus.

Conclusion

The role of iron in hemorrhagic injury and the development of hydrocephalus is a hot topic in current stroke research. It is clear that iron overload is directly related to hydrocephalus, and efforts to specifically address iron in animal models and in *in vitro* experiments have been met with some success. Due to its ability to engage in dangerous Fenton reactions with oxygenated species like hydrogen peroxide, iron can create free radicals and reactive oxygen species capable of causing significant damage to the brain. The mechanism by which these reactions influence hydrocephalus is less well understood. Current hypotheses implicate damage to the ependymal surface and possibly motile cilia in the dysfunction of CSF dynamics. However, additional pathways may exist. Identifying mechanisms of iron-mediated ventriculomegaly is an important goal of hydrocephalus research and is one that holds significant promise with respect to our ability to improve treatment for patients suffering from hydrocephalus.

References

1. Aisen P, Leibman A, Zweier J. Stoichiometric and site characteristics of the binding of iron to human transferrin. J Biol Chem. 1978;253:1930–7.
2. Alayash AI. Haptoglobin: old protein with new functions. Clin Chim Acta. 2011;412:493–8.
3. Bao L, Avshalumov MV, Patel JC, Lee CR, Miller EW, Chang CJ, Rice ME. Mitochondria are the source of hydrogen peroxide for dynamic brain-cell signaling. J Neurosci. 2009;29:9002–10.
4. Biagioli M, Pinto M, Cesselli D, Zaninello M, Lazarevic D, Roncaglia P, Simone R, Vlachouli C, Plessy C, Bertin N, et al. Unexpected expression of alpha- and beta-globin in mesencephalic dopaminergic neurons and glial cells. Proc Natl Acad Sci U S A. 2009;106:15454–9.
5. Borda JT, Alvarez X, Mohan M, Hasegawa A, Bernardino A, Jean S, Aye P, Lackner AA. CD163, a marker of perivascular macrophages, is up-regulated by microglia in simian immunodeficiency virus encephalitis after haptoglobin-hemoglobin complex stimulation and is suggestive of breakdown of the blood-brain barrier. Am J Pathol. 2008;172:725–37.
6. Bradbury MW. Transport of iron in the blood-brain-cerebrospinal fluid system. J Neurochem. 1997;69:443–54.
7. Calabrese V, Lodi R, Tonon C, D'Agata V, Sapienza M, Scapagnini G, Mangiameli A, Pennisi G, Stella AM, Butterfield DA. Oxidative stress, mitochondrial dysfunction and cellular stress response in Friedreich's ataxia. J Neurol Sci. 2005;233:145–62.
8. Cereghetti GM, Stangherlin A, Martins de Brito O, Chang CR, Blackstone C, Bernardi P, Scorrano L. Dephosphorylation by calcineurin regulates translocation of Drp1 to mitochondria. Proc Natl Acad Sci U S A. 2008;105:15803–8.
9. Chen Q, Tang J, Tan L, Guo J, Tao Y, Li L, Chen Y, Liu X, Zhang JH, Chen Z, et al. Intracerebral hematoma contributes to hydrocephalus after intraventricular hemorrhage via aggravating iron accumulation. Stroke. 2015;46:2902–8.
10. Chen-Roetling J, Regan RF. Haptoglobin increases the vulnerability of CD163-expressing neurons to hemoglobin. J Neurochem. 2016;139:586–95.

11. Chen-Roetling J, Chen L, Regan RF. Minocycline attenuates iron neurotoxicity in cortical cell cultures. Biochem Biophys Res Commun. 2009;386:322–6.
12. Cho B, Choi SY, Cho HM, Kim HJ, Sun W. Physiological and pathological significance of dynamin-related protein 1 (drp1)-dependent mitochondrial fission in the nervous system. Exp Neurobiol. 2013;22:149–57.
13. Christian EA, Jin DL, Attenello F, Wen T, Cen S, Mack WJ, Krieger MD, McComb JG. Trends in hospitalization of preterm infants with intraventricular hemorrhage and hydrocephalus in the United States, 2000-2010. J Neurosurg. 2016;17:260–9.
14. Chun HJ, Kim DW, Yi HJ, Kim YS, Kim EH, Hwang SJ, Jwa CS, Lee YK, Ryou H. Effects of statin and deferoxamine administration on neurological outcomes in a rat model of intracerebral hemorrhage. Neurol Sci. 2012;33:289–96.
15. Cui HJ, He HY, Yang AL, Zhou HJ, Wang C, Luo JK, Lin Y, Tang T. Efficacy of deferoxamine in animal models of intracerebral hemorrhage: a systematic review and stratified meta-analysis. PLoS One. 2015;10:e0127256.
16. Etzerodt A, Moestrup SK. CD163 and inflammation: biological, diagnostic, and therapeutic aspects. Antioxid Redox Signal. 2013;18:2352–63.
17. Fagan SC, Waller JL, Nichols FT, Edwards DJ, Pettigrew LC, Clark WM, Hall CE, Switzer JA, Ergul A, Hess DC. Minocycline to improve neurologic outcome in stroke (MINOS): a dose-finding study. Stroke. 2010;41:2283–7.
18. Fruitier I, Garreau I, Lacroix A, Cupo A, Piot JM. Proteolytic degradation of hemoglobin by endogenous lysosomal proteases gives rise to bioactive peptides: hemorphins. FEBS Lett. 1999;447:81–6.
19. Gao C, Du H, Hua Y, Keep RF, Strahle J, Xi G. Role of red blood cell lysis and iron in hydrocephalus after intraventricular hemorrhage. J Cereb Blood Flow Metab. 2014;34:1070–5.
20. Garton T, Keep RF, Hua Y, Xi G. Brain iron overload following intracranial haemorrhage. Stroke Vasc Neurol. 2016;1:172–84.
21. Garton TP, He Y, Garton HJ, Keep RF, Xi G, Strahle JM. Hemoglobin-induced neuronal degeneration in the hippocampus after neonatal intraventricular hemorrhage. Brain Res. 2016;1635:86–94.
22. Garton T, Keep RF, Hua Y, Xi G. CD163, a hemoglobin/haptoglobin scavenger receptor, after intracerebral hemorrhage: functions in microglia/macrophages versus neurons. Transl Stroke Res. 2017;8:612–7.
23. Graversen JH, Madsen M, Moestrup SK. CD163: a signal receptor scavenging haptoglobin-hemoglobin complexes from plasma. Int J Biochem Cell Biol. 2002;34:309–14.
24. Gray NK, Hentze MW. Iron regulatory protein prevents binding of the 43S translation pre-initiation complex to ferritin and eALAS mRNAs. EMBO J. 1994;13:3882–91.
25. Gunshin H, Allerson CR, Polycarpou-Schwarz M, Rofts A, Rogers JT, Kishi F, Hentze MW, Rouault TA, Andrews NC, Hediger MA. Iron-dependent regulation of the divalent metal ion transporter. FEBS Lett. 2001;509:309–16.
26. Guo B, Yu Y, Leibold EA. Iron regulates cytoplasmic levels of a novel iron-responsive element-binding protein without aconitase activity. J Biol Chem. 1994;269:24252–60.
27. Guo J, Chen Q, Tang J, Zhang J, Tao Y, Li L, Zhu G, Feng H, Chen Z. Minocycline-induced attenuation of iron overload and brain injury after experimental germinal matrix hemorrhage. Brain Res. 2015;1594:115–24.
28. Hatakeyama T, Okauchi M, Hua Y, Keep RF, Xi G. Deferoxamine reduces neuronal death and hematoma lysis after intracerebral hemorrhage in aged rats. Transl Stroke Res. 2013;4:546–53.
29. Hill A, Shackelford GD, Volpe JJ. A potential mechanism of pathogenesis for early posthemorrhagic hydrocephalus in the premature newborn. Pediatrics. 1984;73:19–21.
30. Hua Y, Keep RF, Hoff JT, Xi G. Deferoxamine therapy for intracerebral hemorrhage. Acta Neurochir. 2008;105:3–6.
31. Kanat A, Turkmenoglu O, Aydin MD, Yolas C, Aydin N, Gursan N, Tumkaya L, Demir R. Toward changing of the pathophysiologic basis of acute hydrocephalus after subarachnoid hemorrhage: a preliminary experimental study. World Neurosurg. 2013;80:390–5.

32. Ke Y, Qian ZM. Brain iron metabolism: neurobiology and neurochemistry. Prog Neurobiol. 2007;83:149–73.
33. Klein NC, Cunha BA. Tetracyclines. Med Clin North Am. 1995;79:789–801.
34. Kohler E, Prentice DA, Bates TR, Hankey GJ, Claxton A, van Heerden J, Blacker D. Intravenous minocycline in acute stroke: a randomized, controlled pilot study and meta-analysis. Stroke. 2013;44:2493–9.
35. Kuhn LC. Iron regulatory proteins and their role in controlling iron metabolism. Metallomics. 2015;7:232–43.
36. Li L, Holscher C, Chen BB, Zhang ZF, Liu YZ. Hepcidin treatment modulates the expression of divalent metal transporter-1, ceruloplasmin, and ferroportin-1 in the rat cerebral cortex and hippocampus. Biol Trace Elem Res. 2011;143:1581–93.
37. Lisi S, D'Amore M, Sisto M. ADAM17 at the interface between inflammation and autoimmunity. Immunol Lett. 2014;162:159–69.
38. Liu L, Zeng M, Stamler JS. Hemoglobin induction in mouse macrophages. Proc Natl Acad Sci U S A. 1999;96:6643–7.
39. Liu R, Cao S, Hua Y, Keep RF, Huang Y, Xi G. CD163 expression in neurons after experimental intracerebral hemorrhage. Stroke. 2017;48:1369–75.
40. Meng H, Li F, Hu R, Yuan Y, Gong G, Hu S, Feng H. Deferoxamine alleviates chronic hydrocephalus after intraventricular hemorrhage through iron chelation and Wnt1/Wnt3a inhibition. Brain Res. 2015;1602:44–52.
41. Miller JM, McAllister JP 2nd. Reduction of astrogliosis and microgliosis by cerebrospinal fluid shunting in experimental hydrocephalus. Cerebrospinal Fluid Res. 2007;4:5.
42. Moller HJ. Soluble CD163. Scand J Clin Lab Invest. 2012;72:1–13.
43. Nemeth E, Tuttle MS, Powelson J, Vaughn MB, Donovan A, Ward DM, Ganz T, Kaplan J. Hepcidin regulates cellular iron efflux by binding to ferroportin and inducing its internalization. Science. 2004;306:2090–3.
44. O'Brien L, Hosick PA, John K, Stec DE, Hinds TD Jr. Biliverdin reductase isozymes in metabolism. Trends Endocrinol Metab. 2015;26:212–20.
45. Oi S, Di Rocco C. Proposal of "evolution theory in cerebrospinal fluid dynamics" and minor pathway hydrocephalus in developing immature brain. Childs Nerv Syst. 2006;22: 662–9.
46. Okubo S, Strahle J, Keep RF, Hua Y, Xi G. Subarachnoid hemorrhage-induced hydrocephalus in rats. Stroke. 2013;44:547–50.
47. Park J, Lee DG, Kim B, Park SJ, Kim JH, Lee SR, Chang KT, Lee HS, Lee DS. Iron overload triggers mitochondrial fragmentation via calcineurin-sensitive signals in HT-22 hippocampal neuron cells. Toxicology. 2015;337:39–46.
48. Qian ZM, Tang PL, Wang Q. Iron crosses the endosomal membrane by a carrier-mediated process. Prog Biophys Mol Biol. 1997;67:1–15.
49. Qian M, Shen X, Wang H. The distinct role of ADAM17 in APP proteolysis and microglial activation related to Alzheimer's disease. Cell Mol Neurobiol. 2016;36:471–82.
50. Richter F, Meurers BH, Zhu C, Medvedeva VP, Chesselet MF. Neurons express hemoglobin alpha- and beta-chains in rat and human brains. J Comp Neurol. 2009;515:538–47.
51. Rochette L, Gudjoncik A, Guenancia C, Zeller M, Cottin Y, Vergely C. The iron-regulatory hormone hepcidin: a possible therapeutic target? Pharmacol Ther. 2015;146:35–52.
52. Rogers JT, Randall JD, Cahill CM, Eder PS, Huang X, Gunshin H, Leiter L, McPhee J, Sarang SS, Utsuki T, et al. An iron-responsive element type II in the 5′-untranslated region of the Alzheimer's amyloid precursor protein transcript. J Biol Chem. 2002;277:45518–28.
53. Savman K, Nilsson UA, Blennow M, Kjellmer I, Whitelaw A. Non-protein-bound iron is elevated in cerebrospinal fluid from preterm infants with posthemorrhagic ventricular dilatation. Pediatr Res. 2001;49:208–12.
54. Schaer CA, Schoedon G, Imhof A, Kurrer MO, Schaer DJ. Constitutive endocytosis of CD163 mediates hemoglobin-heme uptake and determines the noninflammatory and protective transcriptional response of macrophages to hemoglobin. Circ Res. 2006;99:943–50.

55. Schelshorn DW, Schneider A, Kuschinsky W, Weber D, Kruger C, Dittgen T, Burgers HF, Sabouri F, Gassler N, Bach A, et al. Expression of hemoglobin in rodent neurons. J Cereb Blood Flow Metab. 2009;29:585–95.
56. Schweizer C, Fraering PC, Kuhn LC. Ferritin H gene deletion in the choroid plexus and forebrain results in hydrocephalus. Neurochem Int. 2014;71:17–21.
57. Selim M. Deferoxamine mesylate: a new hope for intracerebral hemorrhage: from bench to clinical trials. Stroke. 2009;40:S90–1.
58. Selim M, Yeatts S, Goldstein JN, Gomes J, Greenberg S, Morgenstern LB, Schlaug G, Torbey M, Waldman B, Xi G, et al. Safety and tolerability of deferoxamine mesylate in patients with acute intracerebral hemorrhage. Stroke. 2011;42:3067–74.
59. Shamoto-Nagai M, Maruyama W, Yi H, Akao Y, Tribl F, Gerlach M, Osawa T, Riederer P, Naoi M. Neuromelanin induces oxidative stress in mitochondria through release of iron: mechanism behind the inhibition of 26S proteasome. J Neural Transm (Vienna). 2006;113:633–44.
60. Siler DA, Berlow YA, Kukino A, Davis CM, Nelson JW, Grafe MR, Ono H, Cetas JS, Pike M, Alkayed NJ. Soluble epoxide hydrolase in hydrocephalus, cerebral edema, and vascular inflammation after subarachnoid hemorrhage. Stroke. 2015;46:1916–22.
61. Slupe AM, Merrill RA, Flippo KH, Lobas MA, Houtman JC, Strack S. A calcineurin docking motif (LXVP) in dynamin-related protein 1 contributes to mitochondrial fragmentation and ischemic neuronal injury. J Biol Chem. 2013;288:12353–65.
62. Strahle JM, Garton T, Bazzi AA, Kilaru H, Garton HJ, Maher CO, Muraszko KM, Keep RF, Xi G. Role of hemoglobin and iron in hydrocephalus after neonatal intraventricular hemorrhage. Neurosurgery. 2014;75:696–705; discussion 706
63. Suzuki H, Muramatsu M, Tanaka K, Fujiwara H, Kojima T, Taki W. Cerebrospinal fluid ferritin in chronic hydrocephalus after aneurysmal subarachnoid hemorrhage. J Neurol. 2006;253:1170–6.
64. Switzer JA, Hess DC, Ergul A, Waller JL, Machado LS, Portik-Dobos V, Pettigrew LC, Clark WM, Fagan SC. Matrix metalloproteinase-9 in an exploratory trial of intravenous minocycline for acute ischemic stroke. Stroke. 2011;42:2633–5.
65. Switzer JA, Sikora A, Ergul A, Waller JL, Hess DC, Fagan SC. Minocycline prevents IL-6 increase after acute ischemic stroke. Transl Stroke Res. 2012;3:363–8.
66. Tan G, Liu L, He Z, Sun J, Xing W, Sun X. Role of hepcidin and its downstream proteins in early brain injury after experimental subarachnoid hemorrhage in rats. Mol Cell Biochem. 2016;418:31–8.
67. Thomsen JH, Etzerodt A, Svendsen P, Moestrup SK. The haptoglobin-CD163-heme oxygenase-1 pathway for hemoglobin scavenging. Oxidative Med Cell Longev. 2013;2013:523652.
68. Tyrrell R. Redox regulation and oxidant activation of heme oxygenase-1. Free Radic Res. 1999;31:335–40.
69. Unno M, Matsui T, Ikeda-Saito M. Crystallographic studies of heme oxygenase complexed with an unstable reaction intermediate, verdoheme. J Inorg Biochem. 2012;113:102–9.
70. Vollmer DG, Hongo K, Ogawa H, Tsukahara T, Kassell NF. A study of the effectiveness of the iron-chelating agent deferoxamine as vasospasm prophylaxis in a rabbit model of subarachnoid hemorrhage. Neurosurgery. 1991;28:27–32.
71. Watchko JF. Bilirubin-induced neurotoxicity in the preterm neonate. Clin Perinatol. 2016;43:297–311.
72. Wetterhall M, Bergquist J, Hillered L, Hjort K, Dahlin AP. Identification of human cerebrospinal fluid proteins and their distribution in an in vitro microdialysis sampling system. Eur J Pharm Sci. 2014;57:34–40.
73. Wicher KB, Fries E. Evolutionary aspects of hemoglobin scavengers. Antioxid Redox Signal. 2010;12:249–59.
74. Wong BX, Tsatsanis A, Lim LQ, Adlard PA, Bush AI, Duce JA. β-Amyloid precursor protein does not possess ferroxidase activity but does stabilize the cell surface ferrous iron exporter ferroportin. PLoS One. 2014;9:e114174.
75. Wu H, Wu T, Xu X, Wang J, Wang J. Iron toxicity in mice with collagenase-induced intracerebral hemorrhage. J Cereb Blood Flow Metab. 2011;31:1243–50.

76. Xie Q, Gu Y, Hua Y, Liu W, Keep RF, Xi G. Deferoxamine attenuates white matter injury in a piglet intracerebral hemorrhage model. Stroke. 2014;45:290–2.
77. Xu H, Tan G, Zhang S, Zhu H, Liu F, Huang C, Zhang F, Wang Z. Minocycline reduces reactive gliosis in the rat model of hydrocephalus. BMC Neurosci. 2012;13:148.
78. Yeatts SD, Palesch YY, Moy CS, Selim M. High dose deferoxamine in intracerebral hemorrhage (HI-DEF) trial: rationale, design, and methods. Neurocrit Care. 2013;19:257–66.
79. Yu Z, Persson HL, Eaton JW, Brunk UT. Intralysosomal iron: a major determinant of oxidant-induced cell death. Free Radic Biol Med. 2003;34:1243–52.
80. Yu Y, Zhao W, Zhu C, Kong Z, Xu Y, Liu G, Gao X. The clinical effect of deferoxamine mesylate on edema after intracerebral hemorrhage. PLoS One. 2015;10:e0122371.
81. Zacharia BE, Vaughan KA, Hickman ZL, Bruce SS, Carpenter AM, Petersen NH, Deiner S, Badjatia N, Connolly ES Jr. Predictors of long-term shunt-dependent hydrocephalus in patients with intracerebral hemorrhage requiring emergency cerebrospinal fluid diversion. Neurosurg Focus. 2012;32:E5.
82. Zhang AS, Enns CA. Iron homeostasis: recently identified proteins provide insight into novel control mechanisms. J Biol Chem. 2009;284:711–5.
83. Zhao F, Hua Y, He Y, Keep RF, Xi G. Minocycline-induced attenuation of iron overload and brain injury after experimental intracerebral hemorrhage. Stroke. 2011;42:3587–93.
84. Zhao J, Chen Z, Xi G, Keep RF, Hua Y. Deferoxamine attenuates acute hydrocephalus after traumatic brain injury in rats. Transl Stroke Res. 2014;5:586–94.
85. Zhao F, Xi G, Liu W, Keep RF, Hua Y. Minocycline attenuates iron-induced brain injury. Acta Neurochir. 2016;121:361–5.
86. Zhou X, Xie Q, Xi G, Keep RF, Hua Y. Brain CD47 expression in a swine model of intracerebral hemorrhage. Brain Res. 2014;1574:70–6.

Cerebrospinal Fluid Biomarkers of Hydrocephalus

3

Albert M. Isaacs and David D. Limbrick Jr.

Introduction

Hydrocephalus is a complex neurological disorder that is characterized by overaccumulation of cerebrospinal fluid (CSF) within the cerebral ventricles, affecting 1 in every 500–1000 individuals worldwide [1, 2]. From an etiological standpoint, there are several forms of hydrocephalus predefined by their respective antecedent neurologic events, including: posthemorrhagic hydrocephalus (PHH), which occurs following severe intraventricular hemorrhage (IVH) in neonates [3, 4]; postinfectious hydrocephalus (PIH), which results from ventriculitis typically in the setting of perinatal sepsis [5, 6], congenital hydrocephalus (CHC), which is associated with a range of genetic aberrations [1, 7–9]; spina-bifida-associated hydrocephalus (SB/HC), which typically occurs in patients myelomeningocele; and idiopathic normal pressure hydrocephalus (iNPH), an adult form with unknown etiology [10]. There are age-related, geographic and environmental differences in the prevalence of hydrocephalus worldwide. For example, in the pediatric population, PIH is the most common globally, predominantly in underdeveloped countries [11], whereas PHH is the most common in North America [12]. In the elderly (>65 years of age), iNPH appears to be the most diagnosed form. However, regardless of the etiology, all forms of hydrocephalus are associated with significant mortality and morbidity, which results

A. M. Isaacs (✉)
Division of Biology and Biomedical Sciences, Washington University in St. Louis, St. Louis, MO, USA

Division of Neurosurgery, Department of Clinical Neuroscience, University of Calgary, Calgary, AB, Canada
e-mail: albert.isaacs@wustl.edu

D. D. Limbrick Jr.
Department of Neurological Surgery, Washington University School of Medicine, St. Louis Children's Hospital, St. Louis, MO, USA

D. D. Limbrick, J. R. Leonard (eds.), *Cerebrospinal Fluid Disorders*,
https://doi.org/10.1007/978-3-319-97928-1_3

from brain injury that is caused by a combination of the antecedent injury, progressive ventricular dilatation, and/or raised intracranial pressure (ICP) [4].

The clinical presentation of hydrocephalus is often related to raised ICP such as tense fontanels and splaying of cranial sutures in infants, and/or generalized headaches, vomiting, papilledema, and seizures in all age groups [4, 13]. Depressed level of consciousness is often an ominous sign that requires prompt relief of the raised ICP through a CSF diversion procedure such as external ventricular drainage, shunting, or endoscopic third ventriculostiomy [14]. iNPH patients typically present with symptoms from a triad of progressive cognitive decline, gait impairment or urinary incontinence, that responds to ventricular shunting [15]. While clinical signs and symptoms may raise the suspicion of hydrocephalus, they are often non-specific, making prompt diagnosis of hydrocephalus challenging, especially in the primary care setting.

In addition to clinical symptoms, current practice guidelines rely heavily on time and changes on neuroimaging and imaging-based measurements, such as the Evan's ratio and the Frontal Occipital Horn Ratio for the diagnosis and/or confirmation of hydrocephalus [16]. However, these metrics are neither sensitive nor specific and do not provide any information on the pathophysiology or natural history of the disease [17]. Therefore, the conventional symptomatologic-radiologic approach often poses diagnostic dilemma in pediatric clinical practice as patients tend to present with large ventricles without clinical signs of hydrocephalus. Also, the conventional approach heavily relies on patient and family compliance to obtain the required imaging and timely follow-up. It is equally important to also note that at the time of diagnosis, especially in the pediatric population, over 80% of the deleterious effects of hydrocephalus are already established and are irremediable by surgery. As such, it is imperative to pursue alternative diagnostic measures that will promote early identification and diagnosis of hydrocephalus, predict treatment efficacy and alert treatment failure in a time-dependent fashion; preferably one that also correlates disease severity and treatment response to facilitate the comparison of treatment modalities in clinical trials. Over the past few decades, CSF proteins have been rigorously investigated as potential biomarkers that can be used independently or to compliment the clinico-radiologic findings of hydrocephalus [18, 19]. Biomarkers would also be valuable in their ability to inform clinicians by providing objective data on the likelihood a patient to develop hydrocephalus following an antecedent injury such as hemorrhage, infection, or trauma.

Pathophysiological Basis of CSF Biomarkers in Hydrocephalus

Interests in pursuing biomarkers of hydrocephalus from CSF stems from a long-standing appreciation that the CSF is an indispensable medium for assessing changes that occur in the brain and periventricular microenvironment. Specifically, in hydrocephalus, it is hypothesized that *the initial injury, intracranial hypertension, ventriculomegaly, and ventricular stretch are all capable of setting off an injurious cascade of hypoxic-ischemic injury, neuroinflammation, axonal disruption and neuronal death that disrupts the micro- and macro-environment of CSF* [12, 20–24]. Consequently, the molecular composition of CSF reflects the neurophysiological status of the neural structures they bathe. In addition, to being a sink for footprint proteins that are involved in the pathogenesis of hydrocephalus, CSF harbors molecular components necessary for neurodevelopment, neuromodulation and neurotransmission which may also be altered by the pathological process of hydrocephalus. While CSF stasis may account for the elevated levels of proteins in many forms of hydrocephalus, other processes such as ependymal layer cellular sloughing, blood products, infectious debris or inflammatory crud may add to the proteome. Impaired glymphatic absorption pathways have also been proposed as potential cause of the hydrodynamic impairments in hydrocephalus and may account for the elevations in CSF proteins due to poor clearance of proteins [25, 26].

Methodological Approaches to CSF Biomarkers

CSF protein analysis for biomarker discovery have been utilized extensively in several neurologic conditions including Alzheimer's disease (AD) [27, 28], amyotropic lateral sclerosis (ALS) [29] and traumatic brain injury (TBI) [30–35]. Conventional methods typically permit the isolation of one protein at a time. However recently, multiplex assays [36, 37] and high throughput "omics" technologies [38–40] have been widely employed to identify arrays of target and novel proteins respectively. These approaches have been adopted to explore biomarkers of hydrocephalus over the past decade [18, 19, 38, 40]. However, it is important to appreciate that the complex proteome of the CSF of hydrocephalus patients present several challenges for biomarker discovery. Specifically, there are a wide range of high abundance proteins present in the CSF of hydrocephalus patients, which makes it challenging to systematically detect putative biomarkers which may be of low-abundance. Nevertheless, adjunctive strategies such as multi-affinity fractionation (MAF) have been developed to deplete high-abundance proteins, thereby enhancing the detection sensitivity of low-abundance proteins, even in complex CSF samples. Morales et al. [40] employed similar techniques to deplete abundant blood-related proteins such as albumin and keratin in the CSF of infants with PHH to increase the yield of detecting low abundance proteins such as cell adhesion molecules, extracellular matrix proteins, and other markers of neurodevelopment [38, 40]. Following proteomics-based detection, it is often necessary to also use targeted protein approaches to confirm and rigorously validate biomarker proteins [40–43].

CSF Biomarkers of Hydrocephalus

Post-hemorrhagic Hydrocephalus

The use of proteomics-based discovery-validation paradigms to detect CSF biomarkers for PHH has recently gained momentum. Presently, the most robust biomarkers of PHH include amyloid precursor protein (*APP*), the APP-related derivative *sAPPα*, neural cell adhesion molecule (*NCAM-1*), L1 neural cell adhesion molecule (*L1-CAM*), *brevican* and total protein (*TP*). Utilizing tandem immunoaffinity proteomics, CSF from preterm neonates with PHH examined by Morales et al. [40] revealed over 400 proteins that are involved with various neurodevelopmental processes including cell adhesion molecules, synaptogenesis, extracellular matrix and cytoskeleton formation and oxidative metabolism. Specifically, APP, NCAM-1, L1-CAM, and brevican were elevated in the CSF of infants who had PHH than matched non-PHH controls [40]. Further, Limbrick et al. [41] utilized ELISAs to analyze lumbar CSF samples obtained from preterm infants with IVH +/− PHH and control CSF from matched infants with Hypoxic-Ischemic Injury and Ventricular enlargement without hydrocephalus [42]. The study confirmed, as well as validated their previous findings that APP and L1-CAM are selectively increased in PHH [42]. In addition, sAPPα and TP were found to be robust biomarkers for PHH. In fact, with an appropriate cut off, sAPPα was 91% sensitive and 95% specific for PHH and had an odds ratio of 200.0 with a relative risk of 46.9 [42]. The utility of these biomarkers has also been clinically monitored, and they have been shown to demonstrate decreasing patterns following CSF diversion interventions. In fact, CSF levels of APP, NCAM-1, and L1CAM correlated with ventricular size following percutaneous ventricular reservoir taps in PHH infants [43].

Congenital Hydrocephalus

Congenital hydrocephalus (CHC) encompasses a heterogeneous group of infantile hydrocephalus conditions that are caused by genetic or epigenetic aberrations in key neurodevelopmental processes including ventricular wall cell junctions proteins [44, 45], ependymal cell differentiation and migration of precursor neural stem cells [46], and cilia polarity [47–50]. Although limited data is available on CSF biomarker studies of CHC, *sAPPα* have been shown to be the most predictive in infants <1 years of age, demonstrating an odds ratio of 528.0 with a sensitivity of 94% and specificity of 97% [41]. Nevertheless, TGF-β1 and aminoterminal propeptide of type I collagen levels have also been shown to be lower in CHC when compared to PHH [51, 52]. In addition, infants with CHC tend to have higher levels of APP, sAPPα, sAPPβ, amyloid-β_{42} ($A\beta_{42}$), total tau (*t-tau*), phosphorylated tau (*p-tau*), L1CAM, and NCAM-1 when compared with controls [41].

Spina Bifida-Associated Hydrocephalus

Over 80% of patients with spina bifida have concomitant hydrocephalus [20–28]. While the CSF of patients with SB/HC has been analyzed, the studies have often included patients with non-SB-related hydrocephalus. To our knowledge only a few studies have compared SB/HC CSF proteomics with other forms of hydrocephalus [53–56]. Nevertheless, myelin basic protein (MBP), glial fibrillary acidic protein (GFAP), vimentin, Fas receptor, vascular endothelial growth factor (VEGF) and stem cell factor (SCF) have all been shown to be elevated in SB/HC [57, 58].

Normal Pressure Hydrocephalus

For a long time, intracranial hypertension was solely implicated for the ventricular distension in hydrocephalus, as well as for the improvement of symptoms following ventricular shunting. However, in the early 1960s, it was observed that a subset of patients who had clinical and radiographic evidence of hydrocephalus, yet an absence of raised intracranial pressure demonstrated symptomatic improvement following shunting. This subtype of hydrocephalus was termed Normal Pressure Hydrocephalus (NPH) and is characterized by as the presence of one or more symptoms of a triad—cognitive impairment, gait difficulties, and urinary incontinence [59]. While some NPH patients have an antecedent cause of their hydrocephalus, others have no identifiable cause. This has led to the subclassification of NPH into secondary (sNPH) and idiopathic (iNPH) NPH, to differentiate the former group from the latter. iNPH is an elderly disease, affecting patients typically over age 65 years old. As such, the diagnosis of iNPH is often challenging as the differential diagnosis always include several other common neurodegenerative conditions of the elderly, such as AD, frontotemporal dementia (FTD) and Parkinson's Disease (PD) [60]. Given the similarities in the clinical phenotype of AD and NPH, majority of NPH CSF biomarker studies have focused on markers of neurodegeneration including Amyloid-beta (Aβ), total tau (t-tau), and phosphorylated (p-tau) [19, 61–66]. The focus on AD-related proteins is probably driven by two major observations: About 40–75% of iNPH patients demonstrate amyloid and/or neurofibrillary tangles in cortical biopsies similar to AD and the dementia that underscores iNPH and AD cannot be reliably distinguished from one other.

A recent meta-analysis [19] of the biomarkers of 10 iNPH CSF biomarkers studies, which included 413 iNPH, 186 AD, and 147 healthy controls concluded that: (1) similar to AD, Aβ-42 (an Aβ isoform) is significantly lowered in iNPH when compared with normal healthy controls. However, the Aβ-42 levels in iNPH tend to be higher than in AD patients; (2) T-tau is significantly lower in iNPH than in AD and normal healthy controls and (3) P-tau is significantly lower in iNPH than in AD and normal healthy controls. However, it is important to note that there is no consensus on the reliability of t-tau and p-tau as a biomarker in iNPH, as other carefully done studies have found conflicting results [67]. In addition to AD-related biomarkers, others that have been explored as potential iNPH biomarkers include neurofilaments [18, 68], VEGF [18, 69], GFAP [18], TNF-α and TGFβ1 [69], and 8-isoprostane [18]; but none has emerged as a robust biomarker for iNPH yet.

Common Pathways of CSF Biomarkers in Hydrocephalus

There are five major categories of CSF biomarkers in hydrocephalus based on their associated physiological processes. While there is significant overlap, biomarkers may be classified as being related to neuroinflammation, cell junctional biology, extracellular matrix and cytoskeleton structure, growth/neurotrophic factors, or neurodegeneration. Primarily, studies of pediatric hydrocephalus tend to focus on neurodevelopment whereas adult studies often direct efforts toward neurodegeneration. Nevertheless, there are some classes of proteins that are ubiquitous across age groups and etiologies of hydrocephalus.

In pediatric hydrocephalus, *APP and APP-related peptides* are of prime importance. APP and its isoforms are associated with neurodevelopment and synaptogenesis [70–72] and their disruption invariably leads to axonal injury [73–77]. As such, the elevated levels of APP and its isoforms in PHH may be attributed to a cascade of axonal disruption caused by the inciting hemorrhagic insult and the ventricular distension [78, 79]. Presumably the reduction of APP levels in the CSF of PHH infants following resolution of ventriculomegaly [43] signals a reversal of the pathologic process. Similarly, *tau protein*, a robust biomarker of CHC likely rises in the setting of neuronal injury. Tau is a microtubule-associated molecule primarily responsible for the stabilization of the axonal cytoskeleton [80] and originates from axons and oligodendrocytes. As such, injury to axons and oligodendrocytes accounts for the elevated levels of *t-tau* in CHC and *p-tau* in PHH. It is important to note, however, that APP and tau are elevated in many other forms of neurologic diseases besides hydrocephalus. Therefore, it is challenging to specifically relate them to CSF hydrodynamics than to axonal or neuronal injury, in general.

In the elderly population, predominantly in iNPH, Aβ appears to be the most robust biomarker to date [19, 61–66]. While the decreased Aβ-42 levels in AD has been shown to be due to Aβ-42 sequestration into the plaques and tangles found on AD histopathology [81], alternative hypotheses have been suggested for iNPH including Aβ-42 shunting via the lymphatic drainage pathways [82], impaired Aβ-42 delivery from the extracellular compartment into CSF due to retrograde CSF flow in iNPH [83, 84], and diminished extracellular fluid space in iNPH [83], which compromises CSF flux and periventricular hypometabolism [61].

Challenges in CSF Biomarker Investigation in Hydrocephalus

The pathophysiology and pathogenesis of hydrocephalus is multifactorial, involving an inciting event, neuroinflammation, progressive ventriculomegaly, and cellular damage, all of which are associated with neurologic injury and release of nonspecific biomarkers into the CSF. Therefore, isolation of a single biomarker from the cesspool of CSF metabolites that will explain the entire syndrome of hydrocephalus is improbable. Perhaps a more prudent approach will be to consider a panel of biomarkers that will complement the clinical and radiographic features of the disease.

Furthermore, the heterogeneity of the different etiologies of hydrocephalus poses significant challenges. In addition to the different forms, the underlying biological process in each subtype is quite variable. For example, there are several distinct generic aberrations that have been implicated in CHC, each of which may be associated with biomarkers that are distinct from one another. Similarly, in PHH, while the underlying etiology is hemorrhage, there is growing literature to suggest that the germinal matrix vascular friability that leads to the hemorrhage results from an antecedent perinatal infection; thereby contaminating the sample with footprints of infection-related markers.

Another major challenge of CSF biomarker studies is the lack of true controls. Given the potential risks associated with CSF collection, majority of the control samples, especially in the pediatric population have come from infants who underwent CSF sampling for suspicion of other forms of CSF pathologies. For example, in PHH, control samples are often obtained from matched preterm infants assessed for intracranial infection, who turn out to have negative CSF cultures. Therefore, one cannot confidently rule out confounding biochemical processes. In addition, premature birth in itself is associated with a wide variety of acute and chronic diseases, such as necrotizing enterocolitis and sepsis, that may affect CSF biomarker levels.

Finally, the comparison of ventricular CSF of hydrocephalic patients with the lumbar CSF of control subjects is an active area of debate, as some studies have reported rostro-caudal protein gradients between the ventricles and the lumbar cisterns [85, 86].

Current Approaches to Improve Generalizability

To circumvent some of these challenges, cross-validation approaches have been utilized to analyze CSF biomarkers. As previously mentioned, targeted approaches such as ELISAs have been used to further validate high throughput proteomics findings [42]. Proteogenomic approaches, which include DNA metagenomics, RNA-seq, and other genomic analyses to cross-validate proteomic data or direct proteomic analysis have gained widespread use [87, 88] and offers substantial promise to fine-tune CSF biomarkers of hydrocephalus. To increase the generalizability of biomarkers, multicenter CSF repositories such as those maintained by the Hydrocephalus Clinical Research Network (HCRN), the Adult Hydrocephalus Clinical Research Network (AHCRN), and the Hydrocephalus Association Network for Discovery Science (HANDS) allow testing of CSF from multiple centers and countries. The repositories offer several relevant biomarkers research advantages: (1) it helps to potentially eliminate the confounding effect of environmental and geographic differences in hydrocephalus and (2) it keeps selection bias to a minimum when comparing treatment efficacy and patient outcomes.

Table 3.1 Published literature on the biomarkers of hydrocephalus in cerebrospinal fluid

Hydrocephalus	Key biomarkers studied	Author	Year	Journal	Title
CH	APP; sAPPα; sAPPβ; Aβ42; tau; pTau; L1CAM; NCAM-1; AQP4; TP	Limbrick et al. [41]	2017	*PLoS One*	Cerebrospinal fluid biomarkers of infantile congenital hydrocephalus.
CH	NGF	Mashayekhi et al. [89]	2005	*European Journal of Neurology*	Expression of nerve growth factor in cerebrospinal fluid of congenital hydrocephalic and normal children.
CH	NGF	Erol et al. [90]	2009	*Pediatric Neurosurgery*	Investigating a correlation between the results of transcranial Doppler and the level of nerve growth factor in cerebrospinal fluid of hydrocephalic infants: clinical study.
Mixed/unspecified	NFL; tau; VIP; NPY; C/S-AR	Tisell et al. [91]	2004	*European Journal of Neurology*	Differences in cerebrospinal fluid dynamics do not affect the levels of biochemical markers in ventricular CSF from patients with aqueductal stenosis and idiopathic normal pressure hydrocephalus.
Mixed/unspecified	Arginine; citrulline; nitrate	Perez-Neri et al. [92]	2007	*Journal of Chromatography*	Arginine, citrulline and nitrate concentrations in the cerebrospinal fluid from patients with acute hydrocephalus.
Mixed/unspecified	tau; 9-HAA	Cengiz et al. [93]	2008	*Pediatric Critical Care Medicine*	Cerebrospinal fluid cleaved-tau protein and 9-hydroxyoctadecadienoic acid concentrations in pediatric patients with hydrocephalus.
Mixed/unspecified	MBP	Sutton et al. [94]	1983	*Journal of Neurosurgery*	Cerebrospinal fluid myelin basic protein in hydrocephalus.
Mixed/unspecified	Calsyntenin-1; Tag1; DJ-1; ICAM5; NCadh; NCAM-1; NCAM-2; NRXN3; Neurocan; NPTX-1; NPTX-2; Neuroserpin; SEMA7A	Waybright et al. [38]	2010	*Journal of Proteomics*	Characterization of the human ventricular cerebrospinal fluid proteome obtained from hydrocephalic patients.
Mixed/unspecified	5-HIAA; HVA	Gopal et al. [95]	2008	*Child's Nervous System*	Comparative evaluation of 5-HIAA (5-hydroxy indoleacetic acid) and HVA (homovanillic acid) in infantile hydrocephalus.

Mixed/ unspecified	VEGF; TNF-α; TGF-β1; tau	Lee et al. [96]	2012	*Medical Science Monitor*	Comparison of cerebrospinal fluid biomarkers between idiopathic normal pressure hydrocephalus and subarachnoid hemorrhage-induced chronic hydrocephalus: a pilot study.
Mixed/ unspecified	TP; FasR; FasL; SCF; HGF; VEGF; IGF-1; TNF-α; IL-6	Naureen et al. [58]	2014	*Child's Nervous System*	Fingerprint changes in CSF composition associated with different aetiologies in human neonatal hydrocephalus: inflammatory cytokines.
Mixed/ unspecified	NGF	Yang et al. [97]	1999	*Clinical Biochemistry*	Increase in CSF NGF concentration is positively correlated with poor prognosis of postoperative hydrocephalic patients.
Mixed/ unspecified	Fas, FasL	Felderhoff-Mueser et al. [98]	2001	*Archives of Disease in Childhood*	Increased cerebrospinal fluid concentrations of soluble Fas (CD95/Apo-1) in hydrocephalus.
Mixed/ unspecified	Tau; pTau; Aβ	de Bont et al. [99]	2008	*European Journal of Paediatric Neurology*	Increased total-Tau levels in cerebrospinal fluid of pediatric hydrocephalus and brain tumor patients.
Mixed/ unspecified	NSE; S-100; CK; CK-BB	Kruse et al. [100]	1991	*Acta Neurochirurgica*	Increases of neuron-specific enolase, S-100 protein, creatine kinase and creatine kinase BB isoenzyme in CSF following intraventricular catheter implantation.
Mixed/ unspecified	Gamma-globulin and alpha 2-globulin	Cerda et al. [101]	1980	*Child's Brain*	Polyacrylamide gel electrophoresis of cerebrospinal fluid proteins in children with nontumoral hydrocephalus.
Mixed/ unspecified	GH; IGLF-I; BP-3	Lopponen et al. [102]	1997	*Archives of Disease in Childhood*	Reduced levels of growth hormone, insulin-like growth factor-I and binding protein-3 in patients with shunted hydrocephalus.
Mixed/ unspecified	5-HT; 5-HIAA	Gopal et al. [103]	2007	*Pediatric Surgery International*	Serotonin and 5-hydroxy indole acetic acid in infantile hydrocephalus.
Mixed/ unspecified	NSE; S-100b; GFAP; MBP	Beems et al. [54]	2003	*Acta Neurochirurgica*	Serum- and CSF-concentrations of brain specific proteins in hydrocephalus.
Mixed/ unspecified	MBP	Longatti et al. [104]	1994	*Child's Nervous System*	The CSF myelin basic protein in pediatric hydrocephalus.

(continued)

Table 3.1 (continued)

Hydrocephalus	Key biomarkers studied	Author	Year	Journal	Title
Mixed/ unspecified	MBP	Longatti et al. [56]	1993	*Journal of Neurosurgical Sciences*	The CSF myelin basic protein: a reliable marker of actual cerebral damage in hydrocephalus.
Mixed/ unspecified	TIMP-4; IL-6; IL-8; MCP-1; MMP-9; TIMP-1; TIMP-2	Killer et al. [105]	2010	*Neurochemical Research*	Cytokine and growth factor concentration in cerebrospinal fluid from patients with hydrocephalus following endovascular embolization of unruptured aneurysms in comparison with other types of hydrocephalus.
NPH	Tf-1; Tf-2	Futakawa et al. [106]	2012	*Neurobiology of Aging*	A unique N-glycan on human transferrin in CSF: a possible biomarker for iNPH.
NPH	Aβ-38, Aβ-40, Aβ-42, sAPP-α; sAPP-β; APLP-1; APLP-1β25; APLP-1β27; APLP-1β28	Jeppsson et al. [107]	2016	*Fluids and Barriers of the CNS*	Amyloid mis-metabolism in idiopathic normal pressure hydrocephalus.
NPH	Aβ-42; tau; pTau	Herukka et al. [108]	2015	*Journal of Alzheimer's Disease*	Amyloid-beta and Tau dynamics in human brain interstitial fluid in patients with suspected normal pressure hydrocephalus.
NPH	LRG; alpha1-antichymotrypsin; apo-D; apo-J; Hp-α1; serum albumin; and alpha-1-microglobulin	Li et al. [62]	2006	*Acta Neurochirurgica*	Analysis of potential diagnostic biomarkers in cerebrospinal fluid of idiopathic normal pressure hydrocephalus by proteomics.
NPH	BDNF	Laske et al. [109]	2007	*Journal of Psychiatric Research*	BDNF serum and CSF concentrations in Alzheimer's disease, normal pressure hydrocephalus and healthy controls.
NPH	sAPP; sAPP-α; Aβ; tTau; pTau	Ray et al. [110]	2011	*Journal of Psychiatric Research*	Biochemical studies in Normal Pressure Hydrocephalus (NPH) patients: change in CSF levels of amyloid precursor protein (APP), amyloid-beta (Abeta) peptide and phospho-tau.

NPH	sAPP; sAPP-α; Aβ-38; Aβ-42; pTau; L-PGDS; cystatin C	Nakajima et al. [30]	2015	*Journal of the Neurological Sciences*	Cerebrospinal fluid biomarkers for prognosis of long-term cognitive treatment outcomes in patients with idiopathic normal pressure hydrocephalus.
NPH	TBAR; SH	Fersten et al. [111]	2004	*Folia Neuropathologica*	Cerebrospinal fluid free-radical peroxidation products and cognitive functioning patterns differentiate varieties of normal pressure hydrocephalus.
NPH	TNF-α; AQP-1	Castaneyra-Ruiz et al. [112]	2016	*Clinical Neurology and Neurosurgery*	Cerebrospinal fluid levels of tumor necrosis factor alpha and aquaporin 1 in patients with mild cognitive impairment and idiopathic normal pressure hydrocephalus.
NPH	tTau; pTau; Aβ42	Kapaki et al. [113]	2007	*European Journal of Neurology*	Cerebrospinal fluid tau, phospho-tau181 and beta-amyloid1-42 in idiopathic normal pressure hydrocephalus: a discrimination from Alzheimer's disease.
NPH	tTau; pTau; Aβ42	Elobeid et al. [114]	2015	*Journal of Neuropathology and Experimental Neurology*	Correlations between mini-mental state examination score, cerebrospinal fluid biomarkers, and pathology observed in brain biopsies of patients with normal-pressure hydrocephalus.
NPH	Sulfatide; NFL; tTau; pTau; Aβ42	Agren-Wilsson et al. [115]	2007	*Acta Neurologica Scandinavica*	CSF biomarkers in the evaluation of idiopathic normal pressure hydrocephalus.
NPH	NFL; GFAP	Tullberg et al. [116]	1998	*Neurology*	CSF neurofilament and glial fibrillary acidic protein in normal pressure hydrocephalus.
NPH	α2HS-glycoprotein; α1-antichimotrypsin; α1β-glycoprotein, GFAP; apo-4; apo-J; apo-E; C-3c; anti-thrombin; α2-antiplasmin; albumin	Scollato et al. [117]	2010	*Neurological Sciences*	CSF proteomic analysis in patients with normal pressure hydrocephalus selected for the shunt: CSF biomarkers of response to surgical treatment.
NPH	Sulfatide	Tullberg et al. [118]	2000	*Journal of Neurology, Neurosurgery, and Psychiatry*	CSF sulfatide distinguishes between normal pressure hydrocephalus and subcortical arteriosclerotic encephalopathy.

(continued)

Table 3.1 (continued)

Hydrocephalus	Key biomarkers studied	Author	Year	Journal	Title
NPH	Homocysteine	Sosvorova et al. [119]	2014	*Physiological Research*	Determination of homocysteine in cerebrospinal fluid as an indicator for surgery treatment in patients with hydrocefalus.
NPH	Aβ-42	Kondo et al. [120]	2013	*The Neuroradiology Journal*	Distribution of amyloid burden differs between idiopathic normal pressure hydrocephalus and Alzheimer's disease.
NPH	tTau; pTau; Aβ-42	Lim et al. [121]	2014	*BMC Neurology*	Evaluation of coexistence of Alzheimer's disease in idiopathic normal pressure hydrocephalus using ELISA analyses for CSF biomarkers.
NPH	LRG; TGF-β1; TGF-β2; TGF-β3; TGF-β2 receptor	Li et al. [63]	2007	*Neuroscience Letters*	Expression of TGF-betas and TGF-beta type II receptor in cerebrospinal fluid of patients with idiopathic normal pressure hydrocephalus.
NPH	GFAP	Albrechtsen et al. [122]	1985	*Journal of the Neurological Sciences*	High cerebrospinal fluid concentration of glial fibrillary acidic protein (GFAP) in patients with normal pressure hydrocephalus.
NPH	Orexin A, HVA, 5-HIAA, MHPG	Kalamatianos et al. [123]	2014	*Peptides*	Higher Orexin A levels in lumbar compared to ventricular CSF: a study in idiopathic normal pressure hydrocephalus.
NPH	tTau; pTau; Aβ-42; Aβ-40; LRG	Jingami et al. [124]	2015	*Journal of Alzheimer's Disease*	Idiopathic normal pressure hydrocephalus has a different cerebrospinal fluid biomarker profile from Alzheimer's disease.
NPH	pTau; Aβ-42	Kang et al. [125]	2014	*Journal of Clinical Neuroscience*	Idiopathic normal-pressure hydrocephalus, cerebrospinal fluid biomarkers, and the cerebrospinal fluid tap test.
NPH	NFL; MBP; Aβ-38; Aβ-40; Aβ42; sAPPα; sAPPβ; tTau, pTau; IL-8; IL-10; MCP-1	Jeppsson et al. [84]	2013	*Neurology*	Idiopathic normal-pressure hydrocephalus: pathophysiology and diagnosis by CSF biomarkers.
NPH	tTau; Aβ-42	Lins et al. [126]	2004	*Journal of Neural Transmission*	Immunoreactivities of amyloid beta peptide ((1-42)) and total tau protein in lumbar cerebrospinal fluid of patients with normal pressure hydrocephalus.

NPH	LRG	Nakajima et al. [127]	2011	*Acta Neurochirurgica*	Leucine-rich alpha-2-glycoprotein is a marker for idiopathic normal pressure hydrocephalus.
NPH	L-PGDS	Mase et al. [128]	2003	*Neuroscience Research*	Lipocalin-type prostaglandin D synthase (beta-trace) in cerebrospinal fluid: a useful marker for the diagnosis of normal pressure hydrocephalus.
NPH	VEGF	Huang et al. [129]	2016	*Neurochemical Research*	Longitudinal metabolite profiling of cerebrospinal fluid in normal pressure hydrocephalus links brain metabolism with exercise-induced VEGF production and clinical outcome.
NPH	Synaptic membrane glycoprotein D2	Sorensen et al. [130]	1983	*Journal of the Neurological Sciences*	Low cerebrospinal fluid concentration of brain-specific protein D2 in patients with normal pressure hydrocephalus.
NPH	β-trace protein; β-2 microglobulin; cystatin C	Brettschneider et al. [131]	2004	*Journal of Neurology, Neurosurgery, and Psychiatry*	Meningeal derived cerebrospinal fluid proteins in different forms of dementia: is a meningopathy involved in normal pressure hydrocephalus?
NPH	tTau; pTau; Aβ-42	Luikku et al. [132]	2016	*Acta Neurochirurgica*	Multimodal analysis to predict shunt surgery outcome of 284 patients with suspected idiopathic normal pressure hydrocephalus.
NPH	TNF-α	Tarkowski et al. [133]	2003	*Neurobiology of Aging*	Normal pressure hydrocephalus triggers intrathecal production of TNF-alpha.
NPH	IL-1β; IL-4; IL-6; IL-10; IL-17A; IL-17F; IL-21; IL-22; IL-23; IL-25; IL-31; IL-33; INF-ɣ; sCD40L; TNF-α	Sosvorova et al. [36]	2014	*Neuro Endocrinology Letters*	Selected pro- and anti-inflammatory cytokines in cerebrospinal fluid in normal pressure hydrocephalus.
NPH	TP; albumin; tTau; pTau (pTau); Aβ-42; Aβ-40; Aβ-42/Aβ-40 ratio	Djukic et al. [134]	2016	*Fluids and Barriers of the CNS*	Small cisterno-lumbar gradient of phosphorylated Tau protein in geriatric patients with suspected normal pressure hydrocephalus.
NPH	sAPP-α; sAPP-β; Aβ-42; tTau; pTau	Miyajima et al. [135]	2013	*European Journal of Neurology*	Soluble amyloid precursor protein alpha in the cerebrospinal fluid as a diagnostic and prognostic biomarker for idiopathic normal pressure hydrocephalus.

(continued)

Table 3.1 (continued)

Hydrocephalus	Key biomarkers studied	Author	Year	Journal	Title
NPH	tTau	Kudo et al. [136]	2000	*Psychiatry and Clinical Neurosciences*	Tau protein is a potential biological marker for normal pressure hydrocephalus.
NPH	sAβPP-α; sAβPP-β; TTR	Laitera et al. [31]	2015	*Journal of Alzheimer's Disease*	The expression of transthyretin and amyloid-beta protein precursor is altered in the brain of idiopathic normal pressure hydrocephalus patients.
NPH	Lactate; 8-isoprostane; VEGF; GFAP; NFH; Aβ-42; tTau	Tarnaris et al. [137]	2009	*Journal of Neurology, Neurosurgery, and Psychiatry*	The longitudinal profile of CSF markers during external lumbar drainage.
NPH	Aβ-42; tTau	Tarnaris et al. [138]	2011	*Journal of Neurosurgery*	Use of cerebrospinal fluid amyloid-beta and total tau protein to predict favorable surgical outcomes in patients with idiopathic normal pressure hydrocephalus.
NPH	Aβ-42	Brandner et al. [86]	2014	*Journal of Alzheimer's Disease*	Ventricular and lumbar cerebrospinal fluid concentrations of Alzheimer's disease biomarkers in patients with normal pressure hydrocephalus and post-traumatic hydrocephalus.
PHH	TGF-β1; TGF-β2; CSPG; NT-CSPG	Chow et al. [139]	2005	*Biology of the Neonate*	Accumulation of transforming growth factor-beta2 and nitrated chondroitin sulfate proteoglycans in cerebrospinal fluid correlates with poor neurologic outcome in preterm hydrocephalus.
PHH	APP; NCAM-1; L1CAM; Brevican	Morales et al. [40]	2012	*Molecular & Cellular Proteomics*	Alterations in protein regulators of neurodevelopment in the cerebrospinal fluid of infants with posthemorrhagic hydrocephalus of prematurity.
PHH	APP; NCAM-1; L1CAM	Morales et al. [43]	2015	*PLoS One*	Cerebrospinal fluid levels of amyloid precursor protein are associated with ventricular size in posthemorrhagic hydrocephalus of prematurity.
PHH	sFas	Schmitz et al. [148]	2011	*Journal of Perinatal Medicine*	Expression of soluble Fas in the cerebrospinal fluid of preterm infants with posthemorrhagic hydrocephalus and cystic white matter damage.

PHH	MMP-9; hepatocyte growth factor	Okamoto et al. [140]	2010	*Early Human Development*	Increased expression of matrix metalloproteinase-9 and hepatocyte growth factor in the cerebrospinal fluid of infants with posthemorrhagic hydrocephalus.
PHH	IL-1β; IL-18; IFN-γ	Schmitz et al. [141]	2007	*Pediatric Research*	Interleukin-1beta, interleukin-18, and interferon-gamma expression in the cerebrospinal fluid of premature infants with posthemorrhagic hydrocephalus—markers of white matter damage?
PHH	APP, sAβPP-α; L1CAM	Morales et al. [42]	2017	*Neurosurgery*	Lumbar cerebrospinal fluid biomarkers of posthemorrhagic hydrocephalus of prematurity: amyloid precursor protein, soluble amyloid precursor protein alpha, and L1 cell adhesion molecule.
PHH	FASL; activated caspase 3	Felderhoff-Mueser et al. [142]	2003	*Pediatric Research*	Soluble Fas (CD95/Apo-1), soluble Fas ligand, and activated caspase 3 in the cerebrospinal fluid of infants with posthemorrhagic and nonhemorrhagic hydrocephalus.
PHH	VEGF; TGF-β1	Heep et al. [51]	2004	*Pediatric Research*	Vascular endothelial growth factor and transforming growth factor-beta1 are highly expressed in the cerebrospinal fluid of premature infants with posthemorrhagic hydrocephalus.
PHH	IL-1α; IL-1β; IL-4; IL-6; IL-8; IL-10; IL-12; TNF-α; TGF-β1; IFN-γ; CXCL-1; CXCL-10; CXCL-11; CXCL-12; CCL-2; CCL-3; CCL-19	Habiyaremye et al. [149]	2017	*Fluids and Barriers of the CNS*	Chemokine and cytokine levels in the lumbar cerebrospinal fluid of preterm infants with posthemorrhagic hydrocephalus.
SAH	TGF-β1	Kitazawa et al. [143]	1994	*Stroke*	Elevation of transforming growth factor-beta 1 level in cerebrospinal fluid of patients with communicating hydrocephalus after subarachnoid hemorrhage.
SAH	TGF-β1; TGF-β2	Douglas et al. [144]	2009	*Journal of Neurology, Neurosurgery, and Psychiatry*	High CSF transforming growth factor-beta levels after subarachnoid hemorrhage: association with chronic communicating hydrocephalus.

(continued)

Table 3.1 (continued)

Hydrocephalus	Key biomarkers studied	Author	Year	Journal	Title
SAH	HMGB-1	Sokol et al. [145]	2015	*Journal of Stroke and Cerebrovascular Diseases*	HMGB1 level in cerebrospinal fluid as a marker of treatment outcome in patients with acute hydrocephalus following aneurysmal subarachnoid hemorrhage.
SAH	S-100	Brandner et al. [146]	2012	*Acta Neurochirurgica. Supplement*	Shunt-dependent hydrocephalus following subarachnoid hemorrhage correlates with increased S100B levels in cerebrospinal fluid and serum.
SAH	TLR-2; TLR-4	Sokol et al. [147]	2016	*PLoS One*	Soluble toll-like receptors 2 and 4 in cerebrospinal fluid of patients with acute hydrocephalus following aneurysmal subarachnoid hemorrhage.

Abbreviations: *5-HIAA* 5-hydroxy indoleacetic acid, *5-HT* serotonin, *9-HAA* 9-hydroxyoctadecadienoic acid, *Aβ-* amyloid beta, *APLP-* amyloid precursor protein like protein, *apo-* apolipoprotein, *APP* amyloid precursor protein, *AQP-* aquaporin, *BDNF* brain-derived neurotrophic factor, *BP-3* binding protein-3, *C-* complement, *C/S-AR* CSF/serum albumin ratio, *CCL-* chemokine (C-C motif) ligand, *CK* creatine kinase, *CK-BB* creatine kinase BB isoenzyme, *CSPG* chondroitin sulfate proteoglycan, *CXCL-* chemokine (C-X-C motif) ligand, *FAs* first apoptosis signal, *FasL* first apoptosis signal ligand, *FasR* first apoptosis signal receptor, *GFAP* glial fibrillary acidic protein, *GH* growth hormone, *GRM4* Glutamate receptor 4, *HGF* hepatocyte growth factor, *HMBG-* high mobility group box, *Hp-* haptoglobin, *HVA* homovanillic acid, *ICAM-* intercellular adhesion molecule, *IGLF-* insulin growth factor, *IL-* interleukin, *INF-* inteferon, *L1CAM* L1 cell adhesion molecule, *L-PGDS* lipocalin-type prostaglandin D synthase, *LRG* leucine-rich alpha-2-glycoprotein, *MBP* myelin basic protein, *MCP-* monocyte chemoattractant protein, *MHPG* 3-methoxy-4-hydroxyphenylglycol, *MMP-* matrix metallopeptidase, *Ncadh* neural cadherin, *NCAM-* neural cell adhesion molecule, *NFH* neurofilament heavy chain protein, *NFL* neurofilament light chain protein, *NGF* nerve growth factor, *NPTX* neuronal pentraxin, *NPY* neuropeptide PYY, *NRXN3* neurexin-3-alpha, *NSE* neuron-specific enolase, *NT-CSPG* nitrated chondroitin sulfate proteoglycan, *pTau* phosphorylated Tau, *S-100* S-100 protein, *sAβPP-* soluble amino-terminal fragment of AbetaPP, *sAPP-* soluble amyloid precursor protein, *sCD40L* soluble CD40-ligand, *SCL* stem cell factor, *SEMA7A* Semaphorin-7A, *SH* protein sulphydryl, *Tag1* contactin-2, *TBAR* thiobarbituric acid-reactive material, *Tf-* transferrin, *TGF* tumor growth factor, *TIMP-4* TIMP metallopeptidase inhibitor, *TLR-* toll-like receptor, *TNF* tumor necrosis factor, *TP* total protein, *tTau* total Tau, *TTR* transthyretin, *VEGF* vascular endothelial growth factor, *VIP* vasoactive intestinal peptide.

Finally, in vitro and in vivo animal models of hydrocephalus offer an unprecedented opportunity to test biomarkers in a controlled environment.

Conclusion

With ongoing efforts, it is possible to identify biomarkers that can be used to improve the outcomes of patients who are debilitated by hydrocephalus worldwide. Biomarkers are essential not only for the diagnosis of hydrocephalus but also for the assessment of treatment outcomes and to predict patients who will develop hydrocephalus following an antecedent event. There are ongoing efforts to streamline the utility, accuracy, and generalizability of CSF biomarkers through cross-validation technologies such as ELISAs, proteogenomics, and multicenter CSF repositories. Consideration of a battery of biomarkers that correlate with clinico-radiographic features of the disease, as opposed to pursuing a single biomarker, is encouraged given the multifactorial pathophysiology and pathogenesis of hydrocephalus (Table 3.1).

References

1. Tully HM, Dobyns WB. Infantile hydrocephalus: a review of epidemiology, classification and causes. Eur J Med Genet. 2014;57(8):359–68.
2. Rekate HL. A contemporary definition and classification of hydrocephalus. Semin Pediatr Neurol. 2009;16(1):9–15.
3. Volpe JJ. Intraventricular hemorrhage and brain injury in the premature infant. Neuropathology and pathogenesis. *Clin Perinatol*. 1989;16(2):361–86.
4. Kahle KT, Kulkarni AV, Limbrick DD Jr, Warf BC. Hydrocephalus in children. Lancet. 2016;387(10020):788–99.
5. Chu SM, Hsu JF, Lee CW, et al. Neurological complications after neonatal bacteremia: the clinical characteristics, risk factors, and outcomes. PLoS One. 2014;9(11):e105294.
6. Li L, Padhi A, Ranjeva SL, et al. Association of bacteria with hydrocephalus in Ugandan infants. J Neurosurg Pediatr. 2011;7(1):73–87.
7. van der Knaap MS, Valk J. Classification of congenital abnormalities of the CNS. AJNR Am J Neuroradiol. 1988;9(2):315–26.
8. Muniz-Talavera H, Schmidt JV. The mouse Jhy gene regulates ependymal cell differentiation and ciliogenesis. PLoS One. 2017;12(12):e0184957.
9. Zhang J, Williams MA, Rigamonti D. Genetics of human hydrocephalus. J Neurol. 2006;253(10):1255–66.
10. Adams RD, Fisher CM, Hakim S, Ojemann RG, Sweet WH. Symptomatic occult hydrocephalus with "normal" cerebrospinal-fluid pressure.A treatable syndrome. N Engl J Med. 1965;273(3):117–26.
11. Warf BC, East African Neurosurgical Research Collaboration. Pediatric hydrocephalus in East Africa: prevalence, causes, treatments, and strategies for the future. World Neurosurg. 2010;73(4):296–300.
12. McAllister JP 2nd, Chovan P. Neonatal hydrocephalus. Mechanisms and consequences. Neurosurg Clin N Am. 1998;9(1):73–93.
13. Wellons JC 3rd, Holubkov R, Browd SR, et al. The assessment of bulging fontanel and splitting of sutures in premature infants: an interrater reliability study by the Hydrocephalus Clinical Research Network. J Neurosurg Pediatr. 2013;11(1):12–4.

14. Murphy BP, Inder TE, Rooks V, et al. Posthaemorrhagic ventricular dilatation in the premature infant: natural history and predictors of outcome. Arch Dis Child Fetal Neonatal Ed. 2002;87(1):F37–41.
15. Relkin N, Marmarou A, Klinge P, Bergsneider M, Black PM. Diagnosing idiopathic normal-pressure hydrocephalus. *Neurosurgery*. 2005;57(3 Suppl):S4–16; discussion ii–v
16. O'Hayon BB, Drake JM, Ossip MG, Tuli S, Clarke M. Frontal and occipital horn ratio: a linear estimate of ventricular size for multiple imaging modalities in pediatric hydrocephalus. Pediatr Neurosurg. 1998;29(5):245–9.
17. Warf B, Ondoma S, Kulkarni A, et al. Neurocognitive outcome and ventricular volume in children with myelomeningocele treated for hydrocephalus in Uganda. J Neurosurg Pediatr. 2009;4(6):564–70.
18. Tarnaris A, Toma AK, Pullen E, et al. Cognitive, biochemical, and imaging profile of patients suffering from idiopathic normal pressure hydrocephalus. Alzheimers Dement. 2011;7(5):501–8.
19. Santangelo R, Cecchetti G, Bernasconi MP, et al. Cerebrospinal fluid amyloid-beta 42, total tau, and phosphorylated tau are low in patients with normal pressure hydrocephalus: analogies and differences with Alzheimer's disease. J Alzheimers Dis. 2017;60:183–200.
20. Del Bigio MR. Cellular damage and prevention in childhood hydrocephalus. Brain Pathol. 2004;14(3):317–24.
21. Williams MA, McAllister JP, Walker ML, et al. Priorities for hydrocephalus research: report from a National Institutes of Health-sponsored workshop. J Neurosurg. 2007;107(5 Suppl):345–57.
22. Del Bigio MR, McAllister JP II. Pathophysiology of hydrocephalus. In: Choux M, DiRocco R, Hockley AD, Walker ML, editors. Pediatric neurosurgery, vol. 4. Philadelphia: Churchill Livingstone; 1999. p. 217–36.
23. Del Bigio MR. Neuropathology and structural changes in hydrocephalus. Dev Disabil Res Rev. 2010;16(1):16–22.
24. McAllister JP 2nd, Williams MA, Walker ML, et al. An update on research priorities in hydrocephalus: overview of the third National Institutes of Health-sponsored symposium "Opportunities for Hydrocephalus Research: Pathways to Better Outcomes". J Neurosurg. 2015;123(6):1427–38.
25. Iliff JJ, Chen MJ, Plog BA, et al. Impairment of glymphatic pathway function promotes tau pathology after traumatic brain injury. J Neurosci Off J Soc Neurosci. 2014;34(49):16180–93.
26. Petraglia AL, Dashnaw ML, Turner RC, Bailes JE. Models of mild traumatic brain injury: translation of physiological and anatomic injury. *Neurosurgery*. 2014;75(suppl_4):S34–49.
27. Fagan AM, Csernansky CA, Morris JC, Holtzman DM. The search for antecedent biomarkers of Alzheimer's disease. J Alzheimers Dis. 2005;8(4):347–58.
28. Fagan AM, Holtzman DM. Cerebrospinal fluid biomarkers of Alzheimer's disease. Biomark Med. 2010;4(1):51–63.
29. Pasinetti GM, Ungar LH, Lange DJ, et al. Identification of potential CSF biomarkers in ALS. Neurology. 2006;66(8):1218–22.
30. Nakajima M, Miyajima M, Ogino I, et al. Cerebrospinal fluid biomarkers for prognosis of long-term cognitive treatment outcomes in patients with idiopathic normal pressure hydrocephalus. J Neurol Sci. 2015;357(1–2):88–95.
31. Laitera T, Kurki MI, Pursiheimo JP, et al. The expression of transthyretin and amyloid-beta protein precursor is altered in the brain of idiopathic normal pressure hydrocephalus patients. J Alzheimers Dis. 2015;48(4):959–68.
32. Sutphen CL, Jasielec MS, Shah AR, et al. Longitudinal cerebrospinal fluid biomarker changes in preclinical Alzheimer disease during middle age. JAMA Neurol. 2015;72(9):1029–42.
33. Tsitsopoulos PP, Marklund N. A delayed spinocutaneous fistula after anterior cervical discectomy and fusion. Spine J. 2015;15(4):783–4.
34. Marklund N, Farrokhnia N, Hanell A, et al. Monitoring of beta-amyloid dynamics after human traumatic brain injury. J Neurotrauma. 2014;31(1):42–55.
35. Steinacker P, Fang L, Kuhle J, et al. Soluble beta-amyloid precursor protein is related to disease progression in amyotrophic lateral sclerosis. PLoS One. 2011;6(8):e23600.

36. Sosvorova L, Vcelak J, Mohapl M, Vitku J, Bicikova M, Hampl R. Selected pro- and anti-inflammatory cytokines in cerebrospinal fluid in normal pressure hydrocephalus. Neuro Endocrinol Lett. 2014;35(7):586–93.
37. Gutierrez-Murgas YM, Skar G, Ramirez D, Beaver M, Snowden JN. IL-10 plays an important role in the control of inflammation but not in the bacterial burden in S. epidermidis CNS catheter infection. *J Neuroinflammation*. 2016;13(1):271.
38. Waybright T, Avellino AM, Ellenbogen RG, Hollinger BJ, Veenstra TD, Morrison RS. Characterization of the human ventricular cerebrospinal fluid proteome obtained from hydrocephalic patients. J Proteome. 2010;73(6):1156–62.
39. Veenstra TD, Conrads TP, Hood BL, Avellino AM, Ellenbogen RG, Morrison RS. Biomarkers: mining the biofluid proteome. Mol Cell Proteomics. 2005;4(4):409–18.
40. Morales DM, Townsend RR, Malone JP, et al. Alterations in protein regulators of neurodevelopment in the cerebrospinal fluid of infants with posthemorrhagic hydrocephalus of prematurity. *Mol Cell Proteomics*. 2012;11(6):M111.011973.
41. Limbrick DD Jr, Baksh B, Morgan CD, et al. Cerebrospinal fluid biomarkers of infantile congenital hydrocephalus. PLoS One. 2017;12(2):e0172353.
42. Morales DM, Silver SA, Morgan CD, et al. Lumbar cerebrospinal fluid biomarkers of posthemorrhagic hydrocephalus of prematurity: amyloid precursor protein, soluble amyloid precursor protein alpha, and L1 cell adhesion molecule. Neurosurgery. 2017;80(1):82–90.
43. Morales DM, Holubkov R, Inder TE, et al. Cerebrospinal fluid levels of amyloid precursor protein are associated with ventricular size in post-hemorrhagic hydrocephalus of prematurity. PLoS One. 2015;10(3):e0115045.
44. Guerra MM, Henzi R, Ortloff A, et al. Cell junction pathology of neural stem cells is associated with ventricular zone disruption, hydrocephalus, and abnormal neurogenesis. J Neuropathol Exp Neurol. 2015;74(7):653–71.
45. Jimenez AJ, Dominguez-Pinos MD, Guerra MM, Fernandez-Llebrez P, Perez-Figares JM. Structure and function of the ependymal barrier and diseases associated with ependyma disruption. Tissue Barriers. 2014;2:e28426.
46. Rodriguez EM, Guerra MM, Vio K, et al. A cell junction pathology of neural stem cells leads to abnormal neurogenesis and hydrocephalus. Biol Res. 2012;45(3):231–42.
47. Ohata S, Alvarez-Buylla A. Planar organization of multiciliated ependymal (E1) cells in the brain ventricular epithelium. Trends Neurosci. 2016;39:543–51.
48. Lee L. Riding the wave of ependymal cilia: genetic susceptibility to hydrocephalus in primary ciliary dyskinesia. J Neurosci Res. 2013;91(9):1117–32.
49. Narita K, Takeda S. Cilia in the choroid plexus: their roles in hydrocephalus and beyond. Front Cell Neurosci. 2015;9:39.
50. Ohata S, Nakatani J, Herranz-Perez V, et al. Loss of Dishevelleds disrupts planar polarity in ependymal motile cilia and results in hydrocephalus. Neuron. 2014;83(3):558–71.
51. Heep A, Stoffel-Wagner B, Bartmann P, et al. Vascular endothelial growth factor and transforming growth factor-beta1 are highly expressed in the cerebrospinal fluid of premature infants with posthemorrhagic hydrocephalus. Pediatr Res. 2004;56(5):768–74.
52. Heep A, Stoffel-Wagner B, Soditt V, Aring C, Groneck P, Bartmann P. Procollagen I C-propeptide in the cerebrospinal fluid of neonates with posthaemorrhagic hydrocephalus. Arch Dis Child Fetal Neonatal Ed. 2002;87(1):F34–6.
53. Hochhaus F, Koehne P, Schaper C, et al. Elevated nerve growth factor and neurotrophin-3 levels in cerebrospinal fluid of children with hydrocephalus. BMC Pediatr. 2001;1:2.
54. Beems T, Simons KS, Van Geel WJ, De Reus HP, Vos PE, Verbeek MM. Serum- and CSF-concentrations of brain specific proteins in hydrocephalus. Acta Neurochir. 2003;145(1):37–43.
55. Koehne P, Hochhaus F, Felderhoff-Mueser U, Ring-Mrozik E, Obladen M, Buhrer C. Vascular endothelial growth factor and erythropoietin concentrations in cerebrospinal fluid of children with hydrocephalus. Childs Nerv Syst. 2002;18(3–4):137–41.
56. Longatti PL, Canova G, Guida F, Carniato A, Moro M, Carteri A. The CSF myelin basic protein: a reliable marker of actual cerebral damage in hydrocephalus. J Neurosurg Sci. 1993;37(2):87–90.

57. Naureen I, Waheed KA, Rathore AW, et al. Fingerprint changes in CSF composition associated with different aetiologies in human neonatal hydrocephalus: glial proteins associated with cell damage and loss. Fluids Barriers CNS. 2013;10(1):34.
58. Naureen I, Waheed Kh A, Rathore AW, et al. Fingerprint changes in CSF composition associated with different aetiologies in human neonatal hydrocephalus: inflammatory cytokines. Childs Nerv Syst. 2014;30(7):1155–64.
59. Krauss JK, Droste DW, Bohus M, et al. The relation of intracranial pressure B-waves to different sleep stages in patients with suspected normal pressure hydrocephalus. Acta Neurochir. 1995;136(3–4):195–203.
60. Williams MA, Relkin NR. Diagnosis and management of idiopathic normal-pressure hydrocephalus. Neurol Clin Pract. 2013;3(5):375–85.
61. Chen Z, Liu C, Zhang J, Relkin N, Xing Y, Li Y. Cerebrospinal fluid Aβ42, t-tau, and p-tau levels in the differential diagnosis of idiopathic normal-pressure hydrocephalus: a systematic review and meta-analysis. Fluids Barriers CNS. 2017;14:13.
62. Li X, Miyajima M, Mineki R, Taka H, Murayama K, Arai H. Analysis of potential diagnostic biomarkers in cerebrospinal fluid of idiopathic normal pressure hydrocephalus by proteomics. Acta Neurochir. 2006;148(8):859–64; discussion 864
63. Li X, Miyajima M, Jiang C, Arai H. Expression of TGF-betas and TGF-beta type II receptor in cerebrospinal fluid of patients with idiopathic normal pressure hydrocephalus. Neurosci Lett. 2007;413(2):141–4.
64. Patel S, Lee EB, Xie SX, et al. Phosphorylated tau/amyloid beta 1-42 ratio in ventricular cerebrospinal fluid reflects outcome in idiopathic normal pressure hydrocephalus. Fluids Barriers CNS. 2012;9(1):7.
65. Tarnaris A, Toma AK, Kitchen ND, Watkins LD. Ongoing search for diagnostic biomarkers in idiopathic normal pressure hydrocephalus. Biomark Med. 2009;3(6):787–805.
66. Tullberg M, Blennow K, Mansson JE, Fredman P, Tisell M, Wikkelso C. Cerebrospinal fluid markers before and after shunting in patients with secondary and idiopathic normal pressure hydrocephalus. Cerebrospinal Fluid Res. 2008;5:9.
67. Blennow K, Hampel H. CSF markers for incipient Alzheimer's disease. Lancet Neurol. 2003;2(10):605–13.
68. Tullberg M, Blennow K, Mansson JE, Fredman P, Tisell M, Wikkelso C. Ventricular cerebrospinal fluid neurofilament protein levels decrease in parallel with white matter pathology after shunt surgery in normal pressure hydrocephalus. Eur J Neurol. 2007;14(3):248–54.
69. Leinonen V, Menon LG, Carroll RS, et al. Cerebrospinal fluid biomarkers in idiopathic normal pressure hydrocephalus. Int J Alzheimers Dis. 2011;2011:312526.
70. Priller C, Bauer T, Mitteregger G, Krebs B, Kretzschmar HA, Herms J. Synapse formation and function is modulated by the amyloid precursor protein. J Neurosci Off J Soc Neurosci. 2006;26(27):7212–21.
71. Kamenetz F, Tomita T, Hsieh H, et al. APP processing and synaptic function. Neuron. 2003;37(6):925–37.
72. Dawkins E, Small DH. Insights into the physiological function of the beta-amyloid precursor protein: beyond Alzheimer's disease. J Neurochem. 2014;129(5):756–69.
73. Roberts GW, Gentleman SM, Lynch A, Murray L, Landon M, Graham DI. Beta amyloid protein deposition in the brain after severe head injury: implications for the pathogenesis of Alzheimer's disease. J Neurol Neurosurg Psychiatry. 1994;57(4):419–25.
74. Gentleman SM, Nash MJ, Sweeting CJ, Graham DI, Roberts GW. Beta-amyloid precursor protein (beta APP) as a marker for axonal injury after head injury. Neurosci Lett. 1993;160(2):139–44.
75. Gorrie C, Oakes S, Duflou J, Blumbergs P, Waite PM. Axonal injury in children after motor vehicle crashes: extent, distribution, and size of axonal swellings using beta-APP immunohistochemistry. J Neurotrauma. 2002;19(10):1171–82.
76. Sherriff FE, Bridges LR, Sivaloganathan S. Early detection of axonal injury after human head trauma using immunocytochemistry for beta-amyloid precursor protein. Acta Neuropathol. 1994;87(1):55–62.

77. Graham DI, Gentleman SM, Nicoll JA, et al. Altered beta-APP metabolism after head injury and its relationship to the aetiology of Alzheimer's disease. Acta Neurochir Suppl. 1996;66:96–102.
78. Rajagopal A, Shimony JS, McKinstry RC, et al. White matter microstructural abnormality in children with hydrocephalus detected by probabilistic diffusion tractography. AJNR Am J Neuroradiol. 2013;34(12):2379–85.
79. Yuan W, McKinstry RC, Shimony JS, et al. Diffusion tensor imaging properties and neurobehavioral outcomes in children with hydrocephalus. AJNR Am J Neuroradiol. 2013;34(2):439–45.
80. Lewczuk P, Esselmann H, Bibl M, et al. Tau protein phosphorylated at threonine 181 in CSF as a neurochemical biomarker in Alzheimer's disease: original data and review of the literature. J Mol Neurosci. 2004;23(1–2):115–22.
81. Olsson B, Lautner R, Andreasson U, et al. CSF and blood biomarkers for the diagnosis of Alzheimer's disease: a systematic review and meta-analysis. Lancet Neurol. 2016;15(7):673–84.
82. Hladky SB, Barrand MA. Mechanisms of fluid movement into, through and out of the brain: evaluation of the evidence. Fluids Barriers CNS. 2014;11(1):26.
83. Graff-Radford NR. Alzheimer CSF biomarkers may be misleading in normal-pressure hydrocephalus. Neurology. 2014;83(17):1573–5.
84. Jeppsson A, Zetterberg H, Blennow K, Wikkelso C. Idiopathic normal-pressure hydrocephalus: pathophysiology and diagnosis by CSF biomarkers. Neurology. 2013;80(15):1385–92.
85. Tarnaris A, Toma AK, Chapman MD, et al. Rostrocaudal dynamics of CSF biomarkers. Neurochem Res. 2011;36(3):528–32.
86. Brandner S, Thaler C, Lelental N, et al. Ventricular and lumbar cerebrospinal fluid concentrations of Alzheimer's disease biomarkers in patients with normal pressure hydrocephalus and posttraumatic hydrocephalus. J Alzheimers Dis. 2014;41(4):1057–62.
87. Sanders WS, Wang N, Bridges SM, et al. The proteogenomic mapping tool. BMC Bioinformatics. 2011;12:115.
88. Ruggles KV, Krug K, Wang X, et al. Methods, tools and current perspectives in proteogenomics. Mol Cell Proteomics. 2017;16(6):959–81.
89. Mashayekhi F, Salehi Z. Expression of nerve growth factor in cerebrospinal fluid of congenital hydrocephalic and normal children. Eur J Neurol. 2005;12(8):632–7.
90. Erol FS, Yakar H, Artas H, Kaplan M, Kaman D. Investigating a correlation between the results of transcranial Doppler and the level of nerve growth factor in cerebrospinal fluid of hydrocephalic infants: clinical study. Pediatr Neurosurg. 2009;45(3):192–7.
91. Tisell M, Tullberg M, Mansson JE, Fredman P, Blennow K, Wikkelso C. Differences in cerebrospinal fluid dynamics do not affect the levels of biochemical markers in ventricular CSF from patients with aqueductal stenosis and idiopathic normal pressure hydrocephalus. Eur J Neurol. 2004;11(1):17–23.
92. Perez-Neri I, Castro E, Montes S, et al. Arginine, citrulline and nitrate concentrations in the cerebrospinal fluid from patients with acute hydrocephalus. J Chromatogr B Analyt Technol Biomed Life Sci. 2007;851(1–2):250–6.
93. Cengiz P, Zemlan F, Ellenbogen R, Hawkins D, Zimmerman JJ. Cerebrospinal fluid cleaved-tau protein and 9-hydroxyoctadecadienoic acid concentrations in pediatric patients with hydrocephalus. Pediatr Crit Care Med. 2008;9(5):524–9.
94. Sutton LN, Wood JH, Brooks BR, Barrer SJ, Kline M, Cohen SR. Cerebrospinal fluid myelin basic protein in hydrocephalus. J Neurosurg. 1983;59(3):467–70.
95. Gopal SC, Pandey A, Das I, et al. Comparative evaluation of 5-HIAA (5-hydroxy indoleacetic acid) and HVA (homovanillic acid) in infantile hydrocephalus. Childs Nerv Syst. 2008;24(6):713–6.
96. Lee JH, Park DH, Back DB, et al. Comparison of cerebrospinal fluid biomarkers between idiopathic normal pressure hydrocephalus and subarachnoid hemorrhage-induced chronic hydrocephalus: a pilot study. Med Sci Monit. 2012;18(12):PR19–25.
97. Yang JT, Chang CN, Hsu YH, Wei KC, Lin TK, Wu JH. Increase in CSF NGF concentration is positively correlated with poor prognosis of postoperative hydrocephalic patients. Clin Biochem. 1999;32(8):673–5.

98. Felderhoff-Mueser U, Herold R, Hochhaus F, et al. Increased cerebrospinal fluid concentrations of soluble Fas (CD95/Apo-1) in hydrocephalus. Arch Dis Child. 2001;84(4):369–72.
99. de Bont JM, Vanderstichele H, Reddingius RE, Pieters R, van Gool SW. Increased total-Tau levels in cerebrospinal fluid of pediatric hydrocephalus and brain tumor patients. Eur J Paediatr Neurol. 2008;12(4):334–41.
100. Kruse A, Cesarini KG, Bach FW, Persson L. Increases of neuron-specific enolase, S-100 protein, creatine kinase and creatine kinase BB isoenzyme in CSF following intraventricular catheter implantation. Acta Neurochir. 1991;110(3–4):106–9.
101. Cerda M, Vielma J, Martinez C, Basauri L. Polyacrylamide gel electrophoresis of cerebrospinal fluid proteins in children with nontumoral hydrocephalus. Childs Brain. 1980;6(3):140–9.
102. Lopponen T, Saukkonen AL, Serlo W, Tapanainen P, Ruokonen A, Knip M. Reduced levels of growth hormone, insulin-like growth factor-I and binding protein-3 in patients with shunted hydrocephalus. Arch Dis Child. 1997;77(1):32–7.
103. Gopal SC, Sharma V, Chansuria JP, Gangopadhyaya AN, Singh TB. Serotonin and 5-hydroxy indole acetic acid in infantile hydrocephalus. Pediatr Surg Int. 2007;23(6):571–4.
104. Longatti PL, Guida F, Agostini S, Carniato B, Carteri A. The CSF myelin basic protein in pediatric hydrocephalus. Childs Nerv Syst. 1994;10(2):96–8.
105. Killer M, Arthur A, Al-Schameri AR, et al. Cytokine and growth factor concentration in cerebrospinal fluid from patients with hydrocephalus following endovascular embolization of unruptured aneurysms in comparison with other types of hydrocephalus. Neurochem Res. 2010;35(10):1652–8.
106. Futakawa S, Nara K, Miyajima M, et al. A unique N-glycan on human transferrin in CSF: a possible biomarker for iNPH. Neurobiol Aging. 2012;33(8):1807–15.
107. Jeppsson A, Holtta M, Zetterberg H, Blennow K, Wikkelso C, Tullberg M. Amyloid mis-metabolism in idiopathic normal pressure hydrocephalus. Fluids Barriers CNS. 2016;13(1):13.
108. Herukka SK, Rummukainen J, Ihalainen J, et al. Amyloid-beta and Tau dynamics in human brain interstitial fluid in patients with suspected normal pressure hydrocephalus. J Alzheimers Dis. 2015;46(1):261–9.
109. Laske C, Stransky E, Leyhe T, et al. BDNF serum and CSF concentrations in Alzheimer's disease, normal pressure hydrocephalus and healthy controls. J Psychiatr Res. 2007;41(5):387–94.
110. Ray B, Reyes PF, Lahiri DK. Biochemical studies in Normal Pressure Hydrocephalus (NPH) patients: change in CSF levels of amyloid precursor protein (APP), amyloid-beta (Abeta) peptide and phospho-tau. J Psychiatr Res. 2011;45(4):539–47.
111. Fersten E, Gordon-Krajcer W, Glowacki M, Mroziak B, Jurkiewicz J, Czernicki Z. Cerebrospinal fluid free-radical peroxidation products and cognitive functioning patterns differentiate varieties of normal pressure hydrocephalus. Folia Neuropathol. 2004;42(3):133–40.
112. Castaneyra-Ruiz L, Gonzalez-Marrero I, Carmona-Calero EM, et al. Cerebrospinal fluid levels of tumor necrosis factor alpha and aquaporin 1 in patients with mild cognitive impairment and idiopathic normal pressure hydrocephalus. Clin Neurol Neurosurg. 2016;146:76–81.
113. Kapaki EN, Paraskevas GP, Tzerakis NG, et al. Cerebrospinal fluid tau, phospho-tau181 and beta-amyloid1-42 in idiopathic normal pressure hydrocephalus: a discrimination from Alzheimer's disease. Eur J Neurol. 2007;14(2):168–73.
114. Elobeid A, Laurell K, Cesarini KG, Alafuzoff I. Correlations between mini-mental state examination score, cerebrospinal fluid biomarkers, and pathology observed in brain biopsies of patients with normal-pressure hydrocephalus. J Neuropathol Exp Neurol. 2015;74(5):470–9.
115. Agren-Wilsson A, Lekman A, Sjoberg W, et al. CSF biomarkers in the evaluation of idiopathic normal pressure hydrocephalus. Acta Neurol Scand. 2007;116(5):333–9.
116. Tullberg M, Rosengren L, Blomsterwall E, Karlsson JE, Wikkelso C. CSF neurofilament and glial fibrillary acidic protein in normal pressure hydrocephalus. Neurology. 1998;50(4):1122–7.
117. Scollato A, Terreni A, Caldini A, et al. CSF proteomic analysis in patients with normal pressure hydrocephalus selected for the shunt: CSF biomarkers of response to surgical treatment. Neurol Sci. 2010;31(3):283–91.

118. Tullberg M, Mansson JE, Fredman P, et al. CSF sulfatide distinguishes between normal pressure hydrocephalus and subcortical arteriosclerotic encephalopathy. J Neurol Neurosurg Psychiatry. 2000;69(1):74–81.
119. Sosvorova L, Bestak J, Bicikova M, et al. Determination of homocysteine in cerebrospinal fluid as an indicator for surgery treatment in patients with hydrocephalus. Physiol Res. 2014;63(4):521–7.
120. Kondo M, Tokuda T, Itsukage M, et al. Distribution of amyloid burden differs between idiopathic normal pressure hydrocephalus and Alzheimer's disease. Neuroradiol J. 2013;26(1):41–6.
121. Lim TS, Choi JY, Park SA, et al. Evaluation of coexistence of Alzheimer's disease in idiopathic normal pressure hydrocephalus using ELISA analyses for CSF biomarkers. BMC Neurol. 2014;14:66.
122. Albrechtsen M, Sorensen PS, Gjerris F, Bock E. High cerebrospinal fluid concentration of glial fibrillary acidic protein (GFAP) in patients with normal pressure hydrocephalus. J Neurol Sci. 1985;70(3):269–74.
123. Kalamatianos T, Markianos M, Margetis K, Bourlogiannis F, Stranjalis G. Higher Orexin A levels in lumbar compared to ventricular CSF: a study in idiopathic normal pressure hydrocephalus. Peptides. 2014;51:1–3.
124. Jingami N, Asada-Utsugi M, Uemura K, et al. Idiopathic normal pressure hydrocephalus has a different cerebrospinal fluid biomarker profile from Alzheimer's disease. J Alzheimers Dis. 2015;45(1):109–15.
125. Kang K, Ko PW, Jin M, Suk K, Lee HW. Idiopathic normal-pressure hydrocephalus, cerebrospinal fluid biomarkers, and the cerebrospinal fluid tap test. J Clin Neurosci. 2014;21(8):1398–403.
126. Lins H, Wichart I, Bancher C, Wallesch CW, Jellinger KA, Rosler N. Immunoreactivities of amyloid beta peptide((1-42)) and total tau protein in lumbar cerebrospinal fluid of patients with normal pressure hydrocephalus. J Neural Transm (Vienna). 2004;111(3):273–80.
127. Nakajima M, Miyajima M, Ogino I, et al. Leucine-rich alpha-2-glycoprotein is a marker for idiopathic normal pressure hydrocephalus. Acta Neurochir. 2011;153(6):1339–46; discussion 1346
128. Mase M, Yamada K, Shimazu N, et al. Lipocalin-type prostaglandin D synthase (beta-trace) in cerebrospinal fluid: a useful marker for the diagnosis of normal pressure hydrocephalus. Neurosci Res. 2003;47(4):455–9.
129. Huang H, Yang J, Luciano M, Shriver LP. Longitudinal metabolite profiling of cerebrospinal fluid in normal pressure hydrocephalus links brain metabolism with exercise-induced VEGF production and clinical outcome. Neurochem Res. 2016;41(7):1713–22.
130. Sorensen PS, Gjerris F, Ibsen S, Bock E. Low cerebrospinal fluid concentration of brain-specific protein D2 in patients with normal pressure hydrocephalus. J Neurol Sci. 1983;62(1–3):59–65.
131. Brettschneider J, Riepe MW, Petereit HF, Ludolph AC, Tumani H. Meningeal derived cerebrospinal fluid proteins in different forms of dementia: is a meningopathy involved in normal pressure hydrocephalus? J Neurol Neurosurg Psychiatry. 2004;75(11):1614–6.
132. Luikku AJ, Hall A, Nerg O, et al. Multimodal analysis to predict shunt surgery outcome of 284 patients with suspected idiopathic normal pressure hydrocephalus. Acta Neurochir. 2016;158(12):2311–9.
133. Tarkowski E, Tullberg M, Fredman P, Wikkelso C. Normal pressure hydrocephalus triggers intrathecal production of TNF-alpha. Neurobiol Aging. 2003;24(5):707–14.
134. Djukic M, Spreer A, Lange P, Bunkowski S, Wiltfang J, Nau R. Small cisterno-lumbar gradient of phosphorylated Tau protein in geriatric patients with suspected normal pressure hydrocephalus. Fluids Barriers CNS. 2016;13(1):15.
135. Miyajima M, Nakajima M, Ogino I, Miyata H, Motoi Y, Arai H. Soluble amyloid precursor protein alpha in the cerebrospinal fluid as a diagnostic and prognostic biomarker for idiopathic normal pressure hydrocephalus. Eur J Neurol. 2013;20(2):236–42.
136. Kudo T, Mima T, Hashimoto R, et al. Tau protein is a potential biological marker for normal pressure hydrocephalus. Psychiatry Clin Neurosci. 2000;54(2):199–202.

137. Tarnaris A, Toma AK, Chapman MD, et al. The longitudinal profile of CSF markers during external lumbar drainage. J Neurol Neurosurg Psychiatry. 2009;80(10):1130–3.
138. Tarnaris A, Toma AK, Chapman MD, Keir G, Kitchen ND, Watkins LD. Use of cerebrospinal fluid amyloid-beta and total tau protein to predict favorable surgical outcomes in patients with idiopathic normal pressure hydrocephalus. J Neurosurg. 2011;115(1):145–50.
139. Chow LC, Soliman A, Zandian M, Danielpour M, Krueger RC Jr. Accumulation of transforming growth factor-beta2 and nitrated chondroitin sulfate proteoglycans in cerebrospinal fluid correlates with poor neurologic outcome in preterm hydrocephalus. Biol Neonate. 2005;88(1):1–11.
140. Okamoto T, Takahashi S, Nakamura E, et al. Increased expression of matrix metalloproteinase-9 and hepatocyte growth factor in the cerebrospinal fluid of infants with posthemorrhagic hydrocephalus. Early Hum Dev. 2010;86(4):251–4.
141. Schmitz T, Heep A, Groenendaal F, et al. Interleukin-1beta, interleukin-18, and interferon-gamma expression in the cerebrospinal fluid of premature infants with posthemorrhagic hydrocephalus--markers of white matter damage? Pediatr Res. 2007;61(6):722–6.
142. Felderhoff-Mueser U, Buhrer C, Groneck P, Obladen M, Bartmann P, Heep A. Soluble Fas (CD95/Apo-1), soluble Fas ligand, and activated caspase 3 in the cerebrospinal fluid of infants with posthemorrhagic and nonhemorrhagic hydrocephalus. Pediatr Res. 2003;54(5):659–64.
143. Kitazawa K, Tada T. Elevation of transforming growth factor-beta 1 level in cerebrospinal fluid of patients with communicating hydrocephalus after subarachnoid hemorrhage. Stroke. 1994;25(7):1400–4.
144. Douglas MR, Daniel M, Lagord C, et al. High CSF transforming growth factor beta levels after subarachnoid haemorrhage: association with chronic communicating hydrocephalus. J Neurol Neurosurg Psychiatry. 2009;80(5):545–50.
145. Sokol B, Wozniak A, Jankowski R, et al. HMGB1 level in cerebrospinal fluid as a marker of treatment outcome in patients with acute hydrocephalus following aneurysmal subarachnoid hemorrhage. J Stroke Cerebrovasc Dis. 2015;24(8):1897–904.
146. Brandner S, Xu Y, Schmidt C, Emtmann I, Buchfelder M, Kleindienst A. Shunt-dependent hydrocephalus following subarachnoid hemorrhage correlates with increased S100B levels in cerebrospinal fluid and serum. Acta Neurochir Suppl. 2012;114:217–20.
147. Sokol B, Wasik N, Jankowski R, Holysz M, Wieckowska B, Jagodzlnski PP. Soluble toll-like receptors 2 and 4 in cerebrospinal fluid of patients with acute hydrocephalus following aneurysmal subarachnoid haemorrhage. *PLoS One*. 2016;11(5):e0156171.
148. Schmitz T, Felderhoff-Mueser U, Sifringer M, Groenendaal F, Kampmann S, Heep A. Expression of soluble Fas in the cerebrospinal fluid of preterm infants with posthemorrhagic hydrocephalus and cystic white matter damage. J Perinat Med. 2011;39(1):83–8.
149. Habiyaremye G, Morales DM, Morgan CD, et al. Chemokine and cytokine levels in the lumbar cerebrospinal fluid of preterm infants with posthemorrhagic hydrocephalus. Fluids Barriers CNS. 2017;14:35.

Intracranial Pulsatility, Cerebrospinal Fluid Flow, and Glymphatic Function in Idiopathic Normal Pressure Hydrocephalus

4

Per Kristian Eide and Geir Ringstad

Abbreviations

Aβ	Amyloid-β
AD	Alzheimer's disease
AQP4	Aquaporin-4
CMI	Chiari malformation type I
CSF	Cerebrospinal fluid
Da	Dalton
Dp71	Dystrophin-71
ICC	Intracranial compliance
ICP	Intracranial pressure
IIH	Intracranial hypertension
iNPH	Idiopathic normal pressure hydrocephalus
MRI	Magnetic resonance imaging
MWA	Mean ICP wave amplitude

Introduction

The pathogenesis behind hydrocephalus is multifactorial. Some important pathophysiological mechanisms are cerebrospinal fluid (CSF) circulation disturbance, alterations in intracranial pressure (ICP) dynamics, and neurodegeneration. How these mechanisms relate is less understood. This chapter addresses how CSF

P. K. Eide (✉)
Oslo University Hospital – Rikshospitalet, Department of Neurosurgery, Oslo, Norway
e-mail: p.k.eide@medisin.uio.no

G. Ringstad
Oslo University Hospital – Rikshospitalet, Department of Radiology, Oslo, Norway

D. D. Limbrick, J. R. Leonard (eds.), *Cerebrospinal Fluid Disorders*,
https://doi.org/10.1007/978-3-319-97928-1_4

circulation disturbances are accompanied with altered intracranial pulsatility, which in turn may be associated with altered CSF flow and glymphatic function in humans. The discussion primarily relates to adult hydrocephalus.

Intracranial Pulsatility in CSF Circulation Disorders

The ICP is usually measured as the absolute pressure difference between the pressure within the cranial compartment and a reference, usually the atmospheric pressure, including assessment of fluctuations in static ICP waves (B waves) [1]. Another component of ICP is the pulsatile ICP, which refers to the pressure changes taking place over the cardiac cycle [2]. While monitoring of ICP in the clinical context is usually synonymous with measurements of static ICP (mean ICP) [3], assessment of pulsatile ICP has not gained widespread clinical use. Reliable measurements of pulsatile ICP require computerized methodology with identification of the single ICP waves [4], and use of single ICP wave analysis has so far only been incorporated in a few clinical practices worldwide.

The pulsatile ICP is characterized by ICP wave features such as the pulse wave amplitude and the pulse wave rise time coefficient [2]. In our experience, we mostly used the mean ICP wave amplitude (MWA) to characterize pulsatile ICP [4], which hereafter is referred to as pulsatile ICP. The exact upper normal thresholds of MWA have not been defined since ICP monitoring is invasive and cannot be done in healthy individuals. To obtain indirect evidence of normal MWA values, we have compared the preoperative MWA values of individuals with CSF circulation disorders who improved/not improved clinically following CSF diversion surgery or who improved spontaneously without shunting (Table 4.1).

The mean ICP wave amplitude (MWA) is a better indicator of the intracranial pressure–volume relationship (intracranial compliance, ICC) than static ICP

Table 4.1 Overview of some studies showing altered pulsatile ICP (illustrated by the parameter MWA) in individuals with CSF circulation disorders

	Average of MWA[a]		
Type of CSF circulation disorder	Clinical responders (mmHg)	Clinical nonresponders (mmHg)	Reference
Pediatrics hydrocephalus	>5	<4	[5–7]
Noncommunicating hydrocephalus	>5	<4	[8]
Idiopathic normal pressure hydrocephalus	>5	<4	[9–11]
Idiopathic intracranial hypertension	>5	<4	[12, 13]
Chiari malformation type I	>5	<4	[13]
Pineal cysts	>4–5	<4	[14, 15]

[a]Average of MWA at group level during a standardized overnight recording time from 11 p.m. to 7 a.m.

(mean ICP) [16, 17]. The ICC refers to the ability of the intracranial contents to adjust to intracranial volume changes [16]. Hence, impaired ICC means that intracranial volume increase is less well tolerated, resulting in increased ICP wave amplitudes. For each cardiac beat, the net intracranial volume increase is normally about 1 ml; the resulting MWA being <4 mmHg. With impaired ICC, MWA typically increases.

In the following, we review data from different CSF circulation disorders that present with impaired ICC and abnormal pulsatile ICP, indicated by raised MWA (Table 4.1).

In idiopathic normal pressure hydrocephalus (iNPH), MWA is elevated to an abnormal level among those individuals showing a clinical improvement following shunt surgery, as compared to those not improving clinically following shunt surgery [9, 10]. Normal MWA is defined as <4 mmHg on average during overnight monitoring and with episodes >5 mmHg in less than 10% of recordings. In iNPH, the elevated MWA is typically reduced to normal levels by CSF diversion (either by extended lumbar drainage or shunt surgery), which is accompanied with clinical improvement [18]. The altered pulsatile ICP cannot be explained by systemic factors such as cardiac output, peripheral vascular resistance, blood pressure, or impaired pressure autoregulation [19]. In iNPH, where mean ICP is within normal range, reduced ICC may be attributed to compromise of CSF and/or venous outflow from the intracranial compartment [2] or even structural changes such as astrogliosis [20].

Elevated MWA may also be seen in noncommunicating hydrocephalus caused by aqueduct stenosis [8]. In these individuals, there was an inverse relationship between MWA and ICC, which was measured as change in volume as related to change in mean ICP. Accordingly, impaired ICC indicative of impaired pressure–volume reserve was accompanied with elevated MWA.

Elevated MWA values seen in adults with either iNPH or noncommunicating hydrocephalus compare well with the elevated MWA seen in pediatric hydrocephalus cases [5]. In our experience, the pulsatile ICP (MWA) is comparable between adult and pediatric individuals though the experience with children less than 2 years is limited [6, 7]. Even though age-dependent differences in pulsatile ICP could have been expected, our observations do not indicate so.

Idiopathic intracranial hypertension (IIH) [12, 13] and Chiari malformation type I (CMI) [13] are other types of CSF circulation disturbances that are characterized by abnormal pulsatile ICP and MWA alterations comparable to that seen in iNPH and noncommunicating hydrocephalus. At MRI, findings of tonsillar ectopy may even overlap [21], and it has been speculated that the two conditions may share a common origin [13]. In IIH, CSF diversion lowered the MWA [12]. Moreover, some individuals with symptomatic, nonhydrocephalic pineal cysts may as well present with abnormal intracranial pulsatility [14], comparable to that seen in IIH. We observed symptom relief following cyst removal in some selected cases, but the role of the pineal cyst per se needs to be further examined [15].

Table 4.1 provides an overview of studies wherein elevated pulsatile ICP has been demonstrated in patients with various forms of hydrocephalus.

Intracranial Pulsatility and CSF Flow

There is some evidence that alterations in pulsatile ICP are accompanied by changes in CSF flow. Phase-contrast magnetic resonance imaging (pcMRI) measurements of CSF flow within the Sylvian aqueduct demonstrated that net flow direction was reversed in iNPH, that is directed upwards and into the supratentorial ventricles [22]. Moreover, it was increased in the downward direction (out of ventricles) following shunt surgery [22]. Most importantly, retrograde CSF flow was a feature typically found in subjects with signs of reduced ICC, that is with higher MWA. Accordingly, it seems as impaired ICC in iNPH is accompanied by redirection of CSF flow into the ventricles. This might be explained by higher resistance to CSF flow at the outer surface of the brain and redirection of CSF flow along pathways of less resistance.

In iNPH, the aqueductal CSF flow rate was −0.56 ml/min (range −12.8 to 0.58 ml/min) before surgery, and following shunting, it increased to 0.06 ml/min (range −4.5 to 1.9 ml/min) [22]. Negative CSF flow rate refers to retrograde flow (inwards to ventricles) and positive to antegrade CSF flow (out of the ventricles) [22]. An absolute CSF production rate of 0.56 ml/min compares with 0.81 l/24 h, while a CSF flow rate of 12.8 ml/min compares with 18.4 l/24 h. These CSF production rates differ profoundly from the traditional concept of ventricular CSF production rate (primarily from choroid plexus) of about 0.3 ml/min (0.43 l/24 h) [23]. However, the traditional understanding of "the third circulation" (from choroid plexus to arachnoid granulations), which practically bypasses present knowledge of CSF flow through brain tissue, have during later years been questioned [24–26].

Net CSF flow into the ventricular system at phase-contrast MRI have been confirmed by studies combining MRI at multiple time points after intrathecal MRI contrast agent administration, utilizing MRI contrast agent as CSF tracer (gMRI) [27]. After intrathecal administration of a CSF tracer in humans, it typically reach the foramen magnum within 20–30 min [27]. While it distributes primarily around the brain surface in reference subjects, the tracer (contrast agent) passes rapidly into, and persists within, the supra-aqueductal ventricular system in iNPH patients [27]. At late scans, sign of transependymal egress of tracer to periventricular brain tissue can be seen. Figure 4.1 shows entry of contrast agent from the cisterna magna and into the brain ventricles of a patient with communicating hydrocephalus (not iNPH), while this was not seen in a reference subject.

Intracranial Pulsatility and Glymphatic Function

It should be noted that the clearance routes for water and larger molecules in the brain may be different. Both CSF and interstitial fluid may mainly be transported and reabsorbed across the blood-brain barrier by simple diffusion and vesicular transport or by co-transport along with substances [28]. The basement membranes surrounding CNS capillaries have furthermore been suggested playing a key role in the bulk transport of fluids and solutes within the CNS [29]. In 1985, Rennels et al. [30] showed that an intrathecal CSF tracer (*horse-radish peroxidase*) distributed

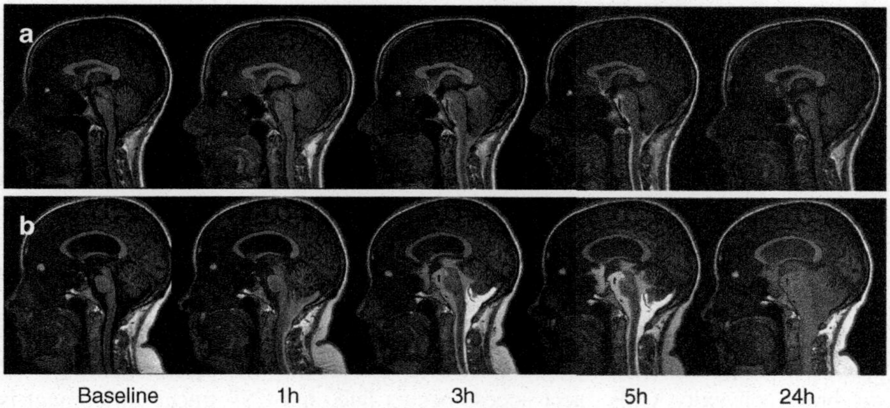

Fig. 4.1 T1 weighted MRI in sagittal plane from MRI at baseline and 1, 3, 5, and 24 h after intrathecal contrast agent administration in (**a**) a 24-year-old reference individual and (**b**) a 32-year-old patient with communicating hydrocephalus. The reference individual underwent MRI for suspected CSF leakage but no leakage was found, and symptoms resolved spontaneously within months. The contrast enhancement was visible within the spinal and basal intracranial subarachnoid spaces and with a marked decline after 24 h (**a**). In the patients with hydrocephalus, contrast enhancement of the subarachnoid and intraventricular spaces was even more evident, with reflux of contrast agent to the third ventricle after 3 h (**b**). After 24 h, clearance of the contrast agent was delayed in the patient with hydrocephalus (**b**) as compared to the reference subject (**a**)

from CSF along arteriolar paravascular spaces of the brain into the extracellular space and finally accumulated around veins. Building on this concept, the *glymphatic system* was described by the Nedergaard group in 2012, referring to a paravascular route for transport and clearance of solutes and brain metabolites from the brain [25]. It was suggested that arterial blood pressure pulsations are instrumental in driving convective transport of CSF and solutes along the brain vessels [25, 31]. The fluid and molecular movement was assumed to occur antegrade along the arteries and arterioles, allowing CSF to freely mix with the interstitial fluid. According to this concept, molecular substances are transported by convective (net) flow from the arterial to the venous side, dependent of aquaporin 4 (AQP4) water channels at the gliavascular interface (astrocytic end feet), and escaping the brain along the veins. Glymphatic clearance of amyloid-β (Aβ) was impaired in AQP4 knockout mice and was therefore suggested as a mechanism behind evolvement of Alzheimer's disease (AD). Among others, it has been shown that glymphatic function declines with increasing age [32], following traumatic brain injury [33], while being dramatically increased during sleep [34] and improved by physical exercise [35].

The current knowledge about glymphatic circulation is primarily based on animal studies, mostly in mice. We studied the glymphatic system by using the MRI contrast agent gadobutrol (molecular weight 604 Da) as CSF tracer (gMRI) [27, 36, 37]. Gadobutrol promotes increased signal intensity of water in MR (T1 weighted) images, and this tracer can therefore be detected, and followed, using consecutive MRI over a prolonged time span (Fig. 4.1). We examined the distribution of CSF tracer to a wide variety of brain regions [27, 36]. The CSF tracer enhancement within the brain parenchyma follows a centripetal pattern from surface to within, and tracer has been detected in all studied locations of the brain [27]. Notably, entry of tracer into the parenchyma is dependent on preceding tracer enrichment of nearby CSF spaces. This provides evidence that the subarachnoid CSF communicates with the paravascular spaces of the human brain. In a recent work, we found delayed clearance of CSF tracer from the entorhinal cortex of iNPH patients [36]. This area of the brain has an important role in cognitive function [38] and entorhinal volume loss typically precedes hippocampal degeneration in AD [39]. Impaired glymphatic clearance and accumulation of Aβ [25] and tau [33] may therefore also be a mechanism behind the dementia seen in iNPH, such as in AD.

After intrathecal CSF tracer injection at the lumbar level, the subarachnoid CSF spaces at the base and lateral fissures of the brain are first enriched (Fig. 4.1). Over the brain convexity, CSF tracer access occurs late, and CSF tracer enrichment is weak along dural sinuses [27]. This suggests that absorption by arachnoid villi plays a minor role, while water exchange within the brain is far more important. Weed, who first proposed that CSF absorption occurs at the arachnoid villi, avoided application of solutions with "diffuse tissue staining" [40], that is, substances that would be resorbed in brain parenchyma. The gMRI studies, however, show that molecular substances of a certain size in the CSF have potential to reach the entire extravascular space of the brain, even deep parts of the brain, before being completely washed out. This opens for new perspectives to how neurological disease at the outside of the blood-brain barrier can be reached, either for diagnostic or therapeutic purposes, or by combination of these two (*theranostics*).

The time course of centripetal CSF tracer distribution suggests convective transport along paravascular spaces and perhaps also along other low-resistance pathways, such as along axons. While diffusion is thought to be the main force behind movement of substances in the interstitial space [41], the glymphatic concept incorporates a role of net convective flow through the interstitial space as well. However, further studies are needed to determine which forces that best account for the reported CSF tracer propagation in human brain parenchyma.

The entry of CSF into the brain is facilitated by pulsations within the paravascular spaces of penetrating arterioles [25, 29, 30]. In line with these findings, we found that CSF tracer primarily enriches antegradely along the major arterial trunks (circle of Willis, anterior, middle, and posterior cerebral arteries) before it is distributed within the entire subarachnoid space [27, 36]. Intriguingly, these areas correspond well with brain structures that have previously been considered part of the "limbic" system. It may therefore seem that these structures are particularly vulnerable to impairment of CSF pulsations and glymphatic flow. Further, the CSF tracer propagates antegradely along arteries. These observations indicate a pivotal role of arterial pulsations for movement of substances along vessels within the subarachnoid and brain paravascular space, which was previously suggested based on animal studies [31]. Moreover, in iNPH patients, evidence of delayed CSF tracer movement along the major arteries was found [27]. This observation in iNPH may be related to restricted arterial pulsations partly because of vascular comorbidity with associated stiffening of arteries but also due to impaired ICC for various reasons (CSF flow stagnation, astrogliosis, etc.), which is expected to impair expansion of arteries and thereby CSF pulsations. Consequently, restricted arterial pulsations may reduce clearance of pathogenic macromolecules such as Aβ. Therefore, the brain interstitial fluid represents a mix of solutes and fluid derived from blood, tissue metabolism, and CSF [42]. In iNPH, the hampered paravascular fluid turnover may contribute to the impaired ICC and enhanced pulsatility seen in these individuals, as well as net CSF flow into the ventricular system.

There are important differences between animals and humans. In animals, peak CSF tracer enhancement occurs after a couple of hours [43], while in humans this typically occurs at 24 h [27, 36]. Rodent brain anatomy differs significantly from the human, and in rodent studies, intrathecal tracer is also typically injected directly into the cisterna magna, which may interfere with the normal pressure physiology within a very tiny intracranial compartment. Observations made in animal studies cannot therefore be readily translated to humans.

Glymphatic Function After Long-Term Shunt Treatment

It is presently unknown how longstanding CSF shunting may affect glymphatic function. We know that shunting decreases the pulsatile ICP, that is normalize MWA [11], and that severe overdrainage may cause a paradoxical change in ICP single waves with slightly elevated MWA [44]. Persistent overdrainage might theoretically affect glymphatic circulation negatively by deteriorating the pulsatile driving force for CSF flow within the subarachnoid space. This topic needs further exploration.

One case is presented (Fig. 4.2). This is a 42-year old man with shunt from 6 years of age. Over time, he had complained of headache, nausea, fatigue, and cognitive impairment (problems with concentration and short-term memory). The indication for shunting had been hydrocephalus and a left temporal arachnoid cyst. Several interesting notes can be made from the gMRI study: There was evidence of noncommunication between the cyst and CSF spaces, as well as delayed clearance of MRI contrast agent (CSF tracer) (Fig. 4.2a). Clearance of CSF tracer from parahippocampal gyrus and subcortical white matter was delayed (Fig. 4.2b), which may have relevance to the cognitive decline seen in this individual. Moreover, it should be noted that ventricular size was markedly increased from baseline at 6 h scanning, while subarachnoid CSF spaces were unaltered, indicating change in brain parenchyma volume at this time (Fig. 4.2c). The brain volume changes over the day/night cycle [45]. These findings may be of important relevance for individuals with CSF circulation problems and in patients with shunt-related problems. Individuals with CSF circulation disorders describe diurnal variation. Like this individual, some patients report increased demand for sleep and are more sensitive to sleep deprivation. In this regard, it is of great interest that there seems to be distinct diurnal variation regarding the function of the glymphatic system [34]. The gMRI of this individual also illustrates how CSF tracer enriches along the large arteries (Fig. 4.2d), and that CSF tracer propagation in the subarachnoid spaces was not restricted by the temporal arachnoid cyst (Fig. 4.2e).

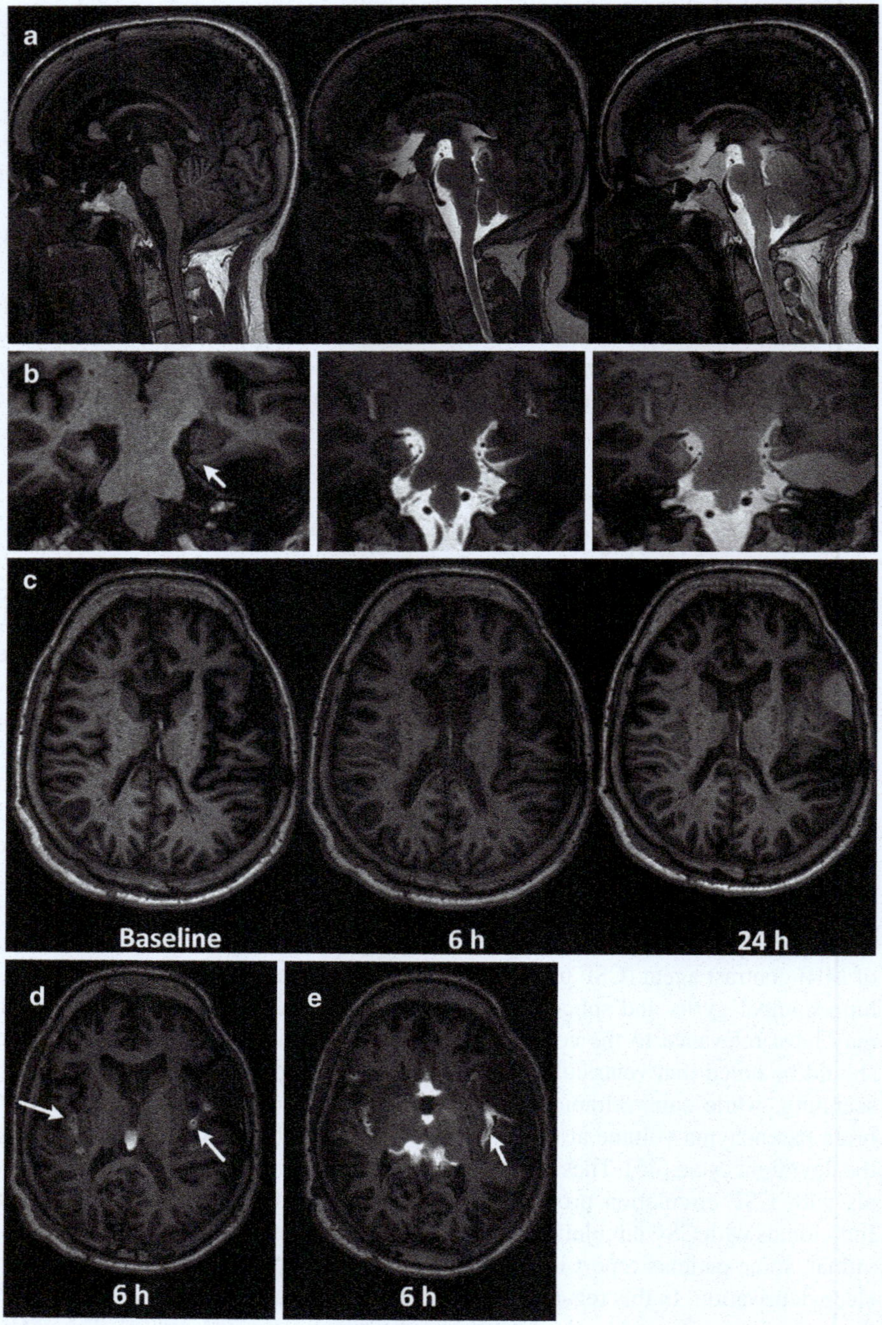
a
b
c
Baseline
6 h
24 h
d
6 h
e
6 h

Fig. 4.2 gMRI from a 42-old-man treated with a ventriculo-peritoneal shunt for 36 years since childhood (age 6 years) due to communicating hydrocephalus of unknown cause and a left temporal arachnoid cyst. Prior to gMRI, he had a history of about 2 years with symptoms characterized by headache, dizziness, fatigue, and cognitive impairment. He was after ICP monitoring diagnosed with overdrainage and therefore underwent a shunt revision. (**a**) Sagittal T1 weighted MRI shows contrast agent serving as CSF tracer, enriching the subarachnoid and ventricular spaces. No enrichment was seen within the CSF over the convexities at any time point. (**b**) The left parahippocampal gyrus was compressed by the cyst and dislocated upward (arrow). Signs of delayed CSF tracer (contrast agent) clearance was found in the left cortex as it revealed increased amounts of remaining CSF tracer at 6 and 24 h (T1 signal unit ratio after 6 h had increased 116% vs. 78% at the left vs. right side, and had after 24 h increased 79% vs. 65% at the left vs. right side. (**c**) At 6 h, the ventricular size was markedly increased despite no alterations in the cortical subarachnoid spaces, which suggests reduction in parenchymal volume, and highlights the dynamic nature of the brain volume. The altered ventricular size cannot be caused by respiration (or Valsalva) since the scan lasts 5–6 min. No movement artifacts can be seen. (**d**) The perivascular contrast enrichment surrounding branches of the middle cerebral artery within the Sylvian fissure was evident (arrows) and was not influenced by the left arachnoid cyst. (**e**) Neither the contrast enrichment within the Sylvian fissure (arrow) was affected by the arachnoid cyst. Hence, in this individual, the arachnoid cyst appeared not to obstruct CSF flow within nearby subarachnoid spaces of the Sylvian fissure

Glymphatic Function and the Water Channel AQP4

The role of AQP4 has mainly been investigated in rodents, where it may cover up to 40% of the astrocytic end foot surrounding the capillary basement membrane [46]. The paravascular space is continuous with CSF [47], and large water fluxes take place across astrocytic end feet throughout the entire brain parenchyma [48]. While water influx to interstitial space is independent of AQP4, its exit is not [49]. Reduced escape of water through AQP4 is expected to increase extracellular water content, as well as extracellular volume fraction, which was demonstrated in AQP4-deficient mice [50]. It has been suggested that the glymphatic circulation is dependent on perivascular AQP4 [25] though others have disputed the role of AQP4 [51].

The role of AQP4 in humans is less well understood. Variations in the APQ4 gene modulate progression of cognitive decline in AD [52], and perivascular AQP4 localization is associated with AD status and Aβ burden [53]. We found that IIH patients presented with astrogliosis and increased perivascular AQP4, which we interpreted as a compensatory response to enhance water efflux. In comparison, a recent study also reported an adaptive response for upregulation of AQP4 aimed at clearing excess brain fluid [54]. In iNPH, on the other hand [55], the ability to upregulate AQP4 seems to be compromised. We recently reported that the expression of perivascular AQP4 and its anchoring molecule, dystrophin-71 (Dp71), is reduced in iNPH [20]. Further, iNPH tissue specimens showed evidence of astrogliosis and also ultrastructural alterations at the capillary level [56]. These findings may provide a patho-anatomic basis for the delayed clearance of CSF tracer from brain parenchyma of iNPH individuals as compared to reference subjects that was most evident after 24 h [27, 36]. Loss of AQP4 along microvessels might cause stagnation of movement of water and solutes and could thereby also explain the typical iNPH finding of reduced ICC. The observations of increased ADC [57] and

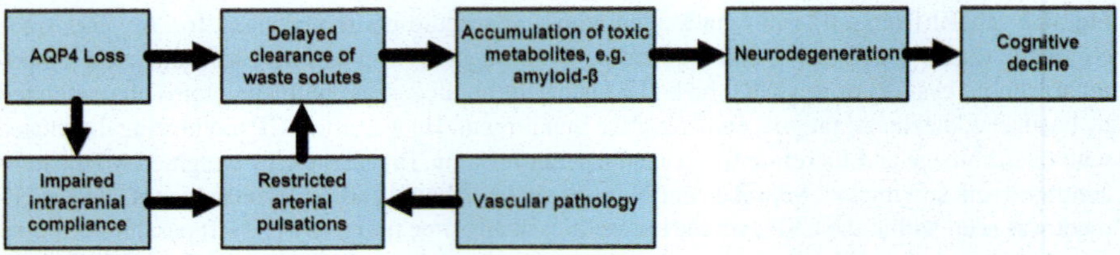

Fig. 4.3 A proposed model of pathogenic events from perivascular AQP4 loss delayed CSF tracer clearance from brain parenchyma, neurodegeneration, and the evolvement of cognitive decline in iNPH

decreased T1 signal [27] in parenchyma of iNPH patients are well in line with these observations at the cellular level, suggesting increased interstitial fluid in these individuals. Therefore, in iNPH, obstruction to CSF flow at the astrocytic end foot may be a key feature that deteriorates intracranial compliance, restricts artery pulsations, and impairs paravascular and glymphatic flow. An overview of possible pathophysiological events in iNPH is given in Fig. 4.3.

Glymphatic Circulation and Cerebral Lymphatic Drainage

It is presently a matter of controversy how fluid and solutes are cleared from the brain, particularly whether the paravascular clearance pathways from the brain are along arteries [58–60] or veins [25, 30, 43]. It has been proposed that molecular clearance occurs along the retrograde direction of arteriolar smooth muscle cells and further along the internal carotid artery [60]. Hence, it is debated how brain solutes like Aβ are transported to cervical neck lymph nodes. A major recent discovery in rodents was the finding of lymphatic vessels lining the dural sinuses [61, 62], which further drained to cervical lymph nodes. More recently, MRI was used to show the existence of dural lymphatic vessels in humans [63]. The efflux routes of molecular substances from the glymphatic system to the extracranial space are presently not clear. We have suggested a direct route from the glymphatic circulation to the extracerebral lymphatic vessels by showing that CSF tracer in brain parenchyma and neck lymph nodes coincided in time [64]. This is in contradistinction to animals studies where lymphatic drainage from the craniospinal compartment occurs directly from CSF. The study of cranial lymphatic drainage in animals and humans is currently a research area of immense interest and important steps forward in finding the link between glymphatics and lymphatics are highly anticipated.

Summary

There is solid evidence that CSF circulation disorders are associated with abnormal pulsatile ICP, indicative of impaired ICC. The underlying cause depends on the particular disease. In iNPH we have found astrogliosis, loss of perivascular AQP4, as well as ultrastructural changes in brain capillaries. Several lines of evidence suggest that impaired ICC may be associated with changes in CSF flow. In iNPH, net CSF flow within the Sylvian aqueduct is retrograde, that is toward the ventricles. Moreover, the antegrade CSF tracer movement along arteries in the CSF is delayed. Further, the clearance of CSF tracer from brain parenchyma is delayed in iNPH patients, indicating that removal of molecules cleared by the same pathways, such as soluble Aβ and tau, may be delayed in these patients. Reduced clearance may lead to accumulation of these proteins in the brain tissue, which is a hallmark of AD. For example, impaired molecular clearance from the entorhinal cortex may underlie impaired cognitive function and entorhinal cortex volume loss, which is seen in early phase of AD. Knowledge about how glymphatic function is impaired in hydrocephalus may have implications for understanding of typically associated but poorly understood symptoms such as cognitive impairment, headache, fatigue, and sleep problems.

References

1. Czosnyka M. Monitoring and interpretation of intracranial pressure. J Neurol Neurosurg Psychiatry. 2004;75:813–21.
2. Wagshul ME, Eide PK, Madsen JR. The pulsating brain: a review of experimental and clinical studies of intracranial pulsatility. Fluids Barriers CNS. 2011;8:5.
3. Harary M, Dolmans RGF, Gormley WB. Intracranial pressure monitoring-review and avenues for development. Sensors (Basel). 2018;18:pii: E465.
4. Eide PK. A new method for processing of continuous intracranial pressure signals. Med Eng Phys. 2006;28:579–87.
5. Eide PK, Egge A, Due-Tonnessen BJ, Helseth E. Is intracranial pressure waveform analysis useful in the management of pediatric neurosurgical patients? Pediatr Neurosurg. 2007;43:472–81.
6. Saehle T, Eide PK. Characteristics of intracranial pressure (ICP) waves and ICP in children with treatment-responsive hydrocephalus. Acta Neurochir. 2015;157:1003–14.
7. Saehle T, Eide PK. Intracranial pressure monitoring in pediatric and adult patients with hydrocephalus and tentative shunt failure: a single-center experience over 10 years in 146 patients. J Neurosurg. 2015;122:1076–86.
8. Eide PK. The pathophysiology of chronic noncommunicating hydrocephalus: lessons from continuous intracranial pressure monitoring and ventricular infusion testing. J Neurosurg. 2018;129:220–33.
9. Eide PK, Sorteberg W. Diagnostic intracranial pressure monitoring and surgical management in idiopathic normal pressure hydrocephalus: a 6-year review of 214 patients. Neurosurgery. 2010;66:80–91.
10. Eide PK, Sorteberg W. Outcome of surgery for idiopathic normal pressure hydrocephalus: role of preoperative static and pulsatile intracranial pressure. World Neurosurg. 2016;86:186–193 e181.
11. Eide PK, Sorteberg W. Changes in intracranial pulse pressure amplitudes after shunt implantation and adjustment of shunt valve opening pressure in normal pressure hydrocephalus. Acta Neurochir. 2008;150:1141–7; discussion 1147.
12. Eide PK, Kerty E. Static and pulsatile intracranial pressure in idiopathic intracranial hypertension. Clin Neurol Neurosurg. 2011;113:123–8.
13. Fric R, Eide PK. Comparative observational study on the clinical presentation, intracranial volume measurements, and intracranial pressure scores in patients with either Chiari malformation Type I or idiopathic intracranial hypertension. J Neurosurg. 2017;126:1312–22.
14. Eide PK, Ringstad G. Increased pulsatile intracranial pressure in patients with symptomatic pineal cysts and magnetic resonance imaging biomarkers indicative of central venous hypertension. J Neurol Sci. 2016;367:247–55.

15. Eide PK, Ringstad G. Results of surgery in symptomatic non-hydrocephalic pineal cysts: role of magnetic resonance imaging biomarkers indicative of central venous hypertension. Acta Neurochir. 2017;159:349–61.
16. Eide PK. The correlation between pulsatile intracranial pressure and indices of intracranial pressure-volume reserve capacity: results from ventricular infusion testing. J Neurosurg. 2016;125:1493–503.
17. Eide PK, Sorteberg W. Association among intracranial compliance, intracranial pulse pressure amplitude and intracranial pressure in patients with intracranial bleeds. Neurol Res. 2007;29:798–802.
18. Eide PK, Stanisic M. Cerebral microdialysis and intracranial pressure monitoring in patients with idiopathic normal-pressure hydrocephalus: association with clinical response to extended lumbar drainage and shunt surgery. J Neurosurg. 2010;112:414–24.
19. Eide PK. Cardiac output in idiopathic normal pressure hydrocephalus: association with arterial blood pressure and intracranial pressure wave amplitudes and outcome of shunt surgery. Fluids Barriers CNS. 2011;8:11.
20. Eide PK, Hansson HA. Astrogliosis and impaired aquaporin-4 and dystrophin systems in idiopathic normal pressure hydrocephalus. Neuropathol Appl Neurobiol. 2018;44:474–90.
21. Aiken AH, Hoots JA, Saindane AM, Hudgins PA. Incidence of cerebellar tonsillar ectopia in idiopathic intracranial hypertension: a mimic of the Chiari I malformation. AJNR Am J Neuroradiol. 2012;33:1901–6.
22. Ringstad G, Emblem KE, Eide PK. Phase-contrast magnetic resonance imaging reveals net retrograde aqueductal flow in idiopathic normal pressure hydrocephalus. J Neurosurg. 2016;124:1850–7.
23. McComb JG. Recent research into the nature of cerebrospinal fluid formation and absorption. J Neurosurg. 1983;59:369–83.
24. Bedussi B, van Lier MG, Bartstra JW, de Vos J, Siebes M, VanBavel E, et al. Clearance from the mouse brain by convection of interstitial fluid towards the ventricular system. Fluids Barriers CNS. 2015;12:23.
25. Iliff JJ, Wang M, Liao Y, Plogg BA, Peng W, Gundersen GA, et al. A paravascular pathway facilitates CSF flow through the brain parenchyma and the clearance of interstitial solutes, including amyloid beta. Sci Transl Med. 2012;4:147ra111.
26. Oreskovic D, Klarica M. A new look at cerebrospinal fluid movement. Fluids Barriers CNS. 2014;11:16.
27. Ringstad G, Vatnehol SAS, Eide PK. Glymphatic MRI in idiopathic normal pressure hydrocephalus. Brain. 2017;140:2691–705.
28. Brinker T, Stopa E, Morrison J, Klinge P. A new look at cerebrospinal fluid circulation. Fluids Barriers CNS. 2014;11:10.
29. Morris AW, Sharp MM, Albargothy NJ, Fernandes R, Hawkes CA, Verma A, et al. Vascular basement membranes as pathways for the passage of fluid into and out of the brain. Acta Neuropathol. 2016;131:725–36.
30. Rennels ML, Gregory TF, Blaumanis OR, Fujimoto K, Grady PA. Evidence for a "paravascular" fluid circulation in the mammalian central nervous system, provided by the rapid distribution of tracer protein throughout the brain from the subarachnoid space. Brain Res. 1985;326:47–63.
31. Iliff JJ, Wang M, Zeppenfeld DM, Venkataraman A, Plog BA, Liao Y, et al. Cerebral arterial pulsation drives paravascular CSF-interstitial fluid exchange in the murine brain. J Neurosci. 2013;33:18190–9.
32. Kress BT, Iliff JJ, Xia M, Wang M, Wei HS, Zeppenfeld D, et al. Impairment of paravascular clearance pathways in the aging brain. Ann Neurol. 2014;76:845–61.
33. Iliff JJ, Chen MJ, Plog BA, Zeppenfeld DM, Soltero M, Yang L, et al. Impairment of glymphatic pathway function promotes tau pathology after traumatic brain injury. J Neurosci. 2014;34:16180–93.
34. Xie L, Kang H, Xu Q, Chen MJ, Liao Y, Thiyagarajan M, et al. Sleep drives metabolite clearance from the adult brain. Science. 2013;342:373–7.

35. von Holstein-Rathlou S, Petersen NC, Nedergaard M. Voluntary running enhances glymphatic influx in awake behaving, young mice. Neurosci Lett. 2018;662:253–8.
36. Eide PK, Ringstad G. Delayed clearance of cerebrospinal fluid tracer from entorhinal cortex in idiopathic normal pressure hydrocephalus: a glymphatic magnetic resonance imaging study. J Cereb Blood Flow Metab. 2018:271678x18760974. https://doi.org/10.1177/0271678X18760974.
37. Eide PK, Ringstad G. MRI with intrathecal MRI gadolinium contrast medium administration: a possible method to assess glymphatic function in human brain. Acta Radiol Open. 2015;4:2058460115609635.
38. Moser MB, Rowland DC, Moser EI. Place cells, grid cells, and memory. Cold Spring Harb Perspect Biol. 2015;7:a021808.
39. Pennanen C, Kivipelto M, Tuomainen S, Hartikainen P, Hanninen T, Laakso MP, et al. Hippocampus and entorhinal cortex in mild cognitive impairment and early AD. Neurobiol Aging. 2004;25:303–10.
40. Weed LH. Studies on Cerebro-Spinal Fluid. No. III: the pathways of escape from the Subarachnoid Spaces with particular reference to the Arachnoid Villi. J Med Res. 1914;31:51–91.
41. Holter KE, Kehlet B, Devor A, Sejnowski TJ, Dale AM, Omholt SW, et al. Interstitial solute transport in 3D reconstructed neuropil occurs by diffusion rather than bulk flow. Proc Natl Acad Sci U S A. 2017;114:9894–9.
42. Abbott NJ. Evidence for bulk flow of brain interstitial fluid: significance for physiology and pathology. Neurochem Int. 2004;45:545–52.
43. Iliff JJ, Lee H, Yu M, Feng T, Logan J, Nedergaard M, et al. Brain-wide pathway for waste clearance captured by contrast-enhanced MRI. J Clin Invest. 2013;123:1299–309.
44. Eide PK, Sroka M, Wozniak A, Saehle T. Morphological characterization of cardiac induced intracranial pressure (ICP) waves in patients with overdrainage of cerebrospinal fluid and negative ICP. Med Eng Phys. 2012;34:1066–70.
45. Elvsashagen T, Zak N, Norbom LB, Pedersen PO, Quraishi SH, Bjornerud A, et al. Evidence for cortical structural plasticity in humans after a day of waking and sleep deprivation. NeuroImage. 2017;156:214–23.
46. Nagelhus EA, Ottersen OP. Physiological roles of aquaporin-4 in brain. Physiol Rev. 2013;93:1543–62.
47. Bedussi B, van der Wel NN, de Vos J, van Veen H, Siebes M, VanBavel E, et al. Paravascular channels, cisterns, and the subarachnoid space in the rat brain: a single compartment with preferential pathways. J Cereb Blood Flow Metab. 2017;37(4):1374–85.
48. Bonomini F, Rezzani R. Aquaporin and blood brain barrier. Curr Neuropharmacol. 2010;8:92–6.
49. Manley GT, Binder DK, Papadopoulos MC, Verkman AS. New insights into water transport and edema in the central nervous system from phenotype analysis of aquaporin-4 null mice. Neuroscience. 2004;129:983–91.
50. Yao X, Hrabetova S, Nicholson C, Manley GT. Aquaporin-4-deficient mice have increased extracellular space without tortuosity change. J Neurosci. 2008;28:5460–4.
51. Smith AJ, Yao X, Dix JA, Jin BJ, Verkman AS. Test of the "glymphatic" hypothesis demonstrates diffusive and aquaporin-4-independent solute transport in rodent brain parenchyma. Elife. 2017;6:pii: e27679. https://doi.org/10.7554/eLife.27679.
52. Burfeind KG, Murchison CF, Westaway SK, Simon MJ, Erten-Lyons D, Kaye JA, et al. The effects of noncoding aquaporin-4 single-nucleotide polymorphisms on cognition and functional progression of Alzheimer's disease. Alzheimers Dement (N Y). 2017;3:348–59.
53. Zeppenfeld DM, Simon M, Haswell J, et al. Association of perivascular localization of aquaporin-4 with cognition and alzheimer disease in aging brains. JAMA Neurol. 2017;74:91–9.
54. Li X, Han Y, Xu H, Sun Z, Zhou Z, Long X, et al. Aquaporin 4 expression and ultrastructure of the blood-brain barrier following cerebral contusion injury. Neural Regen Res. 2013;8:338–45.
55. Eide PK, Eidsvaag VA, Nagelhus EA, Hansson HA. Cortical astrogliosis and increased perivascular aquaporin-4 in idiopathic intracranial hypertension. Brain Res. 2016;1644:161–75.

56. Eidsvaag VA, Hansson HA, Heuser K, Nagelhus EA, Eide PK. Brain capillary ultrastructure in idiopathic normal pressure hydrocephalus: relationship with static and pulsatile intracranial pressure. J Neuropathol Exp Neurol. 2017;76:1034–45.
57. Siasios I, Kapsalaki EZ, Fountas KN, Fotiadou A, Dorsch A, Vakharia K, et al. The role of diffusion tensor imaging and fractional anisotropy in the evaluation of patients with idiopathic normal pressure hydrocephalus: a literature review. Neurosurg Focus. 2016;41:E12.
58. Carare RO, Bernardes-Silva M, Newman TA, Page AM, Nicoll JA, Perry VH, et al. Solutes, but not cells, drain from the brain parenchyma along basement membranes of capillaries and arteries: significance for cerebral amyloid angiopathy and neuroimmunology. Neuropathol Appl Neurobiol. 2008;34:131–44.
59. Engelhardt B, Vajkoczy P, Weller RO. The movers and shapers in immune privilege of the CNS. Nat Immunol. 2017;18:123–31.
60. Weller RO, Djuanda E, Yow HY, Carare RO. Lymphatic drainage of the brain and the pathophysiology of neurological disease. Acta Neuropathol. 2009;117:1–14.
61. Aspelund A, Antila S, Proulx ST, Karlsen TV, Karaman S, Detmar M, et al. A dural lymphatic vascular system that drains brain interstitial fluid and macromolecules. J Exp Med. 2015;212:991–9.
62. Louveau A, Smirnov I, Keyes TJ, Eccles JD, Rouhani SJ, Peske JD, et al. Structural and functional features of central nervous system lymphatic vessels. Nature. 2015;523:337–41.
63. Absinta M, Ha SK, Nair G, Sati P, Luciano NJ, Palisoc M, et al. Human and nonhuman primate meninges harbor lymphatic vessels that can be visualized noninvasively by MRI. Elife. 2017;6:pii: e29738.
64. Eide PK, Vatnehol SAS, Emblem KE, Ringstad G. Magnetic resonance imaging provides evidence of glymphatic drainage from human brain to cervical lymph nodes. Sci Rep. 2018;8:7194. https://doi.org/10.1038/s41598-018-25666-4.

Part II

Clinical Disorders of CSF

Congenital Hydrocephalus

5

Charuta Gavankar Furey, Prince Antwi,
and Kristopher Thomas Kahle

Introduction

Congenital hydrocephalus (CH), with an estimated prevalence of 1 in 1500 births [1], is the most common disease treated by pediatric neurosurgeons and exerts a tremendous burden on patients, caregivers, and healthcare systems worldwide. Characterized by disordered cerebrospinal fluid (CSF) homeostasis, CH often results in clinically significant ventriculomegaly associated with increased intracranial pressure. Symptoms depend on age of onset: infants typically present with progressive macrocephaly [2, 3] whereas older children present with symptoms of intracranial hypertension [4]. CH can disrupt brain development [5], lead to cognitive and motor deficits [6, 7], and if untreated, progress to brain herniation and death.

Evidence indicates genetic factors play a major role in the pathogenesis of congenital hydrocephalus [8, 9], and although results of animal studies have contributed to our understanding of the disorder, our knowledge of genetic determinants and molecular mechanisms of primary (or developmental) hydrocephalus is primitive. Accordingly, the treatment of CH is empiric, symptomatic, and largely achieved with surgical shunting strategies that have not changed in decades [2, 10].

Here, we review the human and nonhuman genetics of CH. Advances in Genetics afford novel opportunities to identify causative genes in this disease that will prove invaluable in elucidating the mechanisms involved in the pathogenesis of the disease. A comprehensive understanding of key genetic drivers and the associated

C. G. Furey · P. Antwi
Department of Neurosurgery, Yale School of Medicine, New Haven, CT, USA

K. T. Kahle (✉)
Departments of Neurosurgery, Pediatrics, and Cellular and Molecular Physiology,
Yale School of Medicine, New Haven, CT, USA
e-mail: kristopher.kahle@yale.edu

D. D. Limbrick, J. R. Leonard (eds.), *Cerebrospinal Fluid Disorders*,
https://doi.org/10.1007/978-3-319-97928-1_5

molecular mechanisms of CH might identify targets for developing novel pharmacotherapeutics.

Classification of Congenital Hydrocephalus

As in other forms of hydrocephalus, several systems have been suggested for classifying CH based on clinical features [8, 11]. We discuss three such systems.

Congenital hydrocephalus is classified as primary or secondary based on etiology. Cases without an apparent external cause are termed primary or developmental. Secondary or acquired congenital hydrocephalus describes those cases due to external causes such as intrauterine infections, hemorrhage, and neoplasm. Based on the CSF flow physiology, CH may be classified as either noncommunicating or communicating. In noncommunicating CH, CSF flow is impeded by discrete lesion(s) along its course through the ventricles and cisterns. In communicating CH, there is no such discrete impediment to CSF flow. Lastly, CH may be classified as syndromic or nonsyndromic based on the presence or absence of other congenital anomalies. In syndromic CH, hydrocephalus is often not the predominant phenotype of the disease that may present with other cerebral or extracerebral anomalies. In nonsyndromic CH, hydrocephalus may be an isolated anomaly, although less prominent clinical features may be present. As you may expect, there is more known about the genetic basis of syndromic CH than is known about nonsyndromic CH.

Genetics of Congenital Hydrocephalus

Genetic factors, including cytogenetic abnormalities and polygenic contributions, are involved in the pathogenesis of both syndromic and nonsyndromic forms of primary CH [12–14]. Population studies clearly demonstrate familial aggregation of primary CH, with significantly increased recurrence risk ratios observed for same-sex twins, and first- and second-degree relatives [15]. These data corroborate earlier epidemiological studies [12, 16, 17]. An estimated 40% of CH associated with aqueductal stenosis is attributed to genetic contributions following Mendelian inheritance patterns [18]. Despite this, an underlying genetic cause is unknown in almost all individuals with nonsyndromic, non-X-linked CH, and 20% of children with syndromic CH [19]. The heterogeneous nature of the disease, an inadequate classification scheme, and the genetic background effects complicate the identification of CH genes. To date, over 50 mutant loci or genes have been linked to hydrocephalus in animal models; however, only six genes have been identified as causative genes in human CH [1, 8, 9].

Human Genetics

Causative Genes in Congenital Hydrocephalus

Mutations in *L1CAM* (OMIM #308840) have been reported to cause X-linked congenital hydrocephalus, contributing to about 30% of X-linked cases of the disease [20, 21]. Mutations in the gene cause both hydrocephalus with stenosis of the aqueduct of Sylvius (HSAS; OMIM #307000) and L1 syndrome (i.e., adducted thumbs, spastic paraplegia, agenesis of corpus callosum, hypoplasia of corticospinal tract, fusion of thalami, and hypoplasia of cerebellar vermis) [22]. There have been more than 200 reported genomic duplications and point mutations in *L1CAM* [23]. *L1CAM* encodes the L1 cell adhesion molecule, a transmembrane glycoprotein that is involved in neurogenesis, neuronal migration, and axon guidance [23, 24]. In neurons developed from human embryonic stem (ES) cells with conditional *L1CAM* loss-of-function mutations, deletion of the gene resulted in impaired arborization of axons and dendrites and generation of action potential [25]. The exact pathomechanism behind congenital hydrocephalus in mutations of *L1CAM* remains to be identified. Suggested hypotheses include: (1) increased CSF pressure and ventricular susceptibility due to decreased elasticity of cortical white matter, (2) narrowed CSF pathway due to abnormal development of midline structures, and (3) thinning of cerebral wall due to formation of poor neuronal connections [9, 26, 27]. It is recommended that males with congenital hydrocephalus be tested for *L1CAM* mutations, especially in the presence of positive family history of adducted thumbs and/or compatible radiographic features [8].

Previously thought to be an example of L1 syndrome, Pettigrew syndrome was described by Strain et al. as a distinct X-linked hydrocephalus with associated features such as intellectual disability, choreoathetosis, fourth ventricular cysts, and deposition of iron or calcium in the basal ganglia [8, 28, 29]. Mutations in *AP1S2* (OMIM #300629) were subsequently identified as causative of congenital hydrocephalus in Pettigrew syndrome [30, 31]. *AP1S2* encodes a subunit of the AP1 adaptin complex, a regulator of vesicular trafficking between the Golgi apparatus and endosomes [32]. Mice with mutations resulting in impaired vesicular trafficking (such as mutations in *Lgl1* and *hyh*) demonstrate severe, and sometimes fatal, hydrocephalus [9, 33]. In *hyh* mutant mice with defective vesicular transport, neuronal progenitor cells prematurely withdraw from the cell cycle resulting in decreased cortical progenitor cells [34]. Males presenting with congenital hydrocephalus, intellectual disability, and iron or calcium deposition on radiographs should be tested for mutations in *AP1S2* [8].

The first reported autosomal recessive gene implicated in congenital hydrocephalus was *CCDC88C* (OMIM #611204), which encodes a Disheveled homolog (DVL)-binding protein DAPLE that negatively regulates the noncanonical Wnt signaling pathway. Using positional cloning in a consanguineous family of nonsyndromic hydrocephalus, Ekici et al. identified a homozygous truncating mutation in *CCDC88C* that resulted in loss of function of the protein and reduced expression of several components of the Wnt pathway [35]. Drieslma et al. subsequently reported truncating mutations in another family with patients afflicted with nonsyndromic hydrocephalus [36]. More recently, using whole exome sequencing, Ruggerri et al. identified homozygous truncating mutations in *CCDC88C* resulting in congenital hydrocephalus [37]. Of note, all reported mutations in *CCDC88C* abolish the PDZ binding domain of DAPLE that is indispensable in its interaction with Disheveled in the Wnt pathway (Fig. 5.1) [9, 37, 38]. Murine models of mutations (such as $Dvl1^{-/-}$ and $3^{+/-}$) in elements of the noncanonical Wnt pathway demonstrate

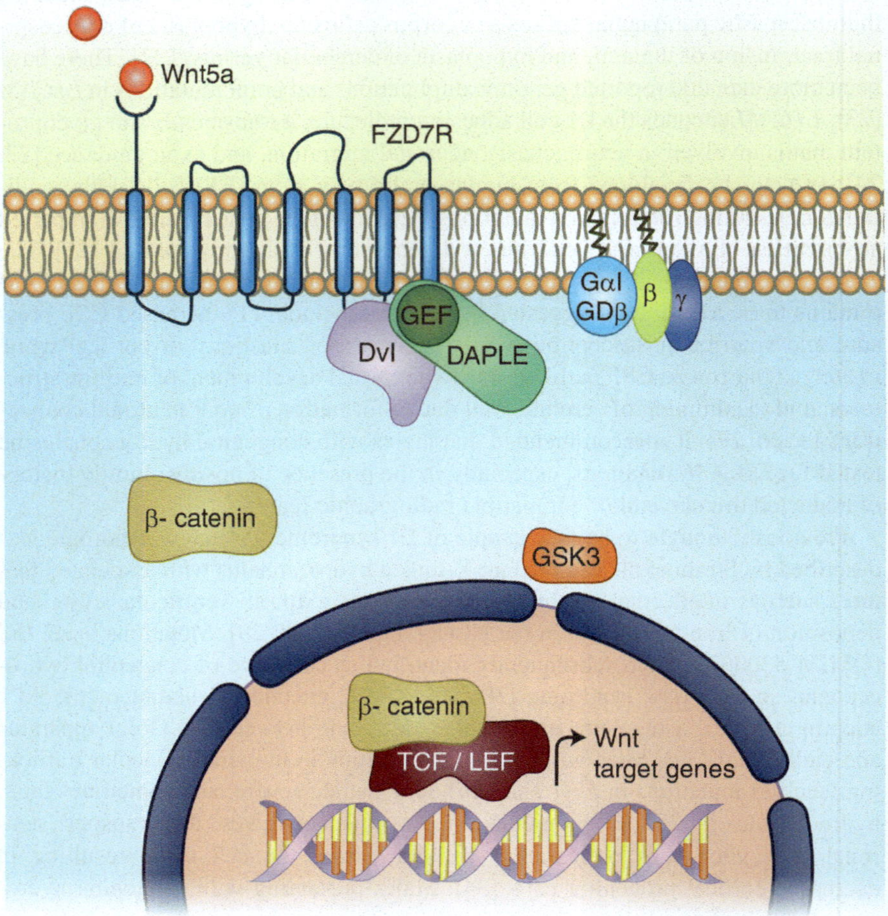

Fig. 5.1 The first autosomal recessive gene identified to cause congenital hydrocephalus was *CCDC88C*, which encodes DAPLE, a negative regulator of the noncanonical Wnt signaling pathway. Mutations that abolish the PDZ binding domain of DAPLE hinder its interaction with Disheveled (Dvl) and are implicated in congenital hydrocephalus

hydrocephalus [39]. Hypothetically, defects in DAPLE's interactions with components of Wnt signaling pathways result in subtly aberrant planar cell polarity and cilia orientation, two pathomechanisms frequently suggested in CH [9, 39].

The second reported autosomal recessive gene implicated in congenital hydrocephalus was *MPDZ* (OMIM #603785), which encodes a tight junction protein known to regulate planar cell polarity. Using autozygosity, linkage analysis, and direct sequencing techniques in a study of families with congenital hydrocephalus, Al-Dosari et al. identified a truncating mutation in *MPDZ* as a cause of CH [40]. As is the case of mutations in other planar cell polarity genes that cause hydrocephalus, mutation in *MPDZ* hypothetically, through a yet-to-be-elucidated mechanism, disrupts ependymal cilia function resulting in hydrocephalus [9, 41]. Mice with global *Mpdz* deletion develop perinatal-onset supratentorial hydrocephalus due to ependymal denudation [42].

In a study employing exome sequencing in families with children afflicted by congenital hydrocephalus, Shaheen et al. identified *EML1* and *WDR81* as causative genes of autosomal recessive congenital hydrocephalus [43]. The patient with homozygous truncating mutation in *EML1* presented with CH, developmental delay, epilepsy, and MRI demonstrating polymicrogyria, band heterotopia, agenesis of corpus callosum, and cerebellar tonsillar herniation. The homozygous truncating mutation in *WDR81* resulted in severe CH and cerebellar hypoplasia or agenesis. *EML1* (OMIM #602033) encodes a microtubule (MT)-associated protein of the EMAP family involved in planar cell polarity. In both humans and mice, mutation of the gene results in neuronal heterotopia [44]; in mice, loss of the gene impairs spindle length and soma shape of neuronal progenitors in the developing cortex [45]. Mutations in *WDR81* have been associated with cerebellar ataxia, mental retardation, and disequilibrium syndrome 2 (CAMRQ2) [46]. WDR81 is localized in mitochondria of Purkinje neurons and is necessary for their survival [47]. Knocking down orthologues of *WDR81* in Drosophila leads to delayed mitotic progression, a hypothetical pathomechanism for microcephaly and cerebellar anomalies associated with mutations in the gene [48]. Independent confirmations of *EML1* and *WDR81* in CH are needed.

Genes Associated with Syndromic Congenital Hydrocephalus

Mutations in more than 100 genes have been identified to cause syndromes whose phenotypes include hydrocephalus. The authors find it profitable to discuss these genes as groups based on their functional processes. This discussion covers only a subset of well-known forms of syndromic congenital hydrocephalus and their related molecular genetics, but a fairly exhaustive list of genes associated with hydrocephalus in humans, mice, zebrafish, and frogs is included for your perusal.

Congenital Hydrocephalus in Neural Tube Defects

Neural tube defects (NTDs) such as spina bifida, anencephaly, encephaloceles, Chiari malformations, and Dandy-Walker malformations, among others, make up a large fraction of congenital malformations involving the nervous system [49]. NTDs are results of impaired neural tube closure during development and many patients with NTDs have hydrocephalus [50, 51]. Cause of NTDs is multifactorial. Environmental factors such as maternal folate intake and medications like valporic acid are implicated in NTDs; there are genetic factors associated with NTDs too [50, 52]. Structurally, it is hypothesized that congenital hydrocephalus in NTDs is due to impedance of CSF flow by a downward displaced cerebellum as a result of tethering during lengthening of the spinal column [9]. Genetically, congenital hydrocephalus in NTDs is often associated with mutations in genes that encode components of the planar cell polarity (or noncanonical Wnt signaling) pathway.

Planar cell polarity, by modulating actin cytoskeleton through activities of GTPases, is indispensable in neural tube closure [53]. Reported mutations in planar cell polarity genes in patients with hydrocephalus include those in *FUZ*, *VANGL1*, *VANGL2*, *CELSR1*, *SCRIB1*, *DVL2*, *GPSM2*, *NOTCH2*, and *PTK7*, most of which are known to be susceptibility genes for NTDs (Table 5.1) [69, 71–76]. Of note, mutations in planar cell polarity genes such as *CELSR2* and the previously discussed *MPDZ* cause hydrocephalus without NTDs [8]. In mice with mutations in *Pkd1* or *Pkd2*, impaired apical localization of Vangl2 in ependymal cilia results in slower ependymal flow and dilatation of the lateral ventricles [91].

Congenital Hydrocephalus in Ciliopathies

In the ependymal model of CSF homeostasis, synchronous beating of ependymal cilia directs CSF flow through the ventricles (Fig. 5.2) [92]. Continuous CSF flow maintains the patency of the aqueduct of Sylvius. Mice with mutation in the anoxemal dynein heavy chain Mdnah5 develop triventricular hydrocephalus secondary to stenosis of the aqueduct due to impaired ependymal flow [92]. In addition to the direction of CSF flow by motile ependymal cilia, the primary (nonmotile) cilia regulate CSF production. Mice with mutations in *E2f5*, impairing activity of the primary cilia, demonstrate hypersecretion of CSF and develop communicating congenital hydrocephalus [93]. Thus, defects in either the motile or nonmotile cilia may result in hydrocephalus. Mutations in several human genes have been reported in ciliopathies whose phenotypes include hydrocephalus. Mutation in *CCNO*, which encodes Cyclin O, a regulator of ciliogenesis and apoptosis, results in congenital mucociliary clearance disorder with reduced generation of motile cilia. Patients with this disorder may present with hydrocephalus and recurrent respiratory infections [94, 95]. Genes with mutations that result in ciliopathies and associated hydrocephalus are listed in Table 5.1. Notable are *DNAH1*, *DNAH5*, *DYX1C1*, *CENPF* mutations in well-known diseases such as Kartagener syndrome, primary ciliary dyskinesia, and Marfan syndrome [60–62, 68]. Less common diseases such as Joubert syndrome and Meckel syndrome may be associated with hydrocephalus [63–67]. Several mice and zebrafish genes known to have mutants resulting in ciliopathies and hydrocephalus are listed in Table 5.2. Recently, Liu et al. demonstrated that mutations in *Ulk4* in mice results in aberrant ciliogenesis leading to dysfunctional subcommissural organs, stenotic aqueduct, and hydrocephalus; *ULK4*, the human homolog of the gene may be a risk factor for neurodevelopmental disorders [168, 169].

Congenital Hydrocephalus in RASopathies

Diseases that are due to germline mutations in genes encoding members of the Ras/mitogen-activated protein kinase (MAPK) pathway are termed RASopathies. The Ras/MAPK pathway, consisting of GTPases, regulates cell growth, proliferation, differentiation, and senescence (Fig. 5.3) [80]. RASopathies associated with hydrocephalus include Noonan syndrome, Costello syndrome, cardio-facio-cutaneous

Table 5.1 Selected syndromes associated with hydrocephalus

Syndrome	Associated features	Gene locus	OMIM ID	(Suggested) pathway	References
L1 syndrome	Adducted thumbs, intellectual disability, corpus callosum agenesis/ atrophy, abnormal gait	*L1CAM*	308840	Neuronal adhesion	Rosenthal et al. [21]
Walker-Warburg syndrome	Intellectual disability, muscular weakness, detached retina, microphthalmia/ anopthalmia	*B3GALNT2*	615181	Dystroglycan modification	van Reeuwijk et al. [54]
		B4GAT1	605517		Shaheen et al. [55]
		FKRP	606596		Bouchet-Seraphin et al. [56]
		FKTN	607440		Bouchet-Seraphin et al. [56]
		GMPPB	615320		Bouchet-Seraphin et al. [56]
		ISPD	614631		Roscioli et al. [57]
		LARGE1	603590		van Reeuwijk et al. [54]
		POMGNT1	606822		Yoshida et al. [58]
		POMGNT2	614828		Bouchet-Seraphin et al. [56]
		POMK	615247		Bouchet-Seraphin et al. [56]
		POMT1	607423		Bouchet-Seraphin et al. [56]
		POMT2	607439		van Reeuwijk et al. [54]
		TMEM5	605862		Bouchet-Seraphin et al. [56]
Peters-plus syndrome	Dwarfism, intellectual disability, ocular anomalies (corneal opacity, cataract, etc.)	*B3GALTL*	610308	Dystroglycan modification	Lesnik Oberstein et al. [59]

(continued)

Table 5.1 (continued)

Syndrome	Associated features	Gene locus	OMIM ID	(Suggested) pathway	References
Primary ciliary dyskinesia	Recurrent respiratory infections, situs inversus, agenesis of corpus callosum, cerebellar hypoplasia	*CENPF*	600236	Ciliogenesis and ciliary function	Waters et al. [60]
Kartagener's syndrome	Dextrocardia, situs inversus, recurrent respiratory infections	*DNAI1*	604366	Ciliogenesis and ciliary function	Pennarun et al. [61]
		DNAH5	603335		Olbrich et al. [62]
Meckel syndrome	Multicystic renal dysplasia, polydactyly, hepatic fibrosis, microcephaly	*TMEM67*	609884	Ciliogenesis and ciliary function	Smith et al. [63]
		MKS1	609883		Kyttala et al. [64]
Bardet-Biedl syndrome	Intellectual disability, postaxial polydactyly, multicystic renal dysplasia, obesity, pigmentary retinopathy	*CEP290*	610142	Ciliogenesis and ciliary function	Kim et al. [65]
Joubert syndrome	Intellectual disability, cerebellar hypoplasia, tachypnea, apnea, ataxia	*TMEM216*	613277	Ciliogenesis and ciliary function	Valente et al. [66]
		CC2D2A	612013		Gorden et al. [67]
Marfan syndrome	Scoliosis, dislocated lens, hyperflexible joints	*FBN1*	134797	Ciliogenesis and ciliary function	Hogue et al. [68]
Chudley-McCullough syndrome	Mental retardation, seizures, sensorineural heaing loss, cerebellar dysplasia, hypoplasia corpus callosum	*GPSM2*	609245	Planar cell polarity	Koenigstein et al. [69]
Adams-Oliver syndrome	Aplasia cutis congenita, calvarial defect, failure thrive, sparse hair	*ARHGAP31*	610911	Planar cell polarity	Caron et al. [70]

Table 5.1 (continued)

Syndrome	Associated features	Gene locus	OMIM ID	(Suggested) pathway	References
Hajdu-Cheney syndrome	Hypertelorism, short stature, thick eyebrow, brachydactyly	*NOTCH2*	600275	Planar cell polarity	Simpson et al. [71]
Susceptibility to neural tube defects	Neural tube defects	*VANGL1*	610132	Planar cell polarity	Kibar et al. [72]
		VANGL2	600533		Kibar et al. [72]
		FUZ	610622		Seo et al. [73]
		PTK7	601890		Wang et al. [74]
		SCRIB1	607733		Pappa et al. [75]
		CELSR1	604523		Allache et al. [76]
Cardio-facio cutaneous syndrome	Coarse facies, intellectual disability, short stature, pulmonic stenosis	*BRAF*	164757	Ras/MAPK signaling pathway	Yoon et al. [77]
Costello syndrome	Spoon-shaped fingernails, failure to thrive, macrocephaly, pulmonic stenosis	*HRAS*	190020	Ras/MAPK signaling pathway	Gripp et al. [78]
Neurofibromatosis 1	Café-au-lait spots, subcutaneous nodules, melanocytic nevus, meningioma	*NF1*	162200	Ras/MAPK signaling pathway	Dincer et al. [79]
Noonan syndrome	Hypertelorism, wide set eyes, aplasia/hypoplasia of abdominal wall musculature, pectus carinatum or excavatum	*PTPN11*	176876	Ras/MAPK signaling pathway	Rauen [80]
		SOS1	182530		Rauen [80]
		RAF1	164760		Rauen [80]
		KRAS	190070		Rauen [80]
		NRAS	164790		Rauen [80]
		SHOC2	602775		Rauen [80]
		CBL	165360		Rauen [80]
Coffin-Lowry syndrome	Intellectual disability, joint hyperflexibility, coarse facies, dysplastic long bones	*RPS6KA3*	300075	MAPK-RPS6KA3 pathway	Tos et al. [81]

(continued)

Table 5.1 (continued)

Syndrome	Associated features	Gene locus	OMIM ID	(Suggested) pathway	References
Apert syndrome	Craniosynostosis, proptosis, conductive deafness	*FGFR2*	176943	Growth factor signaling pathway	Rijken et al. [82]
Achondroplasia	Dwarfism, macrocephaly, hyperlordosis	*FGFR3*	134934	Growth factor signaling pathway	Chen et al. [83]
Campomelic dysplasia	Macrocephaly, hypoplastic or dysplastic long bones, scoliosis	*SOX9*	608160	Growth factor signaling pathway	Matsumoto et al. [84]
Cousin syndrome	Brachydactyly, hypoplastic scapulae, macrocephaly, short stature	*TBX15*	604127	AMPK signaling pathway	Lausch et al. [85]
DiGeorge syndrome	Cardiac defects, hypocalcemia, coarse facies, cleft palate, hypoplastic thymus	*TBX1*	602054	BMP4/SMAD1 signaling pathway	Papangeli and Scambler [86]
Loeys-Dietz syndrome	Aortic aneurysm, high palate, pes planus	*TGFBR1*	190181	TGF-β/SMAD signaling pathway	van Laer et al. [87]
Megalencephaly-polymicrogyria-polydactyly-hydrocephalus syndrome	Macrocephaly, megalencephaly, polymicrogyria, postaxial polydactyly	*PIK3CA*	171834	PI3K-AKT-mTOR pathway	Riviere et al. [88]
		PIK3R2	603157	PI3K-AKT-mTOR pathway	Riviere et al. [88]
		AKT3	611223	PI3K-AKT-mTOR pathway	Riviere et al. [88]
		CCND2	123833	PI3K-AKT-mTOR pathway	Mirzaa et al. [89]
		TBC1D7	612655	PI3K-AKT-mTOR pathway	Capo-chichi et al. [90]

(CFC) syndrome, Coffin-Lowry syndrome, and neurofibromatosis 1 [9, 77, 79, 81]. Hydrocephalus in these syndromes is thought to be due to both genetic defects and ensuing secondary symptoms. Mutations in *PTPN11*, *SOS1*, *RAF1*, *KRAS*, *NRAS*, *SHOC2*, *CBL* have been identified in Noonan syndrome with hydrocephalus [9]. The molecular mechanisms by which these mutations cause hydrocephalus are yet to be elucidated. However, secondary symptoms such as hindbrain herniation and

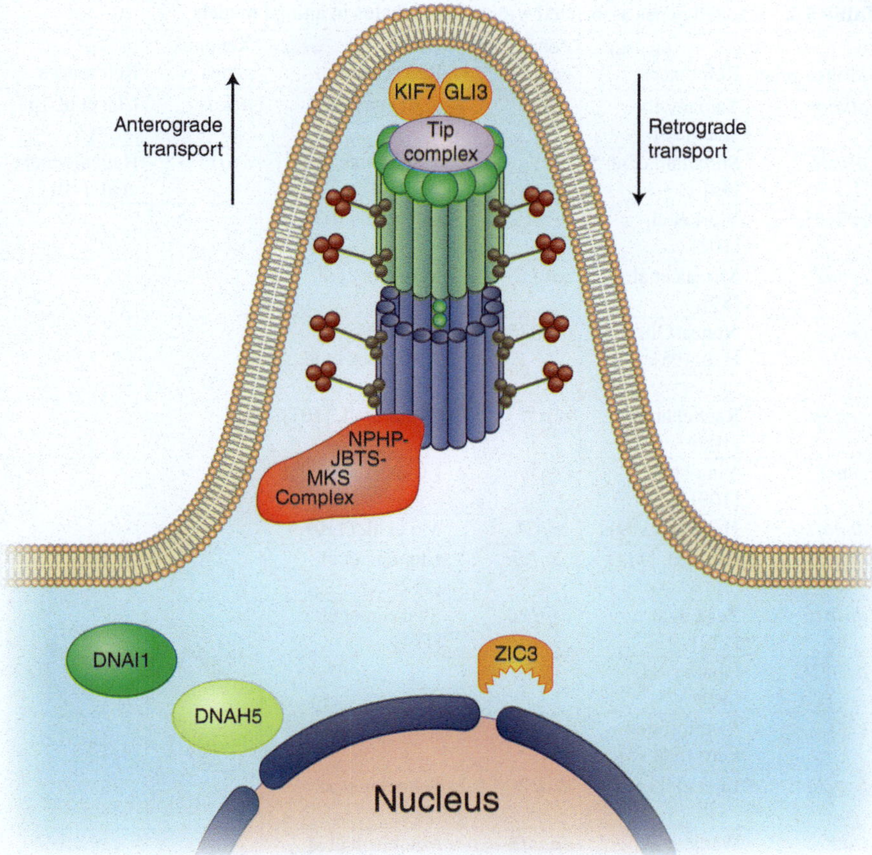

Fig. 5.2 Mutations in genes involved in ciliogenesis, cilia assembly, and/or cilia function are reported in both human and animal models of hydrocephalus. *DNAI1*, *DNAH5*, and *ZIC3* are examples of such genes. The cilium is a complex microtubular structure. The nonmotile primary cilia are involved in CSF production; the motile ependymal cilia regulate CSF flow by beating synchronously, in the bulk flow model of CSF flow

cervical intracord cysts may impede CSF flow [171]. Thompson et al. have reported on a patient with mutation in *RAF1* who presented with Noonan syndrome phenotype with hydrocephalus due to aqueductal stenosis [172]. In four patients with phenotype similar to Noonan syndrome, mutations in *PPP1CB*, a protein phosphatase in the Ras/MAPK pathway, was associated with ventriculomegaly in all patients and cerebellar ectopia and Chiari 1 malformation in some patients [173]. Cerebellar overgrowth likely contributes to hydrocephalus observed in Costello syndrome [78]. Chiari malformations, cervical stenosis, and torticollis in some cases of cardio-facio-cutaneous (CFC) syndrome may obstruct CSF flow in CFC [174]. Hamartomas and brain overgrowth may obstruct CSF flow in neurofibromatosis 1. Tully and Dobyns have hypothesized that increased venous pressures due to hypertrophic cardiomyopathy, a frequent comorbidity in RASopathies, disrupts the pressure

Table 5.2 Selected genes associated with hydrocephalus in animal models

Mouse genes	References	Zebrafish genes	References	Xenopus genes	References
afadin	Yamamoto et al. [96]	*bbs1*	Kim et al. [97]	*foxc1*	Cha et al. [98]
arid1b	Shibutani et al. [99]	*bbs9*	Veleri et al. [100]	*foxj1*	Hagenlocher et al. [101]
ccdc85c	Mori et al. [102]	*betaPix*	Liu et al. [103]		
ccnd2	Mirzaa et al. [89]	*cav1.2*	Muntean et al. [104]		
ccno	Nunez-Olle et al. [95]	*ccdc28b*	Cardenas-Rodriguez et al. [105]		
cep290	Rachel et al. [106]	*ccp1*	Lyons et al. [107]		
cetn2	Ying et al. [108]	*ccp5*	Lyons et al. [107]		
dnaaf1	Ha et al. [109]	*cd164*	Mo et al. [110]		
dnajb13	Oji et al. [111]	*cdc14b*	Clement et al. [112]		
dusp16	Zega et al. [113]	*cep120*	Shaheen et al. [114]		
dvl1/2/3	Ohata et al. [39]				
e2f5	Swetloff and Ferretti [115]				
foxo3a	Li et al. [116]	*dcdc2*	Schueler et al. [117]		
fzd3	Wang et al. [118]	*dnaaf3*	Mitchison et al. [119]		
hydin	Davy et al. [120]	*dyx1c1*	Chandrasekar et al. [121]		
ick	Moon et al. [122]	*ecrg4*	Gonzalez et al. [123]		
idh1	Bardella et al. [124]	*flr*	Pathak et al. [125]		
idh2	Akbay et al. [126]	*gtdc2*	Manzini et al. [127]		
jhy	Muniz-Talavera et al. [128]	*ift46*	Lee et al. [129]		
kidins220	Cesca et al. [130]	*ispd*	Roscioli et al. [57]		
l1cam	Itoh and Fushiki [27]	*kcnb1*	Shen et al. [131]		
lft88	Tong et al. [132]	*kiaa1109*	Gueneau et al. [133]		
lhx9	Yamazaki et al. [134]	*lgi1b*	Teng et al. [135]		

Table 5.2 (continued)

Mouse genes	References	Zebrafish genes	References	Xenopus genes	References
lrrc48	Ha et al. [109]	*lif/lifr*	Hanington et al. [136]		
lrrc6	Inaba et al. [137]	*nestin*	Chen et al. [138]		
myh10	Ridge et al. [139]	*nphp3*	Zhou et al. [140]		
n-wasp	Jain et al. [141]	*nphp7.2*	Kim et al. [97]		
nme5, -7	Vogel et al. [142]	*ofd1*	Ferrante et al. [143]		
pcp4	Raveau et al. [144]	*pank2*	Zizioli et al. [145]		
pkd1	Wodarczyk et al. [146]	*pkd1a/b*	Mangos et al. [147]		
plac1	Fant et al. [148]	*pkd2*	Obara et al. [149]		
pold3	Murga et al. [150]	*psen1*	Nornes et al. [151]		
prdm16	Shimada et al. [152]	*ptk7*	Grimes et al. [153]		
rad50	Roset et al. [154]	*rbpr2*	Shi et al. [155]		
rfx4	Xu et al. [156]	*rpgr*	Ghosh et al. [157]		
rnd3	Lin et al. [158]	*sept7b*	Dash et al. [159]		
scl9a3r1/ scl9a3r2	Ritter-Makinson et al. [160]	*slc41a1*	Hurd et al. [161]		
sox3	Lee et al. [162]	*slc9a3r1*	Treat et al. [163]		
spef2	Lehti et al. [164]	*tcf4*	Brockschmidt et al. [165]		
trp73	Nemajerova et al. [166]	*ttc4, -9c, -36, -39c*	Xu et al. [167]		
ulk4	Liu et al. [168, 169]	*wdr16*	Hirschner et al. [170]		

gradient between the subarachnoid space and the cerebral venous system, thereby hindering absorption of CSF into the systemic circulation [8].

Congenital Hydrocephalus in Skeletal Dysplasias

Hydrocephalus may be associated with syndromes that present with skeletal anomalies as the primary phenotype. In craniosysnostosis and achondroplasia, mutations in *FGFR1*, *FGFR2*, *FGFR3*, and *TGBR1*, among others, affect the growth factor signaling pathway. It is suggested that aberrancy in growth factor signaling partially

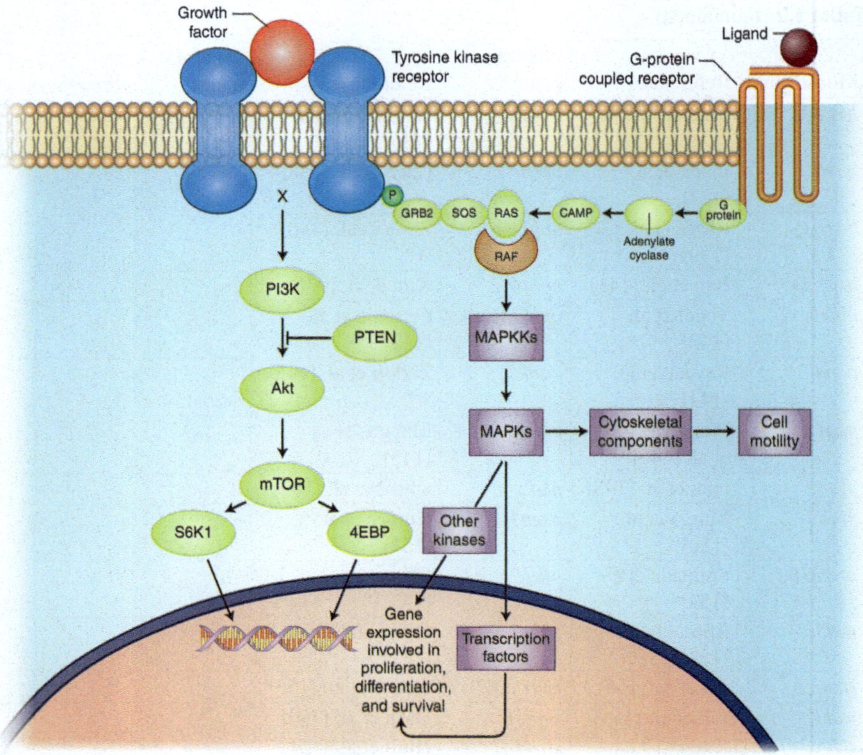

Fig. 5.3 Hydrocephalus may be a phenotypic component of RASopathies and Megalencephaly-associated syndromes. The RAS/MAPK pathway and the PI3K-Akt-mTOR pathway are downstream signaling pathways of growth factor receptors and are both involved in cell proliferation, differentiation and survival. In addition to the genetic alterations in these pathways that may account for hydrocephalus, secondary brain overgrowth in these syndromes contributes to worsening ventriculomegaly

contributes to development of ventriculomegaly, although the exact molecular mechanisms are unknown [9, 70, 82, 83, 87, 175, 176]. Administering *fgf2* to embryonic mouse brains induces hydrocephalus through aberrancy in neuronal differentiation [177]. Aberrant growth factor signaling hypothetically induces brain overgrowth that may obstruct CSF flow in these disorders. Cranial morphology may contribute to hydrocephalus in craniosynostosis and other skeletal anomalies [9, 82, 85, 86]. Increased intracranial venous pressure in these disorders hinder absorption of CSF into systemic circulation, just as is suggested in RASopathies [178]. Fetal and neonatal ventriculomegaly, which may be precursors to congenital hydrocephalus, have been reported in campomelic dysplasia, a rare skeletal dysplasia due to mutations and/or chromosomal rearrangements that affect the expression and activity of SOX9 [179]. SOX9 is a transcription factor involved in craniofacial development and in maintaining neural stem cells [84, 180–182]. In mice, loss of *Sox9* expression resulted in ependymal cells adopting a neuroblast identity with impaired differentiation and ciliation; this could account for ventriculomegaly (and possibly hydrocephalus) in campomelic dysplasia [183].

Congenital Hydrocephalus in Megalencephaly-Associated Syndromes

Megalencephaly syndromes due to mutations in components of the PI3K-Akt-mTOR pathway may present with polymicrogyria, polydactyly, and hydrocephalus [88, 90, 184]. The PI3K-Akt-mTOR pathway integrates environmental stimuli in regulating cell growth and cell proliferation, notably in brain development (Fig. 5.3) [185]. The underlying molecular mechanisms by which mutations in genes encoding components of the PI3K-Akt-mTOR pathway result in megalencephaly syndromes with hydrocephalus remain to be established. In the case of megalencephaly-polymicrogyria-polydactyly-hydrocephalus syndrome 3, which is due to activating mutations in *CCND2*, it has been proposed that increased stability of the mutant *CCND2* in neuronal precursors leads to aberrant expansion of radial glial cells and intermediate progenitor cells that determine brain size [9, 89]. Recent evidence relates hydrocephalus due to aberrancy of the PI3K-Akt-mTOR pathway to ciliogenesis. In primary-cilium-less mice, Foerster et al. observed an abnormal upregulation of the mTOR pathway resulting in enlarged apical domains of radial glial cells and subsequently ventriculomegaly [186]. In addition to the genetic factors that may account for hydrocephalus in megalencephaly syndromes, the secondary symptoms of the syndrome such as brain overgrowth leading to crowded posterior fossa and obstructed CSF flow may contribute to the development of hydrocephalus [8].

Congenital Hydrocephalus in Dystroglycanopathies

Dystroglycanopathies such as Walker-Warburg syndrome, Peters-plus syndrome, and congenital disorder of glycosylation are disorders characterized by defects in glycosylation of α-dystroglycan (Fig. 5.4) [187]. These disorders vary in phenotypic severity, ranging from limb-girdle muscular dystrophy to the largely fatal Walker-Warburg syndrome that presents with cerebral and ocular anomalies and congenital muscular dystrophy. Mutations in genes such as *POMT1*, *POMT2*, *POMGNT1*, *ISPD*, *LARGE*, and *B3GALTL* that encode glycosyltransferases that mediate glycosylation of α-dystroglycan have been reported in these disorders [54–59, 188, 189]. Glycosylated dystroglycans are expressed in many cells of the body and form a link between the extracellular matrix and the intracellular cytoskeleton, mediating cellular processes such as adhesion and signal transduction. It is suggested that in dystroglycanopathies, defects in the link between glycosylated dystroglycan and the extracellular matrix result in aberrant neuronal migration that, in a

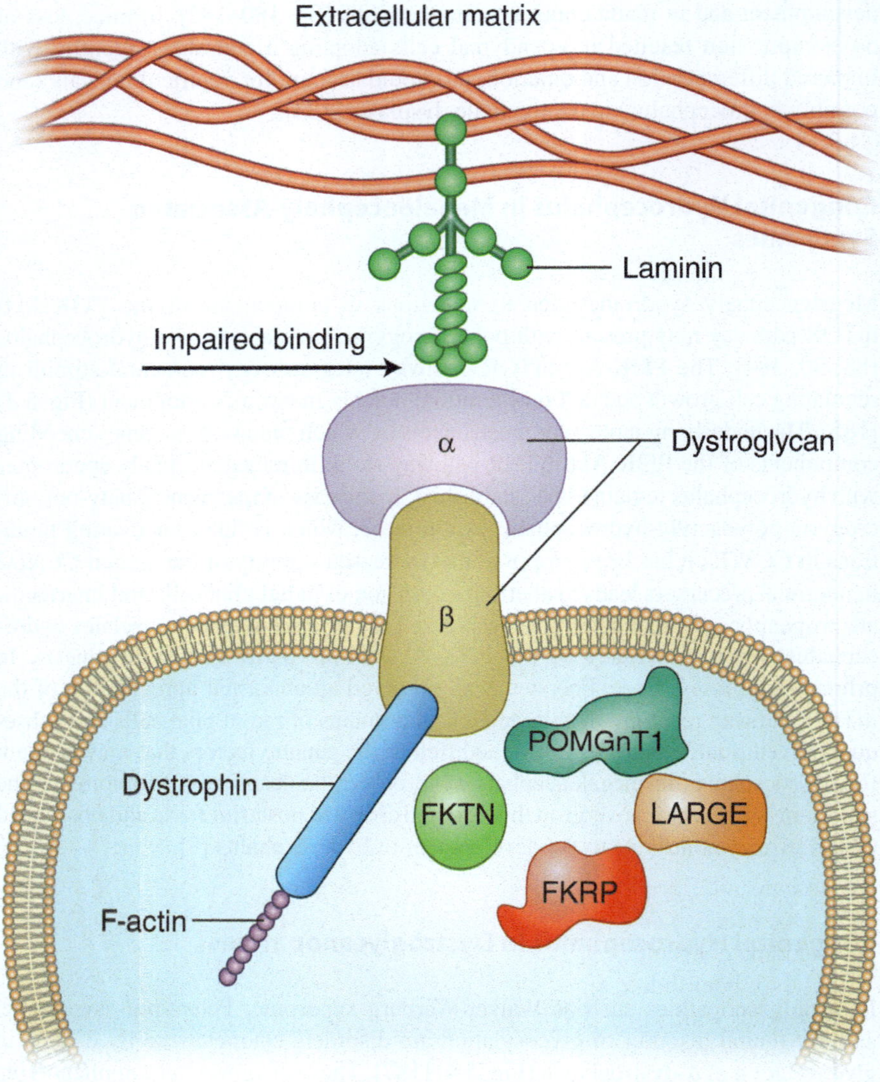

Fig. 5.4 Post-translational modifications of dystroglycans are imperative in their proper function as links between the extracellular matrix and the cell. Mutations in genes involved in modification of dystroglycans result in dystroglycanopathies, which may present with hydrocephalus. *FKTN*, *LARGE*, *FKRP*, and *POMGnT1* have been reported in human syndromic hydrocephalus

yet-to-be-elucidated mechanism, leads to cerebral anomalies such as hydrocephalus in these disorders [190]. Deletion of dystroglycan in the whole brain of mice leads to heterotopia and a cortical morphology that resembles cobblestone lissencephaly, which is associated with hydrocephalus [190]. Further, mice with mutations in *Large*, a glycosyltransferase, show markedly inhibited synaptic transmission,

Table 5.3 Bona fide human congenital hydrocephalus causative genes

Gene locus	OMIM ID	(Suggested) pathways	References
L1CAM	307000	Neuronal adhesion	Rosenthal et al. [21]
AP1S2	304340	Vesicle trafficking	Tarpey et al. [29]
MPDZ	603785	Planar cell polarity	Ishida-Takagishi et al. [38]
CCDC88C	611204	Wnt singaling pathway	Klezovitch et al. [33]
EML1	602033	Planar cell polarity	Shaheen et al. [43]
WDR81	614218	Neuronal differentiation	Shaheen et al. [43]

indicating impairment in long-term potentiation at CA3-CA1 synapses in the hippocampus [190].

Nonhuman Vertebrate Genetics

Animal models have proved invaluable in understanding the genetics and molecular mechanisms underlying both nonsyndromic and syndromic congenital hydrocephalus. A list of selected mouse, zebrafish, and frog genes with mutations that result in hydrocephalus is provided (Table 5.2). There are a few lessons to be taken from studies in animal models of the disease. Firstly, most mutations that cause hydrocephalus in murine models are reported in genes that encode ciliary proteins. These include mutations in *Dyx1c1*, *Ulk4*, and *Spef2* that result in mice with phenotypes resembling well-known human ciliopathies like primary ciliary dyskinesia [142, 168, 169, 191]. This is also true of zebrafish genes like *ift46* and *ttc4/9c/36/39c* and xenopus *foxj1* that may have mutations reported to cause hydrocephalus [101, 129, 167]. That many of these genes encode ciliary proteins highlights the role of synchronous ciliary beating in CSF flow. Secondly, most cases of congenital hydrocephalus are multigenic and depend on existing genetic modifiers, defying the single gene Mendelian inheritance paradigm that had governed previous works in understanding congenital hydrocephalus. This lesson puts into the context the fact that only six bona fide congenital hydrocephalus causative genes are known. In murine models with mutations in *L1cam*, hydrocephalus is observed only in strains with C57BL/6 background [27]. Thirdly, the molecular mechanisms behind congenital hydrocephalus may not be as distinct as previously thought (Table 5.3). For example, primary cilia signaling is associated with cytoskeletal rearrangements and involves both canonical and noncanonical Wnt signaling pathways which are the bases for planar cell polarity [192]. Zebrafish with knockdown of Cav1.2, a voltage-gated calcium channel, develop hydrocephalus; the nonmotile primary cilium regulates this L-type calcium channel through the Wnt signaling pathway [104].

Conclusion

Congenital hydrocephalus make up nearly half of all types of hydrocephalus and represent the most common condition treated by pediatric neurosurgeons [193]. This disorder of CSF homeostasis is due to both genetic and environmental factors that remain largely poorly understood. To date, only six bona fide causative genetic mutations implicated in the disorder have been identified in humans and the molecular pathomechanisms of the disorder need to be further explored. With advances in next generation sequencing and molecular biology, it is very likely that the next years will see identification of several new genes whose mutants cause nonsyndromic and syndromic congenital hydrocephalus. The recent identification of *EML1* and *WDR81* attests to this hope [43]. Molecular biology can then take advantage of these genetic discoveries to elucidate the pathomechanisms of CH. In addition to identifying new causative mutations of CH, future research may explore the relationships between the biological pathways (i.e., neural cell adhesion, Wnt signaling, vesicle transport, planar cell polarity, etc.) that are implicated in congenital hydrocephalus. Understanding these pathways and their relationships to one another may change our current view of congenital hydrocephalus as a disorder of cerebral "plumbing" and potentially establish CH as a neurodevelopmental disorder. Such paradigm shift is needed to move us beyond current therapies such as CSF shunting and endoscopic third ventriculostomy to pharmacotherapies. Lastly, with advancement in knowledge of the molecular genetics of CH, future research may investigate potential biomarkers of CH. Recently, Limbrick et al. measured CSF levels of amyloid precursor protein (APP) and its isoforms (sAPPα, sAPPβ, $A\beta_{42}$), tau, phosphorylated tau, L1CAM, NCAM-1, aquaporin 4 (AQP4), and total proteins in CSF of patients with congenital hydrocephalus [194]. In patients less than a year old, normalized CSF sAPPα threshold of 0.41 predicted congenital hydrocephalus with a sensitivity of 94% and a specificity of 97%. Future studies may identify other biomarkers that will not only improve diagnosis of congenital hydrocephalus but will also prove insightful in understanding the pathogenesis of the disease and in developing pharmacotherapies.

References

1. Zhang J, Williams MA, Rigamonti D. Genetics of human hydrocephalus. J Neurol. 2006;253:1255–66. https://doi.org/10.1007/s00415-006-0245-5.
2. Kahle KT, Kulkarni AV, Limbrick DD, Warf BC. Hydrocephalus in children. Lancet. 2016;387:788–99. https://doi.org/10.1016/s0140-6736(15)60694-8.
3. du Plessis AJ, Robinson S, Volpe JJ. Congenital hydrocephalus. In: Volpe's neurology of the newborn. Philadelphia: Elsevier; 2018. p. 58–72. https://doi.org/10.1016/b978-0-323-42876-7.00003-x.
4. Riva-Cambrin J, et al. Center effect and other factors influencing temporization and shunting of cerebrospinal fluid in preterm infants with intraventricular hemorrhage. J Neurosurg Pediatr. 2012;9:473–81. https://doi.org/10.3171/2012.1.PEDS11292.
5. McAllister JP 2nd. Pathophysiology of congenital and neonatal hydrocephalus. Semin Fetal Neonatal Med. 2012;17:285–94. https://doi.org/10.1016/j.siny.2012.06.004.
6. Lindquist B, Persson EK, Uvebrant P, Carlsson G. Learning, memory and executive functions in children with hydrocephalus. Acta Paediatr. 2008;97:596–601. https://doi.org/10.1111/j.1651-2227.2008.00747.x.
7. Lacy M, Baldassarre M, Nader T, Frim D. Parent ratings of executive functioning in children with shunted hydrocephalus. Pediatr Neurosurg. 2012;48:73–9. https://doi.org/10.1159/000339313.

8. Tully HM, Dobyns WB. Infantile hydrocephalus: a review of epidemiology, classification and causes. Eur J Med Genet. 2014;57:359–68. https://doi.org/10.1016/j.ejmg.2014.06.002.
9. Kousi M, Katsanis N. The genetic basis of hydrocephalus. Annu Rev Neurosci. 2016;39:409–35. https://doi.org/10.1146/annurev-neuro-070815-014023.
10. Wright Z, Larrew TW, Eskandari R. Pediatric hydrocephalus: current state of diagnosis and treatment. Pediatr Rev. 2016;37:478–90.
11. Oi S. Classification of hydrocephalus: critical analysis of classification categories and advantages of "Multi-categorical Hydrocephalus Classification". Childs Nerv Syst. 2011;27:1523–33.
12. Stoll C, Alembik Y, Dott B, Roth MP. An epidemiologic study of environmental and genetic factors in congenital hydrocephalus. Eur J Epidemiol. 1992;8:797–803. https://doi.org/10.1007/bf00145322.
13. Price JR Jr, Horne BM. Family history indicating hereditary factors in hydrocephalus. Ment Retard. 1968;6:40–1.
14. Tipton RE. Familial hydrocephalus. Birth Defects Orig Artic Ser. 1971;7:231.
15. Munch TN, et al. Familial aggregation of congenital hydrocephalus in a nationwide cohort. Brain J Neurol. 2012;135:2409–15. https://doi.org/10.1093/brain/aws158.
16. Fernell E, Hagberg B, Hagberg G, von Wendt L. Epidemiology of infantile hydrocephalus in Sweden. III. Origin in preterm infants. *Acta Paediatr Scand.* 1987;76:418–23.
17. Fernell E, Hagberg B, Hagberg G, von Wendt L. Epidemiology of infantile hydrocephalus in Sweden. II. Origin in infants born at term. *Acta Paediatr Scand.* 1987;76:411–7.
18. Haverkamp F, et al. Congenital hydrocephalus internus and aqueduct stenosis: aetiology and implications for genetic counselling. Eur J Pediatr. 1999;158:474–8.
19. Verhagen JM, et al. Congenital hydrocephalus in clinical practice: a genetic diagnostic approach. Eur J Med Genet. 2011;54:e542–7. https://doi.org/10.1016/j.ejmg.2011.06.005.
20. Finckh U, Schroder J, Ressler B, Veske A, Gal A. *L1CAM* mutations in isolated and familial cases with clinically suspected L1-disease. Am J Med Genet. 2000;92:40–6.
21. Rosenthal A, Jouet M, Kenwrick S. Aberrant splicing of neural cell adhesion molecule L1 mRNA in a family with X-linked hydrocephalus. Nat Genet. 1992;2:107–12.
22. Willems PJ, Brouwer OF, Dijkstra I, Wilmink J. X-linked hydrocephalus. Am J Med Genet. 1987;27:921–8.
23. Adle-Biassette H, et al. Neuropathological review of 138 cases genetically tested for X-linked hydrocephalus: evidence for closely related clinical entities of unknown molecular bases. Acta Neuropathol. 2013;126:427–42. https://doi.org/10.1007/s00401-013-1146-1.
24. Maness PF, Schachner M. Neural recognition molecules of the immunoglobulin superfamily: signal transducers of axon guidance and neuronal migration. Nat Neurosci. 2007;10:19–26.
25. Patzke C, Acuna C, Giam LR, Wernig M, Sudhof TC. Conditional deletion of L1CAM in human neurons impairs both axonal and dendritic arborization and action potential generation. J Exp Med. 2016;213:499–515. https://doi.org/10.1084/jem.20150951.
26. Tully HM, et al. Two hundred thirty-six children with developmental hydrocephalus: causes and clinical consequences. J Child Neurol. 2016;31:309–20. https://doi.org/10.1177/0883073815592222.
27. Itoh K, Fushiki S. The role of L1cam in murine corticogenesis, and the pathogenesis of hydrocephalus. Pathol Int. 2015;65:58–66. https://doi.org/10.1111/pin.12245.
28. Strain L, Wright AF, Bonthron DT. Fried syndrome is a distinct X linked mental retardation syndrome mapping to Xp22. J Med Genet. 1997;34:535–40.
29. Tarpey PS, et al. Mutations in the gene encoding the sigma 2 subunit of the adaptor protein 1 complex, AP1S2, cause X-linked mental retardation. *Am J Hum Genet.* 2006;79:1119–24.
30. Cacciagli P, et al. AP1S2 is mutated in X-linked Dandy-Walker malformation with intellectual disability, basal ganglia disease and seizures (Pettigrew syndrome). Eur J Hum Genet. 2014;22:363–8. https://doi.org/10.1038/ejhg.2013.135.
31. Saillour Y, et al. Mutations in the AP1S2 gene encoding the sigma 2 subunit of the adaptor protein 1 complex are associated with syndromic X-linked mental retardation with hydrocephalus and calcifications in basal ganglia. J Med Genet. 2007;44:739–44. https://doi.org/10.1136/jmg.2007.051334.

32. Reusch U, Bernhard O, Koszinowski U, Schu P. AP-1A and AP-3A lysosomal sorting functions. Traffic. 2002;3:752–61.
33. Klezovitch K, Fernandez TE, Tapscott SJ, Vasioukhin V. Loss of cell polarity causes severe brain dysplasia in *Lgl1* knockout mice. Genes Dev. 2004;18:559–71.
34. Chae TH, Kim S, Marz KE, Hanson PI, Walsh CA. The *hyh* mutation uncovers roles for αSnap in apical protein localization and control of neural cell fate. Nat Genet. 2004;36:264–70.
35. Ekici AB, et al. Disturbed Wnt signalling due to a mutation in CCDC88C causes an autosomal recessive non-syndromic hydrocephalus with medial diverticulum. Mol Syndromol. 2010;1:99–112. https://doi.org/10.1159/000319859.
36. Drielsma A, et al. Two novel CCDC88C mutations confirm the role of DAPLE in autosomal recessive congenital hydrocephalus. J Med Genet. 2012;49:708–12. https://doi.org/10.1136/jmedgenet-2012-101190.
37. Ruggeri G, et al. Bi-allelic mutations of CCDC88C are a rare cause of severe congenital hydrocephalus. Am J Med Genet A. 2018;176:676–81. https://doi.org/10.1002/ajmg.a.38592.
38. Ishida-Takagishi M, et al. The Dishevelled-associating protein Daple controls the non-canonical Wnt/Rac pathway and cell motility. Nat Commun. 2012;3:859. https://doi.org/10.1038/ncomms1861.
39. Ohata S, et al. Loss of Dishevelleds disrupts planar polarity in ependymal motile cilia and results in hydrocephalus. Neuron. 2014;83:558–71. https://doi.org/10.1016/j.neuron.2014.06.022.
40. Al-Dosari MS, et al. Mutation in MPDZ causes severe congenital hydrocephalus. J Med Genet. 2013;50:54–8. https://doi.org/10.1136/jmedgenet-2012-101294.
41. Sotak BN, Gleeson JG. Can't get there from here: cilia and hydrocephalus. Nat Med. 2012;18:1742–3. https://doi.org/10.1038/nm.3011.
42. Feldner A, et al. Loss of Mpdz impairs ependymal cell integrity leading to perinatal-onset hydrocephalus in mice. *EMBO Mol Med.* 2017;9:890–905. https://doi.org/10.15252/emmm.201606430.
43. Shaheen R, et al. The genetic landscape of familial congenital hydrocephalus. Ann Neurol. 2017;81:890–7. https://doi.org/10.1002/ana.24964.
44. Kielar M, et al. Mutations in Eml1 lead to ectopic progenitors and neuronal heterotopia in mouse and human. Nat Neurosci. 2014;17:923–33. https://doi.org/10.1038/nn.3729.
45. Bizzotto S, et al. Eml1 loss impairs apical progenitor spindle length and soma shape in the developing cerebral cortex. Sci Rep. 2017;7:17308. https://doi.org/10.1038/s41598-017-15253-4.
46. Gulsuner S, et al. Homozygosity mapping and targeted genomic sequencing reveal the gene responsible for cerebellar hypoplasia and quadrupedal locomotion in a consanguineous kindred. Genome Res. 2011;21:1995–2003. https://doi.org/10.1101/gr.126110.111.
47. Traka M, et al. WDR81 is necessary for purkinje and photoreceptor cell survival. J Neurosci. 2013;33:6834–44. https://doi.org/10.1523/JNEUROSCI.2394-12.2013.
48. Cavallin M, et al. WDR81 mutations cause extreme microcephaly and impair mitotic progression in human fibroblasts and Drosophila neural stem cells. Brain. 2017;140:2597–609.
49. Shankar P, Zamora C, Castillo M. Congenital malformations of the brain and spine. Handb Clin Neurol. 2016;136:1121–37. https://doi.org/10.1016/B978-0-444-53486-6.00058-2.
50. Copp AJ, Greene ND. Genetics and development of neural tube defects. J Pathol. 2010;220:217–30. https://doi.org/10.1002/path.2643.
51. Mitchell LE. Epidemiology of neural tube defects. Am J Med Genet C Semin Med Genet. 2005;135C:88–94.
52. Balashova OA, Visina O, Borodinsky LN. Folate action in nervous system development and disease. *Dev Neurobiol.* 2018;78:391–402. https://doi.org/10.1002/dneu.22579.
53. Nikolopoulou E, Galea GL, Rolo A, Greene ND, Copp AJ. Neural tube closure: cellular, molecular and biomechanical mechanisms. Development. 2017;144:552–66. https://doi.org/10.1242/dev.145904.
54. van Reeuwijk J, et al. Intragenic deletion in the LARGE gene causes Walker-Warburg syndrome. Hum Genet. 2007;121:685–90. https://doi.org/10.1007/s00439-007-0362-y.

55. Shaheen R, Faqeih E, Ansari S, Alkuraya FS. A truncating mutation in B3GNT1 causes severe Walker-Warburg syndrome. Neurogenetics. 2013;14:243–5. https://doi.org/10.1007/s10048-013-0367-8.
56. Bouchet-Seraphin C, Vuillaumier-Barrot S, Seta N. Dystroglycanopathies: about numerous genes involved in glycosylation of one single glycoprotein. J Neuromuscul Dis. 2015;2:27–38. https://doi.org/10.3233/JND-140047.
57. Roscioli T, et al. Mutations in ISPD cause Walker-Warburg syndrome and defective glycosylation of alpha-dystroglycan. Nat Genet. 2012;44:581–5. https://doi.org/10.1038/ng.2253.
58. Yoshida A, et al. Muscular dystrophy and neuronal migration disorder caused by mutations in a glycosyltransferase, POMGnT1. Dev Cell. 2001;1:717–24.
59. Lesnik Oberstein SA, et al. Peters Plus syndrome is caused by mutations in *B3GALTL*, a putative glycosyltransferase. Am J Hum Genet. 2006;79:562–6.
60. Waters AM, et al. The kinetochore protein, CENPF, is mutated in human ciliopathy and microcephaly phenotypes. J Med Genet. 2015;52:147–56. https://doi.org/10.1136/jmedgenet-2014-102691.
61. Pennarun G, et al. Loss-of-function mutations in a human gene related to *Chlamydomonas reinhardtii* dynein IC78 result in primary ciliary dyskinesia. Am J Hum Genet. 1999;65:1508–19.
62. Olbrich H, et al. Mutations in DNAH5 cause primary ciliary dyskinesia and randomization of left-right asymmetry. Nat Genet. 2002;30:143–4. https://doi.org/10.1038/ng817.
63. Smith UM, et al. The transmembrane protein meckelin (MKS3) is mutated in Meckel-Gruber syndrome and the wpk rat. Nat Genet. 2006;38:191–6. https://doi.org/10.1038/ng1713.
64. Kyttala M, et al. MKS1, encoding a component of the flagellar apparatus basal body proteome, is mutated in Meckel syndrome. Nat Genet. 2006;38:155–7. https://doi.org/10.1038/ng1714.
65. Kim J, Krishnaswami SR, Gleeson JG. CEP290 interacts with the centriolar satellite component PCM-1 and is required for Rab8 localization to the primary cilium. Hum Mol Genet. 2008;17:3796–805. https://doi.org/10.1093/hmg/ddn277.
66. Valente EM, et al. Mutations in TMEM216 perturb ciliogenesis and cause Joubert, Meckel and related syndromes. *Nat Genet*. 2010;42:619–25. https://doi.org/10.1038/ng.594.
67. Gorden NT, et al. CC2D2A is mutated in Joubert syndrome and interacts with the ciliopathy-associated basal body protein CEP290. Am J Hum Genet. 2008;83:559–71. https://doi.org/10.1016/j.ajhg.2008.10.002.
68. Hogue J, et al. Homozygosity for a FBN1 missense mutation causes a severe Marfan syndrome phenotype. Clin Genet. 2013;84:392–3. https://doi.org/10.1111/cge.12073.
69. Koenigstein K, et al. Chudley-McCullough syndrome: variable clinical picture in twins with a novel GPSM2 mutation. Neuropediatrics. 2016;47:197–201.
70. Caron C, et al. CdGAP/ARHGAP31, a Cdc42/Rac1 GTPase regulator, is critical for vascular development and VEGF-mediated angiogenesis. Sci Rep. 2016;6:27485. https://doi.org/10.1038/srep27485.
71. Simpson MA, et al. Mutations in NOTCH2 cause Hajdu-Cheney syndrome, a disorder of severe and progressive bone loss. Nat Genet. 2011;43:303–5. https://doi.org/10.1038/ng.779.
72. Kibar Z, et al. Contribution of VANGL2 mutations to isolated neural tube defects. Clin Genet. 2011;80:76–82.
73. Seo JH, et al. Mutations in the planar cell polarity gene, Fuzzy, are associated with neural tube defects in humans. Hum Mol Genet. 2011;20:4324–33.
74. Wang M, et al. Role of the planar cell polarity gene *Protein tyrosine kinase 7* in neural tube defects in humans. Birth Defects Res A Clin Mol Teratol. 2015;103:1021–7.
75. Pappa L, et al. Exome analysis in an Estonian multiplex family with neural tube defects-a case report. Childs Nerv Syst. 2017;33:1575–81. https://doi.org/10.1007/s00381-017-3491-1.
76. Allache R, De Marco P, Merello E, Capra V, Kibar Z. Role of the planar cell polarity gene CELSR1 in neural tube defects and caudal agenesis. Birth Defects Res A Clin Mol Teratol. 2012;94:176–81. https://doi.org/10.1002/bdra.23002.
77. Yoon G, Rosenberg J, Blaser S, Rauen KA. Neurological complications of cardio-facio-cutaneous syndrome. Dev Med Child Neurol. 2007;49:894–9.

78. Gripp KW, Hopkins E, Doyle D, Dobyns WB. High incidence of progressive postnatal cerebellar enlargement in Costello syndrome: brain overgrowth associated with HRAS mutations as the likely cause of structural brain and spinal cord abnormalities. Am J Med Genet A. 2010;152A:1161–8. https://doi.org/10.1002/ajmg.a.33391.
79. Dincer A, Yener U, Ozek MM. Hydrocephalus in patients with neurofibromatosis type 1: MR imaging findings and the outcome of endoscopic third ventriculostomy. AJNR Am J Neuroradiol. 2011;32:643–6. https://doi.org/10.3174/ajnr.A2357.
80. Rauen KA. The RASopathies. Annu Rev Genomics Hum Genet. 2013;14:355–69. https://doi.org/10.1146/annurev-genom-091212-153523.
81. Tos T, Alp MY, Aksoy A, Ceylaner S, Hanauer A. A familial case of Coffin-Lowry syndrome caused by RPS6KA3 C.898C>T mutation associated with multiple abnormal brain imaging findings. Genet Couns. 2015;26:47–52.
82. Rijken BF, Lequin MH, Van Veelen ML, de Rooi J, Mathijssen IM. The formation of the foramen magnum and its role in developing ventriculomegaly and Chiari I malformation in children with craniosynostosis syndromes. J Craniomaxillofac Surg. 2015;43:1042–8. https://doi.org/10.1016/j.jcms.2015.04.025.
83. Chen CP, et al. Rapid detection of K650E mutation in FGFR3 using uncultured amniocytes in a pregnancy affected with fetal cloverleaf skull, occipital pseudoencephalocele, ventriculomegaly, straight short femurs, and thanatophoric dysplasia type II. Taiwan J Obstet Gynecol. 2013;52:420–5. https://doi.org/10.1016/j.tjog.2013.05.003.
84. Matsumoto A, et al. The presence of diminished white matter and corpus callosal thinning in a case with a SOX9 mutation. Brain and Development. 2017;40:325–9. https://doi.org/10.1016/j.braindev.2017.09.002.
85. Lausch E, et al. TBX15 mutations cause craniofacial dysmorphism, hypoplasia of scapula and pelvis, and short stature in Cousin syndrome. Am J Hum Genet. 2008;83:649–55. https://doi.org/10.1016/j.ajhg.2008.10.011.
86. Papangeli I, Scambler P. The 22q11 deletion: DiGeorge and velocardiofacial syndromes and the role of TBX1. Wiley Interdiscip Rev Dev Biol. 2013;2:393–403. https://doi.org/10.1002/wdev.75.
87. Van Laer L, Dietz H, Loeys B. Loeys-Dietz syndrome. Adv Exp Med Biol. 2014;802:95–105.
88. Riviere JB, et al. De novo germline and postzygotic mutations in AKT3, PIK3R2 and PIK3CA cause a spectrum of related megalencephaly syndromes. Nat Genet. 2012;44:934–40. https://doi.org/10.1038/ng.2331.
89. Mirzaa G, et al. De novo CCND2 mutations leading to stabilization of cyclin D2 cause megalencephaly-polymicrogyria-polydactyly-hydrocephalus syndrome. Nat Genet. 2014;46:510–5. https://doi.org/10.1038/ng.2948.
90. Capo-Chichi JM, et al. Disruption of TBC1D7, a subunit of the TSC1-TSC2 protein complex, in intellectual disability and megalencephaly. J Med Genet. 2013;50:740–4. https://doi.org/10.1136/jmedgenet-2013-101680.
91. Ohata S, et al. Mechanosensory genes Pkd1 and Pkd2 contribute to the planar polarization of brain ventricular epithelium. J Neurosci. 2015;35:11153–68. https://doi.org/10.1523/JNEUROSCI.0686-15.2015.
92. Ibanez-Tallon I, et al. Dysfunction of axonemal dynein heavy chain Mdnah5 inhibits ependymal flow and reveals a novel mechanism for hydrocephalus formation. Hum Mol Genet. 2004;13:2133–41.
93. Banizs B, et al. Dysfunctional cilia lead to altered ependyma and choroid plexus function, and result in the formation of hydrocephalus. Development. 2005;132:5329–39.
94. Wallmeier J, et al. Mutations in CCNO result in congenital mucociliary clearance disorder with reduced generation of multiple motile cilia. Nat Genet. 2014;46:646–51. https://doi.org/10.1038/ng.2961.
95. Nunez-Olle M, et al. Constitutive Cyclin O deficiency results in penetrant hydrocephalus, impaired growth and infertility. Oncotarget. 2017;8:99261–73.

96. Yamamoto H, et al. Genetic deletion of afadin causes hydrocephalus by destruction of adherens junctions in radial glial and ependymal cells in the midbrain. PLoS One. 2013;8:e80356. https://doi.org/10.1371/journal.pone.0080356.
97. Kim YH, et al. A complex of BBS1 and NPHP7 is required for cilia motility in zebrafish. PLoS One. 2013;8:e72549. https://doi.org/10.1371/journal.pone.0072549.
98. Cha JY, et al. The role of FoxC1 in early Xenopus development. Dev Dyn. 2007;236:2731–41.
99. Shibutani M, et al. Arid1b Haploinsufficiency causes abnormal brain gene expression and autism-related behaviors in mice. Int J Mol Sci. 2017;18. https://doi.org/10.3390/ijms18091872.
100. Veleri S, et al. Knockdown of Bardet-Biedl syndrome gene BBS9/PTHB1 leads to cilia defects. PLoS One. 2012;7:e34389. https://doi.org/10.1371/journal.pone.0034389.
101. Hagenlocher C, Walentek P, Muller C, Thumberger T, Feistel K. Ciliogenesis and cerebrospinal fluid flow in the developing Xenopus brain are regulated by foxj1. *Cilia.* 2013;2:e1–e14. https://doi.org/10.1186/2046-2530-2-12.
102. Mori N, et al. Ccdc85c encoding a protein at apical junctions of radial glia is disrupted in hemorrhagic hydrocephalus (hhy) mice. Am J Pathol. 2012;180:314–27. https://doi.org/10.1016/j.ajpath.2011.09.014.
103. Liu J, et al. A betaPix Pak2a signaling pathway regulates cerebral vascular stability in zebrafish. Proc Natl Acad Sci U S A. 2007;104:13990–5. https://doi.org/10.1073/pnas.0700825104.
104. Muntean BS, Jin X, Williams FE, Nauli SM. Primary cilium regulates CaV1.2 expression through Wnt signaling. J Cell Physiol. 2014;229:1926–34. https://doi.org/10.1002/jcp.24642.
105. Cardenas-Rodriguez M, et al. Characterization of CCDC28B reveals its role in ciliogenesis and provides insight to understand its modifier effect on Bardet-Biedl syndrome. Hum Genet. 2013;132:91–105.
106. Rachel RA, et al. CEP290 alleles in mice disrupt tissue-specific cilia biogenesis and recapitulate features of syndromic ciliopathies. Hum Mol Genet. 2015;24:3775–91. https://doi.org/10.1093/hmg/ddv123.
107. Lyons PJ, Sapio MR, Fricker LD. Zebrafish cytosolic carboxypeptidases 1 and 5 are essential for embryonic development. J Biol Chem. 2013;288:30454–62. https://doi.org/10.1074/jbc.M113.497933.
108. Ying G, et al. Centrin 2 is required for mouse olfactory ciliary trafficking and development of ependymal cilia planar polarity. J Neurosci. 2014;34:6377–88. https://doi.org/10.1523/JNEUROSCI.0067-14.2014.
109. Ha S, Lindsay AM, Timms AE, Beier DR. Mutations in Dnaaf1 and Lrrc48 cause hydrocephalus, laterality defects, and sinusitis in mice. G3 (Bethesda). 2016;6:2479–87. https://doi.org/10.1534/g3.116.030791.
110. Mo D, et al. Apical targeting and endocytosis of the sialomucin endolyn are essential for establishment of zebrafish pronephric kidney function. J Cell Sci. 2012;125:5546–54. https://doi.org/10.1242/jcs.111468.
111. Oji A, et al. CRISPR/Cas9 mediated genome editing in ES cells and its application for chimeric analysis in mice. Sci Rep. 2016;6:31666. https://doi.org/10.1038/srep31666.
112. Clement A, Solnica-Krezel L, Gould KL. Functional redundancy between Cdc14 phosphatases in zebrafish ciliogenesis. Dev Dyn. 2012;241:1911–21. https://doi.org/10.1002/dvdy.23876.
113. Zega K, et al. Dusp16 deficiency causes congenital obstructive hydrocephalus and brain overgrowth by expansion of the neural progenitor pool. Front Mol Neurosci. 2017;10:372. https://doi.org/10.3389/fnmol.2017.00372.
114. Shaheen R, et al. A founder CEP120 mutation in Jeune asphyxiating thoracic dystrophy expands the role of centriolar proteins in skeletal ciliopathies. Hum Mol Genet. 2015;24:1410–9. https://doi.org/10.1093/hmg/ddu555.
115. Swetloff A, Ferretti P. Changes in E2F5 intracellular localization in mouse and human choroid epithelium and developmet. Int J Dev Biol. 2005;49:859–65.
116. Li X, et al. Concomitant activation of foxo3a and fancc or fancd2 reveals a two-tier protection from oxidative stress-induced hydrocephalus. Antioxid Redox Signal. 2014;21:1675–92.

117. Schueler M, et al. DCDC2 mutations cause a renal-hepatic ciliopathy by disrupting Wnt signaling. Am J Hum Genet. 2015;96:81–92. https://doi.org/10.1016/j.ajhg.2014.12.002.
118. Wang L, et al. Impaired methylation modifications of FZD3 alter chromatin accessibility and are involved in congenital hydrocephalus pathogenesis. Brain Res. 2014;1569.
119. Mitchison HM, et al. Mutations in axonemal dynein assembly factor DNAAF3 cause primary ciliary dyskinesia. Nat Genet. 2012;44(381–389):S381–2. https://doi.org/10.1038/ng.1106.
120. Davy BE, Robinson ML. Congenital hydrocephalus in hy3 mice is caused by a frameshift mutation in Hydin, a large novel gene. Hum Mol Genet. 2003;12:1163–70.
121. Chandrasekar G, Vesterlund L, Hultenby K, Tapia-Paez I, Kere J. The zebrafish orthologue of the dyslexia candidate gene DYX1C1 is essential for cilia growth and function. PLoS One. 2013;8:e63123. https://doi.org/10.1371/journal.pone.0063123.
122. Moon H, et al. Intestinal cell kinase, a protein associated with endocrine-cerebro-osteodysplasia syndrome, is a key regulator of cilia length and hedgehog signaling. Proc Natl Acad Sci U S A. 2014;111:8541–6. https://doi.org/10.1073/pnas.1323161111.
123. Gonzalez AM, et al. Ecrg4 expression and its product augurin in the choroid plexus- impact on fetal brain development, cerebrospinal fluid homeostasis and neuroprogenitor cell response to CNS injury. Fluids Barriers CNS. 2011;8. https://doi.org/10.1186/2045-8118-8-6.
124. Bardella C, et al. Expression of Idh1(R132H) in the Murine subventricular zone stem cell niche recapitulates features of early Gliomagenesis. Cancer Cell. 2016;30:578–94. https://doi.org/10.1016/j.ccell.2016.08.017.
125. Pathak N, Obara T, Mangos S, Liu Y, Drummond IA. The zebrafish fleer gene encodes an essential regulator of cilia tubulin polyglutamylation. Mol Biol Cell. 2007;18:4353–64. https://doi.org/10.1091/mbc.E07.
126. Akbay EA, et al. D-2-hydroxyglutarate produced by mutant IDH2 causes cardiomyopathy and neurodegeneration in mice. Genes Dev. 2014;28:479–90. https://doi.org/10.1101/gad.231233.113.
127. Manzini MC, et al. Exome sequencing and functional validation in zebrafish identify GTDC2 mutations as a cause of Walker-Warburg syndrome. Am J Hum Genet. 2012;91:541–7. https://doi.org/10.1016/j.ajhg.2012.07.009.
128. Muniz-Talavera H, Schmidt JV. The mouse Jhy gene regulates ependymal cell differentiation and ciliogenesis. PLoS One. 2017;12.
129. Lee MS, et al. IFT46 plays an essential role in cilia development. Dev Biol. 2015;400:248–57. https://doi.org/10.1016/j.ydbio.2015.02.009.
130. Cesca F, et al. Kidins220/ARMS is an essential modulator of cardiovascular and nervous system development. Cell Death Dis. 2011;2:e226. https://doi.org/10.1038/cddis.2011.108.
131. Shen H, Bocksteins E, Kondrychyn I, Snyders D, Korzh V. Functional antagonism of voltage-gated K+ channel alpha-subunits in the developing brain ventricular system. Development. 2016;143:4249–60. https://doi.org/10.1242/dev.140467.
132. Tong CK, et al. Primary cilia are required in a unique subpopulation of neural progenitors. Proc Natl Acad Sci U S A. 2014;111:12438–43. https://doi.org/10.1073/pnas.1321425111.
133. Gueneau L, et al. KIAA1109 variants are associated with a severe disorder of brain development and arthrogryposis. Am J Hum Genet. 2018;102:116–32. https://doi.org/10.1016/j.ajhg.2017.12.002.
134. Yamazaki F, et al. The Lhx9 homeobox gene controls pineal gland development and prevents postnatal hydrocephalus. Brain Struct Funct. 2015;220:1497–509.
135. Teng Y, et al. Loss of zebrafish lgi1b leads to hydrocephalus and sensitization to pentylenetetrazol induced seizure-like behavior. PLoS One. 2011;6:e24596. https://doi.org/10.1371/journal.pone.0024596.
136. Hanington PC, et al. Analysis of leukemia inhibitory factor and leukemia inhibitory factor receptor in embryonic and adult zebrafish (Danio rerio). Dev Biol. 2008;314:250–60. https://doi.org/10.1016/j.ydbio.2007.10.012.
137. Inaba Y, et al. Transport of the outer dynein arm complex to cilia requires a cytoplasmic protein Lrrc6. Genes Cells. 2016;21:728–39. https://doi.org/10.1111/gtc.12380.

138. Chen HL, Yuh CH, Wu KK. Nestin is essential for zebrafish brain and eye development through control of progenitor cell apoptosis. PLoS One. 2010;5:e9318. https://doi.org/10.1371/journal.pone.0009318.
139. Ridge LA, et al. Non-muscle myosin IIB (Myh10) is required for epicardial function and coronary vessel formation during mammalian development. PLoS Genet. 2017;13:e1007068. https://doi.org/10.1371/journal.pgen.1007068.
140. Zhou W, Dai J, Attanasio M, Hildebrandt F. Nephrocystin-3 is required for ciliary function in zebrafish embryos. Am J Physiol Ren Physiol. 2010;299:F55–62. https://doi.org/10.1152/ajprenal.00043.2010.
141. Jain N, et al. Conditional N-WASP knockout in mouse brain implicates actin cytoskeleton regulation in hydrocephalus pathology. Exp Neurol. 2014;254:29–40.
142. Vogel P, et al. Congenital hydrocephalus in genetically engineered mice. Vet Pathol. 2012;49:166–81. https://doi.org/10.1177/0300985811415708.
143. Ferrante MI, et al. Convergent extension movements and ciliary function are mediated by ofd1, a zebrafish orthologue of the human oral-facial-digital type 1 syndrome gene. Hum Mol Genet. 2009;18:289–303. https://doi.org/10.1093/hmg/ddn356.
144. Raveau M, et al. Brain ventriculomegaly in down syndrome mice is caused by Pcp4 dose-dependent cilia dysfunction. Hum Mol Genet. 2017;26:923–31. https://doi.org/10.1093/hmg/ddx007.
145. Zizioli D, et al. Knock-down of pantothenate kinase 2 severely affects the development of the nervous and vascular system in zebrafish, providing new insights into PKAN disease. Neurobiol Dis. 2016;85:35–48. https://doi.org/10.1016/j.nbd.2015.10.010.
146. Wodarczyk C, et al. A novel mouse model reveals that polycystin-1 deficiency in ependyma and choroid plexus results in dysfunctional cilia and hydrocephalus. PLoS One. 2009;4:e7137. https://doi.org/10.1371/journal.pone.0007137.
147. Mangos S, et al. The ADPKD genes pkd1a/b and pkd2 regulate extracellular matrix formation. Dis Model Mech. 2010;3:354–65. https://doi.org/10.1242/dmm.003194.
148. Fant ME, Fuentes J, Kong X, Jackman S. The nexus of prematurity, birth defects, and intrauterine growth restriction: a role for plac1-regulated pathways. Front Pediatr. 2014;2:8. https://doi.org/10.3389/fped.2014.00008.
149. Obara T, et al. Polycystin-2 immunolocalization and function in zebrafish. J Am Soc Nephrol. 2006;17:2706–18. https://doi.org/10.1681/ASN.2006040412.
150. Murga M, et al. POLD3 is Haploinsufficient for DNA replication in mice. Mol Cell. 2016;63:877–83. https://doi.org/10.1016/j.molcel.2016.07.007.
151. Nornes S, et al. Interference with splicing of Presenilin transcripts has potent dominant negative effects on Presenilin activity. Hum Mol Genet. 2008;17:402–12. https://doi.org/10.1093/hmg/ddm317.
152. Shimada IS, Acar M, Burgess RJ, Zhao Z, Morrison SJ. Prdm16 is required for the maintenance of neural stem cells in the postnatal forebrain and their differentiation into ependymal cells. Genes Dev. 2017;31:1134–46. https://doi.org/10.1101/gad.291773.116.
153. Grimes DT, Boswell CW, Morante NF, Henkelman RM, Ciruna B. Zebrafish models of idiopathic scoliosis link cerebrospinal fluid flow defects to spine curvature. Science. 2016;352:1341–3.
154. Roset R, et al. The Rad50 hook domain regulates DNA damage signaling and tumorigenesis. Genes Dev. 2014;28:451–62. https://doi.org/10.1101/gad.236745.113.
155. Shi Y, Obert E, Rahman B, Rohrer B, Lobo GP. The retinol binding protein receptor 2 (Rbpr2) is required for photoreceptor outer segment morphogenesis and visual function in Zebrafish. Sci Rep. 2017;7:16207. https://doi.org/10.1038/s41598-017-16498-9.
156. Xu P, et al. Conditional ablation of the RFX4 isoform 1 transcription factor: allele dosage effects on brain phenotype. PLoS One. 2018;13:e0190561. https://doi.org/10.1371/journal.pone.0190561.
157. Ghosh AK, et al. Human retinopathy-associated ciliary protein retinitis pigmentosa GTPase regulator mediates cilia-dependent vertebrate development. Hum Mol Genet. 2010;19:90–8. https://doi.org/10.1093/hmg/ddp469.

158. Lin X, et al. Genetic deletion of Rnd3 results in aqueductal stenosis leading to hydrocephalus through upregulation of notch signaling. Proc Natl Acad Sci U S A. 2013;110:8236–41.
159. Dash SN, et al. Sept7b is essential for pronephric function and development of left-right asymmetry in zebrafish embryogenesis. J Cell Sci. 2014;127:1476–86. https://doi.org/10.1242/jcs.138495.
160. Ritter-Makinson SL, et al. Group II metabotropic glutamate receptor interactions with NHERF scaffold proteins: implications for receptor localization in brain. Neuroscience. 2017;353:58–75. https://doi.org/10.1016/j.neuroscience.2017.03.060.
161. Hurd TW, et al. Mutation of the Mg2+ transporter SLC41A1 results in a nephronophthisis-like phenotype. J Am Soc Nephrol. 2013;24:967–77. https://doi.org/10.1681/ASN.2012101034.
162. Lee K, et al. Congenital hydrocephalus and abnormal subcommissural organ development in Sox3 transgenic mice. PLoS One. 2012;7:e29041. https://doi.org/10.1371/journal.pone.0029041.
163. Treat AC, et al. The PDZ protein Na+/H+ exchanger regulatory Factor-1 (NHERF1) regulates planar cell polarity and motile cilia organization. PLoS One. 2016;11:e0153144. https://doi.org/10.1371/journal.pone.0153144.
164. Lehti MS, et al. Cilia-related protein SPEF2 regulates osteoblast differentiation. Sci Rep. 2018;8. https://doi.org/10.1038/s41598-018-19204-5.
165. Brockschmidt A, et al. Neurologic and ocular phenotype in Pitt-Hopkins syndrome and a zebrafish model. Hum Genet. 2011;130:645–55. https://doi.org/10.1007/s00439-011-0999-4.
166. Nemajerova A, et al. Non-oncogenic roles of TAp73: from multiciliogenesis to metabolism. Cell Death Differ. 2017;25:144–53. https://doi.org/10.1038/cdd.2017.178.
167. Xu Y, et al. Characterization of tetratricopeptide repeat-containing proteins critical for cilia formation and function. PLoS One. 2015;10:e0124378. https://doi.org/10.1371/journal.pone.0124378.
168. Liu M, et al. Ulk4r is essential for ciliogenesis and CSF flow. J Neurosci. 2016;36:7589–600. https://doi.org/10.1523/JNEUROSCI.0621-16.2016.
169. Liu M, et al. *Ulk4* regulates neural stem cell pool. Stem Cells. 2016;34:2318–31.
170. Hirschner W, et al. Biosynthesis of Wdr16, a marker protein for kinocilia-bearing cells, starts at the time of kinocilia formation in rat, and wdr16 gene knockdown causes hydrocephalus in zebrafish. J Neurochem. 2007;101:274–88. https://doi.org/10.1111/j.1471-4159.2007.04500.x.
171. Heye N, Dunne JW. Noonan's syndrome with hydrocephalus, hindbrain herniation, and upper cervical intracord cyst. J Neurol Neurosurg Psychiatry. 1995;59:338–9.
172. Thompson D, et al. RAF1 variants causing biventricular hypertrophic cardiomyopathy in two preterm infants: further phenotypic delineation and review of literature. *Clin Dysmorphol.* 2017;26:195–9. https://doi.org/10.1097/MCD.0000000000000194.
173. Gripp KW, et al. A novel rasopathy caused by recurrent de novo missense mutations in PPP1CB closely resembles Noonan syndrome with loose anagen hair. Am J Med Genet A. 2016;170:2237–47. https://doi.org/10.1002/ajmg.a.37781.
174. Reinker KA, Stevenson DA, Tsung A. Orthopaedic conditions in Ras/MAPK related disorders. J Pediatr Orthop. 2011;31:599–605.
175. Wilkie AO, et al. Apert syndrome results from localized mutations of *FGFR2* and is allelic with Crouzon syndrome. Nat Genet. 1995;9:165–72.
176. Killer M, et al. Cytokine and growth factor concentration in cerebrospinal fluid from patients with hydrocephalus following endovascular embolization of unruptured aneurysms in comparison with other types of hydrocephalus. Neurochem Res. 2010;35:1652–8. https://doi.org/10.1007/s11064-010-0226-z.
177. Ohmiya M, et al. Administration of FGF-2 to embryonic mouse brain induces hydrocephalic brain morphology and aberrant differentiation of neurons in the postnatal cerebral cortex. J Neurosci Res. 2001;65:228–35.
178. Bristol RE, Lekovic GP, Rekate HL. The effects of craniosynostosis on the brain with respect to intracranial pressure. Semin Pediatr Neurol. 2004;11:262–7.

179. Unger S, Scherer G, Superti-Furga A. Campomelic dysplasia. In: *GeneReviews*. Seattle: University of Washington; 2008. p. 1–17. [updated: 2013].
180. Cheung M, Briscoe J. Neural crest development is regulated by the transcription factor Sox9. Development. 2003;130:5681–93. https://doi.org/10.1242/dev.00808.
181. Lee YH, Saint-Jeannet JP. Sox9 function in craniofacial development and disease. Genesis. 2011;49:200–8. https://doi.org/10.1002/dvg.20717.
182. Gopakumar H, et al. Acampomelic form of campomelic dysplasia with SOX9 missense mutation. Indian J Pediatr. 2014;81:98–100.
183. Scott CE, et al. SOX9 induces and maintains neural stem cells. Nat Neurosci. 2010;13:1181–9. https://doi.org/10.1038/nn.2646.
184. Mirzaa GM, et al. Association of MTOR mutations with developmental brain disorders, including megalencephaly, focal cortical dysplasia, and pigmentary mosaicism. JAMA Neurol. 2016;73:836–45. https://doi.org/10.1001/jamaneurol.2016.0363.
185. Ryskalin L, et al. mTOR-dependent cell proliferation in the brain. Biomed Res Int. 2017;2017:7082696. https://doi.org/10.1155/2017/7082696.
186. Foerster P, et al. mTORC1 signaling and primary cilia are required for brain ventricle morphogenesis. Development. 2017;144:201–10. https://doi.org/10.1242/dev.138271.
187. Godfrey C, et al. Refining genotype phenotype correlations in muscular dystrophies with defective glycosylation of dystroglycan. Brain. 2007;130:2725–35. https://doi.org/10.1093/brain/awm212.
188. van Reeuwijk J, Brunner HG, van Bokhoven H. Glyc-O-genetics of Walker-Warburg syndrome. Clin Genet. 2005;67:281–9.
189. Currier SC, et al. Mutations in *POMT1* are found in a minority of patients with Walker-Warburg syndrome. Am J Med Genet A. 2005;133A:53–7.
190. Satz JS, et al. Brain and eye malformations resembling Walker-Warburg syndrome are recapitulated in mice by dystroglycan deletion in the epiblast. J Neurosci. 2008;28:10567–75. https://doi.org/10.1523/JNEUROSCI.2457-08.2008.
191. Sironen A, et al. Loss of SPEF2 function in mice results in spermatogenesis defects and primary ciliary dyskinesia. Biol Reprod. 2011;85:690–701. https://doi.org/10.1095/biolreprod.111.091132.
192. May-Simera HL, Kelley MW. Cilia, Wnt signaling, and the cytoskeleton. Cilia. 2012;1:7. https://doi.org/10.1186/2046-2530-1-7.
193. Schrander-Stumpel C, Fryns JP. Congenital hydrocephalus: nosologyand guidelines for clinical approach and genetic counselling. Eur J Pediatr. 1998;157:355–62.
194. Limbrick DD Jr, et al. Cerebrospinal fluid biomarkers of infantile congenital hydrocephalus. PLoS One. 2017;12:e0172353. https://doi.org/10.1371/journal.pone.0172353.

Genetics of Hydrocephalus: Causal and Contributory Factors

6

Hannah Tully, Annie Laquerriere, Dan Doherty, and William Dobyns

Introduction

Several mechanisms can cause anatomic or functional derangements of normal CSF flow pathways and lead to hydrocephalus, which we define as progressive ventricular enlargement not explainable by an *ex vacuo* phenomenon. The multifactorial nature of hydrocephalus provides many potential points of influence for genetic factors. For example, mutations in genes responsible for axon guidance can result in brain malformations that directly obstruct CSF flow. Mutations in growth regulating genes can cause crowding within the skull, leading to alterations of CSF and vascular flow that culminate in decreased CSF absorption. Even in hydrocephalus traditionally regarded as acquired, genetic polymorphisms in several pathways could potentially increase susceptibility in the presence of other risk factors.

The Online Mendelian Inheritance in Man (OMIM) database contains over 400 entries associated with hydrocephalus, but in only a few is hydrocephalus the only clinical feature. Hydrocephalus is commonly divided into syndromic and

H. Tully (✉)
Department of Neurology, University of Washington and Seattle Children's Hospital, Center for Integrative Brain Research, Seattle Children's Research Institute, Seattle, WA, USA
e-mail: hmtully@uw.edu

A. Laquerriere
Pathology Laboratory, Rouen University Hospital and Inserm Unit 1245, Team Genetics and Pathophysiology of Neurodevelopmental Disorders, IRIB, Rouen, France

D. Doherty
Department of Pediatrics, University of Washington and Seattle Children's Hospital, Center for Integrative Brain Research, Seattle Children's Research Institute, Seattle, WA, USA

W. Dobyns
Department of Genetics, University of Washington, Center for Integrative Brain Research, Seattle Children's Research Institute, Seattle, WA, USA

D. D. Limbrick, J. R. Leonard (eds.), *Cerebrospinal Fluid Disorders*,
https://doi.org/10.1007/978-3-319-97928-1_6

non-syndromic forms, but the distinction between the two is somewhat arbitrary. For practicality, we will focus first on genetic causes of severe, early-onset forms of hydrocephalus, many of which lack clear distinguishing features beyond the hydrocephalus itself. We will next address syndromes in which hydrocephalus may be an accompanying – but not the primary – clinical feature. Finally, we will touch upon the notion of susceptibility factors – genetic variants that are not pathogenic in themselves, but could increase the likelihood of developing hydrocephalus in the presence of other risk factors.

Part I: Genetic Causes of Severe, Prenatal Onset Hydrocephalus

Prenatal-onset hydrocephalus may be severe, and yet have few distinguishing characteristics. Children who are born with severe hydrocephalus without an obvious extrinsic cause often have obstruction at the level of the aqueduct [1]. Yet aqueductal obstruction can be caused by both genetic and non-genetic factors [2], and therefore may not be a practical feature to guide diagnostic workup.

Despite remarkable advances in genetic technologies, relatively few genes have been directly linked to primary hydrocephalus. Mutations in *L1CAM*, first identified as a cause of X-linked hydrocephalus in 1992 [3], remains the single most common recognized genetic cause. Since 2010, three additional genes have been implicated in primary autosomal recessive hydrocephalus, but their major features and full phenotypic range remain to be elucidated.

***L1CAM*-associated hydrocephalus.** X-linked hydrocephalus associated loss-of-function mutations in *L1CAM* are the most commonly identified heritable form of hydrocephalus. This condition may account for up to 10% of males with isolated idiopathic hydrocephalus [4]. In L1 syndrome, hydrocephalus represents the severe end of a broad spectrum of disease that also includes isolated agenesis of the corpus callosum and X-linked spastic paraplegia (SPG1) [5].

The *L1CAM* gene product plays key roles in neuronal adhesion, neurite outgrowth, axon guidance and synaptogenesis [6]. When mutated, it gives rise to several structural malformations that obstruct CSF flow, most commonly at the level of the aqueduct (Figs. 6.1a–c, 6.2a–c). However, the mechanism by which hydrocephalus develops is unclear and may involve not only direct obstruction but also changes in compliance. On brain imaging, few features distinguish *L1CAM*-associated hydrocephalus from other forms associated with severe, early-onset ventricular dilation, reflecting the observation that no anatomic feature identified on neuropathology is completely sensitive or specific for this condition. In a series of 138 fetal and neonatal autopsy subjects that had clinical features or a family history suggestive of an *L1CAM* mutation [7], 57 (41%) were found to have pathogenic mutations by Sanger sequencing. Of the mutation-positive patients, 98% had abnormalities of the corpus callosum, 90% had aqueductal stenosis (Fig. 6.2b, c), 98% had hypoplasia or aplasia of the corticospinal tracts with absent decussation (2D), and 88% had adducted thumbs. However, among the 79 autopsy subjects

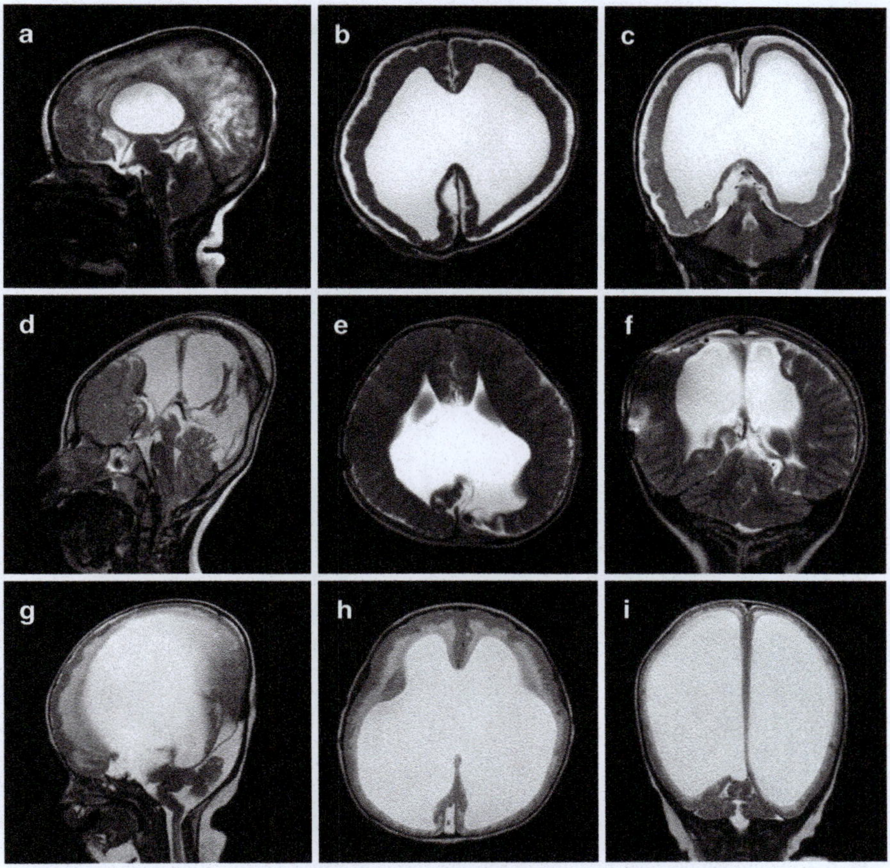

Fig. 6.1 MRI findings in specific forms of severe, prenatal-onset hydrocephalus. (**a**–**c**) *L1CAM*-associated hydrocephalus. T2 mid-sagittal (**a**), axial (**b**) and coronal (**c**) views demonstrate severe dilation of the lateral and third ventricles suggesting obstruction at the level of the aqueduct. Corpus callosum is stretched and white matter volume is reduced, particular posteriorly. These are non-specific findings related to severe hydrocephalus. (**d**–**f**) *CCDC88C*-associated hydrocephalus. T2 mid-sagittal (**a**), axial (**b**) and coronal (**c**) views from MRI performed after shunt placement but before full ventricular decompression demonstrate similar findings to those seen in **a**–**c**. Thickened, brachycephalic skull, cortical infoldings with posterior fossa crowding may be acquired rather than innate features. (**g**–**i**) *POMT1*-associated hydrocephalus. T2 mid-sagittal (**a**) view demonstrates the distinctive retroflexed brainstem with enlarged tectum that characterizes the dystroglycanopathies. Axial (**h**) and coronal (**i**) views show the cobblestone cortex and abnormal white matter that commonly accompany this group of conditions. These features may be relatively subtle on pre- or perinatal scans, or may be difficult to interpret in the setting of severe ventricular dilation

without L1CAM mutations, callosal abnormalities were seen in 73%, corticospinal tract abnormalities in 59%, aqueductal atresia or stenosis in 46%, and adducted thumbs in 27%.

Testing for *L1CAM* mutations should be considered in all individuals whose history suggests X-linked inheritance. However, no consensus has evolved regarding

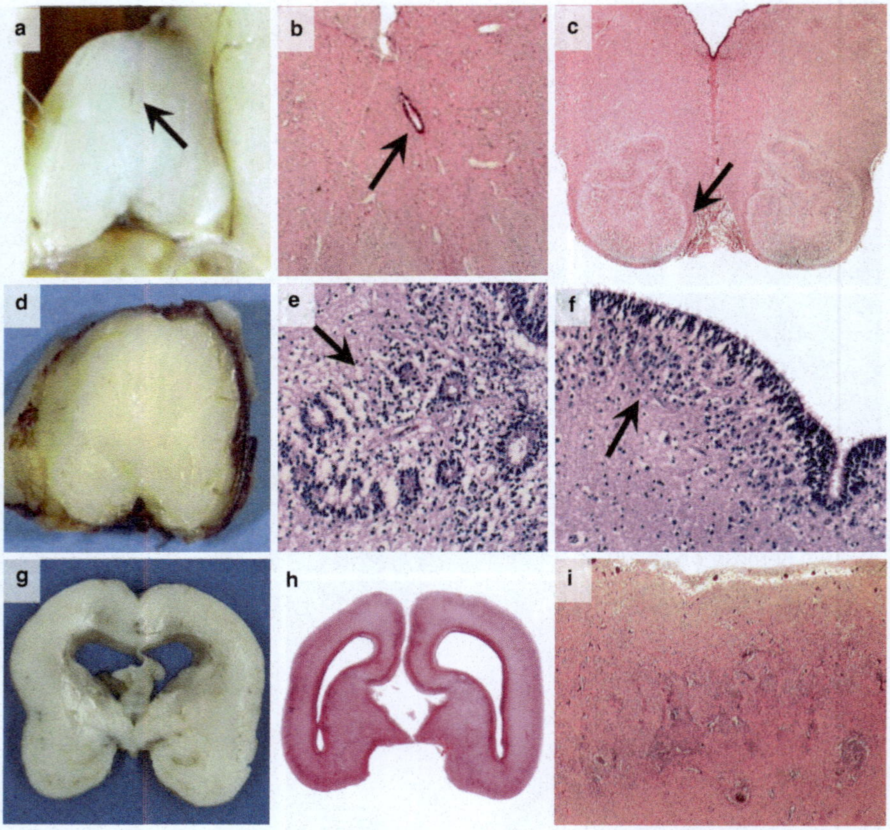

Fig. 6.2 Neuropathological findings in specific forms of severe, prenatal-onset hydrocephalus. (**a–c**) *L1CAM*-associated hydrocephalus. Gross axial view through fetal midbrain (**a**) with corresponding histopathologic section (**b**) demonstrate severe aqueductal narrowing without additional morphologic findings (true stenosis). Histopatholgic section through medulla shows absent descending motor tracts (pyramids). (**d–f**) *MPDZ*-associated hydrocephalus. Gross axial view through fetal midbrain (**d**) demonstrates indiscernible aqueduct. Histopatholgic sections show forking-atresia pattern as opposed to stenosis, characterized by multiple ependymal rosettes in region of aqueduct (**e**) surrounded by immature cells. (**g–i**) *POMT1*-associated dystrocglycanoptahy, commonly associated with hydrocephalus. Gross coronal section of fetal brain demonstrates mildly decreased sulcation relative to gestational age. Corresponding histopatholgic sections (**h**, **i**) shows evidence of abnormal cortical layering and overmigration through the glia limitans

which clinical features should prompt testing in those without a family history. Moreover, though *L1CAM*-associated hydrocephalus is commonly thought to be observed only in males, females may also be affected. Therefore, *L1CAM* testing should also be considered in any individual with severe, early-onset hydrocephalus.

***CCDC88C*-associated hydrocephalus.** Loss-of-function mutations in *CCDC88C* have recently been identified as the cause of autosomal recessive hydrocephalus in Algerian [8], Ashkenazi Jewish [9], Palestinian [9], and Mexican families [10].

CCDC88C encodes DAPLE, a ubiquitously expressed protein that regulates cellular migration through its interaction with disheveled in the non-canonical Wnt pathway [11], but the mechanisms by which loss of gene function leads to hydrocephalus are uncertain. Interestingly, gain-of-function mutations in *CCDC88C* were recently described in association with autosomal dominant spastic paraparesis in a Chinese family [12].

In all affected individuals reported to date, hydrocephalus is associated with severe dilation of the lateral ventricles, implying aqueduct-level obstruction (Fig. 6.1d–f). Other imaging features such as midline cysts have been reported, but these may represent ventricular diverticula, a non-specific finding seen in many forms of severe hydrocephalus. A few reports note schizencephaly or cortical malformations such as polymicrogyria, but these imaging findings may be difficult to distinguish from the collapse pattern seen after decompression of severely dilated ventricles. As such, they may be non-specific, acquired rather than innate features of the hydrocephalus associated with *CCDC88C* mutations.

Few neuropathological studies on affected individuals have been reported, although autopsy on an affected 20-week gestation fetus demonstrated an aqueduct that appeared unremarkable for that stage of development [9].

Testing for *CCDC8C* should be considered for children with otherwise unexplained severe hydrocephalus, particularly when family history suggests the potential for autosomal recessive inheritance.

***MPDZ*-associated hydrocephalus.** Mutations in *MPDZ* were recently implicated as the cause of severe prenatal-onset autosomal recessive hydrocephalus in two Saudi families [13] and three additional unrelated families from France [14]. The *MPDZ* gene product is strongly expressed in embryonic choroid plexus and ependyma, especially in the aqueduct, and is thought to play a role in maintaining the integrity of tight junctions [15].

On most available imaging, the hydrocephalus associated with *MPDZ* appears to be severe, characterized by massive dilation of the lateral ventricles and apparent obstruction at the level of the aqueduct. Several affected individuals are reported to have periventricular nodular heterotopia [16]. The full phenotypic spectrum associated with MPDZ mutations is yet to be defined, however. Recently, compound heterozygous MPDZ mutations were reported in association with mild, non-progressive communication hydrocephalus [17], although clinical and imaging details were limited.

Though imaging features overlap with other forms of hydrocephalus, the neuropathology is distinctive (Fig. 6.2d–f). On autopsy, the affected French fetuses all exhibited hypoplasia of the subcomissural organ and colliculi, a small aqueduct, and a characteristic pattern of multifocal, partially obstructive ependymal rosettes within and distal to the third ventricle [14]. In an animal model, *mpdz*-deficient mice had morphologically normal but functionally abnormal tight junctions, with ependymal denudation, reactive astrogliosis, and aqueductal obstruction [15].

MPDZ testing should be considered for any individual with severe, early-onset hydrocephalus and a family history that suggests autosomal recessive inheritance. Testing should be strongly considered if heterotopia is present; however, this feature may not always be visible on MRI, so its absence should not preclude consideration of this genetic cause.

Part II: Genetic Syndromes in Which Hydrocephalus May Be a Feature

Many clinical and genetic syndromes may sometimes be accompanied by hydrocephalus. For infants with these conditions, diagnosis is usually made on the basis of syndrome-specific clinical findings; however, brain imaging may provide additional clues to diagnosis. When these conditions are accompanied by severe ventricular dilatation, however, even very distinctive clinical and imaging features may be overshadowed.

Alpha-dystroglycanopathy-associated hydrocephalus (Walker-Warburg/Muscle-Eye-Brain disease). Alpha-dystroglycanopthies, caused by a group of 16 genes involved in a-dystroglycan biosynthesis or glycosylation, are classified as muscular dystrophies. However, at the severe end of the spectrum, which encompasses both Warker-Warburg and Muscle-Eye-Brain disease, hydrocephalus may be an early-onset feature that dominates the clinical phenotype, and the additional findings (which provide important clues to diagnosis) may be missed. In the brain, a- dystroglycan is necessary for the proper formation of the glia limitans, and mutations result in defective neuronal binding to the extracellular matrix and defects of the glial limiting membrane [18, 19]. Eye anomalies are a major feature, and may be visible on fetal ultrasound.

On imaging, dystroglycanopathies are typically characterized by a striking Z-shaped brainstem malformation consisting of retroflexion at the medulla, a flattened pons and an enlarged tectum. This may be associated aqueduct-level obstruction, which presumably is the major cause of the severe hydrocephalus that can accompany these conditions (Fig. 6.1g–i). The dystroglycanopathies are also commonly characterized by a cobblestone gyral pattern with abnormal white matter (Fig. 6.2g–i). Pseudo-cystic dysplasia of the cerebellar cortex is another important, though not universal, diagnostic clue. These imaging findings may not be readily appreciated on pre- or perinatal scans [20], particularly if the associated hydrocephalus is severe.

MRIs of children diagnosed with severe, early-onset hydrocephalus should be reviewed for these characteristics but often overlooked imaging features, particularly for the distinctive brainstem malformation. Elevated serum creatine kinase levels and structural eye anomalies can also be useful in establishing a diagnosis.

***AP1S2*-associated hydrocephalus.** Fried syndrome, first described in 1972 [21], was once thought to be an example of L1 syndrome before it was recognized as a separate X-linked disorder [22]. Now known to be caused by mutations in the *AP1S2* gene [23], Fried syndrome is characterized primarily by intellectual disability with prominent basal ganglia iron deposition and/or calcifications [24] on CT scan (which may not be obvious on MRI), and a variable degree of ventricular dilatation. Mutations in the same gene, which encodes a subunit of a protein complex involved in protein sorting in the Golgi complex, have now been recognized as the cause of other overlapping X-linked intellectual disability syndromes [24].

The basal ganglia deposits seen in association with *AP1S2* mutations are well described (if not fully characterized), but the imaging features of the hydrocephalus are not. Some affected individuals have been described as having aqueductal stenosis [21], and others reportedly had retrocerebellar or fourth ventricular cysts [24].

AP1S2 testing should be considered in males with intellectual disability and imaging abnormalities that suggest deposition of iron or calcium with the basal ganglia. Since both iron and calcium may be subtle on basic MRI sequences, these should be evaluated by CT, or by MRI sequences that are particularly sensitive to both iron and calcium (gradient echo or susceptibility-weighted imaging).

Homozygous mutations in *WDR81* were recently reported in two unrelated consanguineous Saudi families with severe hydrocephalus and cerebellar hypoplasia [16]. Mutations in this gene were also reported as the cause of an autosomal recessive cerebellar ataxia syndrome without hydrocephalus (CAMRQ2) [25] and subsequently in a range of brain malformations associated with varying degrees of microcephaly, reduced sulcation and cerebellar hypoplasia. Functional studies showed that WDR81 is essential for mitotic progression of neural stem cells [26].

Mutations in *EML1* were recently identified as the cause of brain heterotopias in mice, and were subsequently implicated as the cause of bilateral giant ribbon-like heterotopia in two unrelated families [27]. Homozygous truncating mutations in this gene were recently reported in an individual in a consanguineous Saudi family with several affected members [16]. Imaging studies from a child with *EML1*-associated hydrocephalus demonstrate severe dilatation of the lateral ventricles, posterior fossa crowding, and extensive cortical and subcortical anomalies consistent with those described in other families without hydrocephalus.

Syndromes associated with intracranial cysts. Intracranial arachnoid cysts are a well-recognized cause of hydrocephalus [28, 29], presumably primarily due to blockage of CSF flow. Small, simple cysts have been attributed to an entrapment of CSF within the meninges [30], which could conceivably be non-genetic in origin. However, simple cysts, usually midline, may be associated with hydrocephalus in the context of Chudley-McCullough syndrome. This condition is caused by mutations in the *GPSM2* gene [31], which plays a role in mitotic spindle orientation in apical progenitor cells [32]. Chudley-McCullough syndrome is also characterized by profound sensorineural hearing loss along with callosal and frontal-predominant gyral abnormalities on imaging, but motor and cognitive development are usually relatively spared.

Several genetic syndromes associated with dysfunction of the primary cilium may be associated with hydrocephalus, presumably due to flow obstruction from the intracranial cysts that commonly occur in these conditions. Primary ependymal dysfunction could conceivably be another factor in ventricular dilation. Oro-facial-digital syndrome type 1 (caused by mutations in the *OFD1* gene) [33], acrocallosal syndrome (*KIF7* and *GLI3*), hydrolethalus syndrome (*HYLS1*) [34], Pallister-Hall syndrome (*GLI3*) [35], and Greig cephalopolysyndactyly (*GLI3*) [36] have overlapping phenotypes. These conditions commonly feature additional physical malformations characteristic of ciliopathies, including cysts in other organs, polydactyly and retinopathy [37].

Craniosynostosis syndromes and skeletal dysplasias. Craniosynostosis syndromes, particularly those causing premature fusion of multiple cranial sutures, are strongly associated with progressive hydrocephalus. In these conditions, mutations in fibroblast growth factor receptor (FGFR) genes cause cranial changes that directly obstruct flow of CSF and reduce absorption into the systemic circulation by increasing venous pressure [38, 39]. Activating mutations in these genes can also cause excessive growth of the brain itself, thereby compounding the problem [40–43]. Interestingly, hydrocephalus can sometimes be seen in FGFR-associated skeletal dysplasias without synostosis, likely reflecting similar underlying mechanisms. Importantly, hydrocephalus is one of the key signs of thanatophoric dysplasia type II.

RASopathies. Mutations in RAS pathway genes cause several overlapping phenotypes including Noonan, cardio-facio-cutaneous and Costello syndromes [44, 45], as well as neurofibromatosis type 1. The hydrocephalus associated with these conditions is likely multifactorial, due to both direct effects of the genetic changes as well as downstream effects from accompanying clinical features. Cerebellar overgrowth is well-documented in Costello syndrome [46]. Chiari I malformations are frequently described in association with both Noonan and CFC syndromes, suggesting cerebellar overgrowth may also be present in those conditions. Noonan, CFC, and Costello are also associated with structural heart disease, so elevated venous pressures may create a pressure gradient that impedes absorption of CSF into the systemic circulation. Hydrocephalus in NF1 is likely due to a combination of brain overgrowth and, in some infants, obstructive hamartomas, particularly at the level of the aqueduct [47].

PI3K-AKT pathway-related megalencephaly syndromes. Mutations in growth-regulating genes within the PI3K-AKT pathway are increasingly recognized as a cause of hydrocephalus [48]. As in the RASopathies, the cause may be multifactorial, related to both direct effects of the genetic defect combined with progressive brain overgrowth that causes posterior fossa crowding and distal obstruction of CSF flow.

Hydrocephalus in the setting of other major brain anomalies. Hydrocephalus can occur as an inconstant accompaniment to several other genetically-based brain malformations and disruptions including holoprosencephaly [49], Fowler syndrome

[50], and lissencephaly (though mostly in the context of severe forms such as X-linked lissencephaly with abnormal genitalia) [51]. The association of VACTERL features with hydrocephalus was first reported in 1984 [52], and was subsequently designated VACTERL-H syndrome. One subset of patients VACTERL-H was found to have X-linked inheritance and Fanconi anemia [53] in association with mutations in *FANCB* [54]. However, another subset of patients with VACTERL-H does not have Fanconi anemia or excess chromosome breakage [55]. Recently, several patients with non-*FANCB*-associated VACTERL-H were noted to have rhombencephalosynapsis [56, 57], a distinctive brain malformation in which the cerebellar vermis is at least partially absent, and the cerebellar hemispheres are continuous across the midline. The genetic causes underlying rhombencephalosynapsis remain unknown.

Other genetic conditions associated with hydrocephalus. Several additional syndromes are associated with hydrocephalus, including the mucopolysaccharidoses [58], Sotos syndrome [58], Peter's Plus syndrome [59], primary ciliary dyskinesia [60, 61], Gorlin syndrome [62], and Rothmund-Thomson syndrome [63]. In addition to these single-gene disorders, many cytogenetic abnormalities have been linked to hydrocephalus, including microdeletion 9q22.3 [64], partial trisomy 1 [65], deletion 6q26q27 [66, 67], terminal duplication of 7q [68], as well as Trisomy 13, 18, 21 and triploidy [69].

Part III: Genetic Points that Could Influence Susceptibility to Hydrocephalus in the Presence of Other Risk Factors

Acquired hydrocephalus is, by definition, the result of extrinsic events acting upon a brain that is structurally normal, at least initially. As a result, acquired hydrocephalus is usually considered to be non-genetic in nature. However, this does not preclude genetic influences that could render some individuals more susceptible to hydrocephalus in the presence of extrinsic risk factors.

Idiopathic normal pressure hydrocephalus. Idiopathic normal pressure hydrocephalus (iNPH) is a condition of elderly adults, characterized by disproportionate ventricular dilatation in association with gait disturbance, urinary incontinence and dementia. Though the clinical and radiographic features of iNPH are well described, its pathogenesis is not fully understood. Epidemiological studies have noted strong associations with vascular risk factors [70]. On specialized imaging studies and on biopsy, comorbid neurodegenerative processes such as Alzheimer disease, frontotemporal dementia, and dementia with Lewy bodies are commonly present [71, 72]. However, it remains unclear whether these accompanying conditions are integral to the pathogenesis of iNPH, are non-causal but compound disease severity, or are biologically unrelated.

Recently, loss of Intron 2 of the *SFMBT1* gene, a variant seen in 4.2% of the normal population, was reported to be present in 26% of elderly Japanese adults with iNPH [73]. This differential copy number variation was recently validated in Nordic populations as well [ref Korhonen, personal correspondence, will update]. *SFMBT1* is involved in epigenetic modification of gene expression [74]. GWAS studies have linked *SFMBT1* to hypertension [75], blood glucose control [76], and serum urate levels [77].

Since iNPH has been linked to multiple vascular risk factors, *SFMBT1* could conceivably mediate the development of iNPH through the metabolic pathways identified in the GWAS studies. However, comparatively little is known about *SFMBT1* function in vivo, or about the effect of intron 2 loss on *SFMBT1* function. Whether this genetic variant could act as a susceptibility factor in other forms of hydrocephalus is similarly unclear.

Post-hemorrhagic hydrocephalus. Post-hemorrhagic hydrocephalus (PHH) is a common consequence of severe intraventricular hemorrhage (IVH), particularly in premature infants. Most research to date has investigated factors that could influence susceptibility to IVH itself. In preclinical studies, variants in proteins associated with vascular integrity [78], angiogenesis [79], and cerebral blood flow [80] confer increased susceptibility to IVH in mice. In human studies, polymophisms in the interleukin gene *IL1B*, which mediates inflammation, and *FV*, which influences coagulation, have both been linked to the development of IVH in premature infants [81].

Comparatively fewer studies have looked at risk factors for the progression to PHH after IVH. In animal models, intraventricular injection of LPA (a blood-borne lipid) led to ependymal disruption and ventricular enlargement [82], a process that may be mediated by dysregulated function of Yap, which maintains ependymal integrity [83]. Intraventricular blood has also been associated with inflammatory pathway-dependent CSF hypersecretion [84]. With antisense oligonucleotide knockdown of SPAK, a kinase that integrates and transduces stress signals [85], CSF hypersecretion was attenuated.

Among a cohort of premature infants with IVH, intraventricular obstruction and relative crowding of the posterior fossa crowding were associated with PHH [86], though the temporal relationship between anatomic findings and the development of PHH was not clear. Taken together, however, these studies underscore the many factors – and the many potential points of genetic influence – that could contribute to the pathogenesis of PHH.

The hydrocephalus that accompanies open spina bifida is commonly regarded as acquired, but it too could be subject to genetic susceptibility factors. Animal models show that chronic intrauterine CSF leakage results in downward herniation of the brainstem and hindbrain (the distinctive Chiari II malformation) [87, 88], which in turn causes obstruction of trans- and intracranial CSF flow. Lending further support for the notion that hydrocephalus is a direct consequence of CSF leakage, in utero surgery to correct the open lesion of spina bifida has been shown to reduce the risk of Chiari and of surgically-treated hydrocephalus [5]. Yet mutations in planar cell polarity genes such as *FUZ* [89], *VANGL1* [90] and *CELSR1* [91] are known to contribute to pathogenesis of NTDs in humans, as well as ependymal cilia organization and CSF flow in mice

[92]. Variations in these genes could therefore conceivably contribute to the severity of hydrocephalus in this clinical setting.

Conclusion

Hydrocephalus, as a multifactorial condition, can be caused or influenced by genetic factors at many levels. The best known genetic causes (though the fewest in number) are mutations in genes such as *L1CAM* that directly and reliably cause hydrocephalus through CSF obstruction. Hydrocephalus may also be a variable feature of many genetic syndromes, such as the congenital muscular dystrophies and the RASopathies. Finally, though evidence is incomplete, acquired or multifactorial forms of hydrocephalus could conceivably be influenced by susceptibility genes in the presence of other risk factors. Future research will help to illuminate additional Mendelian causes of hydrocephalus and further define the complex interplay between environmental and genetically-based risk factors.

References

1. Tully HM, Ishak GE, Rue TC, et al. Two hundred thirty-six children with developmental hydrocephalus: causes and clinical consequences. J Child Neurol. 2016;31:309–20.
2. Lategan B, Chodirker BN, Del Bigio MR. Fetal hydrocephalus caused by cryptic intraventricular hemorrhage. Brain Pathol. 2010;20:391–8.
3. Rosenthal A, Jouet M, Kenwrick S. Aberrant splicing of neural cell adhesion molecule L1 mRNA in a family with X-linked hydrocephalus. Nat Genet. 1992;2:107–12.
4. Schrander-Stumpel C, Vos YJ. L1 syndrome. In: Pagon RA, Adam MP, Bird TD, Dolan CR, Fong CT, Stephens K, editors. GeneReviews. Seattle, WA: University of Washington; 1993.
5. Adzick NS, Thom EA, Spong CY, et al. A randomized trial of prenatal versus postnatal repair of myelomeningocele. N Engl J Med. 2011;364:993–1004.
6. Maness PF, Schachner M. Neural recognition molecules of the immunoglobulin superfamily: signaling transducers of axon guidance and neuronal migration. Nat Neurosci. 2007;10:19–26.
7. Adle-Biassette H, Saugier-Veber P, Fallet-Bianco C, et al. Neuropathological review of 138 cases genetically tested for X-linked hydrocephalus: evidence for closely related clinical entities of unknown molecular bases. Acta Neuropathol. 2013;126:427–42.
8. Ekici AB, Hilfinger D, Jatzwauk M, et al. Disturbed Wnt signalling due to a mutation in CCDC88C causes an autosomal recessive non-syndromic hydrocephalus with medial diverticulum. Mol Syndromol. 2010;1:99–112.
9. Drielsma A, Jalas C, Simonis N, et al. Two novel CCDC88C mutations confirm the role of DAPLE in autosomal recessive congenital hydrocephalus. J Med Genet. 2012;49:708–12.
10. Ruggeri G, Timms AE, Cheng C, et al. Bi-allelic mutations of CCDC88C are a rare cause of severe congenital hydrocephalus. Am J Med Genet A. 2018;176:676–81.
11. Ishida-Takagishi M, Enomoto A, Asai N, et al. The Dishevelled-associating protein Daple controls the non-canonical Wnt/Rac pathway and cell motility. Nat Commun. 2012;3:859.
12. Tsoi H, Yu AC, Chen ZS, et al. A novel missense mutation in CCDC88C activates the JNK pathway and causes a dominant form of spinocerebellar ataxia. J Med Genet. 2014;51:590–5.
13. Al-Dosari MS, Al-Owain M, Tulbah M, et al. Mutation in MPDZ causes severe congenital hydrocephalus. J Med Genet. 2013;50:54–8.
14. Saugier-Veber P, Marguet F, Lecoquierre F, et al. Hydrocephalus due to multiple ependymal malformations is caused by mutations in the MPDZ gene. Acta Neuropathol Commun. 2017;5:36.

15. Feldner A, Adam MG, Tetzlaff F, et al. Loss of Mpdz impairs ependymal cell integrity leading to perinatal-onset hydrocephalus in mice. EMBO Mol Med. 2017;9:890–905.
16. Shaheen R, Sebai MA, Patel N, et al. The genetic landscape of familial congenital hydrocephalus. Ann Neurol. 2017;81:890–7.
17. Al-Jezawi NK, Al-Shamsi AM, Suleiman J, et al. Compound heterozygous variants in the multiple PDZ domain protein (MPDZ) cause a case of mild non-progressive communicating hydrocephalus. BMC Med Genet. 2018;19:34.
18. Dobyns WB, Pagon RA, Armstrong D, et al. Diagnostic criteria for Walker-Warburg syndrome. Am J Med Genet. 1989;32:195–210.
19. Miller G, Ladda RL, Towfighi J. Cerebro-ocular dysplasia--muscular dystrophy (Walker Warburg) syndrome. Findings in 20-week-old fetus. Acta Neuropathol. 1991;82:234–8.
20. Longman C, Mercuri E, Cowan F, et al. Antenatal and postnatal brain magnetic resonance imaging in muscle-eye-brain disease. Arch Neurol. 2004;61:1301–6.
21. Fried K. X-linked mental retardation and-or hydrocephalus. Clin Genet. 1972;3:258–63.
22. Strain L, Wright AF, Bonthron DT. Fried syndrome is a distinct X linked mental retardation syndrome mapping to Xp22. J Med Genet. 1997;34:535–40.
23. Saillour Y, Zanni G, Des Portes V, et al. Mutations in the AP1S2 gene encoding the sigma 2 subunit of the adaptor protein 1 complex are associated with syndromic X-linked mental retardation with hydrocephalus and calcifications in basal ganglia. J Med Genet. 2007;44:739–44.
24. Cacciagli P, Desvignes JP, Girard N, et al. AP1S2 is mutated in X-linked Dandy-Walker malformation with intellectual disability, basal ganglia disease and seizures (Pettigrew syndrome). Eur J Hum Genet. 2014;22:363–8.
25. Gulsuner S, Tekinay AB, Doerschner K, et al. Homozygosity mapping and targeted genomic sequencing reveal the gene responsible for cerebellar hypoplasia and quadrupedal locomotion in a consanguineous kindred. Genome Res. 2011;21:1995–2003.
26. Cavallin M, Rujano MA, Bednarek N, et al. WDR81 mutations cause extreme microcephaly and impair mitotic progression in human fibroblasts and Drosophila neural stem cells. Brain. 2017;140:2597–609.
27. Kielar M, Tuy FP, Bizzotto S, et al. Mutations in Eml1 lead to ectopic progenitors and neuronal heterotopia in mouse and human. Nat Neurosci. 2014;17:923–33.
28. Massimi L, Paternoster G, Fasano T, Di Rocco C. On the changing epidemiology of hydrocephalus. Childs Nerv Syst. 2009;25:795–800.
29. Moritake K, Nagai H, Miyazaki T, Nagasako N, Yamasaki M, Tamakoshi A. Nationwide survey of the etiology and associated conditions of prenatally and postnatally diagnosed congenital hydrocephalus in Japan. Neurol Med Chir (Tokyo). 2007;47:448–52; discussion 52.
30. Westermaier T, Schweitzer T, Ernestus RI. Arachnoid cysts. Adv Exp Med Biol. 2012;724:37–50.
31. Doherty D, Chudley AE, Coghlan G, et al. GPSM2 mutations cause the brain malformations and hearing loss in Chudley-McCullough syndrome. Am J Hum Genet. 2012;90:1088–93.
32. Morin X, Jaouen F, Durbec P. Control of planar divisions by the G-protein regulator LGN maintains progenitors in the chick neuroepithelium. Nat Neurosci. 2007;10:1440–8.
33. Bisschoff IJ, Zeschnigk C, Horn D, et al. Novel mutations including deletions of the entire OFD1 gene in 30 families with type 1 orofaciodigital syndrome: a study of the extensive clinical variability. Hum Mutat. 2013;34:237–47.
34. Putoux A, Thomas S, Coene KL, et al. KIF7 mutations cause fetal hydrolethalus and acrocallosal syndromes. Nat Genet. 2011;43:601–6.
35. Biesecker LG. Pallister-Hall syndrome. In: Pagon RA, Adam MP, Bird TD, Dolan CR, Fong CT, Stephens K, eds. GeneReviews. University of Washington, Seattle); 1993.
36. Biesecker LG. Greig cephalopolysyndactyly syndrome. In: Pagon RA, Adam MP, Bird TD, Dolan CR, Fong CT, Stephens K, editors. GeneReviews. Seattle: University of Washington; 1993.
37. Waters AM, Beales PL. Ciliopathies: an expanding disease spectrum. Pediatr Nephrol. 2011;26:1039–56.

38. Bristol RE, Lekovic GP, Rekate HL. The effects of craniosynostosis on the brain with respect to intracranial pressure. Semin Pediatr Neurol. 2004;11:262–7.
39. Rich PM, Cox TC, Hayward RD. The jugular foramen in complex and syndromic craniosynostosis and its relationship to raised intracranial pressure. AJNR Am J Neuroradiol. 2003;24:45–51.
40. Hevner RF. The cerebral cortex malformation in thanatophoric dysplasia: neuropathology and pathogenesis. Acta Neuropathol. 2005;110:208–21.
41. Thomson RE, Kind PC, Graham NA, et al. Fgf receptor 3 activation promotes selective growth and expansion of occipitotemporal cortex. Neural Dev. 2009;4:4.
42. Khonsari RH, Delezoide AL, Kang W, et al. Central nervous system malformations and deformations in FGFR2-related craniosynostosis. Am J Med Genet A. 2012;158A:2797–806.
43. Hill CA, Martinez-Abadias N, Motch SM, et al. Postnatal brain and skull growth in an Apert syndrome mouse model. Am J Med Genet A. 2013;161A:745–57.
44. Allanson JE, Roberts AE. Noonan syndrome. In: Pagon RA, Adam MP, Bird TD, Dolan CR, Fong CT, Stephens K, editors. GeneReviews. Seattle: University of Washington; 1993.
45. Gripp KW, Lin AE. Costello syndrome. In: Pagon RA, Adam MP, Bird TD, Dolan CR, Fong CT, Stephens K, editors. GeneReviews. Seattle: University of Washington; 1993.
46. Gripp KW, Hopkins E, Doyle D, Dobyns WB. High incidence of progressive postnatal cerebellar enlargement in Costello syndrome: brain overgrowth associated with HRAS mutations as the likely cause of structural brain and spinal cord abnormalities. Am J Med Genet A. 2010;152A:1161–8.
47. Pascual-Castroviejo I, Pascual-Pascual SI, Velazquez-Fragua R, Viano J, Carceller-Benito F. Aqueductal stenosis in the neurofibromatosis type 1. Presentation of 19 infantile patients. Rev Neurol. 2007;45:18–21.
48. Mirzaa GM, Conway RL, Gripp KW, et al. Megalencephaly-capillary malformation (MCAP) and megalencephaly-polydactyly-polymicrogyria-hydrocephalus (MPPH) syndromes: two closely related disorders of brain overgrowth and abnormal brain and body morphogenesis. Am J Med Genet A. 2012;158A:269–91.
49. Plawner LL, Delgado MR, Miller VS, et al. Neuroanatomy of holoprosencephaly as predictor of function: beyond the face predicting the brain. Neurology. 2002;59:1058–66.
50. Williams D, Patel C, Fallet-Bianco C, et al. Fowler syndrome-a clinical, radiological, and pathological study of 14 cases. Am J Med Genet A. 2010;152A:153–60.
51. Kato M, Das S, Petras K, et al. Mutations of ARX are associated with striking pleiotropy and consistent genotype-phenotype correlation. Hum Mutat. 2004;23:147–59.
52. Briard ML, le Merrer M, Plauchu H, et al. Association of VACTERL and hydrocephalus: a new familial entity. Ann Genet. 1984;27:220–3.
53. Porteous ME, Cross I, Burn J. VACTERL with hydrocephalus: one end of the Fanconi anemia spectrum of anomalies? Am J Med Genet. 1992;43:1032–4.
54. McCauley J, Masand N, McGowan R, et al. X-linked VACTERL with hydrocephalus syndrome: further delineation of the phenotype caused by FANCB mutations. Am J Med Genet A. 2011;155A:2370–80.
55. Evans JA, Chodirker BN. Absence of excess chromosome breakage in a patient with VACTERL-hydrocephalus. Am J Med Genet. 1993;47:112–3.
56. Ishak GE, Dempsey JC, Shaw DW, et al. Rhombencephalosynapsis: a hindbrain malformation associated with incomplete separation of midbrain and forebrain, hydrocephalus and a broad spectrum of severity. Brain J Neurol. 2012;135:1370–86.
57. Tully HM, Dempsey JC, Ishak GE, et al. Beyond Gomez-Lopez-Hernandez syndrome: recurring phenotypic themes in rhombencephalosynapsis. Am J Med Genet A. 2012;158A:2393–406.
58. Paciorkowski AR, Greenstein RM. When is enlargement of the subarachnoid spaces not benign? A genetic perspective. Pediatr Neurol. 2007;37:1–7.
59. Schoner K, Kohlhase J, Müller AM, et al. Hydrocephalus, agenesis of the corpus callosum, and cleft lip/palate represent frequent associations in fetuses with Peters' plus syndrome and

B3GALTL mutations. Fetal PPS phenotypes, expanded by Dandy Walker cyst and encephalocele. Prenat Diagn. 2013;33:75–80.
60. Wessels MW, den Hollander NS, Willems PJ. Mild fetal cerebral ventriculomegaly as a prenatal sonographic marker for Kartagener syndrome. Prenat Diagn. 2003;23:239–42.
61. Vieira JP, Lopes P, Silva R. Primary ciliary dyskinesia and hydrocephalus with aqueductal stenosis. J Child Neurol. 2012;27:938–41.
62. Hogge WA, Blank C, Roochvarg LB, Hogge JS, Wulfsberg EA, Raffel LJ. Gorlin syndrome (naevoid basal cell carcinoma syndrome): prenatal detection in a fetus with macrocephaly and ventriculomegaly. Prenat Diagn. 1994;14:725–7.
63. Mitchell EA, Cairns LM, Hodge JL. Rothmund-Thomson syndrome (poikiloderma congenitale) associated with hydrocephalus. Aust Paediatr J. 1980;16:290–1.
64. Muller EA, Aradhya S, Atkin JF, et al. Microdeletion 9q22.3 syndrome includes metopic craniosynostosis, hydrocephalus, macrosomia, and developmental delay. Am J Med Genet A. 2012;158A:391–9.
65. Hwu WL, Kuo PL, Hung YT, Chien YH, Chu SY. Partial trisomy 1 with congenital hydrocephalus and hypogammaglobulinemia: report of one case. Acta paediatrica Taiwanica [Taiwan er ke yi xue hui za zhi]. 2004;45:97–9.
66. Eash D, Waggoner D, Chung J, Stevenson D, Martin CL. Calibration of 6q subtelomere deletions to define genotype/phenotype correlations. Clin Genet. 2005;67:396–403.
67. Bertini V, De Vito G, Costa R, Simi P, Valetto A. Isolated 6q terminal deletions: an emerging new syndrome. Am J Med Genet A. 2006;140:74–81.
68. Morava E, Bartsch O, Czako M, et al. Small inherited terminal duplication of 7q with hydrocephalus, cleft palate, joint contractures, and severe hypotonia. Clin Dysmorphol. 2003;12:123–7.
69. Schrander-Stumpel C, Fryns JP. Congenital hydrocephalus: nosology and guidelines for clinical approach and genetic counselling. Eur J Pediatr. 1998;157:355–62.
70. Jaraj D, Agerskov S, Rabiei K, et al. Vascular factors in suspected normal pressure hydrocephalus: a population-based study. Neurology. 2016;86:592–9.
71. Hiraoka K, Narita W, Kikuchi H, et al. Amyloid deposits and response to shunt surgery in idiopathic normal-pressure hydrocephalus. J Neurol Sci. 2015;356:124–8.
72. Odagiri H, Baba T, Nishio Y, et al. Clinical characteristics of idiopathic normal pressure hydrocephalus with Lewy body diseases. J Neurol Sci. 2015;359:309–11.
73. Kato T, Sato H, Emi M, et al. Segmental copy number loss of SFMBT1 gene in elderly individuals with ventriculomegaly: a community-based study. Intern Med. 2011;50:297–303.
74. Zhang J, Bonasio R, Strino F, et al. SFMBT1 functions with LSD1 to regulate expression of canonical histone genes and chromatin-related factors. Genes Dev. 2013;27:749–66.
75. Yang HC, Liang YJ, Chen JW, et al. Identification of IGF1, SLC4A4, WWOX, and SFMBT1 as hypertension susceptibility genes in Han Chinese with a genome-wide gene-based association study. PLoS One. 2012;7:e32907.
76. Chung RH, Chiu YF, Hung YJ, et al. Genome-wide copy number variation analysis identified deletions in SFMBT1 associated with fasting plasma glucose in a Han Chinese population. BMC Genomics. 2017;18:591.
77. Kottgen A, Albrecht E, Teumer A, et al. Genome-wide association analyses identify 18 new loci associated with serum urate concentrations. Nat Genet. 2013;45:145–54.
78. Gould DB, Phalan FC, Breedveld GJ, et al. Mutations in Col4a1 cause perinatal cerebral hemorrhage and porencephaly. Science. 2005;308:1167–71.
79. McCarty JH, Lacy-Hulbert A, Charest A, et al. Selective ablation of alphav integrins in the central nervous system leads to cerebral hemorrhage, seizures, axonal degeneration and premature death. Development. 2005;132:165–76.
80. Srivastava M, Atwater I, Glasman M, et al. Defects in inositol 1,4,5-trisphosphate receptor expression, Ca(2+) signaling, and insulin secretion in the anx7(+/−) knockout mouse. Proc Natl Acad Sci U S A. 1999;96:13783–8.

81. Ryckman KK, Dagle JM, Kelsey K, Momany AM, Murray JC. Replication of genetic associations in the inflammation, complement, and coagulation pathways with intraventricular hemorrhage in LBW preterm neonates. Pediatr Res. 2011;70:90–5.
82. Yung YC, Mutoh T, Lin ME, et al. Lysophosphatidic acid signaling may initiate fetal hydrocephalus. Sci Transl Med. 2011;3:99ra87.
83. Park R, Moon UY, Park JY, et al. Yap is required for ependymal integrity and is suppressed in LPA-induced hydrocephalus. Nat Commun. 2016;7:10329.
84. Karimy JK, Zhang J, Kurland DB, et al. Inflammation-dependent cerebrospinal fluid hypersecretion by the choroid plexus epithelium in posthemorrhagic hydrocephalus. Nat Med. 2017;23:997–1003.
85. Gagnon KB, Delpire E. Molecular physiology of SPAK and OSR1: two Ste20-related protein kinases regulating ion transport. Physiol Rev. 2012;92:1577–617.
86. Tully HM. Anatomical configurations associated with posthemorrhagic hydrocephalus among premature infants with intraventricular hemorrhage. Neurosurg Focus. 2016;41:E5.
87. McLone DG, Knepper PA. The cause of Chiari II malformation: a unified theory. Pediatr Neurosci. 1989;15:1–12.
88. Sweeney KJ, Caird J, Sattar MT, Allcutt D, Crimmins D. Spinal level of myelomeningocele lesion as a contributing factor in posterior fossa volume, intracranial cerebellar volume, and cerebellar ectopia. J Neurosurg Pediatr. 2013;11:154–9.
89. Seo JH, Zilber Y, Babayeva S, et al. Mutations in the planar cell polarity gene, Fuzzy, are associated with neural tube defects in humans. Hum Mol Genet. 2011;20:4324–33.
90. Bartsch O, Kirmes I, Thiede A, et al. Novel VANGL1 gene mutations in 144 Slovakian, Romanian and German patients with neural tube defects. Mol Syndromol. 2012;3:76–81.
91. Allache R, De Marco P, Merello E, Capra V, Kibar Z. Role of the planar cell polarity gene CELSR1 in neural tube defects and caudal agenesis. Birth Defects Res A Clin Mol Teratol. 2012;94:176–81.
92. Juriloff DM, Harris MJ. A consideration of the evidence that genetic defects in planar cell polarity contribute to the etiology of human neural tube defects. Birth Defects Res A Clin Mol Teratol. 2012;94:824–40.

7 Anatomy and Physiology-Based Magnetic Resonance Imaging in Hydrocephalus

Smruti K. Patel, Shawn M. Vuong, Weihong Yuan, and Francesco T. Mangano

Introduction

Pediatric hydrocephalus is the most common neurosurgical condition treated by pediatric neurosurgeons, accounting for approximately $2 billion in annual health expenditures in the United States [1]. In addition, idiopathic normal pressure hydrocephalus (iNPH) among the elderly continues to be a controversial neuropathological entity with regard to diagnosis and management reaching prevalence from 1% to 5.9% [2]. Neuroimaging with studies such as ultrasound, computed tomography (CT) and magnetic resonance imaging (MRI) play an important role in both the diagnosis and treatment of hydrocephalus. Hydrocephalus is a complex pathologic condition resulting in ventricular enlargement due to a disruption of cerebrospinal fluid (CSF) homeostasis. An increase in intracranial pressure or a change in CSF pulse amplitudes can cause an extensive physical displacement and distortion of the surrounding brain tissue, primarily white matter (WM), alter cerebral blood flow and tissue metabolism, or cause ependymal injury, cortical gliosis, vascular compression, and axonal loss or damage [3–7]. Furthermore, an extensive body of literature has supported that untreated hydrocephalus can often result in axonal disconnections, degeneration, and demyelination as well as impaired neuronal transmission [8, 9]. It is well known that these mechanisms are quite complicated; hydrocephalus may be secondary to several etiologies and its sequelae are

S. K. Patel · S. M. Vuong · F. T. Mangano (✉)
Division of Pediatric Neurosurgery, Cincinnati Children's Hospital Medical Center, Department of Neurological Surgery, University of Cincinnati College of Medicine, Cincinnati, OH, USA
e-mail: Francesco.mangano@cchmc.org

W. Yuan
Department of Radiology, University of Cincinnati, Cincinnati Children's Hospital Medical Center, Cincinnati, OH, USA

D. D. Limbrick, J. R. Leonard (eds.), *Cerebrospinal Fluid Disorders*,
https://doi.org/10.1007/978-3-319-97928-1_7

often multifactorial [9, 10]. In this chapter, we will discuss the utility of various anatomy and physiology-based magnetic resonance imaging (MRI) modalities for the diagnosis and treatment of hydrocephalus including conventional MRI, advanced MRI techniques and analyses, and novel concepts related to diffusion tensor imaging (DTI) as well as emerging imaging modalities such as MR elastography (MRE) and synthetic MRI.

Conventional Magnetic Resonance Imaging

Magnetic resonance imaging is traditionally the study of choice for assessing ventricular anatomy, associated distortion of WM, and for detection of the underlying etiology of congenital hydrocephalus, iNPH, and benign external hydrocephalus (BEH). Conventional T1 and T2 weighted sequences are typically satisfactory for diagnosis, but when considering potential surgical approaches for treatment, a more detailed examination of the CSF pathways and CSF flow is required [11]. When using MRI to evaluate hydrocephalus, it is important to assess basic anatomic parameters such as the size and shape of each of the lateral ventricles, the temporal horns, the absence or presence of any peri-sylvian atrophy, presence of periventricular interstitial edema (more commonly known as transependymal flow), the stretching, thinning, or displacement of the corpus callosum (CC), effacement of the cortical sulci, and/or the absence of CSF flow voids. MRI evaluation of hydrocephalus should include review of imaging for etiology, such as tumor, colloid cyst, aqueductal stenosis, Chiari malformation, or ventricular hemorrhage. Often, contrast-enhanced sequences are helpful in this assessment for identifying and distinguishing between types of mass lesions.

While conventional MRI provides high resolution imaging without exposure to radiation, it is highly susceptible to motion artifact and as a result children often require general anesthesia to obtain the imaging, placing them at an added risk of undergoing anesthesia. For this reason, among others, for patients treated with shunted hydrocephalus who require multiple and ongoing follow-up imaging studies, fast-sequence MRI with ultrafast single-shot sequences (SSh) and turbo-spin echo sequences (TSE) have been developed [12]. These imaging studies are useful for evaluating symptomatic hydrocephalus patients and also have a role for surveillance imaging in asymptomatic patients. Fast-sequence MRI sequences can be obtained in 3–4 min, compared to a 2 min CT acquisition time. These fast acquisition times can allow for children to undergo MRI imaging evaluation without general anesthesia or sedation, which eliminates risks of serious adverse effects [13]. Fast-sequence MRI sequences are T2 based, and allow for strong CSF signal, however, these images are not recommended for evaluation of lesions less than or equal to 5 mm, and are sensitive to imaging artifact at air-tissue or bone-tissue interfaces. Faster scan acquisition times also lead to less gross motion artifact from severely ill, uncooperative, or young patients [14].

3D-Constructive Interference in the Steady State and Phase Contrast MRI

In order to satisfactorily evaluate hydrocephalus patients, a variety of noninvasive refined MR sequences have been developed and investigated including three-dimensional constructive interference in the steady state (3D CISS) and phase contrast (PC-MRI) [15]. 3D CISS consists of a combination of imaging sequences that provide exceptional high spatial resolution to show sharp tissue/fluid distinctions and demonstrate fine morphological details of the CSF pathways and associated membranes. This study is particularly useful, for example, for preoperative review of a patient's ventricular and cisternal anatomy when considering an ETV for treatment of hydrocephalus or for evaluation of multiloculated hydrocephalus. Phase contrast-MRI is a noninvasive technique that allows for the visualization of CSF flow velocity and its directionality during a single cardiac cycle by using a specially designed flow-sensitive gradient echo (GRE) sequence. When used in combination, the 3D CISS and PC-MRI can provide a wealth of information regarding the anatomy and physiology of the CSF pathways, the directionality of flow, areas of obstruction, and potential operative targets for intervention [15–17].

Conventionally, it was thought that hydrocephalus was due to an imbalance between the production and absorption of CSF, otherwise known as the bulk flow theory. This theory has been proven partially inaccurate, predominantly in the case of communicating hydrocephalus, as researchers have shown that most CSF absorption occurs in capillaries and not in the arachnoid granulations as once thought. The modern, hydrodynamic theory subdivides hydrocephalus into acute and chronic or communicating hydrocephalus. It proposes that these latter entities occur due to an increase in pulse pressure in brain capillaries and decreased intracranial compliance, which in turn preserves enlarged ventricular size [18, 19]. In recent years, flow sensitive imaging such as PC-MRI has emerged as an important tool in the assessment of communicating hydrocephalus, particularly in attempts to determine the functionality or success of operative interventions such as the placement of a ventriculoperitoneal shunt (VPS) or ETV [17, 20].

Phase contrast-MRI shows that CSF flow is bidirectional, that is, it flows caudally during systole and cranially during diastole. Classically, this flow is measured as the aqueductal stroke volume (ASV) [20]. Aqueductal stroke volume is defined as the total amount of CSF that is pulsating cranially or caudally through the aqueduct of Sylvius in one cardiac cycle, normally at an aqueductal peak velocity between 3 and 7 cm/s [20]. Using PC-MRI and ASV measurements, researchers have been able to objectively quantify CSF flow as well as confirm patency through ETV stomas or fenestrations [15, 21]. A range of imaging metrics have been analyzed to evaluate the patency of an ETV, including change in ventricular size, flow void signal intensity, MR patency using PC-MRI, aqueductal velocity and velocity ratios, in addition to aqueductal stroke volumes. However, it is unknown if there is a clear-cut connection between CSF flow pulsatility and success of ETV surgery or shunting given the limited number of studies that have evaluated the parameters of stoma patency and CSF pulsatility before and after ETV is performed [22–24].

Time-Spatial Labeling Inversion Pulse

Since the introduction of PC-MRI, a wave of other MR modalities or pulse sequences have been studied for evaluation of CSF in pathophysiologic conditions with some success including, but not limited to, PC balanced steady-state free precession, [25] three-dimensional (3D) MR velocity mapping, [26] Time-spatial labeling inversion pulse (Time-SLIP) and arterial spin labeling (ASL), [17, 25] and 3D-sampling perfection with application optimized contrast (3D-SPACE) [27, 28]. In particular, Time-SLIP and ASL have shown promise with regard to being able to reliably visualize CSF flow in a targeted region when compared to PC-MRI [17]. Time-SLIP is a modified arterial spin labeling technique which is used to show flow in any imaging orientation within a targeted region such as the ventricular or subarachnoid spaces or within cysts [29]. Similar to the way in which traditional ASL magnetically tags blood with radiofrequency pulses and uses blood as its own tracer to create high quality angiograms, Time-SLIP is able to use CSF as its own tracer to generate single shot images over incremental time interval to display CSF movement in both a linear and turbulent fashion [17]. Unlike PC-MRI, Time-SLIP is not cardiac cycle dependent and is able to also demonstrate turbulent CSF reflux flow between the cerebral aqueduct, the third ventricle, through the foramen of Monro, and to the lateral ventricles [29]. Because of these properties, Time-SLIP has truly become a novel way to visualize CSF movement. It is prudent, however, to acknowledge that a thorough understanding of CSF flow disorders requires anatomical data (as provided by sequences such as 3D-CISS) and both quantitative (CSF flow velocities provided by PC-MRI) as well as qualitative information (CSF flow characteristics, pathways, and obstructions provided by Time-SLIP).

MR Ventriculography

MR ventriculography (MRV) has been shown to be a reliable, safe, and effective imaging technique for assessment of CSF flow, sites of obstruction in hydrocephalus and also in evaluating patency of endoscopic third ventriculostomy (ETV) [30, 31]. This technique involves direct injection of contrast into the ventricular system using an external ventricular drain or access device. Once the device is placed, initial T1-weighted MR images are acquired in axial, coronal, and sagittal planes prior to the removal of 2 mL of CSF followed by administration of 2–4 mL of the contrast agent [31]. The child's head is repositioned to facilitate contrast diffusion into the ventricular system and the T1-weighted post contrast images are acquired. While literature regarding this particular technique is limited due to the invasiveness of the method, it appears to provide additional information regarding the ventricular anatomy and has been shown to be particularly useful in cases of complex and multiloculated hydrocephalus [30–32]. This imaging technique is likely to be most effective and informative when used in combination with noninvasive morphological and functional MRI sequences.

Overall, the various MR techniques developed within the last 20 years have been invaluable resources for the noninvasive study of intracranial pulsatility in hydrocephalus. Most studies have consistently shown that hydrocephalus is associated with increased aqueductal flow pulsatility, but a precise association between this and clinical outcomes from surgical interventions is uncertain [22]. It is probable that CSF flow pulsatility only represents one piece of the puzzle regarding the complicated pathophysiology of this disease. Additional noninvasive markers must be investigated to adequately evaluate and predict success with ETV or shunting. Large scale clinical trials with standardized pulsatility parameters are crucial for both clinical use and predicting outcomes in the future.

Current Challenges with Advanced MR Analysis

While morphological and flow-based MRI techniques and CSF specific sequences as described earlier may show ventricular enlargement and can even provide other fine anatomic detail regarding the etiology of the hydrocephalus and CSF flow, they provide limited information about the subtle microstructural pathology and WM integrity related to hydrocephalus. Though the exact pathophysiology of injury in this setting is unknown, hydrocephalus has profound neuropathological effects on the brain, particularly on the WM as a result of physical distortion of WM tracts, impaired cerebral blood flow, ischemia, and can cause axonal and/or myelin damage from abnormal CSF circulation and edema in the periventricular regions, leading to impaired neuronal transmission and perhaps, even irreversible injury [6, 7, 33, 34].

The current treatment for hydrocephalus involves surgical diversion of CSF with shunting from the brain to a distant body cavity, such as the peritoneum (as in a VPS) or with ETV in selected cases such as obstructive hydrocephalus from a tectal glioma or aqueductal stenosis, and has even seen some success in patients with iNPH [10]. ETV has been shown to offer some advantages over ventricular shunting such as lower long-term failure rates and avoiding the need to place shunt hardware [10, 35]. CSF diversion with shunting is typically associated with a smaller post-treatment ventricular size. On the other hand, patients treated with ETV, while asymptomatic, can often have persistently larger than normal post-treatment ventricles. While these surgical interventions are generally effective, many children with hydrocephalus experience persistent delays in cognitive, motor, and physical development and thus, the optimal treatment for hydrocephalus remains controversial [36]. In many studies, neurocognitive outcomes have been shown to be independent of ventricular volume, further suggesting that neither shunting nor ETV is better when using traditional criteria such as improvement in symptoms and ventricular size or volume as indicators of improvement or progress [10, 37–39]. In 2015, Kulkarni et al. showed that large ventricular volume did not correlate with additional WM injury or worse neurocognitive deficits in asymptomatic children with stable, treated hydrocephalus due to obstructive hydrocephalus (i.e., tectal glioma or congenital aqueductal stenosis). Moreover, it challenges the concept that the traditional criteria (e.g., Evans index, ventricular size, ventricular volume) are adequate for predicting cognitive outcomes and suggests that additional metrics must be developed [10]. A recent study shows that brain volume, rather than CSF volume, correlates with improvements in neurocognitive function after surgical treatment, suggesting that brain development or growth may be a better predictor of outcome [40].

Role of Diffusion Tensor Imaging in Hydrocephalus

Over the last decade, there has been increased interest in investigating WM injury as it relates to hydrocephalus and the use of DTI to provide insight into the underlying mechanisms of WM damage and its reversibility with surgical intervention [35, 41–48]. The premise behind the use of DTI arises from the understanding that the diffusion of water in tissue is affected by the microstructure and configuration of WM tracts, thus providing powerful information regarding the effects of disorders that affect the integrity of the WM [41, 42, 49]. DTI is an advanced MRI technique that characterizes the integrity of WM by in vivo quantification of diffusion properties of water in brain tissue. Water diffusion in WM is anisotropic, that is, water diffusion tends to be less restricted in the direction parallel to fiber orientation and is more restricted in the direction perpendicular to fiber orientation. DTI provides the following important parameters within a region of interest (ROI): principal diffusivities (radial [Drad, perpendicular to fibers] or axial [Dax, parallel to fibers]), the mean diffusivity (MD) or overall magnitude of water diffusion, and fractional anisotropy (FA), which is a scalar measure of the preferential restriction in water diffusion. Fractional anisotropy is represented as a value between 0 and 1, where 0 represents unrestricted diffusion or equally restricted in all directions and 1 represents diffusion along only one axis and fully restricted in all other directions [49].

In the past decade, numerous animal and human studies have applied DTI, both in a retrospective and prospective fashion, to investigate WM tracts and results of WM injury in pediatric hydrocephalus [35, 42–48, 50–53]. Some of the most common regions of interest (ROIs) examined in these investigations (Fig. 7.1) included CC, anterior and posterior limb of internal capsule (ALIC, PLIC), corticospinal tract, and superior and inferior longitudinal fasciculus, among others [41, 42, 44, 48, 51, 54, 55]. In 2006, Assaf et al. [41] used DTI parameters to study and compare seven patients (age > 9) with acute hydrocephalus with age-matched healthy control subjects. They showed that FA values were generally increased in hydrocephalic patients in the corona radiata and internal capsule (IC), accompanied by an increase in Dax and decrease in Drad. Conversely, FA values were decreased in the CC, with a reduction in Dax and an increase in Drad. Due to the different patterns of change in the CC and IC, this study raised the original concept that the impact of hydrocephalus on WM might be region specific. After surgical intervention, FA values in the ROIs trended toward those of control values in six of the seven patients [41]. In 2008, Hasan et al. [55] reported their findings with DTI in patients with spina bifida and hydrocephalus (mean age of 12) and showed that these patients had an overall decrease in FA values and increase in Drad in association pathways relative to

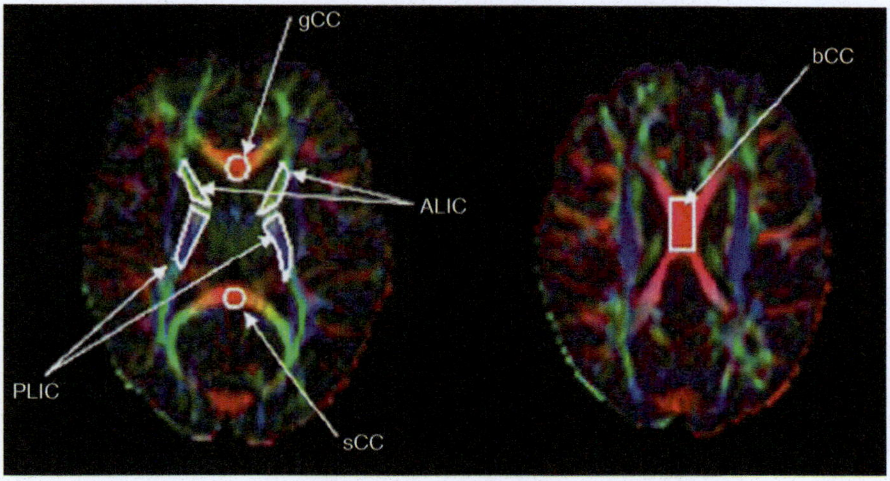

Fig. 7.1 Selected specific regions of interest (ROI) overlaid on representative color-coded FA maps. ROIs include genu (gCC), body (bCC), splenium (sCC) of corpus collosum, anterior (ALIC), and posterior (PLIC) limb of the internal capsule

control subjects. They suggested that these patterns of change in spina bifida patients with hydrocephalus may represent myelination defects or breakdown in the myelin sheath or axonal integrity within these WM tracts [55].

One of the limitations with these early studies was that they only included older children and young adults and there was a lack of DTI data in younger children closer to age of diagnosis of hydrocephalus. Furthermore, the understanding of these indices at the time was limited by the availability of a normative or standard database in healthy pediatric patients [52]. To help address this particular problem, Yuan et al. [42] published a retrospective review of DTI in children with hydrocephalus during early infancy prior to treatment. They showed that infants with hydrocephalus had significantly lower FA and higher MD values in the CC but not in the IC when compared to age-matched controls. In addition, the expected increase in FA with age during normal development (Fig. 7.2) [52, 53, 56] was absent in the CC but was found to be normal in the IC. These discrepancies suggest that WM development in children with hydrocephalus may be affected differently between various locations, with regions closer to the ventricles being more vulnerable under the stress of enlarged ventricles and abnormally elevated ICP [42]. These preoperative region-specific DTI patterns and changes in patients with hydrocephalus were further confirmed by Air el al. in 2010, providing further support that most DTI values normalized after shunt treatment in these patients (Fig. 7.3) [44]. While all the patients with hydrocephalus who received treatment in these retrospective studies showed improvement clinically after surgical intervention, due to the small sample sizes, the predictive power of DTI was deemed to be limited [41, 44].

In 2013, Yuan et al. [47] published the first prospective, multicenter, longitudinal imaging study to quantify the diffusion properties in WM structures in a group of

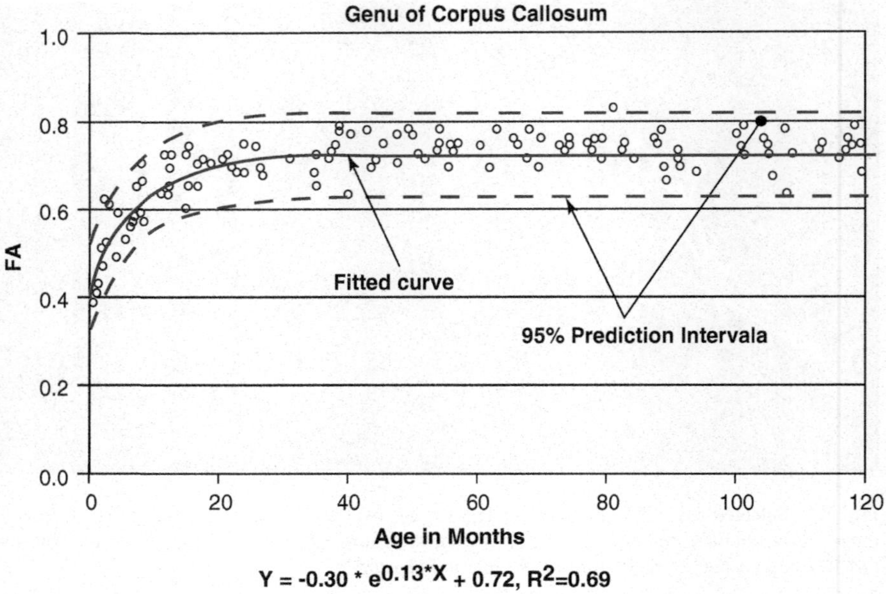

Fig. 7.2 Best-fit exponential function (solid line) and respective 95% prediction interval (dashed lines) overlaid on a scatter plot derived from the raw data of FA values detected in the genu of the corpus callosum (gCC) from individual normal participants with no neurological pathology

children representing the age range and clinical profiles typical of pediatric hydrocephalus. The results reported in the study included 31 patients, 13 patients with hydrocephalus and 18 normal, healthy control subjects. Their key findings included that diffusion properties in children with hydrocephalus were significantly abnormal in several WM regions in the CC and IC. Patients with hydrocephalus had lower FA and higher MD in the genu (gCC) and splenium (sCC) of the corpus callosum. In contrast, the results were more variable in the PLIC and ALIC, where many patients had an abnormally high FA, while others had abnormally low FA values. These findings were consistent with the patterns of DTI indices reported in prior studies. Finally, modest correlations were found between DTI parameters in children with hydrocephalus and caregiver-reported motor deficits on neuropsychological evaluation [47].

DTI Study Based on Probabilistic Diffusion Tractography

The severe deformation in the hydrocephalic brain presents a unique challenge for imaging data processing and analysis. DTI studies of hydrocephalus have been mainly based on analyses of certain ROIs. While ROI-based DTI studies have demonstrated consistent evidence of abnormalities in several key WM regions, the technique used in the delineation of ROIs is typically limited to one or a small fixed number of several slices. A full representation of the WM structure of interest may

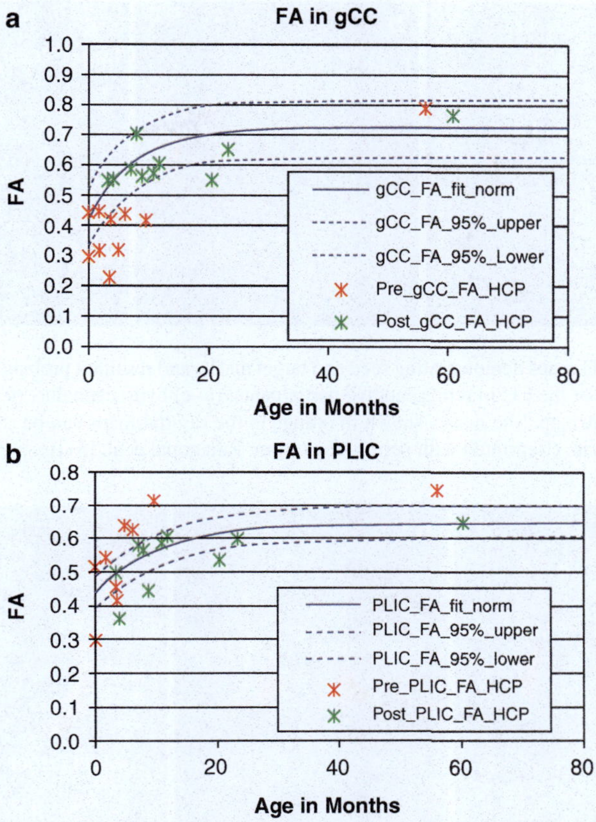

Fig. 7.3 Best-fit exponential function (solid line) and respective 95% prediction interval (dashed lines) overlaid on a scatter plot derived from the raw data of FA values detected in the gCC (**a**) and PLIC (**b**). FA measures yielded abnormal results in several white matter regions of the brain and trended toward normalization following VP shunt placement. (Reprinted with permissions from: Air et al. [44])

be missed. In a study by Rajagopal et al. [51], probabilistic diffusion tractography (PDT), a powerful fiber tracking method that calculates multiple pathways emanating from a seed ROI and from each point along the reconstructed trajectories, was used to generate tract-based connectivity distribution and DTI measures of the gCC (Fig. 7.4) and the corticospinal tracts (Fig. 7.5). This approach avoided the usage of an FA threshold and allowed for tracking to continue through brain regions with significant noise high uncertainty, which is typical in imaging of pediatric hydrocephalic brains with severe distortion, especially in children at a very young age. Based on the tract-based summary measurements, including connectivity index and DTI measures, children with hydrocephalus were found to have a higher percentage of voxels with lower normalized CI values in the gCC and bilateral corticospinal tracts, reflecting disruption in fiber continuity, when compared to controls. Tract-based analyses also showed significant DTI abnormalities in children with hydrocephalus in the WM tracts.

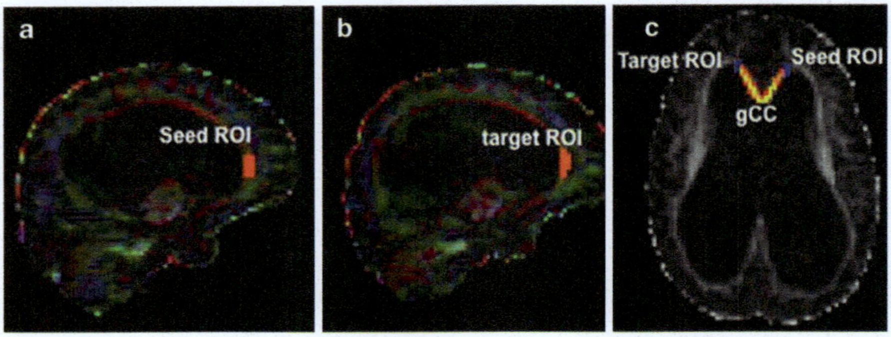

Fig. 7.4 (**a**) DTI maps demonstrating seed and target masks and resultant probabilistic fiber tracking of the genu of the CC in representative participants. (**a–c**) hydrocephalus. (**a**, **b**) Color-coded FA maps. (**c**) FA map. The masks shown in orange in the sagittal maps can be seen as short blue lines on axial map. (Reprinted with permissions from: Rajagopal et al. [51])

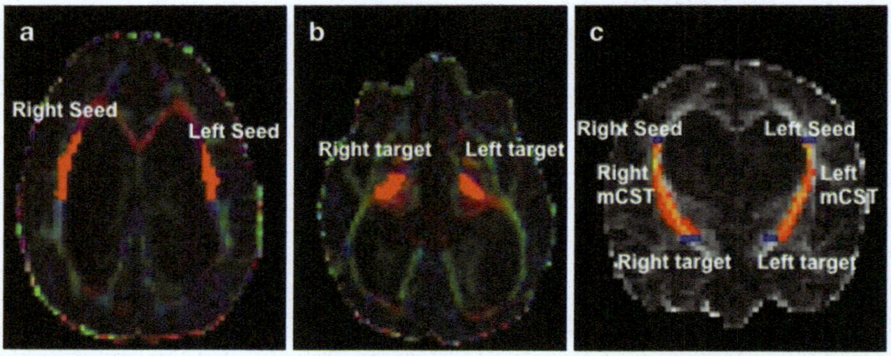

Fig. 7.5 DTI maps demonstrating seed and target masks and resultant probabilistic fiber tracking of the left and right mid-segments of the cortical spinal tracts in representative participants. (**a–c**) Hydrocephalus. (**a**, **b**) Color-coded FA maps. (**c**) FA map. The masks shown in orange on the axial DTI maps can be seen as short blue lines on coronal FA map. (Reprinted with permissions from: Rajagopal et al. [51])

DTI Studies of Structural Connectivity Based on Graph Theory and DTI Tractography

Hydrocephalus is a neurological disorder that may arise from many heterogeneous etiologies. It often presents with regionally specific damage, and this damage is also expected to extend to wider areas throughout the brain and have negative impact on the entire brain. To generate a global quantification for the integrity of the entire brain network and to detect WM abnormalities outside the typical brain regions examined by ROI or tract-based analysis, a novel approach that combined the graph theory and DTI tractography was explored in the study of hydrocephalus [57, 58]. This is a method that has been applied in characterizing the developmental trajectory of network connectivity as well as for investigating the disruption of network connectivity at both global and regional levels in various neurological disorders. Figure 7.6 shows a schematic diagram for the major steps used in the connectivity matrix. When applied to pediatric patients with hydrocephalus, it was found that these patients had significantly lower small-worldness, a global network measure that reflects the competing demand for overall efficiency and regional redundancy. Further analysis showed that patients with hydrocephalus had significant differences in the distribution of network hubs as well as in the regional network indices in some of the hub regions (Fig. 7.7). These differences, in both global and regional network measures, were first identified based on the whole brain network analysis [57]. Furthermore, similar findings were replicated in the network analyses based on the left hemisphere only [58]. The latter study was completed because of a unique situation in the post-surgery hydrocephalus patient population due to MRI artifact from the right-sided placement of a programmable valve that is sometimes implanted. While the structural connectivity analysis based on graph theory and DTI tractography in the study of hydrocephalus is still exploratory, there are significant differences in the network measures, especially when combined with the significant connections found between network measures and future neuropsychological outcomes [58]. This novel approach provides a new avenue for potential diagnostic and prognostic tool for children with hydrocephalus and lends support to the notion about the predictive value of DTI for future clinical and surgical outcomes.

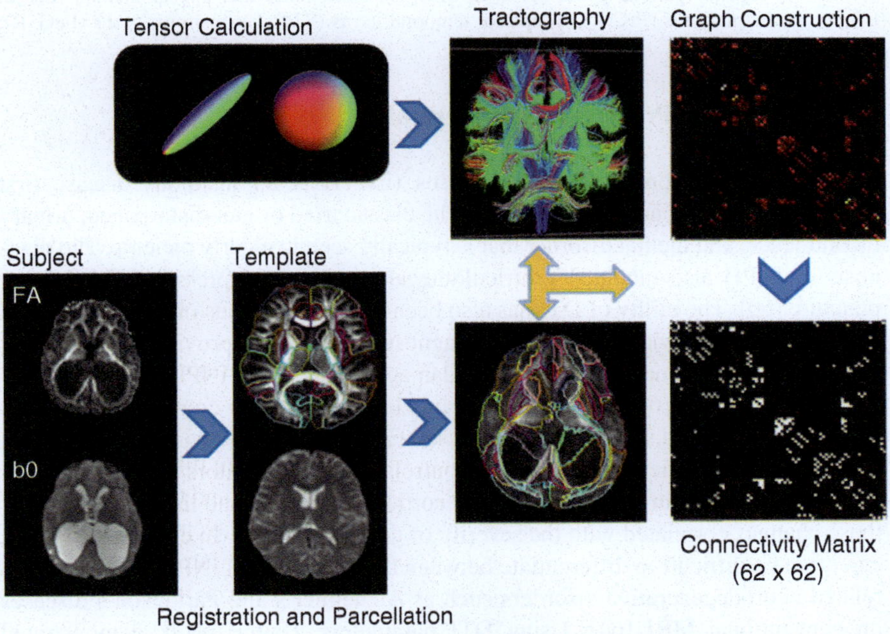

Fig. 7.6 Schematic diagram for constructing a structural connectivity matrix. (Reprinted with permissions from: Yuan et al. [57]. doi: https://doi.org/10.1016/j.nicl.2015.04.015. eCollection 2015)

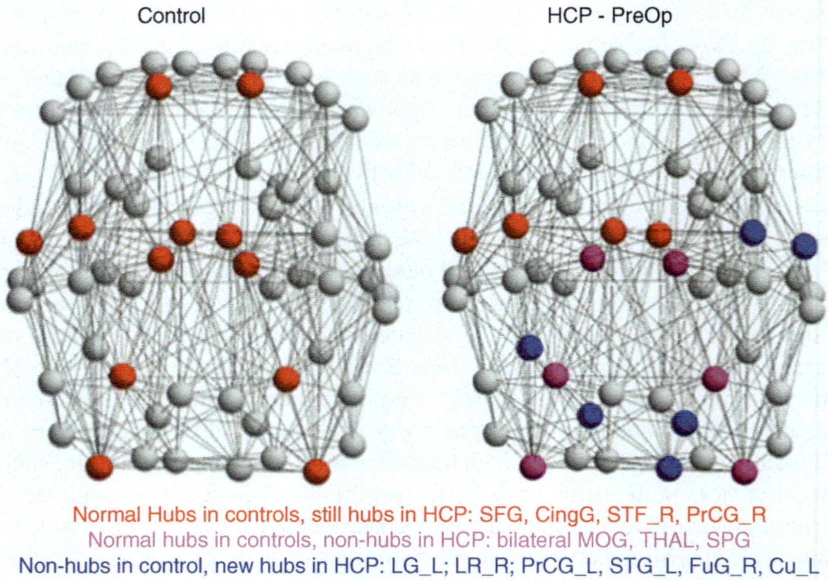

Fig. 7.7 A hub (represented by each single sphere) is a node that has many connections. Therefore, disrupting or removing a hub will cause many disconnections. Nodes found in controls but not as hubs in hydrocephalus are: MOG_L, MOG_R (orbitofrontal gyrus) thalamus (THAL_L; THAL_R); superior parietal gyrus (SPG_L; SPG_R). New nodes that appear include: LG_L; LR_R; precentral gyrus (PrCG_L); superior temporal gyrus (STG_L); fusiform gyrus (FuG_R); cuneate (Cu_L)

DTI and Normal Pressure Hydrocephalus

Idiopathic normal pressure hydrocephalus (iNPH) is an insidious disease first described by Hakim and Adams [59] by the classic triad of gait disturbance, urinary incontinence, and mental disorder that is typically seen in elderly patients. The diagnosis of iNPH also included ventriculomegaly and normal pressure with lumbar puncture [60]. The utility of DTI has also been a particular focus of interest in iNPH with potential to provide a noninvasive diagnostic study and to provide further insight into the underlying mechanisms of WM damage secondary to iNPH [61, 62].

Hattingen et al. [63] compared DTI in 11 iNPH patients compared to normal controls. They found significantly decreased FA values and increased MD values in the CC of iNPH patients compared to controls. The investigators also showed significant differences in FA and MD in the corticospinal tract, and that the severity of these changes correlated with the severity of gait disturbance. In elderly patients, it can often be difficult to differentiate between the diagnoses of iNPH and other age-related neurodegenerative disorders such as Alzheimer's and Parkinson's diseases on conventional MRI [64]. Using DTI parameters, Hattori et al. demonstrated changes in corticospinal tract microstructure sufficient to discriminate iNPH from Alzheimer's and Parkinson's diseases, with a sensitivity of 94% and specificity of 80% [65]. Furthermore, DTI has shown promise in differentiating these disease entities, by measuring microstructural changes in the hippocampus, which have been shown to be more sensitive than volumetric changes in comparing iNPH to dementia [66]. DTI has also shown potential in evaluating the response to shunt placement in iNPH. After shunt surgery, nine patients had a significant decrease in FA of the PLIC compared to a high presurgical baseline. These findings suggest that DTI could further be utilized as a valid, noninvasive diagnostic study as well as to determine treatment-responsiveness in iNPH [67].

DTI and Benign External Hydrocephalus

DTI has also demonstrated clinical value in benign external hydrocephalus (BEH), also known as benign extra-axial fluid of infancy or enlarged subarachnoid spaces. BEH can be accompanied by ventriculomegaly (however, not a requirement for diagnosis) and is a benign, self-limiting condition that often resolves without treatment. It is associated with normal neurological and developmental outcomes [68, 69]. A retrospective review using DTI in children with BEH showed a significant increase in FA and decrease in MD in children with BEH at the time of initial diagnosis when compared to normal children in the gCC and sCC. In longitudinal comparison, these values normalized over time as the brain matured [45]. These results were in parallel with the clinical neurological outcome of these patients, in that BEH resolves spontaneously over time in many of these patients without need for intervention [70].

DTI and Surgically Treated Pediatric Hydrocephalus

In order to further elucidate the use of DTI in the management of childhood hydrocephalus, Mangano et al. [48] recently published the first multicenter, prospective, longitudinal imaging study of pediatric hydrocephalus investigating both imaging and behavioral outcomes at baseline prior to and after surgical management. The study included 54 patients with congenital hydrocephalus who underwent surgery and 64 healthy controls. Both DTI and neurodevelopmental outcome data were collected and analyzed. Patients with hydrocephalus had data collected at baseline prior to intervention, at 3 months after surgical intervention, and at 12 months after surgical intervention. The preoperative data showed that patients with hydrocephalus had abnormal DTI indices, consistent with those found in prior reports (low FA in the gCC and high in PLIC) [44, 47, 54]. Overall, postoperative data showed that gCC abnormalities persisted at 3 and 12 months postoperatively. In contrast, PLIC diffusion abnormalities were significant in studies at 3 months post-treatment but were no longer appreciated at 12 months post-treatment. Further, longitudinal comparison showed that DTI parameters in gCC did not significantly change between the preoperative and 3-month postoperative studies, suggesting that WM injury persists even after CSF diversion at that time point, despite a decrease in ventricular size and improvement in clinical symptoms. Between the 3 and 12 month studies, there was a significant improvement toward normal DTI values. These results correlated with improvement in neuropsychological assessment in the children with hydrocephalus as they performed better on these tests when the DTI measures in the gCC were closer to the normative value.

In 2012, Scheel et al. [71] described similar results in their longitudinal study of 13 adult patients (mean age of 60) with hydrocephalus, 7 with iNPH, 3 with NPH secondary to subarachnoid hemorrhage, and 3 with aqueductal stenosis. They used combined ROI and whole brain voxel-based analysis to compare different DTI parameters and alterations both before and after shunt surgery. They found that while DTI parameters had a trend toward normalization, they remained abnormal in patients who had hydrocephalus several weeks after surgery in comparison to normal control subjects. The findings of these studies further support that DTI is a sensitive noninvasive biomarker for identification of WM abnormalities in patients with hydrocephalus and can serve as a tool for individual patient follow-up and tracking neurological progress post-surgery.

DTI may become an important tool for clinicians who provide long-term care for patients with hydrocephalus. The goal would be to utilize DTI as an objective and noninvasive measure to evaluate patients and serve as a prognostic tool for the future neurocognitive outcomes of postsurgical patients with pediatric hydrocephalus [72]. A recent study published by our group showed that DTI was sensitive in detecting underlying WM changes and correlated highly with improved neurocognitive outcomes after a 6-week iPad application-based occupational therapy intervention in children with surgically treated hydrocephalus [73]. This study further endorses, that when followed longitudinally over time, the DTI parameters would serve to correlate functional outcomes similar to how we currently follow head circumference measurements in infants and toddlers to predict normal development or to predict impending clinical pathology such as shunt malfunction in children [48].

DTI and Animal Studies

In 2010, Yuan et al. demonstrated the feasibility of applying DTI in a kaolin-induced ventriculomegaly rat model and showed various abnormalities in DTI parameters affecting multiple regions of WM. This and other studies have been necessary to evaluate pathologic changes at the cellular level and correlate such changes to imaging and behavior [43]. Kaolin induces an inflammatory response which causes fibrosis in the areas of the subarachnoid space adjacent to the injection site, most commonly the cisterna magna [74, 75]. This preliminary study showed decreased FA and increased MD in the CC and IC in hydrocephalic rats when compared to controls. Furthermore, these DTI findings showed moderate to strong correlations with histopathological data obtained from subjects including GFAP immunoreactivity, astrocytosis, microglial activity, as well as a trend toward decreased myelination in symptomatic animals [43].

In a follow-up study [46], the investigators sought to characterize abnormalities in DTI parameters in various WM ROIs including the genu, body, and splenium of the CC (gCC, bCC, sCC, respectively); anterior, middle, and posterior external capsule (aEC, mEC, and pEC); IC; and fornix (FX). Abnormalities in DTI measures in hydrocephalic rats found in this study were as follows: FA was decreased and MD/Drad was increased in the gCC and bCC; increased Dax in the sCC; FA and Dax were increased in aEC; increased FA in the mEC; increased MD and Drad in the pEC; increased FA and Dax in IC; and increased FA in the FX [46]. No significant correlation was found between the ventricle size based on the local area ratio and any of the DTI parameters in those regions. The results ultimately showed that WM impairment in hydrocephalus is region specific, consistent with prior clinical and experimental studies [41–43].

Kaolin rat model studies have been criticized for causing a severe diffuse inflammatory response like meningitis and therefore, likely do not adequately mimic congenital hydrocephalus [76]. In response to this, Emmert et al. [77] created a rat model of X-linked hydrocephalus using CRISPR which revealed WM abnormalities on DTI compared to controls. Rats in this model were shown to have statistically significant decreases in Dax and FA as well as increased Drad in the CC. The group also found decreased MD and FA levels in the external and IC of these animals. These findings further substantiate that DTI is a sensitive imaging tool in detecting WM abnormalities and supports its use as a noninvasive biomarker for hydrocephalus [78].

While some of the earlier studies identified that WM structures are known to be affected by hydrocephalus on DTI, there remained a lack of insight into which WM regions were more susceptible to ventriculomegaly and how WM injury evolves over time. In order to help fill this knowledge gap, Eskandari et al. [79] used DTI to evaluate various WM structures and quantify their susceptibility to damage and to determine if DTI could be used to assess the mechanisms of injury in a kaolin-induced ventriculomegaly feline model over the course of 12 weeks. They studied DTI indices both before and after placement of a ventricular reservoir during an early and late stage with routine reservoir tapping and removal of CSF. Regions of interest studied in this experiment included the optic chiasm, optic tract, CC, and IC. Ultimately, the results showed that the CC may represent the WM structure that is most susceptible to damage from hydrocephalus and the optic chiasm and tract were the most resilient. A recent animal study by Aojula et al. [80] explored the use of decorin, a TGF-ß antagonist for treatment of communicating hydrocephalus while investigating attenuation of injury-related DTI parameters and cellular changes. They found that decorin decreased myelin damage in the IC and prevents periventricular edema and astrocytosis, and it also prevented the increase in MD seen in the CC. This study also further validates that DTI can act as a surrogate marker of cytopathological changes in hydrocephalus [80].

Emerging Technology and Experimental Imaging

As discussed earlier, MRI acquisition time in pediatric patients can be lengthy and children often require sedation or general anesthesia in order to tolerate the studies [81, 82]. Conventional MRI is mainly qualitative and the signal intensity of the images is related to the specific MR scanner settings making direct comparison of images difficult in terms of absolute image intensity [81, 82]. Synthetic MRI is an emerging tool that allows quantitative measurements of longitudinal T1-relaxation time, transverse T2-relaxation time, and proton density. These physical properties are not scanner or user dependent and provide a quantitative source for individual patient follow-up and comparisons [81]. Researchers are now investigating quantitative or synthetic MRI for rapid, objective, and user-independent assessment of measurements such as intracranial and CSF volumes [83, 84]. A recent study by Virhammar et al. [84] showed that calculation of intracranial volume, CSF volume, and brain parenchymal fraction can provide a rapid, automated index that can be used to monitor ventricular volume, and may serve as another potential noninvasive biomarker for evaluating or monitoring response to treatment for hydrocephalus. Synthetic MRI has tremendous potential to decrease the overall scan time, particularly when multiple contrast-weight images are required, which is typical in the clinical setting and can be helpful, especially in the pediatric population as well as uncooperative patients [85]. While the clinical use of synthetic MRI was limited due to long post-processing times, newer software has been developed that has decreased the post-processing time to less than 1 min [82]. Although synthetic MRI may be a potential acceptable tool for clinical use in hydrocephalus given its benefits, study limitations include inferior overall image quality when compared to conventional images and small number of included subjects.

Further developments are also being made in various advance MR techniques such as MR elastography (MRE) for assessment of brain and ventricular compliance or stiffness in patients with hydrocephalus [86]. MRE is a noninvasive study that evaluates the mechanical properties of tissues in vivo and it has been shown in prior studies that pressure changes that cause changes in tissue elasticity can be detected by MRE [87, 88]. Fattahi et al. [86] reported their study of MRE in adult patients with iNPH, which showed that patients with iNPH have increased brain stiffness when compared with age and sex-matched controls. These results suggested that perhaps MRE can serve as a novel diagnostic and surveillance tool in pediatric hydrocephalus. A recent animal study conducted by Pong et al. evaluating changes in brain tissue mechanical properties between adult and juvenile rats with kaolin-induced hydrocephalus showed that brain tissue stiffness did not change significantly in adult rats when compared to juvenile rats [89]. Moreover, they also found that there is a regional and temporal variation in brain tissue stiffness during hydrocephalus development in juvenile rats [90]. Their results suggest that these changes that occur in brain mechanical properties during hydrocephalus are more complex than just due to brain tissue deformation. Further studies regarding the complex interactions between brain tissue stiffness (characterized by MRE), deformation, edema, and neuronal or WM damage (characterized by DTI) are necessary before MRE can be utilized as a biomarker to track changes in brain biomechanics in the setting of hydrocephalus.

Conclusion

Neuroimaging techniques for the evaluation of cerebrospinal fluid disorders have progressed remarkably over the last century. Currently, conventional CT and MRI remain the most common imaging studies used to evaluate and monitor pediatric hydrocephalus. While these studies allow for adequate gross structural and anatomical assessment, they do not provide sufficient information regarding complex pathophysiological mechanisms, microstructural neuropathology, or brain tissue biomechanics that may occur because of hydrocephalus, particularly within the white matter. Diffusion tensor imaging and tractography have emerged as powerful and sensitive biomarkers to quantify these white matter abnormalities and have shown potential as predictive tools for neurobehavioral outcomes in patients with hydrocephalus. Furthermore, coupling novel imaging sequences such as MRE and synthetic MRI with more sophisticated methods of analyses of data retrieved from these imaging studies provide a future avenue in the diagnosis and prognosis of hydrocephalus.

References

1. Simon TD, Riva-Cambrin J, Srivastava R, Bratton SL, Dean JM, Kestle JR, et al. Hospital care for children with hydrocephalus in the United States: utilization, charges, comorbidities, and deaths. J Neurosurg Pediatr. 2008;1(2):131–7.
2. Siasios I, Kapsalaki EZ, Fountas KN, Fotiadou A, Dorsch A, Vakharia K, et al. The role of diffusion tensor imaging and fractional anisotropy in the evaluation of patients with idiopathic normal pressure hydrocephalus: a literature review. Neurosurg Focus. 2016;41(3):E12.
3. Del Bigio MR. Neuropathology and structural changes in hydrocephalus. Dev Disabil Res Rev. 2010;16(1):16–22.
4. Del Bigio MR. Cellular damage and prevention in childhood hydrocephalus. Brain Pathol. 2004;14(3):317–24.
5. Del Bigio MR. Pathophysiologic consequences of hydrocephalus. Neurosurg Clin N Am. 2001;12(4):639–49, vii.
6. Del Bigio MR, da Silva MC, Drake JM, Tuor UI. Acute and chronic cerebral white matter damage in neonatal hydrocephalus. Can J Neurol Sci. 1994;21(4):299–305.
7. Khan OH, Enno TL, Del Bigio MR. Brain damage in neonatal rats following kaolin induction of hydrocephalus. Exp Neurol. 2006;200(2):311–20.
8. Del Bigio MR, Zhang YW. Cell death, axonal damage, and cell birth in the immature rat brain following induction of hydrocephalus. Exp Neurol. 1998;154(1):157–69.
9. McAllister JP. Getting to the root of hydrocephalus. Sci Transl Med. 2011;3(99):99fs4.
10. Kahle KT, Kulkarni AV, Limbrick DD Jr, Warf BC. Hydrocephalus in children. Lancet. 2016;387(10020):788–99.
11. Drake JM. The surgical management of pediatric hydrocephalus. Neurosurgery. 2008;62(Suppl 2):633–40; discussion 40–2.
12. Koral K, Blackburn T, Bailey AA, Koral KM, Anderson J. Strengthening the argument for rapid brain MR imaging: estimation of reduction in lifetime attributable risk of developing fatal cancer in children with shunted hydrocephalus by instituting a rapid brain MR imaging protocol in lieu of Head CT. AJNR Am J Neuroradiol. 2012;33(10):1851–4.
13. Patel DM, Tubbs RS, Pate G, Johnston JM Jr, Blount JP. Fast-sequence MRI studies for surveillance imaging in pediatric hydrocephalus. J Neurosurg Pediatr. 2014;13(4):440–7.
14. Patel MR, Klufas RA, Alberico RA, Edelman RR. Half-fourier acquisition single-shot turbo spin-echo (HASTE) MR: comparison with fast spin-echo MR in diseases of the brain. AJNR Am J Neuroradiol. 1997;18(9):1635–40.
15. Dincer A, Ozek MM. Radiologic evaluation of pediatric hydrocephalus. Childs Nerv Syst. 2011;27(10):1543–62.
16. Battal B, Kocaoglu M, Bulakbasi N, Husmen G, Tuba Sanal H, Tayfun C. Cerebrospinal fluid flow imaging by using phase-contrast MR technique. Br J Radiol. 2011;84(1004):758–65.
17. Yamada S, Tsuchiya K, Bradley WG, Law M, Winkler ML, Borzage MT, et al. Current and emerging MR imaging techniques for the diagnosis and management of CSF flow disorders: a review of phase-contrast and time-spatial labeling inversion pulse. AJNR Am J Neuroradiol. 2015;36(4):623–30.

18. Greitz D. Paradigm shift in hydrocephalus research in legacy of Dandy's pioneering work: rationale for third ventriculostomy in communicating hydrocephalus. Childs Nerv Syst. 2007;23(5):487–9.
19. Greitz D. The hydrodynamic hypothesis versus the bulk flow hypothesis. Neurosurg Rev. 2004;27(4):299–300.
20. Wagshul ME, Chen JJ, Egnor MR, McCormack EJ, Roche PE. Amplitude and phase of cerebrospinal fluid pulsations: experimental studies and review of the literature. J Neurosurg. 2006;104(5):810–9.
21. Greitz D. Radiological assessment of hydrocephalus: new theories and implications for therapy. Neurosurg Rev. 2004;27(3):145–65; discussion 66–7.
22. Wagshul ME, Eide PK, Madsen JR. The pulsating brain: a review of experimental and clinical studies of intracranial pulsatility. Fluids Barriers CNS. 2011;8(1):5.
23. Stivaros SM, Sinclair D, Bromiley PA, Kim J, Thorne J, Jackson A. Endoscopic third ventriculostomy: predicting outcome with phase-contrast MR imaging. Radiology. 2009;252(3):825–32.
24. Bargallo N, Olondo L, Garcia AI, Capurro S, Caral L, Rumia J. Functional analysis of third ventriculostomy patency by quantification of CSF stroke volume by using cine phase-contrast MR imaging. AJNR Am J Neuroradiol. 2005;26(10):2514–21.
25. McCormack EJ, Egnor MR, Wagshul ME. Improved cerebrospinal fluid flow measurements using phase contrast balanced steady-state free precession. Magn Reson Imaging. 2007;25(2):172–82.
26. Brandner S, Buchfelder M, Eyuepoglu IY, Luecking H, Doerfler A, Stadlbauer A. Visualization of CSF flow with time-resolved 3D MR velocity mapping in aqueductal stenosis before and after endoscopic third ventriculostomy: a feasibility study. Clin Neuroradiol. 2018;28(1):69–74.
27. Algin O. Prediction of endoscopic third ventriculostomy (ETV) success with 3D-SPACE technique. Neurosurg Rev. 2015;38(2):395–7.
28. Algin O, Ucar M, Ozmen E, Borcek AO, Ozisik P, Ocakoglu G, et al. Assessment of third ventriculostomy patency with the 3D-SPACE technique: a preliminary multicenter research study. J Neurosurg. 2015;122(6):1347–55.
29. Yamada S, Miyazaki M, Kanazawa H, Higashi M, Morohoshi Y, Bluml S, et al. Visualization of cerebrospinal fluid movement with spin labeling at MR imaging: preliminary results in normal and pathophysiologic conditions. Radiology. 2008;249(2):644–52.
30. Gandhoke GS, Frassanito P, Chandra N, Ojha BK, Singh A. Role of magnetic resonance ventriculography in multiloculated hydrocephalus. J Neurosurg Pediatr. 2013;11(6):697–703.
31. Joseph VB, Raghuram L, Korah IP, Chacko AG. MR ventriculography for the study of CSF flow. AJNR Am J Neuroradiol. 2003;24(3):373–81.
32. Singh I, Haris M, Husain M, Husain N, Rastogi M, Gupta RK. Role of endoscopic third ventriculostomy in patients with communicating hydrocephalus: an evaluation by MR ventriculography. Neurosurg Rev. 2008;31(3):319–25.
33. Del Bigio MR. Neuropathological changes caused by hydrocephalus. Acta Neuropathol. 1993;85(6):573–85.
34. Del Bigio MR, Cardoso ER, Halliday WC. Neuropathological changes in chronic adult hydrocephalus: cortical biopsies and autopsy findings. Can J Neurol Sci. 1997;24(2):121–6.
35. Buckley RT, Yuan W, Mangano FT, Phillips JM, Powell S, McKinstry RC, et al. Longitudinal comparison of diffusion tensor imaging parameters and neuropsychological measures following endoscopic third ventriculostomy for hydrocephalus. J Neurosurg Pediatr. 2012;9(6):630–5.
36. Mataro M, Junque C, Poca MA, Sahuquillo J. Neuropsychological findings in congenital and acquired childhood hydrocephalus. Neuropsychol Rev. 2001;11(4):169–78.
37. Kulkarni AV, Donnelly R, Mabbott DJ, Widjaja E. Relationship between ventricular size, white matter injury, and neurocognition in children with stable, treated hydrocephalus. J Neurosurg Pediatr. 2015;16(3):267–74.
38. Warf B, Ondoma S, Kulkarni A, Donnelly R, Ampeire M, Akona J, et al. Neurocognitive outcome and ventricular volume in children with myelomeningocele treated for hydrocephalus in Uganda. J Neurosurg Pediatr. 2009;4(6):564–70.

39. Azab WA, Mijalcic RM, Nakhi SB, Mohammad MH. Ventricular volume and neurocognitive outcome after endoscopic third ventriculostomy: is shunting a better option? A review. Childs Nerv Syst. 2016;32(5):775–80.
40. Mandell JG, Kulkarni AV, Warf BC, Schiff SJ. Volumetric brain analysis in neurosurgery: Part 2. Brain and CSF volumes discriminate neurocognitive outcomes in hydrocephalus. J Neurosurg Pediatr. 2015;15(2):125–32.
41. Assaf Y, Ben-Sira L, Constantini S, Chang LC, Beni-Adani L. Diffusion tensor imaging in hydrocephalus: initial experience. AJNR Am J Neuroradiol. 2006;27(8):1717–24.
42. Yuan W, Mangano FT, Air EL, Holland SK, Jones BV, Altaye M, et al. Anisotropic diffusion properties in infants with hydrocephalus: a diffusion tensor imaging study. AJNR Am J Neuroradiol. 2009;30(9):1792–8.
43. Yuan W, Deren KE, McAllister JP 2nd, Holland SK, Lindquist DM, Cancelliere A, et al. Diffusion tensor imaging correlates with cytopathology in a rat model of neonatal hydrocephalus. Cerebrospinal Fluid Res. 2010;7:19.
44. Air EL, Yuan W, Holland SK, Jones BV, Bierbrauer K, Altaye M, et al. Longitudinal comparison of pre- and postoperative diffusion tensor imaging parameters in young children with hydrocephalus. J Neurosurg Pediatr. 2010;5(4):385–91.
45. Sun M, Yuan W, Hertzler DA, Cancelliere A, Altaye M, Mangano FT. Diffusion tensor imaging findings in young children with benign external hydrocephalus differ from the normal population. Childs Nerv Syst. 2012;28(2):199–208.
46. Yuan W, McAllister JP 2nd, Lindquist DM, Gill N, Holland SK, Henkel D, et al. Diffusion tensor imaging of white matter injury in a rat model of infantile hydrocephalus. Childs Nerv Syst. 2012;28(1):47–54.
47. Yuan W, McKinstry RC, Shimony JS, Altaye M, Powell SK, Phillips JM, et al. Diffusion tensor imaging properties and neurobehavioral outcomes in children with hydrocephalus. AJNR Am J Neuroradiol. 2013;34(2):439–45.
48. Mangano FT, Altaye M, McKinstry RC, Shimony JS, Powell SK, Phillips JM, et al. Diffusion tensor imaging study of pediatric patients with congenital hydrocephalus: 1-year postsurgical outcomes. J Neurosurg Pediatr. 2016;18(3):306–19.
49. Alexander AL, Lee JE, Lazar M, Field AS. Diffusion tensor imaging of the brain. Neurotherapeutics. 2007;4(3):316–29.
50. Yuan Y, Zhu H, Styner M, Gilmore JH, Marron JS. Varying coefficient model for modeling diffusion tensors along white matter tracts. Ann Appl Stat. 2013;7(1):102–25.
51. Rajagopal A, Shimony JS, McKinstry RC, Altaye M, Maloney T, Mangano FT, et al. White matter microstructural abnormality in children with hydrocephalus detected by probabilistic diffusion tractography. AJNR Am J Neuroradiol. 2013;34(12):2379–85.
52. Cancelliere A, Mangano FT, Air EL, Jones BV, Altaye M, Rajagopal A, et al. DTI values in key white matter tracts from infancy through adolescence. AJNR Am J Neuroradiol. 2013;34(7):1443–9.
53. Yuan W, McAllister JP, Mangano FT. Neuroimaging of white matter abnormalities in pediatric hydrocephalus. J Pediatr Neuroradiol. 2013;2:119–28.
54. Ben-Sira L, Goder N, Bassan H, Lifshits S, Assaf Y, Constantini S. Clinical benefits of diffusion tensor imaging in hydrocephalus. J Neurosurg Pediatr. 2015;16(2):195–202.
55. Hasan KM, Eluvathingal TJ, Kramer LA, Ewing-Cobbs L, Dennis M, Fletcher JM. White matter microstructural abnormalities in children with spina bifida myelomeningocele and hydrocephalus: a diffusion tensor tractography study of the association pathways. J Magn Reson Imaging. 2008;27(4):700–9.
56. Mukherjee P, Miller JH, Shimony JS, Philip JV, Nehra D, Snyder AZ, et al. Diffusion-tensor MR imaging of gray and white matter development during normal human brain maturation. AJNR Am J Neuroradiol. 2002;23(9):1445–56.
57. Yuan W, Holland SK, Shimony JS, Altaye M, Mangano FT, Limbrick DD, et al. Abnormal structural connectivity in the brain networks of children with hydrocephalus. Neuroimage Clin. 2015;8:483–92.

58. Yuan W, Meller A, Shimony JS, Nash T, Jones BV, Holland SK, et al. Left hemisphere structural connectivity abnormality in pediatric hydrocephalus patients following surgery. Neuroimage Clin. 2016;12:631–9.
59. Adams RD, Fisher CM, Hakim S, Ojemann RG, Sweet WH. Symptomatic occult hydrocephalus with "normal" cerebrospinal-fluid pressure. A treatable syndrome. N Engl J Med. 1965;273:117–26.
60. Hakim S, Adams RD. The special clinical problem of symptomatic hydrocephalus with normal cerebrospinal fluid pressure. Observations on cerebrospinal fluid hydrodynamics. J Neurol Sci. 1965;2(4):307–27.
61. Keong NC, Price SJ, Gillard JH, Pickard JD. DTI profiles in NPH. Br J Neurosurg. 2012;26(5):600.
62. Keong NC, Pena A, Price SJ, Czosnyka M, Czosnyka Z, DeVito EE, et al. Diffusion tensor imaging profiles reveal specific neural tract distortion in normal pressure hydrocephalus. PLoS One. 2017;12(8):e0181624.
63. Hattingen E, Jurcoane A, Melber J, Blasel S, Zanella FE, Neumann-Haefelin T, et al. Diffusion tensor imaging in patients with adult chronic idiopathic hydrocephalus. Neurosurgery. 2010;66(5):917–24.
64. Ivkovic M, Liu B, Ahmed F, Moore D, Huang C, Raj A, et al. Differential diagnosis of normal pressure hydrocephalus by MRI mean diffusivity histogram analysis. AJNR Am J Neuroradiol. 2013;34(6):1168–74.
65. Hattori T, Yuasa T, Aoki S, Sato R, Sawaura H, Mori T, et al. Altered microstructure in corticospinal tract in idiopathic normal pressure hydrocephalus: comparison with Alzheimer disease and Parkinson disease with dementia. AJNR Am J Neuroradiol. 2011;32(9):1681–7.
66. Hong YJ, Yoon B, Shim YS, Cho AH, Lim SC, Ahn KJ, et al. Differences in microstructural alterations of the hippocampus in Alzheimer disease and idiopathic normal pressure hydrocephalus: a diffusion tensor imaging study. AJNR Am J Neuroradiol. 2010;31(10):1867–72.
67. Kim MJ, Seo SW, Lee KM, Kim ST, Lee JI, Nam DH, et al. Differential diagnosis of idiopathic normal pressure hydrocephalus from other dementias using diffusion tensor imaging. AJNR Am J Neuroradiol. 2011;32(8):1496–503.
68. Girard NJ, Raybaud CA. Ventriculomegaly and pericerebral CSF collection in the fetus: early stage of benign external hydrocephalus? Childs Nerv Syst. 2001;17(4–5):239–45.
69. Smith R, Leonidas JC, Maytal J. The value of head ultrasound in infants with macrocephaly. Pediatr Radiol. 1998;28(3):143–6.
70. Kumar R. External hydrocephalus in small children. Childs Nerv Syst. 2006;22(10):1237–41.
71. Scheel M, Diekhoff T, Sprung C, Hoffmann KT. Diffusion tensor imaging in hydrocephalus–findings before and after shunt surgery. Acta Neurochir. 2012;154(9):1699–706.
72. Patel SK, Yuan W, Mangano FT. Advanced Neuroimaging Techniques in Pediatric Hydrocephalus. Pediatr Neurosurg. 2017;52:436.
73. Yuan W, Harpster K, Jones BV, Shimony JS, McKinstry RC, Weckherlin N, et al. Changes of white matter diffusion anisotropy in response to a 6-week iPad application-based occupational therapy intervention in children with surgically treated hydrocephalus: a pilot study. Neuropediatrics. 2016;47(5):336–40.
74. Hatta J, Hatta T, Moritake K, Otani H. Heavy water inhibiting the expression of transforming growth factor-beta1 and the development of kaolin-induced hydrocephalus in mice. J Neurosurg. 2006;104(4 Suppl):251–8.
75. Slobodian I, Krassioukov-Enns D, Del Bigio MR. Protein and synthetic polymer injection for induction of obstructive hydrocephalus in rats. Cerebrospinal Fluid Res. 2007;4:9.
76. Cohen AR, Leifer DW, Zechel M, Flaningan DP, Lewin JS, Lust WD. Characterization of a model of hydrocephalus in transgenic mice. J Neurosurg. 1999;91(6):978–88.
77. Emmert AS, Goto J, Shula C, Qin S, Hu Y, Mangano FT, editors. CRISPR/cas9-based development of novel transgenic rat model of x-linked hydrocephalus. Joint Congress of the International Children's Continence Society (ICCS) and The Society For Research Into Hydroephalus And Spina Bifida (SRHSB); 2017; St. Louis, MO.

78. Emmert A, Vuong S, Shula C, Hu Y, Goto J, Mangano FT, editors. CRISPR/Cas9-based development of novel transgenic rat model of X-linked hydrocephalus: diffusion tensor imaging provides mild white abnormalities in a CRISPR/Cas9-Generated [Abstract]. 46th Annual AANS/CNS Section on Pediatric Neurological Surgery Meeting; 2017; Houston, TX.
79. Eskandari R, Abdullah O, Mason C, Lloyd KE, Oeschle AN, McAllister JP 2nd. Differential vulnerability of white matter structures to experimental infantile hydrocephalus detected by diffusion tensor imaging. Childs Nerv Syst. 2014;30(10):1651–61.
80. Aojula A, Botfield H, McAllister JP 2nd, Gonzalez AM, Abdullah O, Logan A, et al. Diffusion tensor imaging with direct cytopathological validation: characterisation of decorin treatment in experimental juvenile communicating hydrocephalus. Fluids Barriers CNS. 2016;13(1):9.
81. Betts AM, Leach JL, Jones BV, Zhang B, Serai S. Brain imaging with synthetic MR in children: clinical quality assessment. Neuroradiology. 2016;58:1017.
82. Blystad I, Warntjes JB, Smedby O, Landtblom AM, Lundberg P, Larsson EM. Synthetic MRI of the brain in a clinical setting. Acta Radiol. 2012;53(10):1158–63.
83. Ambarki K, Lindqvist T, Wahlin A, Petterson E, Warntjes MJ, Birgander R, et al. Evaluation of automatic measurement of the intracranial volume based on quantitative MR imaging. AJNR Am J Neuroradiol. 2012;33(10):1951–6.
84. Virhammar J, Warntjes M, Laurell K, Larsson EM. Quantitative MRI for rapid and user-independent monitoring of intracranial CSF volume in hydrocephalus. AJNR Am J Neuroradiol. 2016;37(5):797–801.
85. Hagiwara A, Warntjes M, Hori M, Andica C, Nakazawa M, Kumamaru KK, et al. SyMRI of the brain: rapid quantification of relaxation rates and proton density, with synthetic MRI, automatic brain segmentation, and myelin measurement. Investig Radiol. 2017;52(10):647–57.
86. Fattahi N, Arani A, Perry A, Meyer F, Manduca A, Glaser K, et al. MR elastography demonstrates increased brain stiffness in normal pressure hydrocephalus. AJNR Am J Neuroradiol. 2016;37(3):462–7.
87. Hirsch S, Beyer F, Guo J, Papazoglou S, Tzschaetzsch H, Braun J, et al. Compression-sensitive magnetic resonance elastography. Phys Med Biol. 2013;58(15):5287–99.
88. Mousavi SR, Fehlner A, Streitberger KJ, Braun J, Samani A, Sack I. Measurement of in vivo cerebral volumetric strain induced by the Valsalva maneuver. J Biomech. 2014;47(7):1652–7.
89. Pong AC, Juge L, Bilston LE, Cheng S. Development of acute hydrocephalus does not change brain tissue mechanical properties in adult rats, but in juvenile rats. PLoS One. 2017;12(8):e0182808.
90. Juge L, Pong AC, Bongers A, Sinkus R, Bilston LE, Cheng S. Changes in rat brain tissue microstructure and stiffness during the development of experimental obstructive hydrocephalus. PLoS One. 2016;11(2):e0148652.

Posthemorrhagic Hydrocephalus

8

Jonathan A. Pindrik and Mark Halverson

Abbreviations

AF	Anterior fontanelle
AVM	Arteriovenous malformation
CP	Cerebral palsy
CSF	Cerebrospinal fluid
EI	Evans index
ELBW	Extremely low birth weight
ETV	Endoscopic third ventriculostomy
ETV/CPC	Endoscopic third ventriculostomy with choroid plexus cauterization
EVD	External ventricular drain
FOR	Frontal/occipital horn ratio
g	Grams
GA	Gestational age
GMH	Germinal matrix hemorrhage
HC	Head circumference
HCRN	Hydrocephalus Clinical Research Network
ICP	Intracranial pressure
IVH	Intraventricular hemorrhage
kg	Kilograms
LP	Lumbar puncture
MDI	Mental Developmental Index
ml	Milliliters

J. A. Pindrik (✉)
Division of Pediatric Neurosurgery, Department of Neurological Surgery, Nationwide Children's Hospital, The Ohio State University College of Medicine, Columbus, OH, USA
e-mail: jonathan.pindrik@nationwidechildrens.org

M. Halverson
Department of Radiology, Nationwide Children's Hospital, Columbus, OH, USA

D. D. Limbrick, J. R. Leonard (eds.), *Cerebrospinal Fluid Disorders*,
https://doi.org/10.1007/978-3-319-97928-1_8

MRI	Magnetic resonance imaging
NICU	Neonatal intensive care unit
OR	Odds ratio
PDI	Psychomotor Development Index
PHH	Posthemorrhagic hydrocephalus
PHVD	Posthemorrhagic ventricular dilation
PVHI	Periventricular hemorrhagic infarction
PVL	Periventricular leukomalacia
RBC	Red blood cell
TGF-β	Transforming growth factor-β
US	Ultrasound
VAD	Ventricular access device
VAS	Ventriculoatrial shunt
VBR	Ventricular-brain ratio
VPS	Ventriculoperitoneal shunt
VSGS	Ventriculo-subgaleal shunt
VLBW	Very low birth weight

Terminology

Intraventricular hemorrhage (IVH) indicates the abnormal presence of acute or chronic blood products within the intracranial ventricular system. Routine cerebrospinal fluid (CSF) flow may distribute blood breakdown products diffusely or discretely between the ventricular, cisternal, and subarachnoid compartments. Following IVH, radiographic enlargement of the ventricular system may occur, reflecting posthemorrhagic ventricular dilation (PHVD) (Fig. 8.1). As an early or late feature, posthemorrhagic hydrocephalus (PHH) develops in a subset of patients with IVH. Hydrocephalus entails progressive enlargement of the ventricular system (ventriculomegaly or PHVD) with clinical signs of elevated intracranial pressure (ICP), due to an imbalance between CSF production and absorption. Preterm infants with IVH may also develop ventriculomegaly due to cystic periventricular leukomalacia (PVL), reflecting hydrocephalus ex-vacuo due to parenchymal volume loss (Fig. 8.2). In the context of IVH, communicating hydrocephalus results from impaired CSF absorption through the subarachnoid spaces and at the level of arachnoid villi or granulations (among other pathophysiologic mechanisms, see Pathophysiology Section below), while obstructive hydrocephalus occurs due to mechanical blockage of CSF flow through the ventricular system. The occurrence of PHH depends on multiple factors (see Epidemiology and Pathophysiology sections below) including the severity of IVH. This chapter focuses on PHH as a consequence of IVH related to prematurity, defined as birth prior to 37 weeks gestational age (GA).

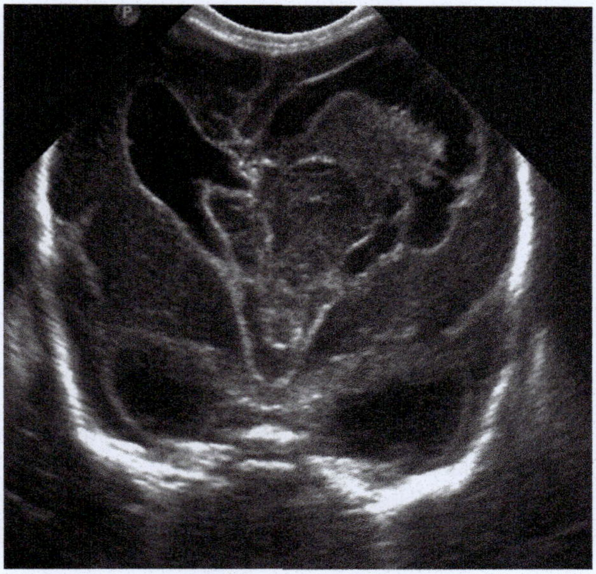

Fig. 8.1 Posthemorrhagic ventricular dilation (PHVD). This coronal view of a head ultrasound demonstrates the appearance of PHVD in a 3-week-old neonate with a history of prematurity and Grade IV IVH

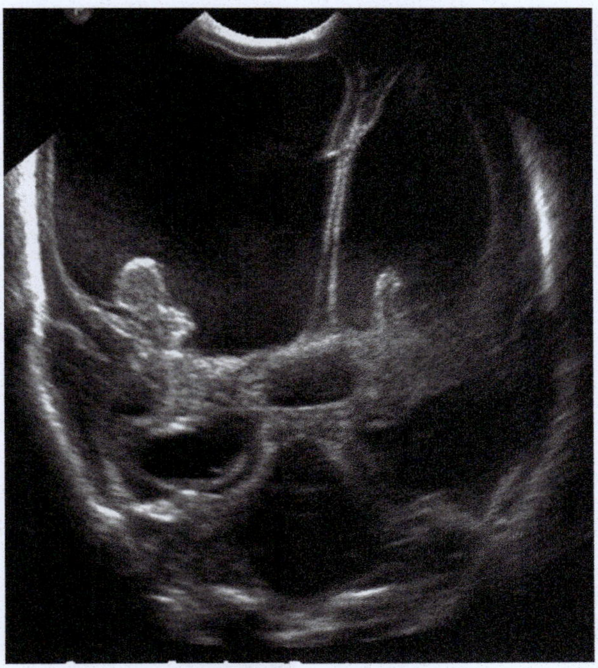

Fig. 8.2 Marked volume loss following Grade IV IVH. This coronal view of a head ultrasound shows cystic periventricular leukomalacia (PVL) and marked cerebral parenchymal volume loss in a 2.5-month-old neonate with history of prematurity and extensive periventricular hemorrhagic infarction (PHVI) or Grade IV IVH

Grading

The extent or severity of IVH can be summarized and communicated effectively by the Papile grading system and/or the Volpe modified classification [1–3]. These grading systems stratify IVH severity based on the estimated percent of ventricular involvement (with laterality dichotomized), the presence of ventricular dilation, and the presence of parenchymal involvement [1, 3, 4]:

Papile Grading System for Intraventricular Hemorrhage (IVH)

- Grade I IVH: Hemorrhage restricted to the germinal matrix zone (sub-ependymal parenchyma) and/or involving <10% of the ventricle (Fig. 8.3).
- Grade II IVH: Hemorrhage involving > = 10% but <= 50% of the ventricle, without ventricular dilation (Fig. 8.4).
- Grade III IVH: Hemorrhage involving >50% of the ventricle, and/or causing ventricular dilation (Fig. 8.5).
- Grade IV IVH or periventricular hemorrhagic infarction (PVHI): Hemorrhage extending to the adjacent parenchyma, likely reflecting venous infarct with hemorrhagic conversion (Fig. 8.6).

The IVH grading system possesses utility in predicting risk for the development of PHH and offers prognostication regarding late sequelae of IVH, including cerebral palsy and neurocognitive impairment.

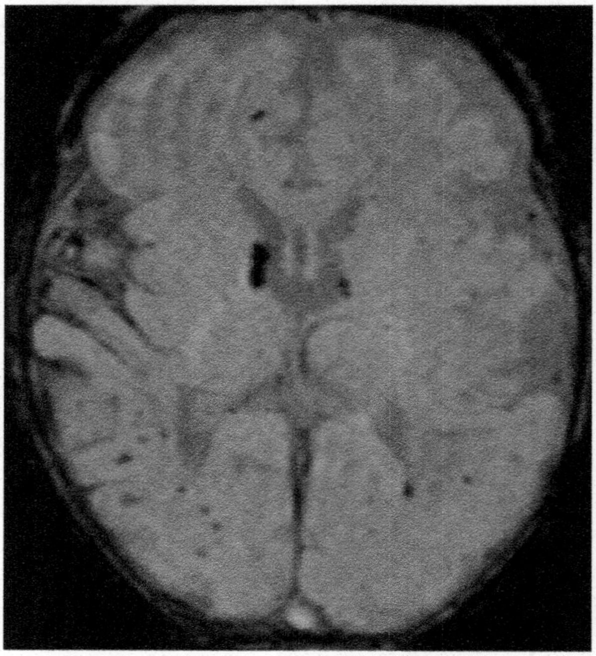

Fig. 8.3 Grade I IVH. This axial view of a magnetic resonance imaging (MRI) susceptibility weighted sequence demonstrates evidence of prior hemorrhage along bilateral (right greater than left) caudothalamic grooves, consistent with germinal matrix hemorrhage (GMH). This, along with the negligible amount of blood located within the dependent portion of the left lateral ventricular occipital horn, satisfies criteria for Grade I IVH

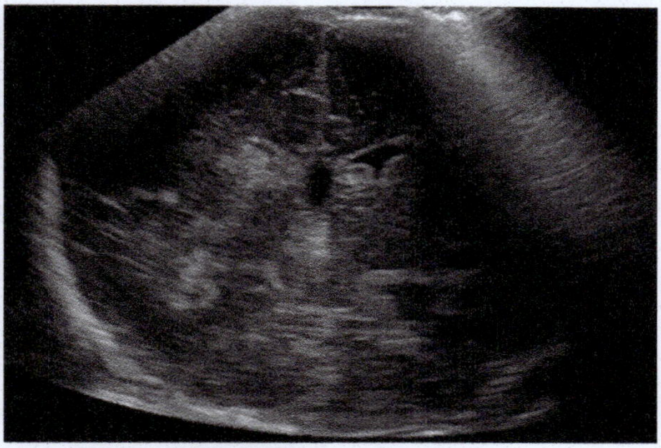

Fig. 8.4 Grade II IVH. This coronal view of a head ultrasound demonstrates moderate IVH occupying the lateral and third ventricles without ventricular dilation, consistent with Grade II IVH. Subsequent imaging on this same patient demonstrated resolution of the IVH without ventricular enlargement

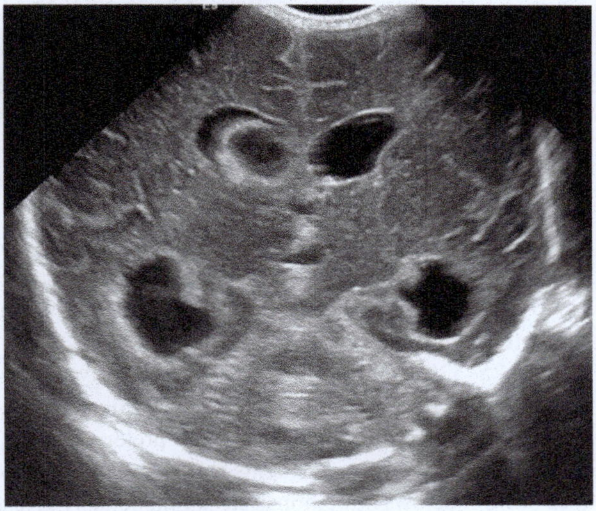

Fig. 8.5 Grade III IVH. This coronal view of a head ultrasound illustrates the appearance of bilateral IVH (also involving the third ventricle) with ventricular enlargement, consistent with Grade III IVH

Epidemiology

Although not unique to the neonatal period, IVH and subsequent PHH represent common and potentially debilitating conditions within premature infants, especially those with very low birth weight (VLBW; Birth weight < 1500 grams [g]). Several population-based studies have reported incidence rates of IVH and subsequent PHH within preterm infants. With enhanced survival rates of VLBW and extremely low birth weight (ELBW; birth weight <= 1000 g) preterm infants, the incidence rates of severe IVH have remained stable (around 11–16%) despite recent declines in the overall incidence of IVH [2, 3, 5–8]. Multiple studies have shown an inverse relationship between GA, birth weight, and the incidence of IVH, such that more extreme degrees of prematurity and VLBW predict higher rates of IVH, especially Grade II-IV IVH [1–3, 5, 8–11].

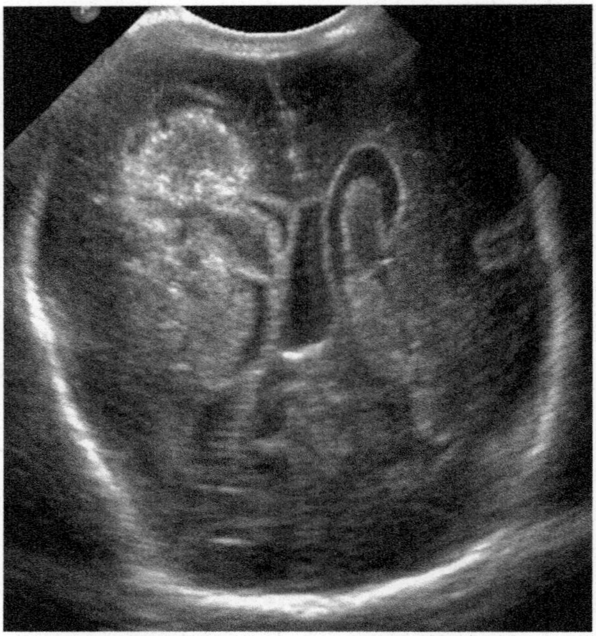

Fig. 8.6 Grade IV IVH. This coronal view of a head ultrasound depicts significant right intraparenchymal hemorrhage reflecting periventricular hemorrhagic infarction (PVHI), consistent with Grade IV IVH. The evolution of this extensive PVHI can be seen in Fig. 8.8.2, acquired from the same patient 2 months later

Within the USA and similarly developed countries, recent data has suggested an overall incidence rate of IVH in preterm infants around 10–20%, increasing slightly to 15–23% in preterm VLBW infants, and escalating up to 33% in the context of prematurity and ELBW [1, 3–7, 9, 10, 12–17]. Among patients with IVH, approximately 25–33% will develop ventriculomegaly or PHVD without progression or clinical signs of elevated ICP [10, 12]. Similarly, progressive PHVD or PHH will develop in approximately 21–30% of preterm infants with IVH [1, 10, 12, 13]. While up to 60% of these patients may respond adequately to temporizing measures (see section below) or demonstrate spontaneously arrested hydrocephalus, approximately 40% will require permanent CSF diversion [1, 10, 16]. Overall, approximately 10–15% of preterm infants with IVH will require definitive treatment for PHH [1, 5, 9, 10, 17]. Greater IVH severity (Grade III or IV) predicts a higher rate (up to 29%) of progressive PHH requiring permanent CSF diversion [1, 5, 10, 13, 18]. Stratified further, patients with Grade III IVH have demonstrated higher rates of progression to PHVD and PHH (likely due to greater amounts of intraventricular blood and better survival) as compared to those with Grade IV IVH [18].

Other population-based studies reflect similar or slightly divergent trends depending on nationality. Based on data obtained from the Israel National VLBW Infant Database, approximately 22% of preterm infants between 24 and 28 weeks GA with at least Grade II IVH developed PHH [3]. Additionally, moderate IVH severity (unilateral Grade III or Grade IV IVH) suggested modest increase in the odds ratio (OR) for developing PHH (OR 3.5 and OR 3.8, respectively), while greater IVH severity (bilateral Grade III or unilateral Grade 3 with contralateral Grade IV IVH) implied higher risk for developing PHH (OR 12.2 and OR 13.7, respectively) [3]. Similar to American trends, approximately 42% of these patients with PHH required definitive therapy with ventriculoperitoneal shunt (VPS) insertion, representing 9% of patients with at least Grade II IVH [3].

Findings from other population-based studies reflect geographic variation in rates of IVH due to prematurity. A Korean-based population study reported a 42% overall incidence rate of IVH in VLBW infants, differing from American incidence rates described above [2]. The distribution of IVH Grades within the Korean VLBW population also differed from American trends. For instance, a higher proportion of Grade I (59%) and lower proportions of Grade III (11%) and Grade IV (13%) IVH patients were identified in the Korean VLBW population as compared to those reported in a prior American population-based study (Grade I, 48%; Grade III, 15%; Grade IV, 19%) [2, 10]. Given these differences, the rate of IVH progression to PHH requiring temporizing or permanent interventions for CSF diversion was expectedly lower in the Korean VLBW population (8.5%) as compared to the American VLBW population (9–10%) [2, 10]. Other population-based studies from Sweden, Netherlands, and Germany also have reported lower incidence rates (5–6%) of severe IVH in VLBW infants [5, 18].

Pathophysiology

The exact pathophysiologic mechanisms accounting for the development of IVH in the setting of prematurity and subsequent PHH remain unclear. Multiple theories have been proposed to explain the occurrence of each event. Germinal matrix hemorrhage (GMH) likely results from immaturity and fragility of vasculature within the proliferative zone of neural and glial precursor cells located between the ventricular wall and caudate nucleus within the caudothalamic groove [1, 4, 5] (Fig. 8.3). The germinal matrix undergoes involution starting after 24 weeks gestation and completing by 34–37 weeks gestation [4, 5]. Birth prior to completion of precursor cell migration and germinal matrix involution (37 weeks, term) fosters the presence of thin-walled vessels lacking muscularis mucosa and fully competent basal laminae. While structurally deficient, these vessels also may encounter endothelial cell death and vasodilation due to hypoxia in the setting of systemic hypotension, a frequent occurrence during prematurity. These factors result in impaired compliance and autoregulatory capacity, heightening risk of vascular damage or rupture during elevations in cerebral perfusion pressure [1, 4, 5, 11]. These and other stressors (hypertension, increased venous pressure, coagulopathy) account for the high risk of GMH within the first 72 hours of birth in the setting of prematurity [4, 19]. Consequent hemorrhage in the germinal matrix zone may extend to the ventricle through the ependyma, leading to IVH of varying degrees.

Ventricular size and the development of hydrocephalus rely upon the balance between CSF production and absorption. Choroid plexus accounts for the majority (~80%) of CSF production. The remainder (~20%) occurs via transependymal flow to the ventricular system from the brain parenchyma [14]. Following circulation through the ventricular system and subarachnoid space, CSF enters the venous system primarily through arachnoid villi and granulations [4, 14] (Fig. 8.7). However, arachnoid granulations do not achieve full maturity or competency during the neonatal stage and there remains a paucity of evidence to support the theory of

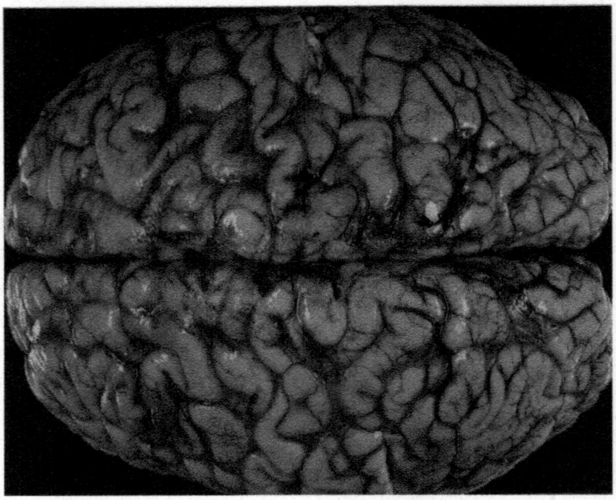

Fig. 8.7 Arachnoid villi and granulations, cadaver specimen. As shown in this cadaver specimen, arachnoid villi and granulations protrude through the dura into dural venous sinuses and are consolidated mostly along the midline superior sagittal sinus

arachnoid obstruction leading to PHH from IVH during prematurity [4]. Therefore, accessory pathways of CSF resorption likely play critical roles in normal and pathologic states of CSF dynamics in premature neonates with IVH [4, 16]. Imbalances between CSF production and absorption may result in ventricular volume changes and pathologic progression to hydrocephalus.

Progressive ventricular dilation (either PHVD or PHH) following IVH may occur via several mechanisms. Intraventricular clots may impede CSF flow at critical anatomic locations (Cerebral Aqueduct of Sylvius, Foramen of Monro, fourth ventricular outlets) causing an obstructive form of hydrocephalus [1, 4, 5, 13, 14, 20]. This mechanism likely accounts for more acute progression of PHH [16]. Reduction of CSF absorptive capacity represents an alternative etiology of PHH with a more prolonged or indolent course. Thromboembolic obstruction, deposition of hemorrhagic debris, or inflammation within arachnoid villi and granulations directly impairs CSF resorption into dural venous sinuses [1, 4, 14]. Additionally, intraventricular blood breakdown products and hemorrhagic debris may induce an inflammatory response leading to ependymitis, arachnoiditis, and gliosis [16, 17]. Prompted by an inflammatory cascade involving transforming growth factor-β (TGF-β) and other cytokines, the ensuing subarachnoid scarring, fibrosis, and adhesion formation impedes routine CSF flow and absorption [3–5, 9, 13, 14, 20, 21]. Gliosis and extracellular matrix deposition around the ventricular ependymal lining further impair CSF reabsorption through transependymal channels [5, 13, 20].

Diagnosis

While the diagnosis of IVH and/or PHVD relies solely on imaging data, the designation of PHH incorporates both clinical and radiographic criteria. Head ultrasound (US) typically represents the initial and most frequently utilized imaging modality to evaluate for the presence of IVH. While obviating diagnostic radiation exposure (as compared to head computed tomography [CT]) and requiring less time for completion (as compared to magnetic resonance imaging [MRI]), Head US can be performed at the bedside and limits transport of patients from the neonatal intensive care unit (NICU). Serial studies offer time-dependent examination of ventricular size and IVH burden, to confirm the diagnosis of PHVD and assess the evolution of intraventricular blood products. Importantly, the presence of cystic PVL may contribute to ventricular dilation due to an ex-vacuo effect, thereby confounding the radiographic determination of progressive PHVD. Multiple radiographic measures have been used to confirm the presence of abnormal ventricular dilation, including ventricular volume, ventricular-brain ratio (VBR), Evans ratio or index (EI), and frontal/occipital horn ratio (FOR) (Table 8.1) [12, 22–25]. Various studies have confirmed the relative superiority of the FOR in correlating with true ventricular volume, as compared to other linear indices [22, 25, 26].

Following Head US, more definitive imaging studies (Brain MRI, Head CT) may provide enhanced visualization of the ventricular system, IVH burden, and surrounding cerebral parenchyma. Additionally, these imaging modalities may be used as adjuncts for surgical planning, including intraoperative frameless stereotaxis to augment ventricular catheter placement. Progressive PHVD demonstrated on serial imaging studies raises concern for the development of PHH in the appropriate clinical context.

Table 8.1 Radiographic measures of ventricular size

Radiographic measure	Definition	Quantity stratification	Advantages, disadvantages
Ventricular volume	Computed three-dimensional volume of ventricular system	–	Highly accurate More complex method; computerized technique Requires magnetic resonance imaging Less practical
Ventricular-brain ratio (VBR)	(Cross-sectional area of ventricular system)/(Cross-sectional area of total brain)[a]	~5 Normal ~7 Equivocal >10 Abnormal	Correlates well with ventricular volume More complex method; computerized technique
Evans ratio or index (EI)	(Maximum frontal horn width)/(Maximum biparietal diameter)	<0.3 Normal >0.3 Ventricular enlargement	Linear technique Applicable on multiple imaging modalities Correlates less accurately with ventricular volume
Frontal/occipital horn ratio (FOR)	[(Maximum frontal horn width) + (Maximum occipital horn width)]/[2 * (Maximum biparietal diameter)]	0.37 Normal >0.37 Ventricular enlargement	Linear technique Applicable on multiple imaging modalities Correlates well with ventricular volume

[a]Cross-sectional areas measured at the level of the body of the lateral ventricle. Information from: 1. O'Hayon et al. [22]. 2. Sari et al. [23]. 3. Synek and Reuben [24]. 4. Ragan et al. [25].

The diagnosis of PHH requires the combination of radiographic findings described above and clinical signs or symptoms suggesting elevated ICP. Clinical symptoms that may reflect elevated ICP in premature neonates include:

- Somnolence or lethargy.
- Excessive irritability or fussiness.
- Frequent emesis or inability to tolerate oral intake.

Physical exam findings that may reflect elevated ICP include:

- Vital sign abnormalities including episodes of bradycardia, desaturation, or apnea.
- Increasing head circumference (HC) across percentiles.
- Splitting or splaying of the cranial sutures.
- Elevation and/or firmness of the anterior fontanelle.
- Vertical upgaze palsy or paresis (often described as ocular "sun-downing").
- Prominence of scalp veins (typically late finding).

Treatment

The development of PHH reflects an imbalance between CSF production and absorption that typically requires surgical treatment via CSF diversion. Indications for operative intervention include progressive ventriculomegaly on serial imaging studies, increasing frontal-occipital head circumference (HC) across percentiles (without subsequent plateau), fullness of the anterior fontanelle (AF) with or without splitting or splaying of the cranial sutures, vital sign changes, including episodes of apnea or bradycardia, upgaze palsy, or other clinical signs suggesting elevated ICP [27]. Patients requiring surgical intervention may fulfill one or more of these criteria depending on the clinical scenario. Following the decision to treat, further planning involves timing of intervention and the specific type of surgical intervention employed.

Temporizing Measures

Prior to definitive therapy, patients may require temporizing measures due to inadequate body weight, immature immune systems, or concurrent medical comorbidities (infection, sepsis, oscillator requirements) that preclude operative intervention. The risks of skin breakdown, infection, inadequate absorption within the intraperitoneal space, necrotizing enterocolitis, or mechanical obstruction of shunt components by intraventricular blood breakdown products warrant postponing definitive therapy [7, 28]. Prior studies investigating early shunt insertion in the setting of prematurity and PHH have shown high rates of shunt failure due to malfunction or infection, further justifying the delay of permanent shunt insertion until adequate body weight and reduction of CSF blood or protein levels [5].

Despite the lack of evidence-based guidelines for timing of definitive therapy, many pediatric centers employ a threshold of at least 2.0 kilograms (kg) body weight before considering VPS insertion [1, 5, 12, 21, 29, 30]. In a prospective study, the Hydrocephalus Clinical Research Network (HCRN) developed a set of rubrics or guidelines regarding management of PHH (based on ventricular size, body weight, and clinical signs), which have been implemented by multiple centers [31]. Premature infants with lower body weight (<1800–2000 g) or other contraindications to definitive therapy may benefit from temporizing measures that relieve intracranial pressure through temporary removal or diversion of CSF. Evidence-based guidelines do not support the use of nonsurgical temporizing measures, including intraventricular thrombolytic agents (tissue plasminogen activator, urokinase, streptokinase), acetazolamide, or furosemide to reduce rates of PHH requiring definitive therapy [5, 14, 17, 18, 20, 29, 31]. Additionally, a previous multicenter randomized controlled trial showed that a combination strategy involving intraventricular drainage, irrigation, and fibrinolytic therapy ("DRIFT") did not significantly reduce rates of death or permanent shunting as compared to standard therapy with lumbar puncture (LP) and ventricular access device (VAD) insertion [20]. This proposed treatment modality was abandoned after causing higher rates of secondary IVH (35%) leading to greater frequency of blood transfusions and permanent shunt insertion [5, 17, 18, 20]. However, a longer-term (2 year) follow-up study demonstrated reduced rates of mortality and severe cognitive disability following DRIFT as compared to standard therapy (LPs, VAD insertion) [17].

Procedures and Surgical Temporizing Measures

Procedural or surgical temporizing measures include LP, trans-fontanelle ventricular tap, external ventricular drain (EVD) placement, or insertion of a ventriculosubgaleal shunt (VSGS) or VAD. The former interventions (LP, ventricular tap) allow acute relief of elevated ICP in patients medically unfit for the surgical theatre. Additionally, LP or trans-fontanelle ventricular tap allows sampling of CSF to investigate the presence of meningitis prior to VSGS or VAD insertion, in the appropriate clinical context. However, evidence-based guidelines do not support the routine use of serial LPs to halt the progression of PHH or to avoid permanent CSF diversion [20, 29, 32]. Additionally, trans-fontanelle ventricular taps should be used sparingly due to risks of intraparenchymal hemorrhage, subdural hemorrhage, or iatrogenic frontal lobe porencephaly (Fig. 8.8) [7].

Insertion of an EVD may be performed at bedside in the neonatal intensive care unit (NICU) or preferably within the more controlled and sterile setting of the operating room. Following ventriculostomy through a frontal approach into the frontal horn of the lateral ventricle, CSF drainage may be controlled at a rate of 10–20 ml/kg per day [5]. However, this approach presents several potential challenges, including risks of skin breakdown around the externalized catheter and logistical challenges of EVD management in the NICU. Furthermore, risks of CSF leakage and infection mandate strict adherence to infection-prevention protocols [5]. Previously

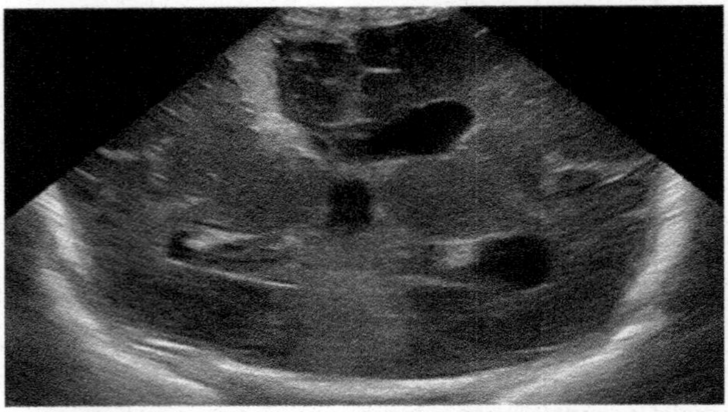

Fig. 8.8 Complications following trans-fontanelle ventricular tap. Complications following a trans-fontanelle ventricular tap may include intraparenchymal hemorrhage along the tract and extra-axial hemorrhage, both depicted in this coronal view of a head ultrasound

published rates of infection following EVD insertion reached as high as 60% [11]. With similar rates of permanent shunt placement as compared to VSGS or VAD insertion [5, 21, 28], EVD insertion typically does not represent first-line therapy for temporary CSF diversion in premature infants with PHH at most major pediatric academic neurosurgical centers.

As alternative measures, VSGS or VAD insertion allow displacement of CSF from the ventricular compartment into a contained subgaleal pocket below the scalp (VSGS) or to the external environment via percutaneous aspiration (VAD). Assuming patency of the subgaleal pocket, VSGS insertion reduces the need for serial percutaneous CSF aspirations in comparison to VAD insertion [12]. Reducing the number of percutaneous exposures may decrease the risk of infection, CSF leakage, and skin breakdown that may complicate up to 5–15% of VAD insertions [5, 12, 28, 29, 33]. In contrast, VAD insertion offers theoretical advantages of evacuating intraventricular blood breakdown products and challenging or promoting CSF absorptive capacity [28, 31]. Percutaneous aspirations may be performed daily, with removal of 10–20 ml CSF/kg (body weight) per day [5]. Close attention must be directed toward serum sodium levels and overall fluid status following serial aspirations due to the risk of hyponatremia, often requiring fluid replacement with saline [5]. Both VAD and VSGS insertion appear preferable to EVD placement. In addition to lower morbidity and mortality rates reported with the use of VADs as opposed to EVDs, VSGS or VAD insertion avoids many of the logistical challenges present with EVD management [29, 34].

Given the lack of superiority demonstrated with either approach, the decision between VAD and VSGS insertion typically relies upon training and surgeon preference. Various retrospective and prospective studies have compared specific outcome measures following VSGS and VAD insertion with mixed results. While one multicenter study demonstrated a significantly lower rate of conversion to permanent CSF diversion following VAD (69%) than VSGS (86%) insertion, a subsequent large single institution study showed no statistically significant difference between VAD (75%) and VSGS (67%) insertion regarding future shunt dependence [21, 28]. Neither study demonstrated statistically significant differences in the rates of device (VAD or VSGS) infection or shunt infection during the initial 6 months following permanent shunt insertion [21, 28]. In a prospective study performed by the HCRN,

Wellons et al. found no significant difference in rates of permanent shunting or infection between VSGS and VAD cohorts, while demonstrating high (90%) compliance rates with surgical decision-making protocols [31]. A separate single-institution retrospective study demonstrated longer time intervals before and greater mean body weights at the time of permanent shunt placement in PHH patients undergoing VSGS as opposed to VAD insertion, potentially reflecting better surgical candidacy for definitive therapy in the VSGS cohort [12]. While suggesting a nonsignificant trend for more frequent positive CSF cultures in the VAD cohort, this study demonstrated no significant differences in rates of device (VSGS or VAD) infection, VP shunt insertion, or early VP shunt infection following definitive therapy [12].

Ventricular Shunt Insertion

Following close observation or temporizing measures, a subset of patients with IVH and subsequent PHVD will continue to exhibit radiographic and clinical signs of PHH. As discussed above, permanent modes of intervention typically require a threshold body weight greater than or equal to 2.0–2.5 kg [5, 12, 20, 21, 29, 30, 35]. Increasing HC, progressive ventricular dilation, and/or clinical evidence of elevated ICP following conservative management or temporizing measures suggest the need for definitive therapy. VPS insertion represents the typical permanent treatment strategy for premature infants with IVH and subsequent PHH [10]. However, contraindications (history of necrotizing enterocolitis, extensive abdominal surgery, or prior intraperitoneal infection) to intraperitoneal insertion of the distal catheter warrant consideration of other distal termini, including the internal jugular vein leading ultimately to the superior vena cava and right atrial junction (ventriculoatrial shunt [VAS]). A VPS contains multiple components, including the ventricular catheter, reservoir (may or may not be present, depending on surgeon preference), shunt valve, and distal catheter (Fig. 8.9). Adjunctive measures may be used to augment ventricular catheter insertion, including intraoperative frameless stereotaxis or intraoperative ultrasound.

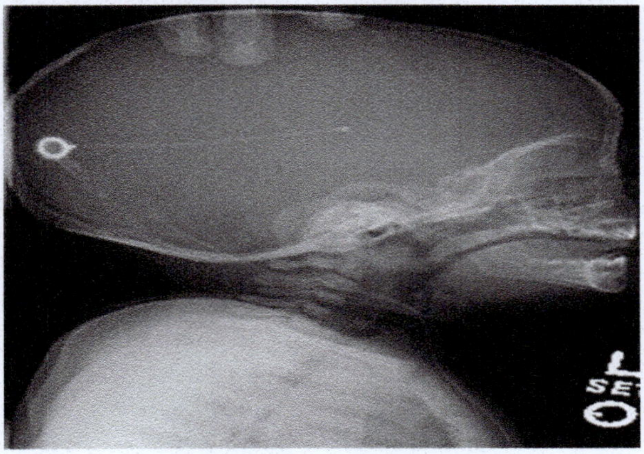

Fig. 8.9 Components of ventriculoperitoneal shunt (VPS). This postoperative lateral shunt series X-ray demonstrates the multiple components of a standard VPS, including ventricular catheter, reservoir, valve, and distal catheter

Since their introduction in the 1950s, VPS and shunt valve designs have reduced hydrocephalus related mortality significantly. However, patients with permanent indwelling shunt systems (VPS, VAS, etc.) remain at risk for shunt failure and/or infection during their lifetime. Unfortunately, premature infants with IVH and PHH exhibit increased susceptibility to shunt infection and malfunction due to immature immune systems, poor skin quality, increased epidermal bacterial colonization, previous episodes of infection or sepsis, elevated CSF protein levels, and increased CSF viscosity [10, 28, 30, 31]. A large prospective observational study performed by the HCRN identified three significant risk factors for shunt failure (malfunction or infection) in children following initial shunt insertion—age younger than 6 months at the time of insertion, use of neuroendoscopy to augment placement, and cardiac comorbidity [36]. This study reported a 33.2% rate of shunt failure with overall shunt infection rate of 7.6% over a 3-year period in children undergoing first-time definitive ventricular shunt insertion [36]. A separate study by the HCRN demonstrated an 18% risk reduction in time to first shunt failure for children undergoing insertion at one of the seven original HCRN centers (2008–2012) as compared to historical controls from the 1990s [37]. Despite this improvement in shunt survival, shunt failure remains a paramount concern for hydrocephalic patients, families, and care-providers.

The potential morbidity and burden created by instances of shunt malfunction or infection impact patients' lives significantly. Rates of shunt failure or infection requiring operative revision may reach as high as 45–50% within the first 2 years after shunt insertion [10, 13]. Simon et al. reported 1-year per-patient and per-procedure shunt infection rates of 21% and 10%, respectively, in a large single-center retrospective cohort study [38]. Despite showing higher per-patient risks of shunt infection (typically 6–8% in published literature), this study demonstrated externally consistent findings of time to shunt infection (median 3 weeks) following surgery [38]. The risk of shunt infection (4–13%, per procedure) remains greatest during the first 6 months following insertion (especially during the first 2 months), with subsequent decline in risk [13, 21, 28, 30, 36, 38–42]. Young patient age (0–6 months) and the presence of a gastrostomy tube at the time of shunt insertion independently increase the risk of shunt infection [38, 41]. Furthermore, one (3- to 4-fold higher) or multiple (6- to 13-fold higher) shunt revisions significantly increase the risk for future shunt infections [38, 41, 43]. Shunt infections typically result from gram-positive organisms, mainly staphylococcal species (80–90%), but may result from gram-negative organisms as well [39, 40].

Multiple techniques have been developed and adopted to reduce the frequency of shunt failure by infection or obstruction. Sterile aseptic surgical technique and preoperative antibiotics represent standard measures to decrease risk of infection in shunt (and most other) neurosurgical procedures [10, 30, 42, 44]. Standardized protocols for CSF shunt insertion have been developed and explored in multiple studies, with consistent results demonstrating lower infection rates in compliant as compared to noncompliant procedures [42, 44]. In separate studies organized by the HCRN, Kestle et al. reported significantly decreased infection rates for shunt insertion and revision (8.8% to 5.7%, 2011; 8.7% to 5.0%, 2016) through protocol compliance at multiple HCRN centers (with an overall compliance rate of 75–77%) [42, 44]. In addition to prior algorithms, antibiotic-impregnated catheters (AICs) have been investigated retrospectively and prospectively, with consistent results demonstrating decreased shunt infection rates [39, 40]. This benefit extends to permanent shunt insertion within hydrocephalic infants, including those with prematurity and PHH [30]. Engineered with Clindamycin and Rifampin (bactericidal agents), AICs attempt to reduce shunt infection from colonized skin flora (mainly gram-positive staphylococcal species) from the time of shunt insertion [30, 39, 40]. Interestingly, addition of AICs to the previous HCRN standardized protocol did not reduce infection risk further in an updated HCRN study (6.0% vs. 5.7%) [44].

Endoscopic Third Ventriculostomy (ETV) with/without Choroid Plexus Cauterization (ETV/CPC)

As an alternative to ventricular shunt insertion, endoscopic third ventriculostomy (ETV) represents a treatment modality for CSF diversion that avoids insertion of permanent hardware. Traditionally, ETV had been used selectively in children or adults with obstructive hydrocephalus, especially those with aqueductal stenosis. Given low rates of ETV success in patients with IVH and PHH, especially premature infants below age 6–12 months, choroid plexus cauterization (CPC) has been added as an adjunct to augment success rates [10, 13, 45–47]. Through cauterization of choroid plexus within the bodies and temporal horns of both lateral ventricles, CPC attempts to enhance endoscopic treatment of hydrocephalus by reducing bulk CSF production and blunting the amplitude of periodic CSF pulsations [46]. Prospective studies in Uganda and North America have demonstrated encouraging overall success rates (52–66%) of ETV/CPC in infants with hydrocephalus [46–48]. Studies focusing more specifically on premature infants with PHH have demonstrated lower success rates (37%) with ETV/CPC [13].

Several factors increase the risk of ETV/CPC failure, including previous meningitis or ventriculitis with postinfectious hydrocephalus; more severe IVH (Grade IV); age less than 6 months; history of prior CSF diversion with ventricular shunting; and prepontine cistern scarring, adhesions, or narrowing [13, 46]. Absence of these risk factors may appreciably increase ETV/CPC success rates to warrant strong consideration of this treatment modality in appropriate patients [46, 47].

Survival, Outcomes, and Neurocognitive Development

Intraventricular hemorrhage represents a significant cause of morbidity and mortality in the premature neonatal population. Largely due to improvements in obstetric and neonatal care, mortality rates for prematurity and IVH have declined since the early 1980s [10]. Severity of IVH represents a primary determining factor of survival, with higher grades (Grade III and IV IVH) conferring a greater risk of mortality. Previous retrospective studies have reported overall mortality rates of up to 20% for IVH, with rates as high as 59% for patients with Grade IV IVH [1, 2]. A recent retrospective study in the Netherlands reported improved but persistently high mortality rates for premature infants with Grade III (28%) and Grade IV (37%) IVH [18]. The development of PHH further exacerbates rates of mortality. In contrast, patients with lower grade IVH (Grade I or II) have demonstrated lower rates of mortality in retrospective studies, between 2% and 20% [1].

Despite increased survival rates of premature infants with VLBW or ELBW and successful treatments for PHH, patients may still experience severe medical comorbidities and long-term disability [1–3, 5, 9, 17]. Neurocognitive outcomes for many patients with history of prematurity, IVH, and PHH remain poor despite advancements in neonatal and neurosurgical care [13, 15, 17]. Severity of IVH (especially the presence of Grade IV IVH and the extent of intraparenchymal hemorrhagic infarction) remains a strong predictor of survival, cognitive and motor outcomes, and seizure risk for preterm infants with PHH [1, 7, 11, 17]. Many patients with prematurity and IVH remain at high risk for developing cerebral palsy (CP) and epilepsy as well [1, 9, 10, 15, 18, 49]. The presence of PVHI (Grade IV IVH), especially bilateral PVHI, dictates an especially high risk for developing CP (up to 49–53%) in contrast to the remaining grades of IVH [10, 18, 35]. Notably, the combination of prematurity with low grade GMH or IVH (Grade I-II) did not adversely impact neurocognitive development at corrected age 2 years within a retrospective case-control study [49]. Similarly, 56% of patients with Grade I IVH demonstrated good outcomes (without obvious neurological deficits) in retrospective studies with more prolonged follow-up (up to 15 years) [1].

In contrast, higher grade IVH (Grade III–IV) portends a worse prognosis regarding motor and cognitive developmental outcomes and functional independence [9, 1, 3, 5, 10]. Severe IVH, with or without PHH requiring shunt insertion, represents a significant risk factor for neurodevelopmental impairment as assessed by the Bayley Scales of Infant Development IIR, including the Mental Development Index (MDI) and Psychomotor Development Index (PDI) [9]. Premature infants with PHH requiring shunt insertion exhibit further deficits in motor and cognitive performance based on MDI and PDI assessments at 18–22 months corrected age [9]. Retrospective studies using other measures of neurodevelopmental outcomes, including the Griffiths' Mental Developmental Scale (GMDS), have shown similarly poor outcomes for premature infants with Grade IV IVH and PHVD requiring intervention [18]. Ultimately, this may lead to moderate or severe neurocognitive impairment and poor neurodevelopmental outcomes during early childhood [1, 3, 9]. With prolonged follow-up into adolescence, patients with history of severe IVH similarly show high rates of neurological disability. Up to 70% of these patients may exhibit signs of mental retardation while greater than 90% may require augmented school services [9].

Complications of treatment for PHH may further exacerbate neurocognitive impairment. For instance, shunt infection portends a worse prognosis for cognitive development and academic performance, while increasing the risk of seizures and psychomotor retardation [39, 40]. While difficult to quantify, the occurrence of shunt malfunctions and associated surgical revisions may also impact neurocognitive development given transient increases in ICP, multiple anesthetic settings, and disruptions to school performance. These presumed effects may impact many patients with hydrocephalus, as shunt malfunction occurs in up to 80% of patients with a VPS in prolonged follow-up [13]. However, some retrospective studies have failed to show any significant differences in long-term functional outcomes between IVH patients with or without VP shunt insertion (and multiple surgical revisions) after prolonged follow-up [1]. Despite overall grim forecasts for neurocognitive development, recent studies have demonstrated some improvement in neurological development for premature infants with IVH, largely due to improved neonatal care [10, 18]. For instance, a recent small retrospective study in the Netherlands demonstrated encouraging results for premature infants with severe IVH and PHH requiring intervention, with nearly 60% of patients lacking major cognitive or motor impairments on prolonged follow-up (age 5–8 years) [35].

Current Research

Current research endeavors involving PHH focus on the pathophysiologic mechanism of IVH occurrence and PHH development along with potential neuroprotective strategies to prevent consequent neurocognitive impairment. Several studies have investigated the role of inflammatory mediators in the evolution of PHH. The following inflammatory cytokines have been studied and found to be elevated in CSF from premature infants with PHH: interleukin-1β (IL-1β), IL-6, IL-8, IL-18, interferon-γ, tumor necrosis factor α, and TGF-β [9, 14, 16]. While the exact role of these inflammatory mediators remains unknown, their potential contribution to the development of PHH offers exciting research opportunities focusing on the diagnosis, prevention, and treatment of PHH. Based on current literature, TGF-β appears to offer potential as a CSF biomarker with diagnostic and prognostic utility in PHH [16]. Additional research endeavors have focused on the potential role of other CSF biomarkers as adjuncts to physical exam and imaging parameters in the diagnosis and management of PHH. For instance, CSF levels of amyloid precursor protein, and neural cell adhesion molecule-L1 to a lesser extent, have shown strong association with ventricular size (as measured by FOR) throughout the course of PHH diagnosis and treatment [15].

Research involving neuroprotective or restorative strategies has targeted caffeine, erythropoietin, and stem cells as potential agents of therapy for patients with IVH and PHH. Based on its activity as a pluripotent cytokine that promotes neural cell survival and differentiation, erythropoietin has shown encouraging results in animal studies and smaller clinical trials with effects of reducing histological brain damage and improving neurological outcome measures [10]. Similarly, umbilical cord stem cells or induced pluripotent stem cells may help promote neural cell growth and differentiation by reducing local inflammation and secreting neurotrophic factors [10]. Investigations into antenatal and postnatal treatments have resulted in two findings—maternal administration of corticosteroids and neonatal administration of indomethacin—that may reduce the risk of IVH in prematurity [4].

Multiple different animal models have been explored to mimic the development of GMH and PHH in premature infants. Among the different species trialed (dogs, pigs, rabbits, sheep, mice, rats), neonatal rats injected with various agents (autologous blood, collagenase, hemoglobin, iron) have shown the most encouraging results to model the development of PHH and subsequent neurological sequelae [4, 14, 19]. These animal models allow for the trial of various agents theorized to prevent the progression of IVH to PHH. For instance, intraventricular thrombolytic therapy remains a potential research strategy despite previous safety concerns with tissue plasminogen activator (tPA). More recent rat models have shown improved functional recovery following intraventricular injection of urokinase-type plasminogen activator (uPA) without complications related to inflammation associated with tPA [14]. Enhancing early red blood cell (RBC) phagocytosis and preventing RBC lysis through complement inhibition represent other potential methods of PHH prevention by reducing intraventricular hemoglobin release [4, 14]. Recognizing the contribution of hemoglobin, iron, and oxygen free radicals in the development of PHH has offered multiple potential therapeutic targets through iron chelation (deferoxamine, minocycline) and free-radical scavenging (edaravone) [4, 14]. The important roles of TGF-β and subarachnoid fibrosis in pathologic CSF flow dynamics have offered other potential avenues for PHH prevention through cytokine inhibition and subarachnoid fibrinolysis [14].

References

1. Vassilyadi M, Tataryn Z, Shamji MF, Ventureyra EC. Functional outcomes among premature infants with intraventricular hemorrhage. Pediatr Neurosurg. 2009;45(4):247–55.
2. Ahn SY, Shim SY, Sung IK. Intraventricular hemorrhage and post hemorrhagic hydrocephalus among very-low-birth-weight infants in Korea. J Korean Med Sci. 2015;30(Suppl 1):S52–8.
3. Klinger G, Osovsky M, Boyko V, Sokolover N, Sirota L, Lerner-Geva L, et al. Risk factors associated with post-hemorrhagic hydrocephalus among very low birth weight infants of 24-28 weeks gestation. J Perinatol. 2016;36(7):557–63.
4. Strahle J, Garton HJ, Maher CO, Muraszko KM, Keep RF, Xi G. Mechanisms of hydrocephalus after neonatal and adult intraventricular hemorrhage. Transl Stroke Res. 2012;3(Suppl 1):25–38.
5. Ellenbogen JR, Waqar M, Pettorini B. Management of post-haemorrhagic hydrocephalus in premature infants. J Clin Neurosci. 2016;31:30–4.
6. Lemons JA, Bauer CR, Oh W, Korones SB, Papile LA, Stoll BJ, et al. Very low birth weight outcomes of the National Institute of Child health and human development neonatal research network, January 1995 through December 1996. NICHD Neonatal Research Network. Pediatrics. 2001;107(1):E1.
7. Christian EA, Melamed EF, Peck E, Krieger MD, McComb JG. Surgical management of hydrocephalus secondary to intraventricular hemorrhage in the preterm infant. J Neurosurg Pediatr. 2016;17(3):278–84.
8. Stoll BJ, Hansen NI, Bell EF, Shankaran S, Laptook AR, Walsh MC, et al. Neonatal outcomes of extremely preterm infants from the NICHD Neonatal Research Network. Pediatrics. 2010;126(3):443–56.

9. Adams-Chapman I, Hansen NI, Stoll BJ, Higgins R. Neurodevelopmental outcome of extremely low birth weight infants with posthemorrhagic hydrocephalus requiring shunt insertion. Pediatrics. 2008;121(5):e1167–77.
10. Robinson S. Neonatal posthemorrhagic hydrocephalus from prematurity: pathophysiology and current treatment concepts. J Neurosurg Pediatr. 2012;9(3):242–58.
11. Levy ML, Masri LS, McComb JG. Outcome for preterm infants with germinal matrix hemorrhage and progressive hydrocephalus. Neurosurgery. 1997;41(5):1111–7. discussion 7-8
12. Wang JY, Amin AG, Jallo GI, Ahn ES. Ventricular reservoir versus ventriculosubgaleal shunt for posthemorrhagic hydrocephalus in preterm infants: infection risks and ventriculoperitoneal shunt rate. J Neurosurg Pediatr. 2014;14(5):447–54.
13. Chamiraju P, Bhatia S, Sandberg DI, Ragheb J. Endoscopic third ventriculostomy and choroid plexus cauterization in posthemorrhagic hydrocephalus of prematurity. J Neurosurg Pediatr. 2014;13(4):433–9.
14. Chen Q, Feng Z, Tan Q, Guo J, Tang J, Tan L, et al. Post-hemorrhagic hydrocephalus: recent advances and new therapeutic insights. J Neurol Sci. 2017;375:220–30.
15. Morales DM, Holubkov R, Inder TE, Ahn HC, Mercer D, Rao R, et al. Cerebrospinal fluid levels of amyloid precursor protein are associated with ventricular size in post-hemorrhagic hydrocephalus of prematurity. PLoS One. 2015;10(3):e0115045.
16. Merhar S. Biomarkers in neonatal posthemorrhagic hydrocephalus. Neonatology. 2012;101(1):1–7.
17. Whitelaw A, Jary S, Kmita G, Wroblewska J, Musialik-Swietlinska E, Mandera M, et al. Randomized trial of drainage, irrigation and fibrinolytic therapy for premature infants with posthemorrhagic ventricular dilatation: developmental outcome at 2 years. Pediatrics. 2010;125(4):e852–8.
18. Brouwer A, Groenendaal F, van Haastert IL, Rademaker K, Hanlo P, de Vries L. Neurodevelopmental outcome of preterm infants with severe intraventricular hemorrhage and therapy for post-hemorrhagic ventricular dilatation. J Pediatr. 2008;152(5):648–54.
19. Lekic T, Manaenko A, Rolland W, Krafft PR, Peters R, Hartman RE, et al. Rodent neonatal germinal matrix hemorrhage mimics the human brain injury, neurological consequences, and post-hemorrhagic hydrocephalus. Exp Neurol. 2012;236(1):69–78.
20. Whitelaw A, Evans D, Carter M, Thoresen M, Wroblewska J, Mandera M, et al. Randomized clinical trial of prevention of hydrocephalus after intraventricular hemorrhage in preterm infants: brain-washing versus tapping fluid. Pediatrics. 2007;119(5):e1071–8.
21. Limbrick DD Jr, Mathur A, Johnston JM, Munro R, Sagar J, Inder T, et al. Neurosurgical treatment of progressive posthemorrhagic ventricular dilation in preterm infants: a 10-year single-institution study. J Neurosurg Pediatr. 2010;6(3):224–30.
22. O'Hayon BB, Drake JM, Ossip MG, Tuli S, Clarke M. Frontal and occipital horn ratio: a linear estimate of ventricular size for multiple imaging modalities in pediatric hydrocephalus. Pediatr Neurosurg. 1998;29(5):245–9.
23. Sari E, Sari S, Akgun V, Ozcan E, Ince S, Babacan O, et al. Measures of ventricles and evans' index: from neonate to adolescent. Pediatr Neurosurg. 2015;50(1):12–7.
24. Synek V, Reuben JR. The ventricular-brain ratio using planimetric measurement of EMI scans. Br J Radiol. 1976;49(579):233–7.
25. Ragan DK, Cerqua J, Nash T, McKinstry RC, Shimony JS, Jones BV, et al. The accuracy of linear indices of ventricular volume in pediatric hydrocephalus: technical note. J Neurosurg Pediatr. 2015;15(6):547–51.
26. Mandell JG, Kulkarni AV, Warf BC, Schiff SJ. Volumetric brain analysis in neurosurgery: Part 2. Brain and CSF volumes discriminate neurocognitive outcomes in hydrocephalus. J Neurosurg Pediatr. 2015;15(2):125–32.
27. Adzick NS, Thom EA, Spong CY, Brock JW 3rd, Burrows PK, Johnson MP, et al. A randomized trial of prenatal versus postnatal repair of myelomeningocele. N Engl J Med. 2011;364(11):993–1004.
28. Wellons JC, Shannon CN, Kulkarni AV, Simon TD, Riva-Cambrin J, Whitehead WE, et al. A multicenter retrospective comparison of conversion from temporary to permanent cerebro-

spinal fluid diversion in very low birth weight infants with posthemorrhagic hydrocephalus. J Neurosurg Pediatr. 2009;4(1):50–5.
29. Mazzola CA, Choudhri AF, Auguste KI, Limbrick DD Jr, Rogido M, Mitchell L, et al. Pediatric hydrocephalus: systematic literature review and evidence-based guidelines. Part 2: Management of posthemorrhagic hydrocephalus in premature infants. J Neurosurg Pediatr. 2014;14(Suppl 1):8–23.
30. Sciubba DM, Noggle JC, Carson BS, Jallo GI. Antibiotic-impregnated shunt catheters for the treatment of infantile hydrocephalus. Pediatr Neurosurg. 2008;44(2):91–6.
31. Wellons JC 3rd, Shannon CN, Holubkov R, Riva-Cambrin J, Kulkarni AV, Limbrick DD Jr, et al. Shunting outcomes in posthemorrhagic hydrocephalus: results of a Hydrocephalus Clinical Research Network prospective cohort study. J Neurosurg Pediatr. 2017;20(1):19–29.
32. Whitelaw A. Repeated lumbar or ventricular punctures in newborns with intraventricular hemorrhage. Cochrane Database Syst Rev. 2001;1:CD000216.
33. Lam HP, Heilman CB. Ventricular access device versus ventriculosubgaleal shunt in post hemorrhagic hydrocephalus associated with prematurity. J Matern Fetal Neonatal Med. 2009;22(11):1097–101.
34. Gurtner P, Bass T, Gudeman SK, Penix JO, Philput CB, Schinco FP. Surgical management of posthemorrhagic hydrocephalus in 22 low-birth-weight infants. Childs Nerv Syst. 1992;8(4):198–202.
35. Brouwer AJ, van Stam C, Uniken Venema M, Koopman C, Groenendaal F, de Vries LS. Cognitive and neurological outcome at the age of 5-8 years of preterm infants with post-hemorrhagic ventricular dilatation requiring neurosurgical intervention. Neonatology. 2012;101(3):210–6.
36. Riva-Cambrin J, Kestle JR, Holubkov R, Butler J, Kulkarni AV, Drake J, et al. Risk factors for shunt malfunction in pediatric hydrocephalus: a multicenter prospective cohort study. J Neurosurg Pediatr. 2016;17(4):382–90.
37. Kulkarni AV, Riva-Cambrin J, Butler J, Browd SR, Drake JM, Holubkov R, et al. Outcomes of CSF shunting in children: comparison of Hydrocephalus Clinical Research Network cohort with historical controls: clinical article. J Neurosurg Pediatr. 2013;12(4):334–8.
38. Simon TD, Whitlock KB, Riva-Cambrin J, Kestle JR, Rosenfeld M, Dean JM, et al. Revision surgeries are associated with significant increased risk of subsequent cerebrospinal fluid shunt infection. Pediatr Infect Dis J. 2012;31(6):551–6.
39. Sciubba DM, Stuart RM, McGirt MJ, Woodworth GF, Samdani A, Carson B, et al. Effect of antibiotic-impregnated shunt catheters in decreasing the incidence of shunt infection in the treatment of hydrocephalus. J Neurosurg. 2005;103(2 Suppl):131–6.
40. Govender ST, Nathoo N, van Dellen JR. Evaluation of an antibiotic-impregnated shunt system for the treatment of hydrocephalus. J Neurosurg. 2003;99(5):831–9.
41. Simon TD, Butler J, Whitlock KB, Browd SR, Holubkov R, Kestle JR, et al. Risk factors for first cerebrospinal fluid shunt infection: findings from a multi-center prospective cohort study. J Pediatr. 2014;164(6):1462–8.e2.
42. Kestle JR, Riva-Cambrin J, Wellons JC 3rd, Kulkarni AV, Whitehead WE, Walker ML, et al. A standardized protocol to reduce cerebrospinal fluid shunt infection: the Hydrocephalus Clinical Research Network Quality Improvement Initiative. J Neurosurg Pediatr. 2011;8(1):22–9.
43. George R, Leibrock L, Epstein M. Long-term analysis of cerebrospinal fluid shunt infections. A 25-year experience. J Neurosurg. 1979;51(6):804–11.
44. Kestle JR, Holubkov R, Douglas Cochrane D, Kulkarni AV, Limbrick DD Jr, Luerssen TG, et al. A new Hydrocephalus Clinical Research Network protocol to reduce cerebrospinal fluid shunt infection. J Neurosurg Pediatr. 2016;17(4):391–6.
45. Kulkarni AV, Drake JM, Mallucci CL, Sgouros S, Roth J, Constantini S. Endoscopic third ventriculostomy in the treatment of childhood hydrocephalus. J Pediatr. 2009;155(2):254–9.e1.
46. Stone SS, Warf BC. Combined endoscopic third ventriculostomy and choroid plexus cauterization as primary treatment for infant hydrocephalus: a prospective North American series. J Neurosurg Pediatr. 2014;14(5):439–46.

47. Kulkarni AV, Riva-Cambrin J, Browd SR, Drake JM, Holubkov R, Kestle JR, et al. Endoscopic third ventriculostomy and choroid plexus cauterization in infants with hydrocephalus: a retrospective Hydrocephalus Clinical Research Network study. J Neurosurg Pediatr. 2014;14(3):224–9.
48. Warf BC. Comparison of endoscopic third ventriculostomy alone and combined with choroid plexus cauterization in infants younger than 1 year of age: a prospective study in 550 African children. J Neurosurg. 2005;103(6 Suppl):475–81.
49. Reubsaet P, Brouwer AJ, van Haastert IC, Brouwer MJ, Koopman C, Groenendaal F, et al. The impact of low-grade germinal matrix-intraventricular hemorrhage on neurodevelopmental outcome of very preterm infants. Neonatology. 2017;112(3):203–10.

Multiloculated Hydrocephalus: Diagnosis, Treatment, and Clinical Implications

9

Eric Anthony Sribnick

Introduction

Multiloculated hydrocephalus continues to represent a relatively rare but cumbersome surgical challenge which frequently requires repeat operations. This chapter covers multiloculated hydrocephalus from several perspectives, including diagnosis and evaluation, risk factors/etiology, treatment, and outcomes. Essential to discussing multiloculated hydrocephalus is defining the disease pattern. While terms like "loculated hydrocephalus" have been used to refer to both uniloculated and multiple loculations, this chapter focuses on cases with multiple isolated compartments. This is in contrast to single isolated compartments (e.g., as seen in patients with an entrapped ventricle). While the two disease processes may appear related, patients with single loculations may be more likely to tolerate treatment without the use of a cerebrospinal fluid (CSF) shunt, may present with a more benign clinical course, and tend to respond better to interventions [1–5]. In short, while cases of multiloculated hydrocephalus are rare, a discussion of this specific population is important because they tend to present with poorer neurological function, tend to require more frequent procedures, and are more likely to require a shunt. Much of the neurosurgical literature has used various terminologies in describing patients, and subsequently many of the studies presented do not discriminate between uniloculated and multiloculated hydrocephalus. Future studies could perhaps improve this situation by following a standard nomenclature in describing patients with ventricular loculation(s) [6].

E. A. Sribnick
Division of Neurosurgery, Nationwide Children's Hospital, Department of Neurosurgery, The Ohio State University College of Medicine, Columbus, OH, USA
e-mail: eric.sribnick@nationwidechildrens.org

D. D. Limbrick, J. R. Leonard (eds.), *Cerebrospinal Fluid Disorders*,
https://doi.org/10.1007/978-3-319-97928-1_9

History

In review of the literature, loculated hydrocephalus may have first been referenced by Harvey Cushing in 1908 [7]. In 1973, examination of the pathology revealed septations described as "filmy, translucent membranes" and microscopic analysis showed "fibroglial elements, ...polymorphonuclear cells" and "small areas of denuded ependymal and glial tufts extending through the denuded ependymal into the ventricular lumen" [8]. Additionally, they noted aqueductal stenosis secondary to inflammation and debris [8].

Epidemiology

While the prevalence of multiloculated hydrocephalus in the general population has not been directly addressed, there are data to suggest that it is rare. For instance, in the long-term follow-up (minimum 1 year) to the shunt design trial, loculated ventricles were noted in 2% of the population [9]. Again, in the multicenter prospective cohort study of the Strata valve, approximately 2% of patients were noted to have shunt malfunction secondary to loculated ventricles [10].

Risk Factors

Several factors have been associated with multiloculated hydrocephalus. Some of the first modern reports of multiloculated hydrocephalus were noted in patients with a history of neonatal meningitis [8, 11]. This finding is thought to be due to the propensity of neonates to develop ventriculitis with resultant intraventricular gliosis [12]. In at least two early reports of ventriculitis-related multiloculated hydrocephalus in neonates, authors describe that the septations are generally seen to divide the ventricles transversely [13, 14]. In this population, synechiae have also been described between the skull and dura mater [13]. In one study of patients with neonatal meningitis, septations in the ventricles were seen in 23% of patients examined by ventriculography [15].

Intraventricular hemorrhage in the neonate is another recognized risk factor for the subsequent development of multiloculated hydrocephalus [16]. In a single center study examining posthemorrhagic hydrocephalus over a 14-year period, 76 patients were identified with more than 6 months of follow-up, and 11 of those patients (approximately 14%) were noted to have ventricular loculation requiring further intervention [16]. Interestingly, 5 of the 11 had a history of ventriculitis [16]. While the small number of patients in this study makes it difficult to use for statistical analysis, there was no evidence that gender, estimated gestational age at birth, or use of a ventricular reservoir before placement of a final ventricular shunt correlated with later development of loculated hydrocephalus [16].

Spinal dysraphism is not typically recognized as a risk factor for multiloculated hydrocephalus; however, a single center study on myelomeningocele patients over a 10-year period noted 11 occurrences of loculated ventricles in 189 patients [17]. Again, in this specific patient population, shunt infection was noted to be much higher in first time shunt malfunctions (approximately 24%) [17] than seen in other shunt studies examining a more diverse patient population [9, 10].

Congenital disease can also lead to multiloculated hydrocephalus. Agenesis of the corpus callosum can be accompanied by cyst formation and potentially multiloculated hydrocephalus (Fig. 9.1) [18]. Neurosarcoidosis has also reportedly led to ventricular loculations [19].

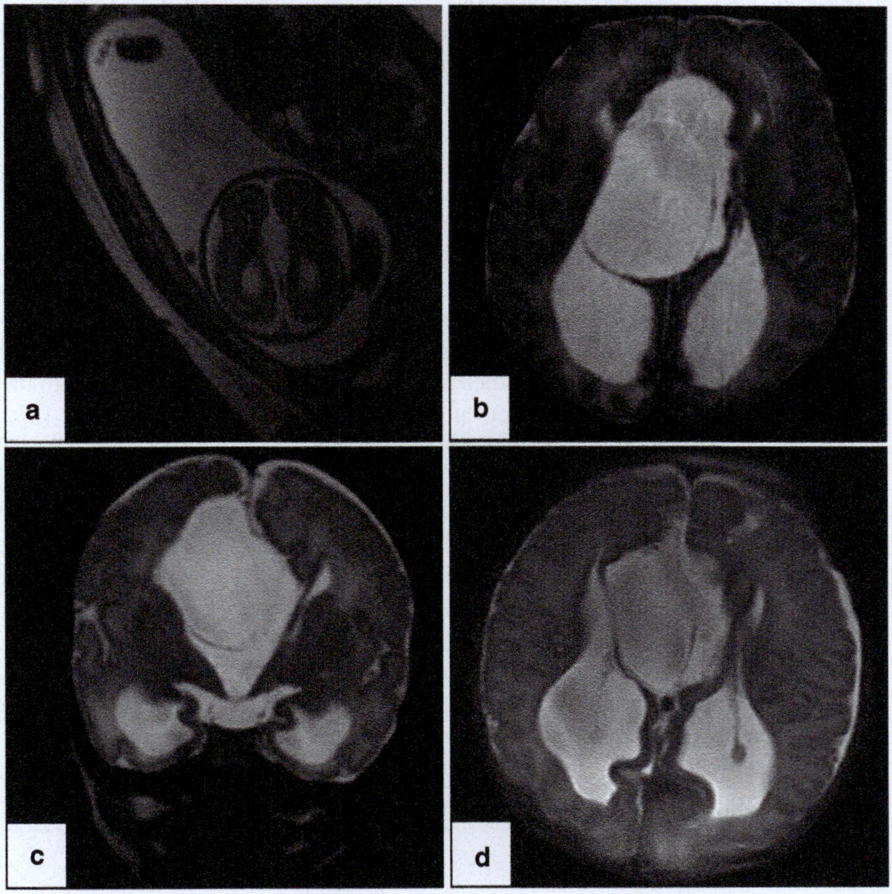

Fig. 9.1 MRI, T2 weighted images, demonstrate a neonate with agenesis of the corpus callosum and multiloculated hydrocephalus before and after surgery. (**a**) A prenatal MRI demonstrates a midline cyst, colpocephalic lateral ventricles, and agenesis of the corpus callosum. (**b**, **c**) Preoperative MRI images in the axial and coronal plane, respectively, demonstrate two midline cysts. (**d**) Surgery consisted of fenestration of the midline cysts into the posterior horn of the right lateral ventricle. Imaging on postoperative day 1 demonstrates reduction in volume of the lateral ventricles and the midline cysts

Diagnosis

Multiloculated hydrocephalus is a radiographic diagnosis which has been aided by the evolution of neuroradiographic techniques. Early studies evaluated multiloculated hydrocephalus by air ventriculography [8]. The utility of computed tomography (CT) was quickly recognized to demonstrate the complex and evolving anatomy of multiloculated hydrocephalus [11]. Early reports noted that the septae of multiloculated hydrocephalus may not initially be recognized on CT [11].

The development of magnetic resonance imaging (MRI) has added techniques particularly useful for studying multiloculated hydrocephalus. Constructive interference in steady-state, three-dimensional, Fourier transformation (CISS) MRI is a commonly used imaging technique which highlights detailed anatomy within fluid spaces, and CISS MRI can be used for both preoperative planning and for confirmation of fenestrations postoperatively [20]. Another MRI technique that can be applied to multiloculated hydrocephalus is phase-contrast imaging, which allows for observation of cerebrospinal fluid (CSF) flow dynamics by contrasting stationary and dynamic nuclei through pulsations from the cardiac cycle [21]. Phase contrast can be used to assess patency at natural ostia such as the foramen of Monro, Sylvian aqueduct, or the fourth ventricular outlets [22]. It can also be used to examine whether cysts communicate with the ventricular system, whether fenestrations are patent, and patency within a shunt system [22].

Other imaging techniques that are useful include CT contrast ventriculography, and contrast can be administered either by an intraventricular technique or into the lumbar intrathecal space if patency at the posterior fossa is in question [23]. Documented steps for this method of ventricular injection include aspiration of 15–20 mL of CSF; introduction of 5 mL of nonionic low osmolar contrast agent; introduction of 2 mL of the aspirated CSF as flush; and then 15–20 minutes of elevating, lowering, and rotating the patient's head prior to imaging [23].

The use of air in a diagnostic procedure for multiloculated hydrocephalus has recently been reintroduced. Using an endoscope and intraoperative ultrasound, one group described utilizing small amounts of air by cannulating the intended ventricular compartment, injecting 5 mL of air, and using the air as a marker with intraoperative ultrasound to fenestrate into the correct compartment [24]. A similar technique has been described using an intraoperative ultrasound to visualize jets of saline delivered by a ventricular catheter to document flow between compartments [25].

Treatment

As alluded to in the introduction, the treatment of multiloculated hydrocephalus can involve multiple surgeries. Prior to the introduction of the neuroradiographic and neuroendoscopic techniques that are commonplace in modern neurosurgery, multiloculated hydrocephalus was associated with a high mortality rate [14].

Placement of multiple shunts is one technique for treatment of multiloculated hydrocephalus, and this has been described in a case series describing nine patients with eight having two proximal catheters and one having three proximal catheters [26]. In this series, the mean follow-up time was 2.5 years, and there were six reported shunt revisions [26]. For those using multiple proximal catheters, the author did suggest that a single valve is preferable over multiple valves for "better equilibration of different pressures" [26].

Craniotomy has been used to fenestrate loculations with a goal of reducing the number of ventricular catheters or maintaining a shunt with a single ventricular catheter [5, 27]. One series documented using a parietal craniotomy and a 2–3 cm corticectomy, and the majority of patients were able to tolerate having a single proximal catheter [5]. Complications from this approach did include a greater than 10% infection rate, and the majority of patients required multiple fenestration surgeries [5]. Transcallosal fenestration has also been described, and in the six patients where this technique was described, there was a reduction in the number of shunt revisions following craniotomy when compared to the revision rate in the same patients prior to the craniotomy [27].

Neuroendoscopy may provide a less invasive method for cyst fenestration while accomplishing the same goal as craniotomy. In a series describing 34 patients with either multiloculated or uniloculated hydrocephalus, the authors noted a reduction in shunt revisions per year in both groups of patients; however, patients with multiloculated hydrocephalus still frequently required at least one shunt and often required multiple endoscopic procedures for fenestration of cysts [25]. Similarly, in another series describing the use of endoscopic fenestration in children less than 1-year-old, one patient had multiple loculations secondary to a neonatal infection, and the authors were able to successfully treat her with one shunt, but she required three separate fenestrations [2]. Treatment with neuroendoscopy and shunting versus shunting alone has been compared in a single center with a larger patient volume (127 children total), and study results demonstrated a reduction in the average number of procedures per year in patients treated utilizing neuroendoscopic fenestrations [3].

Endoscopic-assisted placement of a ventricular catheter was not shown to reduce the rate of malfunctions in shunt patients in general [28]. However, there has been suggestion that in patients with loculations, endoscopic assistance may be useful in proximal catheter placement [29].

In our own clinical experience, we have treated multiloculated hydrocephalus with the use of neuroendoscopy to attempt to reduce the number of required shunt catheters. We typically use thin-slice three-dimensional MRI sequences to study the anatomy preoperatively and for use with neuronavigation during surgery. Electromagnetic navigation using a flexible stylet (Medtronic AxiEM, Minneapolis, MN) allows for placement of the stylet through one of the working channels on the endoscope, allowing for real-time neuronavigation of the endoscope. Such a technique of using simultaneous neuronavigation and endoscopic visualization has been described previously [30], but with newer designs, there is no longer a need to affix a reference frame to the cranium. We use a technique of making multiple perforations in the cyst wall: first cauterizing the cyst wall, puncturing with a blunt or sharp instrument, making additional small fenestrations in the surrounding area, and then

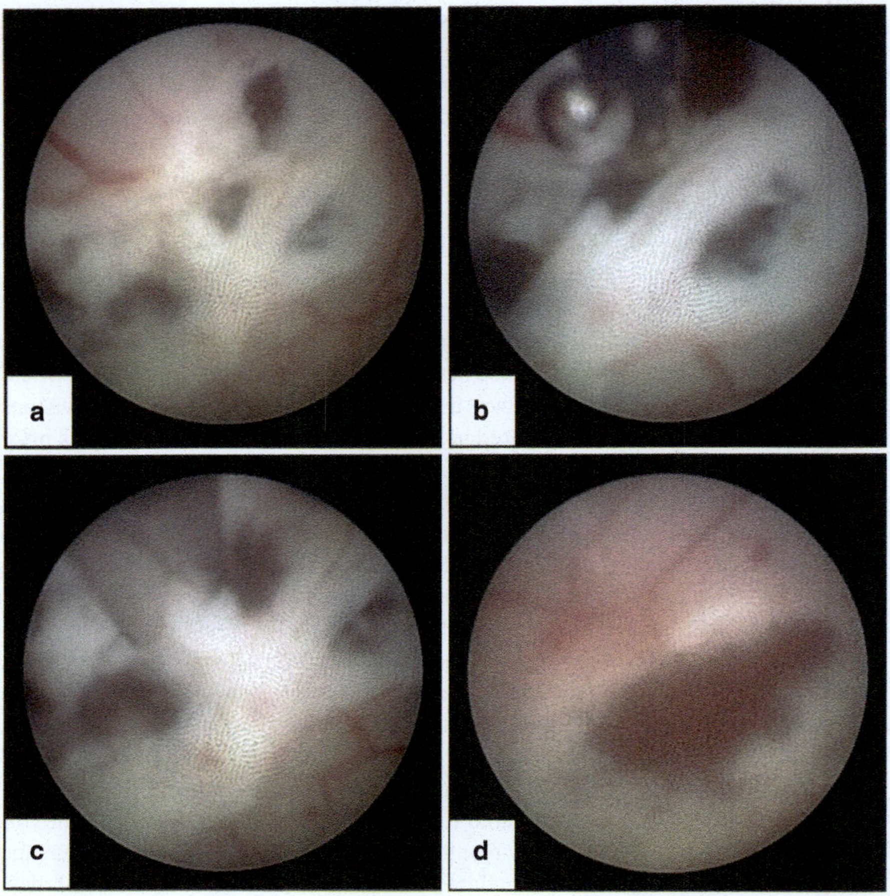

Fig. 9.2 Images from a neuroendoscopy case with fenestration of a cyst wall. (**a**) Multiple punctate fenestrations are made in the cyst wall. (**b**) The tissue between the fenestrations are cauterized. (**c**) Scissors are used to connect the fenestrations (**d**) creating a larger opening in the cyst wall

finally cauterizing the area between the fenestrations and connecting the fenestrations using scissors to enlarge the final opening (Fig. 9.2). Other groups have advocated for fenestrations in the cyst wall to be at least 1 cm wide and that the cyst wall should be devascularized, if possible [25].

Outcomes

While surgical outcomes (e.g., requirements for shunt placement, shunt revision, and further surgeries) have been well documented in this patient population, functional outcomes have not been as closely reported. Long-term functional outcome data, including the use of validated cognitive and neurodevelopmental metrics, are lacking, and this may be an area of interest for future research. Such information could inform clinicians on how to counsel parents regarding neurodevelopmental expectations.

Nonetheless, there are some relevant data in this area. Earlier studies reported a high mortality rate, even with surgical management. A retrospective study from 1973 examined seven patients: five died prior to 36 months (71% of the total) and the remaining two were noted to have spastic quadriplegia and moderate to severe mental retardation [8]. Another retrospective study from 1981 examined five patients: three died at or prior to 3 years of age (60% of the total) and two were noted to be either moderately or severely disabled [13].

More recent works have shown better rates of survival for these patients. A retrospective study from 2005 examined outcomes in patients who underwent open fenestration and included 33 patients [5]. They noted 1 patient death (3% of the total), 4 patients (12%) with mild neurological deficits, and 28 patients (85%) with significant neurological deficits [5]. A 2003 retrospective study compared the efficacy of neuroendoscopic fenestration and shunting with shunting alone, and they also reported functional outcomes [3]. On analysis of the 127 patients studied, there were 20 reported deaths (16%), 19 patients in a persistent vegetative state (15% of total), 69 patients (54%) who were severely disabled, 16 patients (13%) who were moderately disabled, and 3 (2%) who were mildly disabled [3]. Again, while survival rates have improved, survivors are still likely to have significant neurological deficits and cognitive/developmental delay.

Prevention

While more attention has focused on treatment of multiloculated hydrocephalus, there have been studies examining techniques that could potentially result in reducing loculation formation in high-risk groups. Direct ventricular irrigation using an endoscope has been examined in the treatment of adults with ventriculitis [31]. While the number of patients in the study was small ($n = 14$), the group treated with direct ventricular irrigation using an endoscope showed a significant decrease in the number of days a postoperative drainage catheter was required [31].

Urokinase has also been used in one case report of a 2-month-old with a *Citrobacter* abscess with ventriculitis, and the authors describe using the intraventricular urokinase specifically to prevent subsequent loculation [32]. Similar treatments have been used in neonates with intraventricular hemorrhage of prematurity; however, streptokinase was not recommended as a therapy in a Cochrane systematic review [33].

Conclusions

Although rare, patients with multiloculated hydrocephalus continue to present a challenge for pediatric neurosurgeons. Advances in MRI have allowed for better understanding of complex ventricular and cyst anatomy. Neuroendoscopy has provided a relatively less invasive method for fenestrating cysts. However, despite these advances, patients with multiloculated hydrocephalus still often require multiple surgical procedures, often require shunting, and have poorer neurological outcomes than patients without loculated hydrocephalus. To date, no therapy has been shown to successfully prevent formation of loculations in at-risk patients.

Funding Source This project was done with no specific funding support.

Financial Disclosure Statement The author has no financial relationships to disclose regarding this manuscript.

Conflict of Interest Statement The author has no conflicts of interests to report regarding this manuscript.

References

1. Akbari SH, Holekamp TF, Murphy TM, Mercer D, Leonard JR, Smyth MD, et al. Surgical management of complex multiloculated hydrocephalus in infants and children. Childs Nerv Syst. 2015;31(2):243–9.
2. Fritsch MJ, Mehdorn M. Endoscopic intraventricular surgery for treatment of hydrocephalus and loculated CSF space in children less than one year of age. Pediatr Neurosurg. 2002;36(4):183–8.
3. Nowoslawska E, Polis L, Kaniewska D, Mikolajczyk W, Krawczyk J, Szymanski W, et al. Effectiveness of neuroendoscopic procedures in the treatment of complex compartmentalized hydrocephalus in children. Childs Nerv Syst. 2003;19(9):659–65.
4. Oi S, Hidaka M, Honda Y, Togo K, Shinoda M, Shimoda M, et al. Neuroendoscopic surgery for specific forms of hydrocephalus. Childs Nerv Syst. 1999;15(1):56–68.
5. Sandberg DI, McComb JG, Krieger MD. Craniotomy for fenestration of multiloculated hydrocephalus in pediatric patients. Neurosurgery. 2005;57(1 Suppl):100–6; discussion 106.
6. Andresen M, Juhler M. Multiloculated hydrocephalus: a review of current problems in classification and treatment. Childs Nerv Syst. 2012;28(3):357–62.
7. Cushing H. Surgery of the head. In: Keen WW, editor. Surgery, its principles and practice, vol. 3. Philadelphia: W.B. Saunders; 1912. p. 17–276.
8. Schultz P, Leeds NE. Intraventricular septations complicating neonatal meningitis. J Neurosurg. 1973;38(5):620–6.
9. Kestle J, Drake J, Milner R, Sainte-Rose C, Cinalli G, Boop F, et al. Long-term follow-up data from the shunt design trial. Pediatr Neurosurg. 2000;33(5):230–6.
10. Kestle JR, Walker ML, Strata I. A multicenter prospective cohort study of the strata valve for the management of hydrocephalus in pediatric patients. J Neurosurg. 2005;102(2 Suppl):141–5.
11. Brown LW, Zimmerman RA, Bilaniuk LT. Polycystic brain disease complicating neonatal meningitis: documentation of evolution by computed tomography. J Pediatr. 1979;94(5):757–9.
12. Berman PH, Banker BQ. Neonatal meningitis. A clinical and pathological study of 29 cases. Pediatrics. 1966;38(1):6–24.
13. Albanese V, Tomasello F, Sampaolo S. Multiloculated hydrocephalus in infants. Neurosurgery. 1981;8(6):641–6.
14. Kalsbeck JE, DeSousa AL, Kleiman MB, Goodman JM, Franken EA. Compartmentalization of the cerebral ventricles as a sequela of neonatal meningitis. J Neurosurg. 1980;52(4):547–52.
15. Handler LC, Wright MG. Postmeningitic hydrocephalus in infancy. Ventriculography with special reference to ventricular septa. Neuroradiology. 1978;16:31–5.

16. Christian EA, Melamed EF, Peck E, Krieger MD, McComb JG. Surgical management of hydrocephalus secondary to intraventricular hemorrhage in the preterm infant. J Neurosurg Pediatr. 2016;17(3):278–84.
17. Tuli S, Drake J, Lamberti-Pasculli M. Long-term outcome of hydrocephalus management in myelomeningoceles. Childs Nerv Syst. 2003;19(5–6):286–91.
18. Barkovich AJ, Simon EM, Walsh CA. Callosal agenesis with cyst: a better understanding and new classification. Neurology. 2001;56(2):220–7.
19. Schlitt M, Duvall ER, Bonnin J, Morawetz RB. Neurosarcoidosis causing ventricular loculation, hydrocephalus, and death. Surg Neurol. 1986;26(1):67–71.
20. Aleman J, Jokura H, Higano S, Akabane A, Shirane R, Yoshimoto T. Value of constructive interference in steady-state three-dimensional, Fourier transformation magnetic resonance imaging for the neuroendoscopic treatment of hydrocephalus and intracranial cysts. Neurosurgery. 2001;48(6):1291–5; discussion 5–6.
21. Nitz WR, Bradley WG Jr, Watanabe AS, Lee RR, Burgoyne B, O'Sullivan RM, et al. Flow dynamics of cerebrospinal fluid: assessment with phase-contrast velocity MR imaging performed with retrospective cardiac gating. Radiology. 1992;183(2):395–405.
22. Battal B, Kocaoglu M, Bulakbasi N, Husmen G, Tuba Sanal H, Tayfun C. Cerebrospinal fluid flow imaging by using phase-contrast MR technique. Br J Radiol. 2011;84(1004):758–65.
23. Roth J, Ben-Sira L, Udayakumaran S, Constantini S. Contrast ventriculo-cisternography: an auxiliary test for suspected fourth ventricular outlet obstruction. Childs Nerv Syst. 2012;28(3):453–9.
24. Padayachy L, Fieggen GAG. 176 Microbubble assisted ultrasound guidance for assessing the adequacy of endoscopic membrane fenestration in multiloculated hydrocephalus in children. Neurosurgery. 2014;61(CN_suppl_1):218.
25. Lewis AI, Keiper GL Jr, Crone KR. Endoscopic treatment of loculated hydrocephalus. J Neurosurg. 1995;82(5):780–5.
26. Kaiser G. The value of multiple shunt systems in the treatment of nontumoral infantile hydrocephalus. Childs Nerv Syst. 1986;2(4):200–5.
27. Nida TY, Haines SJ. Multiloculated hydrocephalus: craniotomy and fenestration of intraventricular septations. J Neurosurg. 1993;78(1):70–6.
28. Kestle JR, Drake JM, Cochrane DD, Milner R, Walker ML, Abbott R 3rd, et al. Lack of benefit of endoscopic ventriculoperitoneal shunt insertion: a multicenter randomized trial. J Neurosurg. 2003;98(2):284–90.
29. Roth J, Constantini S. Selective use of intra-catheter endoscopic-assisted ventricular catheter placement: indications and outcome. Childs Nerv Syst. 2012;28(8):1163–9.
30. Mangano FT, Limbrick DD Jr, Leonard JR, Park TS, Smyth MD. Simultaneous image-guided and endoscopic navigation without rigid cranial fixation: application in infants: technical case report. Neurosurgery. 2006;58(4 Suppl 2):ONS-E377; discussion ONS-E.
31. Terada Y, Mineharu Y, Arakawa Y, Funaki T, Tanji M, Miyamoto S. Effectiveness of neuroendoscopic ventricular irrigation for ventriculitis. Clin Neurol Neurosurg. 2016;146:147–51.
32. Martinez-Lage JF, Martinez-Lage Azorin L, Almagro MJ, Bastida ME, Reyes S, Tellez C. Citrobacter koseri meningitis: a neurosurgical condition? Eur J Paediatr Neurol. 2010;14(4):360–3.
33. Whitelaw A, Odd DE. Intraventricular streptokinase after intraventricular hemorrhage in newborn infants. Cochrane Database Syst Rev. 2007;4:CD000498.

Hydrocephalus Secondary to Spina Bifida

10

Michael C. Dewan, John C. Wellons III, and Robert P. Naftel

Spina Bifida

Spina bifida is a spinal abnormality considered to be the most common nonfatal congenital anomaly of the central nervous system, affecting nearly 1 out of every 4000 infants [3]. The term falls under the umbrella of spinal dysraphism, which denotes a spectrum of conditions resulting from aberrant formation of the neural tube during early embryogenesis. The most common variant is also the most severe: myelomeningocele (MM). This subtype of dysraphism consists of an open neural tube defect whereby neural structures and their surrounding meninges extrude beyond a bony defect in the midline spinal column (Fig. 10.1). While other dysraphism variants exist, including lipomyelomeningocele, split cord malformation, and dermal sinus tract, among others, – myelomeningocele is uniquely associated with hydrocephalus, and thus constitutes the focus of this chapter [10].

Spina Bifida-associated Hydrocephalus

Hydrocephalus is the most important neurological sequelae effecting neonates with MM (Fig. 10.2). Not only does it dictate early diagnostic and therapeutic interventions, but hydrocephalus also has been shown to be the primary predictor of long-term functional outcomes in MM, as will be discussed later in this chapter. Historically, between 70% and 85% of children born with MM will develop

M. C. Dewan
Vanderbilt University Medical Center, Monroe Carell Jr. Children's Hospital at Vanderbilt, Department of Neurological Surgery, Nashville, TN, USA

J. C. Wellons III · R. P. Naftel (✉)
Monroe Carell Jr. Children's Hospital at Vanderbilt, Neurological Surgery, Division of Pediatric Neurosurgery, Nashville, TN, USA
e-mail: robert.p.naftel@vanderbilt.edu

D. D. Limbrick, J. R. Leonard (eds.), *Cerebrospinal Fluid Disorders*,
https://doi.org/10.1007/978-3-319-97928-1_10

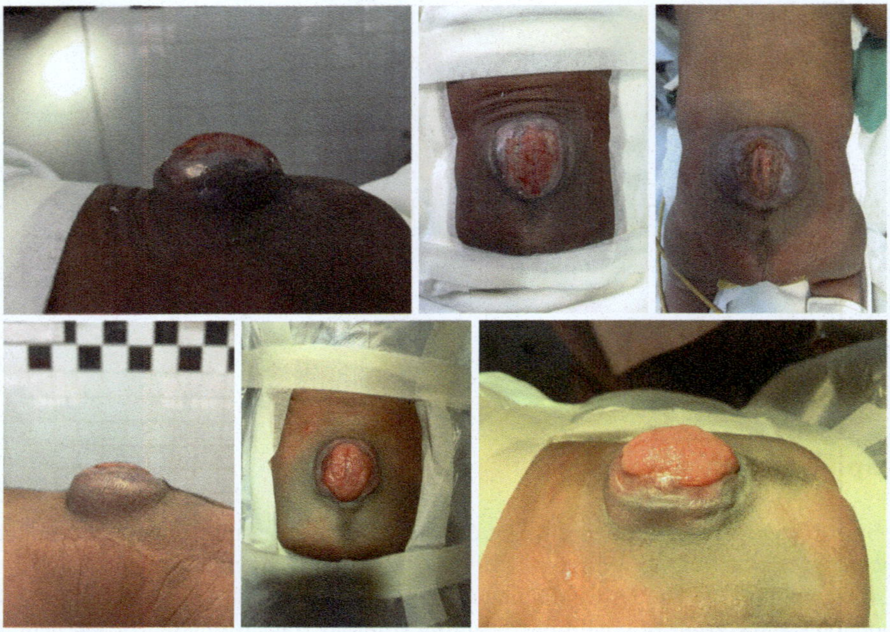

Fig. 10.1 Typical appearance of lumbar myelomeningocele in three patients prior to defect closure

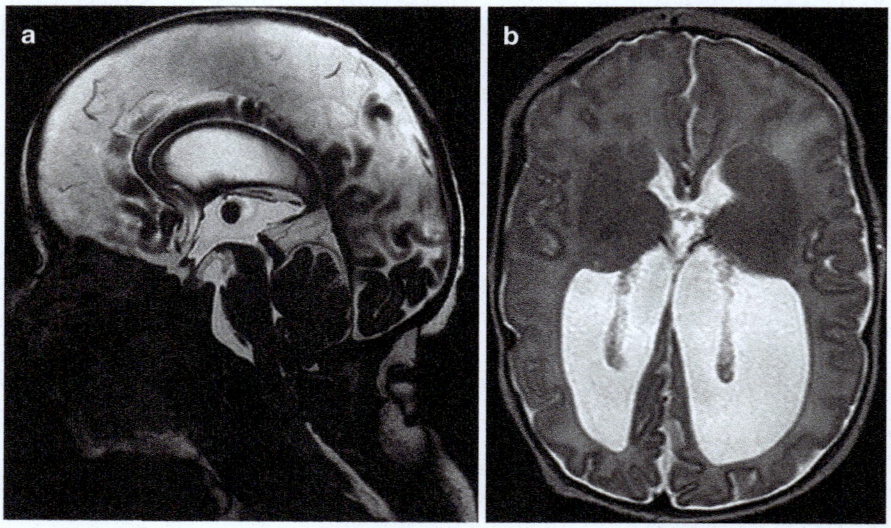

Fig. 10.2 Mid-sagittal (**a**) MRI in a patient with MM demonstrating characteristic radiographic findings, including enlarged third ventricle, prominent interthalamic adhesion, small posterior fossa with resultant hindbrain herniation downward through the foramen magna. Axial (**b**) image in the same patient with occipital horn dilation out of proportion to dilation observed in the frontal horns

hydrocephalus requiring the need for permanent CSF diversion [23, 37]. Among all forms of early childhood hydrocephalus, myelomeningocele accounts for approximately one third [35, 53]. In parts of the developing world where maternal malnutrition and folate deficiency boost MM incidence, the burden of hydrocephalus secondary to MM is likely greater [57].

Pathophysiology of Myelomeningocele-Related Hydrocephalus

The precise mechanistic cause of hydrocephalus in MM remains a topic of debate, but likely involves a dynamic interaction between differential pressure and flow of CSF in about three compartments: the intraventricular space, the posterior fossa and fourth ventricle, and the CSF compartment created by the pathologic neural outpouching. Central in most theories is the presence of the Chiari II malformation: tonsillar descent and foramen magnum crowding in MM (Fig. 10.3). In a unifying theory proposed by Williams et al. [59] the vertebral dysgenesis and subsequent development of spina bifida results in a relative state of low intraspinal pressure. As a consequence, the posterior fossa contents—particularly the cerebellar tonsils—are drawn caudally to dorsally abut the superior cervical spine [29]. Surrounded by the relatively fixed circumference of the bony foramen magnum, the ventricular outlet foramen are obstructed along with the myelencephalic cisternal spaces. Outlet foraminal obstruction prevents CSF egress from the ventricles into the perispinal space, raising intracranial pressure and resulting in hydrocephalus. Meanwhile, blockage of the cisternal spaces at the craniocervical junction prevents movement of CSF back into the cranial compartment where it would otherwise be reabsorbed by the arachnoid villi. This results in increased intraspinal pressure,

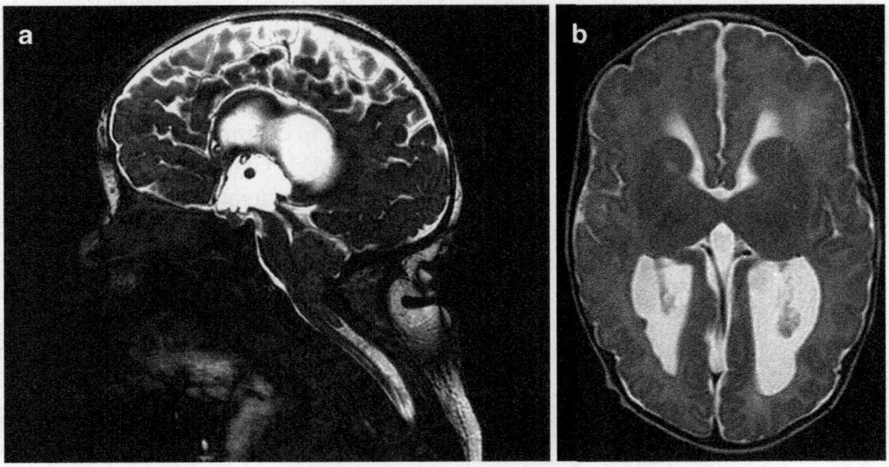

Fig. 10.3 MRI in a patient with severe hindbrain malformation related to MM with a severely condensed posterior fossa, and tonsillar and cerebellar herniation (**a**). Colpocephaly—select enlargement of the occipital horns—is demonstrated (**b**)

further exacerbating the spina defect and potentially leading to syrinx formation [59]. This unifying theory was founded on work reported by McLone and Knepper in 1989. They suggested that insufficient mesenchymal induction in the embryonal posterior fossa secondary to CSF loss through the spinal defect resulted in underdevelopment of the bony posterior fossa, which caused hindbrain herniation [29]. The related theories are supported by observations following intrauterine spinal defect repair, whereby elimination of the large spinal CSF compartment, and therefore the pathologically low intraspinal pressure, reduces the incidence of both Chiari II malformation and hydrocephalus postnatally. Others have proposed a genetic contribution to the hydrocephalus that accompanies MM, independent of structural disruptions along CSF pathways [50].

While further laboratory investigations are needed to establish a definitive pathophysiologic mechanism, the close relationship between the spinal defect, abnormal tonsillar descent, posterior fossa crowding, and ventriculomegaly ensures the treatment of one of these entities influences the nature of one or more of the others.

Presentation and Diagnosis

Hydrocephalus in spina bifida develops early, as ventriculomegaly is often observed during routine screening ultrasonography early in the second trimester [9]. After delivery, patients are closely monitored for the development of progressive hydrocephalus. As with other variants of infant hydrocephalus, three clinical parameters are measured and evaluated for change over time: fontanel status, head circumference, and ventricle size. Ventricle size can be evaluated by ultrasound, magnetic resonance imaging, and if necessary, computed tomography (CT) (Figs 10.2 and 10.3). The frontal and occipital horn ratio (FOHR) and Evan's ratio are both valid and reliable metrics to follow ventricle size. In a large single center series, the mean FOHR in patients without hydrocephalus was 0.45, while in those requiring CSF diversion the value was 0.55 [37]. In the spina bifida population, in particular, the lateral ventricle atrium (LVA) has also gained particular traction [30]. The LVA is a convenient way for obstetricians and neurosurgeons to communicate regarding the ventricular volume in the fetus and neonate with MM. Generally, an LVA width ≥15 mm indicates sufficient ventriculomegaly to warrant treatment [30].

Meanwhile, daily measurement of the occipital frontal circumference (OFC) is essential and should be charted on a standard growth chart appropriate for the patient's gestational age. Often, the absolute OFC in a child with myelomeningocele-related hydrocephalus (MM-HC) is within normal limits, thus focus should remain on the OFC trajectory over time rather than any individual measurement. An OFC that crosses percentile lines in the days or weeks after delivery could indicate progressive hydrocephalus and deserves evaluation for possible CSF diversion [37].

Next, routine fontanel assessment remains an essential piece of information to guide surgical decision-making. Recently, the status of the fontanel, more than any other clinical or radiographic metric, was shown to be a more specific indicator of progressive hydrocephalus in young infants, including those with MM [14]. Indeed, a secondary analysis of the Management of Myelomeningocele Study (MOMS) (described in detail below) showed that neurosurgeons were hesitant to place a shunt in the absence of a bulging fontanel, split sutures, or sun-setting eyes, even when the OFC was crossing percentiles or the ventricles were considered larger than normal [52]. Finally, clinical signs and symptoms should be routinely monitored in the newborn MM infant. Apneic and bradycardic spells may be a harbinger for critically elevated ICP, while dysphagia, aspiration, and other bulbar signs may represent foramen magnum crowding secondary to a Chiari II malformation.

Delayed development of hydrocephalus in the infant with MM is rare [18]. Rather, the vast majority of patients who develop hydrocephalus will demonstrate clinical features of elevated ICP within the first 2 months of life and therefore mandate treatment early [48]. The exception involves patients who have no or compensated ventriculomegaly as an infant but later develop worsening, uncompensated hydrocephalus as a child or young adult in the setting of worsening CIIM. Of note, stable mild or moderate ventriculomegaly may be acceptable in MM so long as all signs of elevated ICP are absent. In a single center study by Warf et al., neurocognitive outcomes were shown to be superior in patients who avoided CSF diversion; meanwhile, greater ventricular volume did not correlate with worse neurocognitive scores [58].

Surgical Management of Hydrocephalus Secondary to Myelomeningocele

Ventriculoperitoneal Shunting

The treatment of hydrocephalus in this population has undergone a significant evolution over the last several decades. The rate of VPS insertion has diminished significantly for several reasons. First, establishment of a definitive role for folate in neural tube development has led to massively successful nutritional supplementation campaigns for women of childbearing age worldwide, particularly in high and upper middle-income countries [13, 39]. Second, the number of children in high-resourced countries born with MM is probably waning partly as a result of prenatal diagnosis and subsequent elective termination [34]. While the spinal defect alone may not trigger disruption of pregnancy, sonographic evidence of severe ventriculomegaly or other significant cerebral malformation may. As a result, fewer women are giving birth to babies with MM. Third, the perception of CSF shunts in this population has changed among the neurosurgical community, both in relation to shunt-related complications and also to differing theories regarding the indications for CSF diversion in these infants.

As with other forms of hydrocephalus, catheter-based CSF shunting has been the mainstay for hydrocephalus management since shunts were popularized more than half a century ago. The rate of VPS insertion in MM infants ranges from 78% to 86% in older series [6, 33, 40, 43, 54]. This relatively high rate of shunting is the consequence of three concepts. First, it became evident with other variants of hydrocephalus that insertion of a VPS was followed by a reliable and immediate decrease in ventricle size. Thus, when a child with MM was noted to be developing progressive ventriculomegaly, the instinctual treatment algorithm led the surgeon to recommend a shunt be inserted. Over time, as shunt-related morbidity, including the risks associated with shunting and the need for revisions became more apparent, this paradigm was reevaluated. Second, the third ventriculostomy, while developed even prior to the VPS, had fallen out of favor in the decades following the advent of shunt catheters. As pediatric neurosurgeons became more comfortable with the endoscope, the ETV came to be recognized as a safe, minimally invasive alternative to VPS for select patients [4]. The utility of ETV for MM-HC is discussed later in this chapter. Finally a high rate of VPS insertion in the MM population reflected an effort by surgeons to avoid CSF leakage, infection, and wound breakdown at the site of the spinal defect repair. Rather than wait for the patient to develop true refractory elevated intracranial pressure following MM repair, surgeons frequently placed a VPS "prophylactically" to ensure that spinal intrathecal hypertension would not compromise the integrity of the defect closure [2, 28]. In the discussion that follows, the timing of CSF diversion in relation to MM repair is discussed, including the pros, cons, and current consensus on the topic. Today, the rate of VPS insertion in patients with MM-HC has decreased as a result of changing surgical perceptions as well as the maturation of long-term clinical outcomes data. Nonetheless, even some recent series still describe a high rate of VPS insertion (85%), suggesting either that the included patients have disproportionately severe hydrocephalus or that some neurosurgeons do not share the perception that VPS can be avoided by either patient selection or alternative treatments [23].

Surgical Complications of VPS

Myelomeningocele patients with VPS experience higher complication rates than many of their counterparts with non-MM-related causes of hydrocephalus, particularly infectious complications. In a single center long-term follow-up study, Gmeiner et al. reported a lifetime VPS infection rate of 29%, with approximately 10% of patients experiencing at least two shunt infections requiring extended hospitalization and shunt revision [20]. In a 25-year institutional experience, Clemmensen and authors report a 31% infection rate among all MM patients treated with VPS. Among patients who presented to the hospital with CSF leakage from the spinal defect, over half of patients (56%) developed at least one CSF infection mandating VPS removal and reinsertion [11]. Dupepe et al. describe one of the largest studies to date on this topic, including 519 MM patients followed for more than 17 years postoperatively [16]. The risk of shunt revision in the first year of life was 23% and fell each year thereafter, except for the early teenage years when a modest spike (11–12% per year) was observed. Among 417 patients requiring primary VPS insertion, a total of 682 VPS revisions were performed between ages 0 and 43. Others have described more modest rates of shunt complications in MM patients approaching 20% [18]. Of note, most cases of shunt infection in MM patients occur in the first year following VPS insertion, while obstructions often occur years later. In the following section, the relationship between the timing of CSF diversion and infectious complications is elaborated upon. Excluding the presence of CSF leakage at presentation and the temporal relationship between defect closure and VPS, few predictors of shunt infection have been identified in the MM population. Prophylactic administration of antibiotics in the perinatal period is commonplace, albeit supported by low-level evidence [11]. Among MM patients undergoing VPS, neither the type of valve (e.g., adjustable vs. flow control vs. fixed pressure) nor the type of catheter (antibiotic impregnated vs. standard) influence the rate of shunt infection. While further study is warranted, neonatal-design or ultra-small valves may be associated with a lower risk of early shunt complications [24].

Timing of CSF Diversion

In general, for the infant with concomitant hydrocephalus and MM, hydrocephalus can be treated at one of two points in time: simultaneously with the MM repair or in a delayed fashion days or weeks after the back closure. The rationale for simultaneous treatment resides in the notion that relieving CSF pressure with VPS insertion creates a more suitable environment for spinal wound healing, therefore decreasing the rate of CSF leak or wound breakdown. Some authors employ this strategy as a matter of routine [18, 28], while others only perform simultaneous surgery in patients with severe hydrocephalus as birth [23]. In a small, single institutional series, the rate of VPS infection and that of delayed wound healing were both 9%, leading the authors to conclude this was an acceptable risk profile [28].

Opponents of this treatment strategy point to data demonstrating unacceptable rates of catheter-related morbidity, including infection and obstruction. Arslan et al. describe a 12% infection rate if the closure and VPS insertion are performed simultaneously within 48 h of delivery and over 30% if the simultaneous surgeries occur between 3 and 15 days after delivery [2]. Accordingly, this strategy has been abandoned by most surgeons. Moreover, there would likely be a subgroup who would have gone on to not need CSF diversion for more agreed upon reasons as detailed above and therefore would have undergone VPS insertion unnecessarily.

Rarely, a neonate with severe ventriculomegaly and symptoms of decompensating hydrocephalus (e.g., bradycardia, bulbar dysfunction) may warrant urgent CSF diversion prior to MM closure. In the authors' opinion, however, this strategy should be rarely employed due to the risk of foreseeable VPS complications in the wake of the spinal defect repair.

Endoscopic Third Ventriculostomy

ETV for hydrocephalus in the myelomeningocele patient has been utilized with greater frequency over the past two decades, as the technique has undergone revisions and the understanding of patient selection evolves. The applicability of ETV for MM-HC rests on the principle that hydrocephalus is primarily obstructive in nature, resulting from blockage of the fourth ventricular outlet foramina by C2M or from congenital aqueductal stenosis. Initially, however, ETV was largely reserved for older patients who had experienced a VPS malfunction. In a report by Teo et al.

describing an ETV experience between 1978 and 1995, the procedure was successful in 72% of older spina bifida patients diagnosed with shunt obstruction [49]. The anomalous intraventricular architecture in MM, including a thickened tuber cinereum and large interthalamic adhesion, had discouraged surgeons from using this technique. But creating an adequate stoma while avoiding disruption of nearby eloquent structures is possible in most patients [19], and similar successful results have been well described. Nonetheless, a favorable success profile appears limited to patients aged 1 year or older [36]. Success of ETV requires that CSF diverted directly from the third ventricle into the cisternal spaces is matched by an absorptive mechanism capable of accommodating the CSF burden. However, for reasons that remain ill defined, the CSF absorptive capacity is immature or otherwise insufficient. Thus, ETV alone is an unsatisfactory means of primary treatment for young MM infants with hydrocephalus.

Endoscopic Third Ventriculostomy with Choroid Plexus Cauterization

As outlined earlier, hydrocephalus in this population develops early and definitive CSF diversion is typically required in the first 2 months of life. Thus, while ETV alone may have a role in older patients who fail shunt therapy, a shunt-free option for primary treatment is necessary. A potential solution was offered when Benjamin Warf, MD, began describing his experience with ETV and choroid plexus cauterization (ETV/CPC) for infants in a rural hospital in East Africa [55]. In this procedure, following creation of the stoma at the third ventricle floor, the choroid plexus in the lateral ventricles is obliterated with electrocautery. The use of a flexible endoscope permits access to the choroid plexus in the temporal horns bilaterally, with creation of a septostomy if necessary. While its mechanism of function remains unclear, intersections of ETV/CPC with the bulk flow and hydrodynamic models of hydrocephalus have been described [15, 56]. Through either reduction in CSF production, alterations in pulsatility, or still alternative mechanisms, the destruction of choroid plexus may provide sufficient supplementation of the ETV to deliver a more favorable treatment success rate in infants with hydrocephalus. In 2008, Warf and Cambell described their initial experience with ETV/CPC in patient with MM-HC. Among 93 patients (median age 2 months) undergoing the combined procedure, 76% enjoyed treatment success at a median follow-up period of 19 months. Of note, the vast majority of failures occurred within 6 months and no infections were described. Successful results were replicated in a French cohort wherein a 72% success rate for ETV/CPC was described for patients treated at a median 9 days of life [4]. In this study, the Kaplan-Meier analysis demonstrated a more durable treatment outcome for ETV/CPC than for either VPS alone or ETV with VPS. The durability of ETV/CPC in very young infants with MM-HC has now been demonstrated in several North American cohorts [14, 27, 44]. At the authors' institution, treatment with ETV/CPC has become the first-line treatment for MM patients who develop hydrocephalus in the first year of life, regardless of age.

Fetal Surgery

Intrauterine MM repair has impacted the rate at which patients require CSF diversion for symptomatic MM-HC. Primary and secondary analyses of the Management of Myelomeningocele Study (MOMS), described below, have shed light on ventricle and cerebral changes that may occur following fetal repair. While many lessons are gleaned from the MOMS results, the influence of IUSBR on hydrocephalus and its treatment is most relevant to this text. While the rate of shunt implantation was less than half among prenatally treated infants, the difference in formal rates of hydrocephalus was less dramatic. Based upon prespecified criteria (crossing head circumference percentiles, bulging fontanel, ventriculomegaly with symptomatic Chiari II, etc.), 68% of patients in the prenatal cohort were diagnosed with hydrocephalus relative to 98% in the standard group. The disparity between ratios is a result of surgeons relying on overt clinical signs of hydrocephalus to determine need for VPS rather than prespecified measurement cutoffs. Secondary analysis of the MOMS population offered important information about ventricle size and the implications for patient selection. If ventricle size (measured by axial dimension of the lateral ventricle atrium) was less than 10 mm at time of initial screening, the probability of needing a shunt was 0.2. A fetus with a measurement of between 10 and 15 mm displayed a probability of 0.45 [52]. Conversely, ventricle size of ≥ 15 mm was associated with a 0.79 risk of needing a shunt. Consequently, in a fetus with an LVA measurement of ≥15 mm, prenatal surgery may not offer an overall benefit, particularly in light of the risk profile associated with intrauterine surgery.

Since the first intrauterine spina bifida repair (IUSBR) was performed in 1997, more than 1000 fetuses have undergone the procedure, and there exists Level I evidence to demonstrate its superiority to postnatal repair in select patients. The path taken between clinical hypothesis and the routine conduction of prenatal MM repair at numerous specialty centers follows an elegant scientific course rarely observed for a modern surgical procedure.

The rationale for prenatal repair rests on two important observations. First, lower extremity leg function in the fetus with myelomeningocele diminishes progressively throughout gestation [25]. It has been hypothesized that beyond the innate insult from the structural spinal anomaly, exposure of nerve roots to the intrauterine compartment is toxic and causes neuronal dysfunction [42]. This has been labeled the "two-hit hypothesis" and has gained traction in the last decades [1, 32]. Second, hindbrain herniation—the Chiari II malformation—becomes more progressive as the fetal brain develops in-utero [46]. In animal models, prenatal coverage of the spinal defect correlated not only with improved neurologic function, but also demonstrated a correction in the hindbrain malformation, thereby lending credence to both theories [5, 31].

By the early 2000s, hundreds of babies had undergone IUSBR at select high-volume centers. Early results from modest human series mirrored findings from laboratory and animal studies. Serial MRIs performed in fetuses following defect repair demonstrated near normalization of the hindbrain malformation which persisted throughout gestation and early infancy [46]. The same group showed that lower extremity function may be improved in patients selected for IUSBR as compared to their postnatal repair counterparts [12]. Tulipan et al. described a lower rate of shunt-dependent hydrocephalus in patients undergoing fetal repair [51]. Despite these encouraging results, intrauterine repair was associated with increased maternal risk (preterm labor, uterine damage) and fetal risk (preterm birth, spontaneous abortion). The need for a randomized clinical trial to compare relevant risks and benefits was needed, thus the MOMS trail (Management of Myelomeningocele Study) ensued. Women with a fetus diagnosed with myelomeningocele were randomized to undergo fetal repair prior to 26 weeks gestation or postnatal repair. Enrollment terminated early for efficacy and four key observations were made: (1) 40% of patients in the prenatal cohort underwent VPS insertion relative to 82% in the postnatal cohort; (2) mental development and motor function at 30 months was improved in the prenatal group; (3) hindbrain herniation at 12 months and ambulation by 30 months was also improved in the prenatal cohort; and (4) the risk of preterm delivery and uterine dehiscence was greater in those treated with IUSBR [1]. Overall, composite outcomes for the prenatal group were more favorable than for the postnatal group, thus establishing a new standard of care for select women [21].

For those patients who undergo prenatal repair and subsequently develop progressive hydrocephalus postnatally, the treatment rationale is similar to other MM patients. Most of the literature describes shunt placement in this population, as the experience with ETV (+/− CPC) is thin and the data immature. In a single center series of 60 IUSBR patients, ETV alone was successful in 46% of patients [17]. Similar to shunt, predictors of ETV failure included ventricle size ≥15 mm and age < 6 months at time of ETV. The incorporation of ETV in the treatment armamentarium resulted in a shunt dependency rate of 35%—slightly lower that what was described in MOMS. Combined ETV/CPC following IUSBR has not been formally studied, but may be a viable and promising treatment alternative to VPS.

Quality of Life and Survival

As the management of MM-related infections, deformities, and hydrocephalus have improved, between 70% and 80% of patients are living into young adulthood [7, 47]. Once a congenital malformation resulting in childhood disability and death, MM has become a chronic health condition in many parts of the world. Understanding quality of life, therefore, becomes increasingly important and simultaneously challenging. Myelomeningocele-related hydrocephalus is a secondary manifestation of a primary developmental insult that causes downstream insults affecting organ systems beyond just the central nervous system. This differs from other variants of hydrocephalus such as congenital idiopathic hydrocephalus or posthemorrhagic hydrocephalus, wherein direct effects are limited primarily to the CNS. Accordingly, measuring quality of life in a patient with MM-HC is necessarily tethered to entities like bowel function and ambulation, not simply cognitive or neuropsychiatric function.

Patients with myelomeningocele and hydrocephalus score more poorly on physical, emotional, and social quality of life measures than do patients with other forms of hydrocephalus [45]. Similarly, neuropsychiatric scores are generally worse for MM-HC than other forms of infantile hydrocephalus [22]. Certainly, a much greater proportion of patients with MM-HC require ambulatory assistance (e.g., wheelchair, bracing) [35]. However, rates of epilepsy and need for speech therapy are lower in MM-HC than in other HC variants [53].

Moreover, patients with myelomeningocele and hydrocephalus fare worse than patients with myelomeningocele without hydrocephalus. The coexistence of hydrocephalus results in worse functional and quality of life outcomes for myelomeningocele patients than if hydrocephalus is absent. In a study by Kulkarni et al. myelomeningocele children with hydrocephalus demonstrated significantly poorer health-related quality of life across most fields than their shunt-free counterparts [26]. Similarly, others have reported that a history of shunt treatment and Chiari decompression correlate worse quality of life [41]. Importantly, among all comorbidities and complications that may affect patients with myelomeningocele, hydrocephalus is the single most important barrier to attaining adult milestones [8].

Today, for patients surviving beyond the neonatal time period, the median overall survival is 40 years—a number which has more than quadrupled over the last 50 years following the advent of shunts and clean intermittent catheterization [6, 38]. While sepsis, respiratory failure, and pulmonary embolism account for the majority of adult mortality, hydrocephalus and shunt failure remain an important cause of death for older patients with myelomeningocele. As we look to a future in which more children with spina bifida continue to survive longer into adulthood, it is critical that our field understand the role of transitioning care to adult providers or congenital specialists, trained in the relevant issues detailed in this chapter but with links to adult disease processes. It would be a great victory to 1 day find these patients, having maximized their neurologic function and quality of life through interactions with innovative care during their formative years, now aging well into their older years and finding themselves battling the same medical conditions as any other septuagenarian.

References

1. Adzick NS, Thom EA, Spong CY, Brock JW, Burrows PK, Johnson MP, et al. A randomized trial of prenatal versus postnatal repair of myelomeningocele. N Engl J Med. 2011;364:993–1004.
2. Arslan M, Eseoglu M, Gudu BO, Demir I, Kozan A, Gokalp A, et al. Comparison of simultaneous shunting to delayed shunting in infants with myelomeningocele in terms of shunt infection rate. Turk Neurosurg. 2010;21:1–6.
3. Barkovich J, Koch BL, Moore KR. Diagnostic imaging: pediatric neuroradiology. 2nd ed. Philadelphia: Elsevier; 2014.
4. Beuriat P-A, Szathmari A, Grassiot B, Plaisant F, Rousselle C, Mottolese C. Role of endoscopic third ventriculostomy in the management of myelomeningocele-related hydrocephalus: a retrospective study in a single French institution. World Neurosurg. 2016;87:484–93.
5. Bouchard S, Davey MG, Rintoul NE, Walsh DS, Rorke LB, Adzick NS. Correction of hindbrain herniation and anatomy of the vermis after in utero repair of myelomeningocele in sheep. J Pediatr Surg. 2003;38:451–8.

6. Bowman RM, McLone DG, Grant JA, Tomita T, Ito JA. Spina bifida outcome: a 25-year prospective. Pediatr Neurosurg. 2001;34:114–20.
7. Bowman RM, Boshnjaku V, McLone DG. The changing incidence of myelomeningocele and its impact on pediatric neurosurgery: a review from the Children's Memorial Hospital. Childs Nerv Syst. 2009;25:801–6.
8. Cope H, McMohan K, Heise E, Eubanks S, Garett M, Gregory S, et al. Outcome and life satisfaction of adults with myelomeningocele. Disabil Health J. 2013;6:236–43.
9. Cavalheiro S, da Costa MDS, Mendonça JN, Dastoli PA, Suriano IC, Barbosa MM, et al. Antenatal management of fetal neurosurgical diseases. Childs Nerv Syst. 2017;28: 568–617.
10. Chance A, Sandberg DI. Hydrocephalus in patients with closed neural tube defects. Childs Nerv Syst. 2014;31:329–32.
11. Clemmensen D, Rasmussen MM, Mosdal C. A retrospective study of infections after primary VP shunt placement in the newborn with myelomeningocele without prophylactic antibiotics. Childs Nerv Syst. 2010;26:1517–21.
12. Danzer E, Gerdes M, Bebbington MW, Sutton LN, Melchionni J, Adzick NS, et al. Lower extremity neuromotor function and short-term ambulatory potential following in utero myelomeningocele surgery. Fetal Diagn Ther. 2009;25:47–53.
13. De Wals P, Tairou F, Van Allen MI, Uh S-H, Lowry RB, Sibbald B, et al. Reduction in neural-tube defects after folic acid fortification in Canada. N Engl J Med. 2007;357:135–42.
14. Dewan MC, Lim J, Morgan CD, Gannon SR, Shannon CN, Wellons JC III, et al. Endoscopic third ventriculostomy with choroid plexus cauterization outcome: distinguishing success from failure. J Neurosurg Pediatr. 2016;18:1–8.
15. Dewan MC, Naftel RP. The global rise of endoscopic third ventriculostomy with choroid plexus cauterization in pediatric hydrocephalus. Pediatr Neurosurg. 2016;0:1–8.
16. Dupepe EB, Hopson B, Johnston JM, Rozzelle CJ, Jerry Oakes W, Blount JP, et al. Rate of shunt revision as a function of age in patients with shunted hydrocephalus due to myelomeningocele. Neurosurg Focus. 2016;41:E6.
17. Elbabaa SK, Gildehaus AM, Pierson MJ, Albers JA, Vlastos EJ. First 60 fetal in-utero myelomeningocele repairs at Saint Louis Fetal Care Institute in the post-MOMS trial era: hydrocephalus treatment outcomes (endoscopic third ventriculostomy versus ventriculo-peritoneal shunt). Childs Nerv Syst. 2017;33:1–12.
18. Elgamal E. Natural history of hydrocephalus in children with spinal open neural tube defect. Surg Neurol Int. 2012;3:112–6.
19. Giordano F, Spacca B, Danti A, Taverna M, Losi S, Stagi S, et al. Amenorrhea after endoscopic third ventriculostomy for a failed shunt in spina bifida: case report and review of the literature. Pediatr Neurosurg. 2016;51:35–41.
20. Gmeiner M, Wagner H, Zacherl C, Polanski P, Auer C, Ouwerkerk WJR, et al. Long-term mortality rates in pediatric hydrocephalus—a retrospective single-center study. Childs Nerv Syst. 2017;33:1–9.
21. Grivell RM, Andersen C, Dodd JM. Prenatal versus postnatal repair procedures for spina bifida for improving infant and maternal outcomes. Cochrane Database Syst Rev. 2014;10:CD008825.
22. Hampton LE, Fletcher JM, Cirino P, Blaser S, Kramer LA, Dennis M. Neuropsychological profiles of children with aqueductal stenosis and Spina Bifida myelomeningocele. J Int Neuropsychol Soc. 2013;19:127–36.
23. Januschek E, Röhrig A, Kunze S, Fremerey C, Wiebe B, Messing-Jünger M. Myelomeningocele—a single institute analysis of the years 2007 to 2015. Childs Nerv Syst. 2016;32:1–7.
24. Kahilogullari G, Etus V, Tugba Morali G, Hakan K, Agahan U. Does shunt selection affect the rate of early shunt complications in neonatal myelomeningocele-associated hydrocephalus? A multi-center report. Turk Neurosurg. 2016;28:303–6.
25. Korenromp MJ, van Gool JD, Bruinese HW, Kriek R. Early fetal leg movements in myelomeningocele. Lancet. 1986;1:917–8.

26. Kulkarni AV, Cochrane DD, McNeely PD, Shams I. Medical, social, and economic factors associated with health-related quality of life in Canadian children with hydrocephalus. J Pediatr. 2008;153:689–95.
27. Kulkarni AV, Riva-Cambrin J, Browd SR, Drake JM, Holubkov R, Kestle JRW, et al. Endoscopic third ventriculostomy and choroid plexus cauterization in infants with hydrocephalus: a retrospective Hydrocephalus Clinical Research Network study. J Neurosurg Pediatr. 2014;14:224–9.
28. Machado HLR, Santos de Oliveira R. Simultaneous repair of myelomeningocele and shunt insertion. Childs Nerv Syst. 2004;20:107–9.
29. McLone DG, Knepper PA. The cause of Chiari II malformation: a unified theory. Pediatr Neurosci. 1989;15:1–12.
30. Melo JRT, Pacheco P, de Melo EN, Vasconcellos Â, Passos RK. Clinical and ultrasonographic criteria for using ventriculoperitoneal shunts in newborns with myelomeningocele. Arq Neuropsiquiatr. 2015;73:759–63.
31. Meuli M, Meuli-Simmen C, Hutchins GM, Yingling CD, Hoffman KM, Harrison MR, et al. In utero surgery rescues neurological function at birth in sheep with spina bifida. Nat Med. 1995;1:342–7.
32. Meuli M, Moehrlen U. Fetal surgery for myelomeningocele: a critical appraisal. Eur J Pediatr Surg. 2013;23:103–9.
33. Mirzai H, Erşahin Y, Mutluer S, Kayahan A. Outcome of patients with meningomyelocele: the Ege University experience. Childs Nerv Syst. 1998;14:120–3.
34. Olde Scholtenhuis MAG, Cohen-Overbeek TE, Offringa M, Barth PG, Stoutenbeek P, Gooskens RH, et al. Audit of prenatal and postnatal diagnosis of isolated open spina bifida in three university hospitals in The Netherlands. Ultrasound Obstet Gynecol. 2003;21:48–52.
35. Paulsen AH, Lundar T, Lindegaard K-F. Pediatric hydrocephalus: 40-year outcomes in 128 hydrocephalic patients treated with shunts during childhood. Assessment of surgical outcome, work participation, and health-related quality of life. J Neurosurg Pediatr. 2015;16:633–41.
36. Perez da Rosa S, Millward CP, Chiappa V, Martinez de Leon M, Ibáñez Botella G, Ros López B. Endoscopic third ventriculostomy in children with myelomeningocele: a case series. Pediatr Neurosurg. 2015;50:113–8.
37. Phillips BC, Gelsomino M, Pownall AL, Ocal E, Spencer HJ, O'Brien MS, et al. Predictors of the need for cerebrospinal fluid diversion in patients with myelomeningocele. J Neurosurg Pediatr. 2014;14:167–72.
38. Piatt JH. Treatment of myelomeningocele: a review of outcomes and continuing neurosurgical considerations among adults. J Neurosurg Pediatr. 2010;6:515–25.
39. Ray JG, Meier C, Vermeulen MJ, Boss S, Wyatt PR, Cole DEC. Association of neural tube defects and folic acid food fortification in Canada. Lancet. 2002;360:2047–8.
40. Rintoul NE, Sutton LN, Hubbard AM, Cohen B, Melchionni J, Pasquariello PS, et al. A new look at myelomeningoceles: functional level, vertebral level, shunting, and the implications for fetal intervention. Pediatrics. 2002;109:409–13.
41. Rocque BG, Bishop ER, Scogin MA, Hopson BD, Arynchyna AA, Boddiford CJ, et al. Assessing health-related quality of life in children with spina bifida. J Neurosurg Pediatr. 2015;15:144–9.
42. Sival DA, Begeer JH, Staal-Schreinemachers AL, Vos-Niël JM, Beekhuis JR, Prechtl HF. Perinatal motor behaviour and neurological outcome in spina bifida aperta. Early Hum Dev. 1997;50:27–37.
43. Steinbok P, Irvine B, Cochrane DD, Irwin BJ. Long-term outcome and complications of children born with meningomyelocele. Childs Nerv Syst. 1992;8:92–6.
44. Stone SSD, Warf BC. Combined endoscopic third ventriculostomy and choroid plexus cauterization as primary treatment for infant hydrocephalus: a prospective North American series. J Neurosurg Pediatr. 2014;14:439–46.
45. Sumpter R, Dorris L, Brannan G, Carachi R. Quality of life and behavioural adjustment in childhood hydrocephalus. Scott Med J. 2012;57:18–25.

46. Sutton LN, Adzick NS, Bilaniuk LT, Johnson MP, Crombleholme TM, Flake AW. Improvement in hindbrain herniation demonstrated by serial fetal magnetic resonance imaging following fetal surgery for myelomeningocele. JAMA. 1999;282:1826–31.
47. Talamonti G, D'Aliberti G, Collice M. Myelomeningocele: long-term neurosurgical treatment and follow-up in 202 patients. J Neurosurg. 2007;107:368–86.
48. Tamburrini G, Frassanito P, Iakovaki K, Pignotti F, Rendeli C, Murolo D, et al. Myelomeningocele: the management of the associated hydrocephalus. Childs Nerv Syst. 2013;29:1569–79.
49. Teo C, Jones R. Management of hydrocephalus by endoscopic third ventriculostomy in patients with myelomeningocele. Pediatr Neurosurg. 1996;25:57–63; discussion 63
50. Tissir F, Qu Y, Montcouquiol M, Zhou L, Komatsu K, Shi D, et al. Lack of cadherins Celsr2 and Celsr3 impairs ependymal ciliogenesis, leading to fatal hydrocephalus. Nat Neurosci. 2010;13:700–7.
51. Tulipan N, Sutton LN, Bruner JP, Cohen BM, Johnson M, Adzick NS. The effect of intrauterine myelomeningocele repair on the incidence of shunt-dependent hydrocephalus. Pediatr Neurosurg. 2003;38:27–33.
52. Tulipan N, Wellons JC, Thom EA, Gupta N, Sutton LN, Burrows PK, et al. Prenatal surgery for myelomeningocele and the need for cerebrospinal fluid shunt placement. J Neurosurg Pediatr. 2015;16:613–20.
53. Tully HM, Ishak GE, Rue TC, Dempsey JC, Browd SR, Millen KJ, et al. Two hundred thirty-six children with developmental hydrocephalus. J Child Neurol. 2016;31:309–20.
54. Wakhlu A, Ansari NA. The prediction of postoperative hydrocephalus in patients with spina bifida. Childs Nerv Syst. 2004;20:104–6.
55. Warf BC. Comparison of endoscopic third ventriculostomy alone and combined with choroid plexus cauterization in infants younger than 1 year of age: a prospective study in 550 African children. J Neurosurg. 2005;103:475–81.
56. Warf BC. Congenital idiopathic hydrocephalus of infancy: the results of treatment by endoscopic third ventriculostomy with or without choroid plexus cauterization and suggestions for how it works. Childs Nerv Syst. 2013;29:935–40.
57. Warf BC. Hydrocephalus associated with neural tube defects: characteristics, management, and outcome in sub-Saharan Africa. Childs Nerv Syst. 2011;27:1589–94.
58. Warf B, Ondoma S, Kulkarni A, Donnelly R, Ampeire M, Akona J, et al. Neurocognitive outcome and ventricular volume in children with myelomeningocele treated for hydrocephalus in Uganda. J Neurosurg Pediatr. 2009;4:564–70.
59. Williams H. A unifying hypothesis for hydrocephalus, Chiari malformation, syringomyelia, anencephaly and spina bifida. Cerebrospinal Fluid Res. 2008;5:7.

Hydrocephalus and Brain Tumors

11

Jonathan Roth and Shlomi Constantini

Introduction

Hydrocephalus, an imbalance between production and clearing of cerebrospinal fluid (CSF), is associated with brain tumors. Many factors may contribute to tumor-associated hydrocephalus, including overproduction of CSF, obstruction of CSF pathways, and reduced absorption. Hydrocephalus may be linked to surgical decisions, affecting prioritization of treatments, surgical techniques, and risks. Additionally, hydrocephalus may develop following tumor resection in selected locations, being obstructive or nonobstructive in nature.

In this chapter, we present a general overview of the clinical and treatment-related aspects of hydrocephalus and brain tumors.

Mechanisms of Hydrocephalus

Tumor-associated hydrocephalus may occur secondary to several conditions; it may be obstructive and/or nonobstructive. In the following sections, we discuss the various mechanisms.

CSF Pathway Obstruction

Tumors at or near the ventricular or CSF pathways often present only once they have reached a sufficient size to obstruct the CSF pathway, leading to classic obstructive hydrocephalus and triggering symptoms secondary to increased intracranial pressure.

J. Roth (✉) · S. Constantini
Dana Children's Hospital, Tel-Aviv Medical Center, Pediatric Neurosurgery, Tel Aviv, Israel

D. D. Limbrick, J. R. Leonard (eds.), *Cerebrospinal Fluid Disorders*,
https://doi.org/10.1007/978-3-319-97928-1_11

Apart from typical tumors at specific locations at or near the ventricular system (such as fourth ventricular medulloblastomas or tectal gliomas), other processes (gliomas, metastasis, or lymphomas) may occur anywhere in the CNS and periventricular regions, and should always be considered based on clinical and radiological findings.

Hydrocephalus may occur secondary to inner pathway obstruction, such as a colloid cyst (CC) or a subependymal giant cell astrocytoma (SEGA, in Tuberous Sclerosis Complex) that obstructs the foramen of Monro or a fourth ventricular tumor. Hydrocephalus may also occur secondary to an outer pathway lesion. Outer pathway lesions may be intra-axial (such as a thalamic tumor that compresses the CSF pathways leading to an obstruction) or extra-axial (such as a pineal region tumor that compresses the pathway secondary to compressed but uninvolved neural tissue). Tumors located in the posterior fossa, even extra-axial tumors, may also lead to compression of cerebellar tissue and fourth ventricle, leading to CSF obstruction.

Thus, hydrocephalus may accompany any intracranial tumor, be it intra- or extraventricular, intra- or extra-axial, once the lesion is large enough to affect the CSF pathways.

Prior surgery may also lead to obstructive hydrocephalus. For example, removal of a fourth ventricular tumor may lead to local scarring and obstruction of the fourth ventricular outlet.

Nonobstructive (Absorptive) Causes of Hydrocephalus

Certain tumors are associated with protein secretion, which may interfere with absorption. A typical example is a vestibular schwannoma (Fig. 11.1) [9, 33]. Leptomeningeal spread may also lead to CSF malabsorption and hydrocephalus.

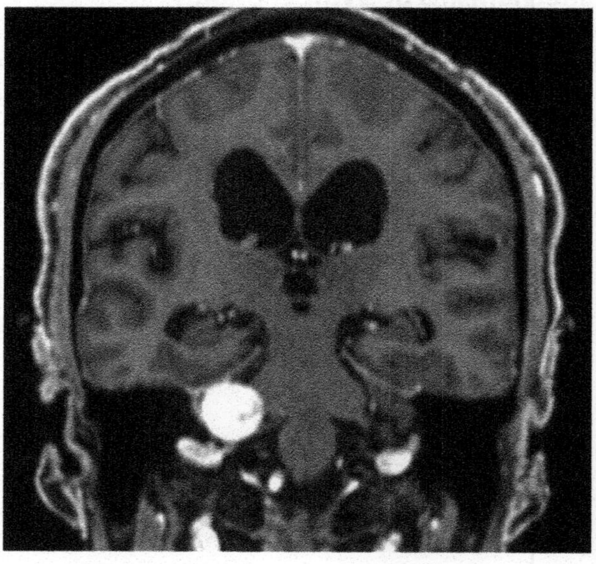

Fig. 11.1 Coronal T1-Gad MRI showing a right vestibular schwannoma in a 62-year-old presenting with symptoms suggestive of normal pressure hydrocephalus. The tumor was treated with radiosurgery and a shunt was placed

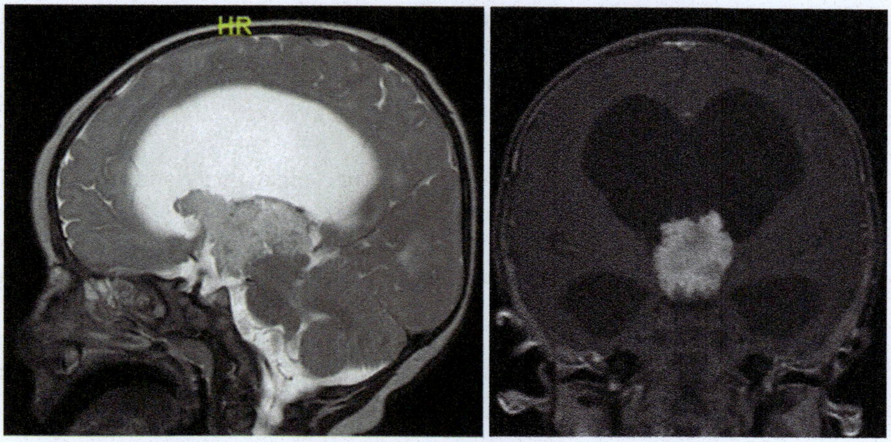

Fig. 11.2 Sagittal T2 and axial T1-Gad showing a third ventricular choroid plexus papilloma in a 5-month-old baby. The tumor was resected and a shunt was placed

Prior surgery may contribute to hydrocephalus by scarring along the CSF pathways, some of which may be at the cerebral convexity, often leading to a "nonobstructive"-like pattern.

CSF Overproduction

CSF overproduction is a rare condition and associated with two pathologies—choroid plexus hyperplasia (CPH; not a true tumor) and choroid plexus papilloma (CPP; typical or atypical)—both presenting in early childhood. Note that choroid plexus carcinoma (CPC) is not associated with CSF overproduction, probably because the cells lose their native ability to produce CSF. CPP may produce up to 5 liters of CSF per day [1, 8, 21], often with a high protein level. Thus, CPP may lead to hydrocephalus secondary to several causes: CSF overproduction, CSF pathway obstruction, and CSF malabsorption (Fig. 11.2).

Presentation of Hydrocephalus Related to Tumor Diagnosis

Hydrocephalus is the most typical reason for diagnosis of certain tumors, at certain ages, and is closely linked to the treatment strategy of tumors at certain locations.

Symptoms depend mostly on the age of the patient as well as the rate of hydrocephalus development; however, other more specific symptoms may accompany specific tumors. Thus, complimentary medical evaluations are needed. For example:

- Hypothalamic region may be associated with various endocrinopathies (over- and/or underproduction of pituitary-related hormones).

- Diabetes insipidus may present with germ cell tumors as well as follow treatment of craniopharyngiomas.
- Chiasmatic region tumors may lead to visual field compromise.
- Pineal region tumors, as well as other obstructive hydrocephalic conditions, may lead to Parinaud syndrome.
- Specific tumor locations may compress corticospinal tracts and cause focal motor deficits (such as thalamic or basal ganglia).
- Certain tumors are associated with specific syndromes, such as tuberous sclerosis, NF1, Li-Fraumeni, and Torcut. Thus, genetic consultations are advised in selected cases.
- Certain tumors are associated with a typical set of multiple locations, which may cause related symptoms (such as bifocal tumors and trilateral retinoblastoma).

Typical Tumor-Related Hydrocephalic Scenarios

Tectal Gliomas

These usually benign tumors are frequently associated with hydrocephalus secondary to obstruction of the aqueduct of Sylvius [12]. Often present in teenaged children, they cause increased ICP symptoms, usually presenting with acute hydrocephalus.

Tectal gliomas have a typical radiological appearance, with hyperintense T2 signal, isointense T1 signal, and no enhancement or restriction. Their diagnosis is usually radiological, and no tissue biopsy is needed (Fig. 11.3).

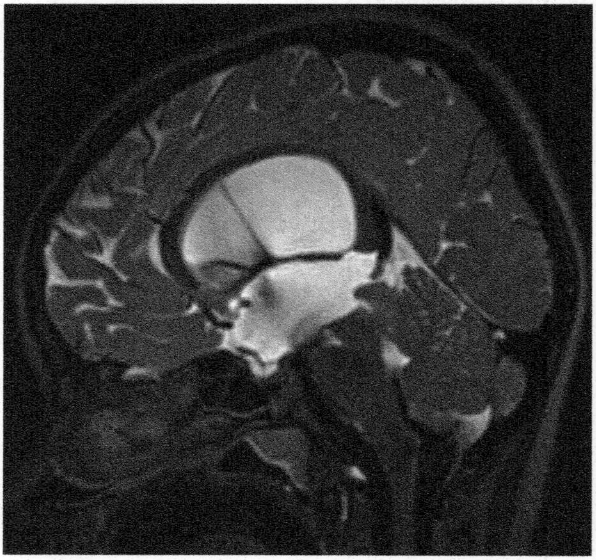

Fig. 11.3 Tectal glioma: Sagittal T2 SPACE MRI showing a tectal glioma and obstructive hydrocephalus in a 30-year-old. An ETV was performed and patient is followed

Care must be taken to differentiate these tumors from other closely located lesions, such as pineal and aqueductal tumors (ATs), which often necessitate a tissue biopsy. Also, atypical appearances such as tumor enhancement or restriction should prompt a tissue biopsy.

Pineal (Region) Tumors

Pineal tumors may overlap radiologically with adjacent originating tumors, such as aqueductal, tectal, and quadrigeminal cistern tumors. These tumors may cause aqueductal obstruction, and often, if truly of pineal origin, may also cause posterior third ventricular obstruction (Fig. 11.4).

Pineal region tumors involve a large differential diagnosis, such as germ cell tumors, primary pineal tumors (pineocytoma, pineoblastoma, papillary tumor pineal region, pineal parenchymal tumor), gliomas, and meningiomas. As treatment is dictated by the histopathological nature of these tumors, the primary treatment will often include an endoscopic third ventriculostomy (ETV) to solve the hydrocephalic condition, concurrently with testing of CSF cytology and markers (such as AFP, BHCG), and often an endoscopic biopsy from the tumor [19, 27].

Aqueductal Tumors

Closely located to the pineal region, and sometimes difficult to differentiate, this relatively rarely described entity causes aqueductal obstruction [26]. The main anatomical difference between aqueductal tumors (ATs) and other adjacent tumors is that ATs are epicentered **within** the aqueduct (Fig. 11.5). Thus, surgical resection

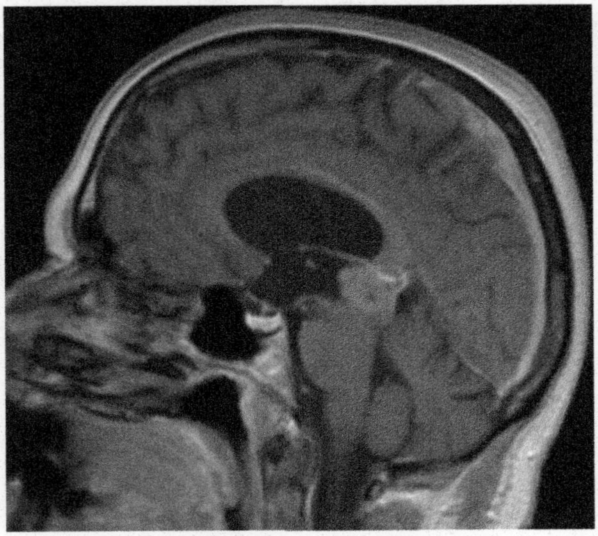

Fig. 11.4 Pineal tumor: Sagittal T1-Gad MRI showing a pineal region tumor in a 58-year-old. The patient underwent an ETV and endoscopic biopsy. Pathology was pineal parenchymal tumor of intermediate differentiation. The tumor was resected

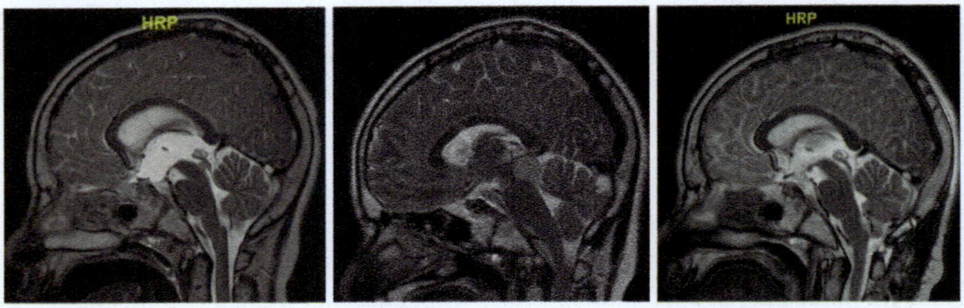

Fig. 11.5 Aqueductal tumor: A 12-year-old boy with neurofibromatosis type 2 presented with a small aqueductal tumor and hydrocephalus. He underwent an ETV. Two years later, the boy underwent a resection of the aqueductal tumor that grew. Pathology was ependymoma grade II

should involve approaches along the aqueduct, either from below (via the fourth ventricle) or from above (via the third ventricle) and not from posterior regions (thus risking the tectal plate).

ATs involve a large differential diagnosis, and as they present with obstructive hydrocephalus, we recommend a concurrent ETV and endoscopic biopsy [26].

Colloid Cysts

This is a benign tumor, typically located at the anterior third ventricle, connected to the anterior part of the tela choroidea and adjacent to both foramen of Monro (Fig. 11.6). Other locations have been described such as within the septum pellucidum or elsewhere in the ventricular system.

The cyst often presents with hydrocephalic-related symptoms secondary to obstruction of the foramen of Monro. Neurocognitive symptoms may occur, secondary to hydrocephalus and possibly compression of the fornix. Diagnosis is usually based on radiological appearance. Rarely, other pathologies may mimic CC.

Lateral Ventricular Lesion

The differential diagnosis of lateral ventricular tumors includes several typical pathologies such as central neurocytomas, subependymal giant cell astrocytomas (SEGA; associated with tuberous sclerosis complex), choroid plexus tumors, ependymomas, and others (Figs 11.7 and 11.8). These tumors often obstruct the foramen of Monro, leading to unilateral hydrocephalus. However, often, the septum pellucidum is shifted to the contralateral side, and the contralateral foramen of Monro may also become distorted and occluded.

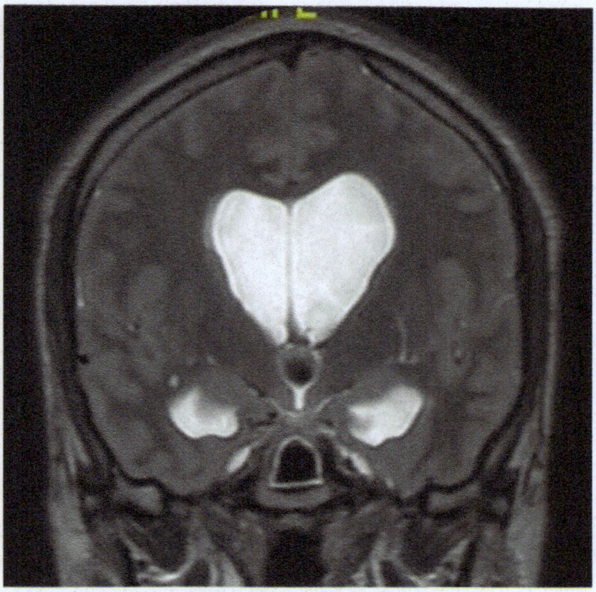

Fig. 11.6 Colloid cyst: Coronal T2 MRI showing a third ventricular colloid cyst in a 36-year-old presenting with acute hydrocephalus. The cyst was endoscopically removed

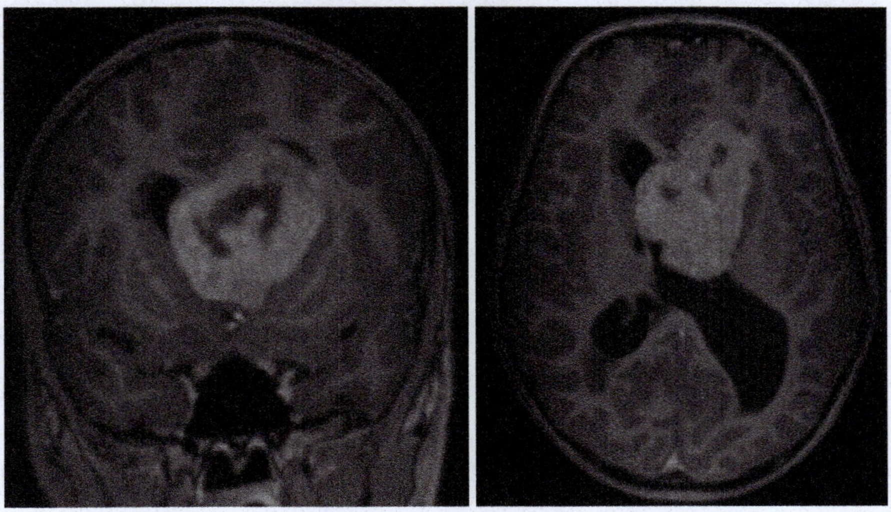

Fig. 11.7 Subependymal giant cell astrocytoma in lateral ventricle: Axial and coronal T1-Gad MRI showing a left ventricular SEGA in a 7-year-old boy with tuberous sclerosis. The tumor was resected, followed by a shunt

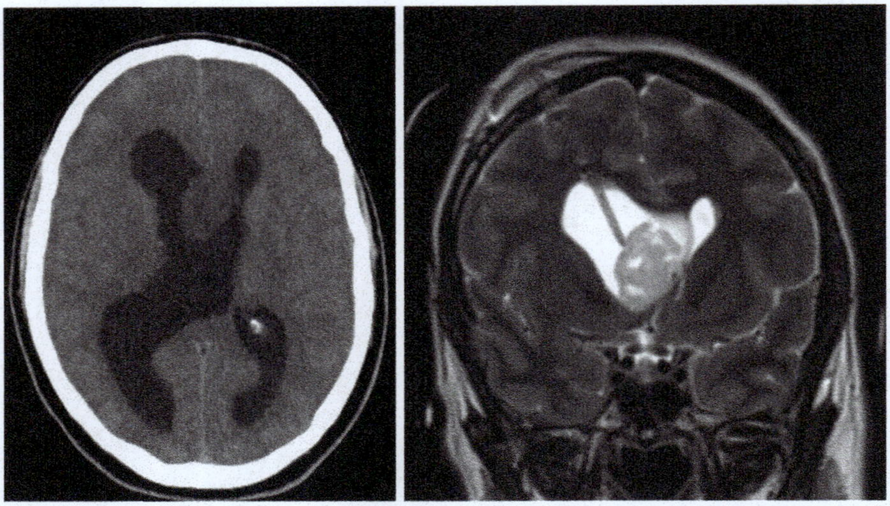

Fig. 11.8 Lateral ventricle subependymoma: A CT scan showing a right ventricular tumor in a 34-year-old presenting with acute hydrocephalus. An EVD was placed, followed by an MRI (coronal T2). The tumor was endoscopically resected, avoiding the need for permanent CSF diversion. Pathology was subependymoma

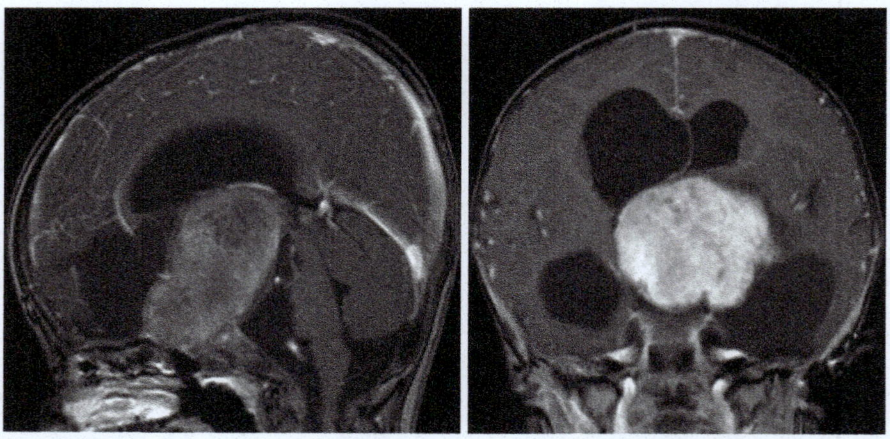

Fig. 11.9 Optic pathway glioma: Sagittal and coronal T1-Gad MRI showing a large chiasmatic-hypothalamic glioma in a 16-month-old. The tumor was subtotally resected, followed by a shunt and chemotherapy

Anterior Third Ventricular Tumors

A long list of pathologies may be located at this location, often occluding the foramen of Monro. Typically, these include high chiasmatic-hypothalamic gliomas (often referred to as optic pathway gliomas (OPG)) and other intraventricular pathologies (Fig. 11.9). However, tumors arising from the sella turcica, or below the

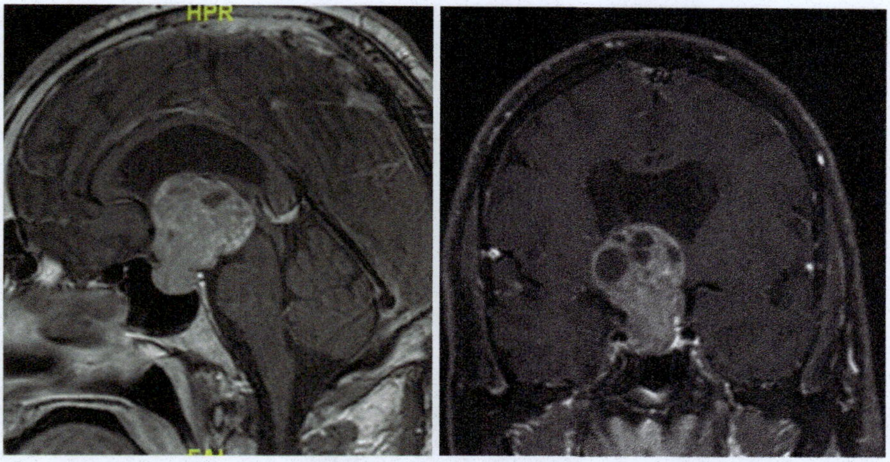

Fig. 11.10 Pituitary adenoma: Sagittal and coronal T1-Gad MRI showing a giant nonfunctioning pituitary adenoma with obstructive hydrocephalus in a 55-year-old. The tumor was resected via a transcallosal approach

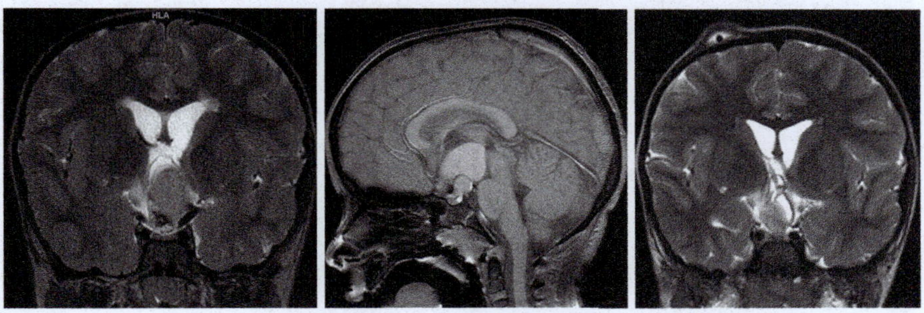

Fig. 11.11 Craniopharyngioma: A coronal T2, sagittal T1 MRI showing a craniopharyngioma in a 6-year-old. The child underwent an endoscopic placement of an ommaya and intracystic catheter, followed by radiotherapy

tuber cinereum, may grow upward, elevating the third ventricular floor and acting like any other intraventricular tumor, causing obstructive hydrocephalus (Figs 11.10 and 11.11). It is important to maximize use of diagnostic modalities such as CT scans (often demonstrating calcifications in craniopharyngiomas), tumor markers (AFP, BHCG, mAP), and endocrine and ophthalmological status.

Fourth Ventricular Tumors

Typically occurring at childhood (but not exclusively), these tumors include medulloblastomas, ependymomas, pilocytic astrocytomas, ATRT, and choroid plexus tumors (Fig. 11.12). As some of these tumors (especially medulloblastomas and

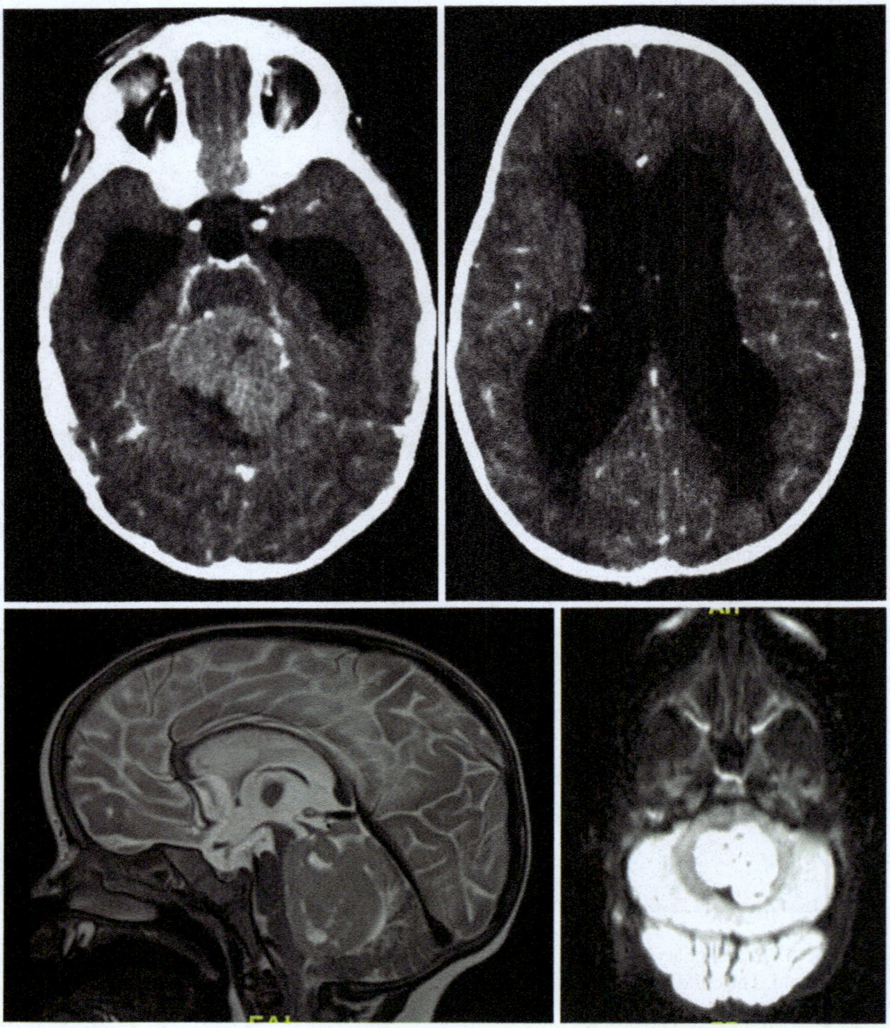

Fig. 11.12 Medulloblastoma: CT scan of a 14-month-old boy presenting in a deteriorated condition secondary to hydrocephalus secondary to a posterior fossa tumor. The child was shunted. Sagittal T2 and axial diffusion MRI showing a fourth ventricle medulloblastoma. The tumor was resected

ependymomas) may present with a metastatic disease, it is important to perform a full spinal MRI prior to surgical resection, as treatment paradigms may differ depending on the metastatic status.

The *Canadian Preoperative Prediction Rule for Hydrocephalus* (CPPRH) is a validated score that estimates the risk for postoperative hydrocephalus following resection of a posterior fossa tumor in children [7, 23]. The score lists five variables, including age, presence of papilledema prior to surgery, presence of significant hydrocephalus prior to resection, metastatic status, and histopathology. Each

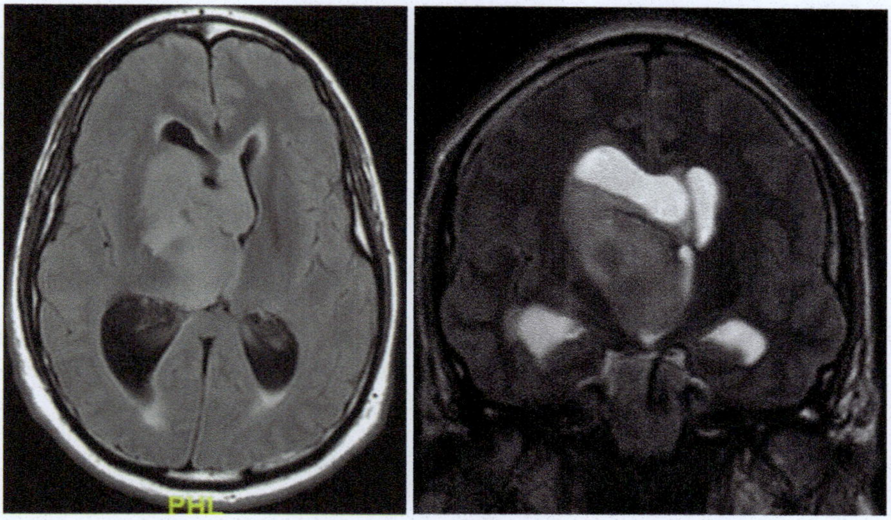

Fig. 11.13 Basal ganglia tumor: Axial FLAIR and coronal T2 MRI showing a right basal ganglia and forniceal tumor in a 29-year-old. The patient underwent an endoscopic septostomy—biopsy and a shunt. Pathology was an anaplastic astrocytoma. Patient was treated with chemotherapy and radiation

variable has a certain "weight" affecting the total score. For example, based on this score, it has been shown that children younger than 2 years with a medulloblastoma, presenting with significant hydrocephalus, have a greater than 80% chance of having postoperative hydrocephalus.

Thalamic and Basal Ganglia Tumors

These are rare tumors, including mostly gliomas of various grades (Fig. 11.13). The cause of hydrocephalus is usually obstructive—either by compression of the posterior third ventricle and aqueduct of Sylvius (associated with thalamic tumors) or by compression of the foramen of Monro and anterior third ventricle (associated with basal ganglia tumors) [28].

These tumors are of grades I–IV. Depending on the exophytic aspect to the ventricle, decisions regarding the ability to safely resect these tumors should be tailored per case.

Treatment of Hydrocephalus Associated with Brain Tumors

Treatment of tumor-associated hydrocephalus is a broad topic, and the patient-pathology strategy should be tailored. Generally, decision-making should focus on several goals:

1. Reducing treatment-related risks:
   The entire clinical scenario should be evaluated, not only the images.
   How old is the patient, what is the general and oncological condition, and what are the current symptoms attributed to?
   Often, treatment of the hydrocephalus entails a more limited procedure compared to surgery aimed at removing the causative pathology. A shunt, ETV, or septostomy may improve the symptoms even when not addressing the tumor.
2. Solve the life-threatening condition:
   Hydrocephalus may present as an acute life-threatening event, often necessitating an immediate response.
   Tumor-related mass effect (in the context of hydrocephalus) usually does not lead to a life-threatening condition apart from the hydrocephalus, and its treatment may be delayed and planned at a later stage.
   This is not to recommend that as a standard; tumors should not routinely be treated upfront, but rather judicious judgment should be exercised.
3. Solve the oncological condition:
   The treatment plan must focus on the tumor. Thus, depending on patient factors as well as tumor location, presumed diagnosis, and optional treatment paradigms, tumor-related surgical options can be planned, whether resection, biopsy, or testing CSF cytology and markers.

   To implement these goals, the following points must be considered:

1. Prioritization of treatment.
2. Treatment options for hydrocephalus: Shunt vs. endoscopy and technical considerations.
3. Treatment options for the tumor: Follow, biopsy, resect, and technical considerations.

In the following sections, we present several typical clinical scenarios and discuss treatment options.

Tectal Gliomas

This is probably the prototypical case of tumor-associated hydrocephalus. Since tectal gliomas obstructs the aqueduct and have an indolent oncological course, treatment consists of an endoscopic third ventriculostomy (ETV). No routine tumor biopsy is needed. Long-term ETV success is estimated to be greater than 80%. Enhancing lesions are an indicator for an endoscopic biopsy concurrently with the ETV [3, 22].

Pineal Region Tumors

These often present with obstructive hydrocephalus and are also associated with excellent long-term success following an ETV. However, as the differential diagnosis of such lesions includes germ cell tumors (especially in children and young adults) as well as many other tumors, CSF samples for cytology and markers should be checked. Ideally, a tissue sample should be supplied too.

Performing an ETV and an endoscopic biopsy (EBX) concurrently for a posterior third ventricular lesion necessitates two separate trajectories, both through the foramen of Monro: an anterior trajectory for the ETV and a posterior trajectory for the EBX. The anterior trajectory (for the ETV) is planned more or less parallel to the basilar artery (to avoid vascular injury), while the posterior trajectory (for the EBX) enables a clear view and access to the posterior-located tumor. Often, especially with relatively small and posterior located tumors, there is a large angle between both trajectories. This large angle limits the ability to use a single "ideal" entry for both ETV and EBX [19, 27]. To overcome these limitations, various techniques have been applied, each with its pros and cons:

- Drilling one *compromised* burr hole, midway between both "ideal" entry sites: This will impose some (but probably of limited clinical importance) pressure on the fornix (when performing the ETV) and on the posterior border of the foramen of Monro (when performing the EBX). In this technique, a rigid endoscope is used. This technique is applicable, especially when the tumor is not located extremely posteriorly or when it is larger than about 2 cm. Morgenstern et al. suggested the use of Massa intermedia (MI) as an anatomical border and recommended applying two burr holes for lesions situated behind the MI and one burr hole for lesions extending anterior to the MI [19].
- Drilling two separate burr holes, each one planned for a separate trajectory: The ETV entry is usually at the mid-pupillary line, about 1–2 cm anterior to the foramen of Monro, while the EBX entry is placed more anterior, at the hairline. Navigation is applied to identify the "ideal" locations of these entry sites. Usually, a rigid endoscope is used for both procedures. The major downside is the need for two burr holes and two separate transcortical passes.
- Drilling one burr hole but using a flexible endoscope: The flexible endoscope may be flexed anteriorly and posteriorly to reach the tuber cinereum or the tumor site, and may be used to perform both the ETV and the EBX.
- Drilling one entry hole (located as per the "ideal" trajectory for an ETV): You would then use a rigid endoscope for anatomical inspection, evaluation of tumor spread, and performing an ETV; and use a flexible endoscope for performing the EBX [27].

Interestingly, beyond the actual technique described, in cases with germ cell tumors, a fine ependymal staining of tumor deposits ("sugar coating") not visible on MRI scans may be seen intraoperatively when using an endoscope.

Colloid Cysts

Although benign in nature, these may lead to significant morbidity and mortality if not treated in a timely fashion once patients present with hydrocephalus. Once treated exclusively by an "open" resection (either transcortically or interhemispherically)

[20], today many surgeons are experienced with endoscopic resection of these lesions, with good results and low morbidity [11]. Several technical nuances should be noted:

1. A septostomy is recommended as a safety measure, taking into account potential tumor recurrence.
2. The entry point should be located relatively anterior, to achieve good control on the venous attachment of the CC.
3. The rate of cyst recurrence is probably low, even if some of the cyst capsule is not removed and is coagulated.

In cases of acute presentation, a unilateral (preferably with a septostomy) or bilateral external ventricular drain (EVD) may save the patient; a semi-elective surgery for tumor resection may be performed at a later stage.

For elderly patients or for patients with small cysts, a shunt coupled with a septostomy is a valid alternative.

Third Ventricular Tumors

Tumors occupying the anterior region of the third ventricle preclude the option of an ETV. Some of these tumors (such as giant pituitary adenomas which are non-prolactinomas and ependymomas) are resected. Others, such as cystic craniopharyngiomas, may be treated endoscopically by draining a large cyst and decompressing the obstruction (followed by intracystic treatments or radiation) [31]. Large chiasmatic-hypothalamic tumors may be treated by a multimodality approach, including some combination of surgery, chemotherapy, and radiation. In such cases, a shunt (with or without a septostomy) may solve the hydrocephalus. Interestingly, shunt-related ascites has been described treating OPG-related hydrocephalus, possibly secondary to a higher protein load in the CSF [10].

Thalamic and Basal Ganglia Tumors

Posterior thalamic tumors are good candidates for ETV and endoscopic biopsy of the tumor. Anterior thalamic and basal ganglia tumors may distort the regions of the foramen of Monro and anterior third ventricle, thus sometimes they may be treated with an ETV (possibly leaving a stent through the Monro) or a shunt [28].

It is important to carefully analyze the images, as adjustments in technique and use of navigation may be crucial in maintaining patient safety.

Lateral Ventricular Tumors

Depending on the acuteness of presentation and clinical context, several treatment approaches may be utilized. Endoscopic resections may be appropriate for relatively small and avascular lesions [2, 13]. Open approaches, either transcortical or interhemispheric/transcallosal, may be used as well. Often, removing the offending mass may solve the hydrocephalic condition with no need for additional CSF-related procedures. Generally, it is advised to perform a septostomy while treating the tumor, as postresection adhesions or tumor recurrence may lead to obstruction of the Monro.

Posterior Fossa Tumors

This is a broad topic which includes several tumor types and locations. Generally, a cerebellar hemispheric tumor causing mass effect with secondary hydrocephalus presents with a chronic condition, and thus should be resected upfront (Fig. 11.14). This eliminates the need for upfront CSF-related surgery (unless patient presents in an acute setting). In addition, a pre-resection treatment of the hydrocephalus with a shunt may pose a potential risk for upward herniation and intratumoral hemorrhage, although this is extremely rare [6].

Posterior fossa tumors in children pose a unique group. As indicated by the CPPRH score, young children presenting with significant hydrocephalus have a high risk for developing postoperative hydrocephalus [7, 23]. Sainte-Rose et al. suggested performing an ETV in children with posterior fossa tumor-related hydrocephalus before treating the tumor itself. This "prophylactic" ETV significantly reduced the rate of postoperative hydrocephalus from 27% to 6% [30]. However, this topic is debated, and many surgeons prefer to first address the tumor itself and treat the hydrocephalus later, only if necessary [6].

Placement of an EVD prior to tumor resection is highly recommended for patients presenting with acute hydrocephalus or for small children with a high

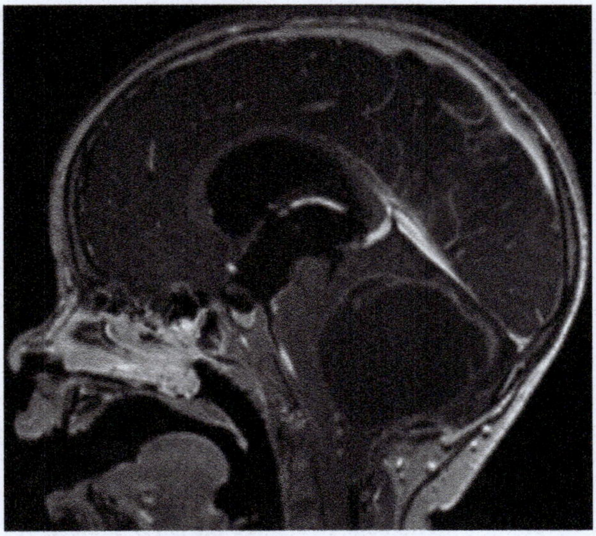

Fig. 11.14 Posterior fossa pilocytic astrocytoma: Sagittal T1-Gad MRI showing a posterior fossa pilocytic astrocytoma in a 3-year-old. Tumor was resected

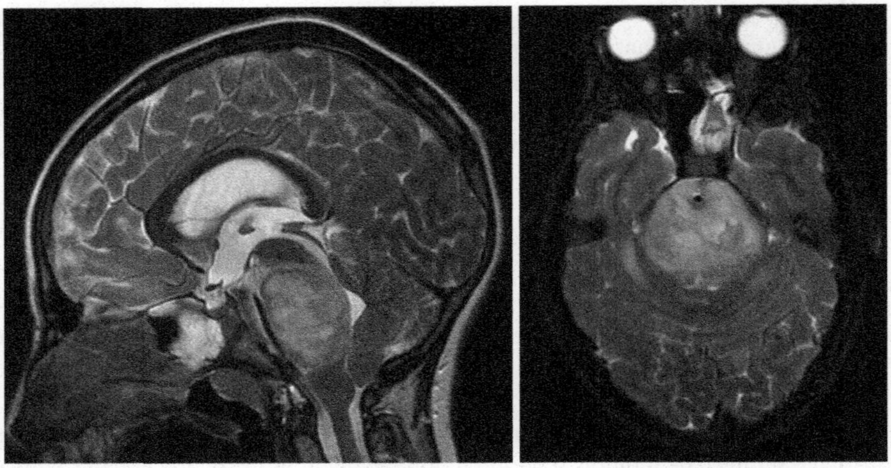

Fig. 11.15 Diffuse intrinsic pontine glioma: Sagittal and axial T2 MRI showing a DIPG and hydrocephalus in a 10-year-old. A shunt was placed

CPPRH score [16]. The EVD serves to reduce ICP during tumor resection as well as serve as a safety measure until the child has fully recovered and the ICP is under control while the EVD is closed [16].

Hydrocephalus following resection of posterior fossa tumors may often be related to fourth ventricle outlet obstruction (FVOO) secondary to local adhesions. These patients are thus candidates for an ETV or a shunt. In a recent systemic review, ETVs were associated with a higher short-term failure rate compared to shunts; however, they were associated with a higher long-term treatment durability compared to shunts [4].

Brainstem-related hydrocephalus is common in children with diffuse intrinsic pontine gliomas (DIPG). As the prognosis is poor and the brainstem tumor displaces the basilar artery anteriorly, we recommend avoiding ETV and placing a shunt (Fig. 11.15) [29].

Instrumentation

Shunt and Drain Related

In recent years, the main advancement in shunt and drain instrumentation has been the implementation of antibiotic impregnated catheters (AIC). It has been shown in several randomized trials that the use of AIC EVD has significantly reduced drain-related infections [25]. Despite the lack of randomized trials for shunt catheters, many extrapolate the results from the EVD literature and use AIC for shunts too [15].

We have recently published our experience converting EVDs to shunts (many of the patients underwent tumor-related surgeries). We found a low rate of failure or infection, with no need to change the EVD catheter [32].

Regarding the valves, there are many models in the market and there is no "ideal" valve. However, it is important to acknowledge that many of these patients undergo routine MRI scans for tumor follow-up. Programmable valves may cause artifacts on the scans, and some may need to be reprogrammed following an MRI scan.

Endoscopy

There are many endoscopes by many companies. Choosing a suitable endoscope depends on the actual planned procedure, and the need for more robust instrumentations, be it larger tumor forceps, good irrigation abilities, ability to aspirate blood clots, use of endoscopic aspirators (see below), need for a flexible endoscope, etc. For instance, smaller endoscopes with smaller working channels may suffice for an ETV; however, endoscopes with larger working channels are needed for insertion of larger instruments or aspirators.

Endoscopic Aspirators

Over recent years, several devices have been employed to assist purely endoscopic removal of intraventricular tumors. One device uses a "side cutter" that shaves and aspirates tissue [5, 14, 17, 18, 24]. Other devices are based on a Cavitron ultrasonic aspirator (CUSA) [2]. These systems are not widely used and experience is limited. The main limitations using such aspirators are related to the size and vascularity of the tumor. Several surgeons advise limiting use of an aspirator to small lesions, up to about 2–2.5 cm. Additionally, vascular lesions cause staining of the ambient fluid, limiting visualization and potentially risking the patient. Thus, careful patient selection is essential and the surgeon must be prepared to convert to an "open" surgery, if needed.

Risk Avoidance in Treating Tumor-Related Hydrocephalus

As discussed earlier, the topic of tumor-associated hydrocephalus is broad and there are no simple guidelines for treatment. However, careful radiological analysis of the lesion, good understanding of the clinical aspects, and a meticulous surgical technique, utilizing the appropriate technologies, are the basis for avoiding complications.

Follow-Up

As for any other hydrocephalic patient and even more so since the cause is tumor-related, long-term clinical and radiological follow-ups are warranted, preferably with MRI.

If prior treatment included an ETV, flow sensitive sequences such as T2 SPACE should be performed to enhance flow demonstration through the stoma.

Conclusion

Tumor-related hydrocephalus is often the leading cause of presenting symptoms and may lead to significant morbidity and mortality. Treatment of patients with tumor-related hydrocephalus should relate to acuteness of symptoms, pathophysiological cause of the hydrocephalus, tumor-related factors (such as location, presumed diagnosis, metastatic status), and availability of endoscopic instrumentations.

In certain cases, treatment of the hydrocephalus may be the main surgical treatment needed, preceding any other surgical and oncological treatment.

References

1. Cataltepe O, Liptzin D, Jolley L, Smith TW. Diffuse villous hyperplasia of the choroid plexus and its surgical management. J Neurosurg Pediatr. 2010;5:518–22.
2. Cinalli G, Imperato A, Mirone G, Di Martino G, Nicosia G, Ruggiero C, et al. Initial experience with endoscopic ultrasonic aspirator in purely neuroendoscopic removal of intraventricular tumors. J Neurosurg Pediatr. 2017;19:325–32.
3. Daglioglu E, Cataltepe O, Akalan N. Tectal gliomas in children: the implications for natural history and management strategy. Pediatr Neurosurg. 2003;38:223–31.
4. Dewan MC, Lim J, Shannon CN, Wellons JC 3rd. The durability of endoscopic third ventriculostomy and ventriculoperitoneal shunts in children with hydrocephalus following posterior fossa tumor resection: a systematic review and time-to-failure analysis. J Neurosurg Pediatr. 2017;19:578–84.
5. Dlouhy BJ, Dahdaleh NS, Greenlee JD. Emerging technology in intracranial neuroendoscopy: application of the NICO Myriad. Neurosurg Focus. 2011;30:E6.
6. El-Gaidi MA, El-Nasr AH, Eissa EM. Infratentorial complications following preresection CSF diversion in children with posterior fossa tumors. J Neurosurg Pediatr. 2015;15:4–11.
7. Foreman P, McClugage S 3rd, Naftel R, Griessenauer CJ, Ditty BJ, Agee BS, et al. Validation and modification of a predictive model of postresection hydrocephalus in pediatric patients with posterior fossa tumors. J Neurosurg Pediatr. 2013;12:220–6.
8. Fujimura M, Onuma T, Kameyama M, Motohashi O, Kon H, Yamamoto K, et al. Hydrocephalus due to cerebrospinal fluid overproduction by bilateral choroid plexus papillomas. Childs Nerv Syst. 2004;20:485–8.
9. Fukuda M, Oishi M, Kawaguchi T, Watanabe M, Takao T, Tanaka R, et al. Etiopathological factors related to hydrocephalus associated with vestibular schwannoma. Neurosurgery. 2007;61:1186–92; discussion 1192–93
10. Gil Z, Beni-Adani L, Siomin V, Nagar H, Dvir R, Constantini S. Ascites following ventriculoperitoneal shunting in children with chiasmatic-hypothalamic glioma. Childs Nerv Syst. 2001;17:395–8.
11. Greenlee JD, Teo C, Ghahreman A, Kwok B. Purely endoscopic resection of colloid cysts. Neurosurgery. 2008;62:51–5; discussion 55–6
12. Griessenauer CJ, Rizk E, Miller JH, Hendrix P, Tubbs RS, Dias MS, et al. Pediatric tectal plate gliomas: clinical and radiological progression, MR imaging characteristics, and management of hydrocephalus. J Neurosurg Pediatr. 2014;13:13–20.
13. Harter DH, Omeis I, Forman S, Braun A. Endoscopic resection of an intraventricular dysembryoplastic neuroepithelial tumor of the septum pellucidum. Pediatr Neurosurg. 2006;42:105–7.

14. Hidalgo ET, Ali A, Weiner HL, Harter DH. Resection of intraventricular tumors in children by purely endoscopic means. World Neurosurg. 2016;87:372–80.
15. Klimo P Jr, Thompson CJ, Baird LC, Flannery AM. Pediatric Hydrocephalus Systematic R, Evidence-Based Guidelines Task F: pediatric hydrocephalus: systematic literature review and evidence-based guidelines. Part 7: antibiotic-impregnated shunt systems versus conventional shunts in children: a systematic review and meta-analysis. J Neurosurg Pediatr. 2014;14(Suppl 1):53–9.
16. Lin CT, Riva-Cambrin JK. Management of posterior fossa tumors and hydrocephalus in children: a review. Childs Nerv Syst. 2015;31:1781–9.
17. Mohanty A, Thompson BJ, Patterson J. Initial experience with endoscopic side cutting aspiration system in pure neuroendoscopic excision of large intraventricular tumors. World Neurosurg. 2013;80(655):e615–21.
18. Moore RJ, Scherer A, Fulkerson DH. Frontal burr hole approach for neuroendoscopic resection of craniopharyngioma with the NICO Myriad device: report of two cases. Childs Nerv Syst. 2017;33:659–64.
19. Morgenstern PF, Souweidane MM. Pineal region tumors: simultaneous endoscopic third ventriculostomy and tumor biopsy. World Neurosurg. 2013;79(S18):e19–3.
20. Nair S, Gopalakrishnan CV, Menon G, Easwer HV, Abraham M. Interhemispheric transcallosal transforaminal approach and its variants to colloid cyst of third ventricle: technical issues based on a single institutional experience of 297 cases. Asian J Neurosurg. 2016;11: 292–7.
21. Nimjee SM, Powers CJ, McLendon RE, Grant GA, Fuchs HE. Single-stage bilateral choroid plexectomy for choroid plexus papilloma in a patient presenting with high cerebrospinal fluid output. J Neurosurg Pediatr. 2010;5:342–5.
22. Oka K, Kin Y, Go Y, Ueno Y, Hirakawa K, Tomonaga M, et al. Neuroendoscopic approach to tectal tumors: a consecutive series. J Neurosurg. 1999;91:964–70.
23. Riva-Cambrin J, Detsky AS, Lamberti-Pasculli M, Sargent MA, Armstrong D, Moineddin R, et al. Predicting postresection hydrocephalus in pediatric patients with posterior fossa tumors. J Neurosurg Pediatr. 2009;3:378–85.
24. Rodgers SD, Bassani L, Weiner HL, Harter DH. Stereotactic endoscopic resection and surgical management of a subependymal giant cell astrocytoma: case report. J Neurosurg Pediatr. 2012;9:417–20.
25. Root BK, Barrena BG, Mackenzie TA, Bauer DF. Antibiotic impregnated external ventricular drains: meta and cost analysis. World Neurosurg. 2016;86:306–15.
26. Roth J, Chaichana KL, Jallo G, Mirone G, Cinalli G, Constantini S. True aqueductal tumors: a unique entity. Acta Neurochir. 2015;157:169–77.
27. Roth J, Constantini S. Combined rigid and flexible endoscopy for tumors in the posterior third ventricle. J Neurosurg. 2015;122:1341–6.
28. Roth J, Ram Z, Constantini S. Endoscopic considerations treating hydrocephalus caused by basal ganglia and large thalamic tumors. Surg Neurol Int. 2015;6:56.
29. Roujeau T, Di Rocco F, Dufour C, Bourdeaut F, Puget S, Rose CS, et al. Shall we treat hydrocephalus associated to brain stem glioma in children? Childs Nerv Syst. 2011;27:1735–9.
30. Sainte-Rose C, Cinalli G, Roux FE, Maixner R, Chumas PD, Mansour M, et al. Management of hydrocephalus in pediatric patients with posterior fossa tumors: the role of endoscopic third ventriculostomy. J Neurosurg. 2001;95:791–7.
31. Shukla D. Transcortical transventricular endoscopic approach and Ommaya Reservoir Placement for Cystic Craniopharyngioma. Pediatr Neurosurg. 2015;50:291–4.
32. Soleman J, Benvenisti H, Constantini S, Roth J. Conversion of external ventricular drainage to ventriculo-peritoneal shunt: to change or not to change the proximal catheter? Childs Nerv Syst. 2017;33:1947.
33. Taniguchi M, Nakai T, Kohta M, Kimura H, Kohmura E. Communicating hydrocephalus associated with small- to medium-sized vestibular schwannomas: clinical significance of the tumor apparent diffusion coefficient map. World Neurosurg. 2016;94:261–7.

Idiopathic Normal Pressure Hydrocephalus

12

Albert M. Isaacs, Mark G. Hamilton, and Michael A. Williams

Introduction

Hydrocephalus is characterized by overaccumulation of cerebrospinal fluid (CSF) within the cerebral ventricles due to a mismatch between CSF production and CSF resorption into systemic circulation [1]. While many forms of hydrocephalus are associated with raised intracranial pressure (ICP) [2, 3], some patients have clinical and radiologic signs of hydrocephalus in the presence of low-to-normal ICP. This form of hydrocephalus was described in the 1960s by Salomon Hakim, who called it normal pressure hydrocephalus (NPH) [4–6]. The patients that Hakim described had an antecedent cause of hydrocephalus such as hemorrhage, trauma, or infection; however, patients were later found to have the NPH syndrome in the absence of known risk factors, which was designated idiopathic normal pressure hydrocephalus (iNPH), which now constitutes the majority of cases [7]. Thus, NPH can be either idiopathic or secondary to known risk factors [8–10]. iNPH is primarily observed in adult patients (age ≥65 years) and is clinically characterized by the presence of neurologic gait impairment plus additional features of a symptom triad—cognitive impairment and urinary incontinence [11].

A. M. Isaacs (✉)
Division of Biology and Biomedical Sciences, Washington University in St. Louis, St. Louis, MO, USA

Division of Neurosurgery, Department of Clinical Neuroscience, University of Calgary, Calgary, AB, Canada
e-mail: albert.isaacs@wustl.edu

M. G. Hamilton
Division of Neurosurgery, Department of Clinical Neuroscience, University of Calgary, Calgary, AB, Canada

M. A. Williams
Departments of Neurology and Neurological Surgery, University of Washington School of Medicine, Seattle, WA, USA

D. D. Limbrick, J. R. Leonard (eds.), *Cerebrospinal Fluid Disorders*,
https://doi.org/10.1007/978-3-319-97928-1_12

Epidemiology

The global epidemiology of iNPH is not known. Published regional studies have reported highly variable rates of prevalence, ranging from 10/100,000 to 5900/100,000 [12, 13]. In some groups of patients, prevalence rates are higher than the general population. For example, the prevalence among dementia patients and those with cerebrovascular disease are 5380/100,000 [14] and 4000/100,000 [15], respectively. Among the elderly residing in care facilities, iNPH prevalence may be up to 14,000/100,000 [16]. Studies on the incidence of iNPH are uncommon. In a pooled population-based study of people ≥65 years old, an incidence rate of 120 new cases per 100,000 was found [17]. The variability in reported prevalence and incidence rates may be attributed to differences in the diagnostic criteria used among studies. In a recent systematic review by Martin-Laez et al. (2015), iNPH diagnoses in over half of the studies were not guidelines based [18]. In addition, a majority of those studies included only few patients, with heterogeneity in the age cut off for inclusion [18]. This underscores the need for robust epidemiological studies, more research, and diagnostic guidance in iNPH care.

Pathophysiology

Recent evidence for the pathophysiology of iNPH implicates a combined effect of disrupted CSF flow dynamics, impaired brain metabolism, grey and white matter microstructural changes, dysregulated CSF biochemistry, and cerebrovascular compromise [19–24]. From a symptoms perspective, the gait impairment has been attributed to several mechanisms, including reduced cerebral blood flow in subcortical regions [25], disruption of the midbrain cytoarchitecture [25–27], cortical and subcortical circuit disruption [25–28], disinhibited corticospinal excitability [27, 29], and postural disturbance [27, 30]. The cognitive dysfunction is believed to be due to diffuse cortical and subcortical dysfunction, which may be attributed to mechanical disruption by the enlarged ventricles [31–33], CSF metabolic and neurochemical derangements [33–35], and reduced regional cerebral perfusion, especially in the frontal and anterior temporal lobes [33–36]. The urinary incontinence is attributed to disinhibition of the central micturition centers [37, 38], blunting of the spinobulbospinal reflex [38], detrusor overactivity, and reduced bladder capacity [38, 39]. A unifying pathophysiological mechanism of the reversible neuronal and glial dysfunction responsible for iNPH symptoms has not yet been identified. Thus, the mechanism by which shunting restores neurologic function is not fully understood and may be multifactorial [26, 40].

Risk Factors

Cerebrovascular, cardiovascular, and peripheral vascular diseases are often comorbidities of iNPH, and they have also been reported as risk factors [15, 41]. In fact, cerebrovascular disease has been implicated as the most common cause of death in iNPH [42]. Other associated comorbidities of iNPH include diabetes, low high-density lipoprotein levels, depression, apathy, sleep disturbance, and a history of stroke or transient ischemic attack [7, 22, 43, 44]. This does raise the question of whether risk factor modification strategies can reduce the risk of developing iNPH [15].

Natural History

By definition, iNPH is a disease of the elderly (age ≥65 years old) and the majority of patients present with gait impairment [44, 45]. As a general rule, iNPH is considered to be a progressive disorder, but the rate of progression is difficult to predict. Although many patients and families describe a sudden onset of symptoms, careful review often reveals that the patient has had insidiously developing symptoms for weeks or months that did not come to attention until a specific event (such as a fall) or hospitalization. The symptoms of iNPH are often preceded by a period of asymptomatic progressive ventricular dilatation that may last several years [44]. The syndrome of patients who present with enlarged ventricles without any signs or symptoms of iNPH have been termed asymptomatic ventriculomegaly with features of iNPH on MRI (AVIM). These patients have an increased risk of developing dementia [46, 47]. No clinical consensus exists with respect to treating or monitoring patients with AVIM while they are asymptomatic.

On the other hand, patients who have been diagnosed with iNPH by the recommendations and guidelines described below should be treated [48, 49], as delay of iNPH treatment even for 3–6 months may lead to poorer outcomes [50, 51]. Untreated hydrocephalus is associated with a 5-year mortality risk of 87% [52], which has been attributed to heart disease, cerebrovascular disease, dementia, and injury [42, 53–55].

Clinical Examination

The diagnosis of iNPH requires thorough history taking, physical examination, review of imaging, and exclusion of other diagnoses that would explain the patient's symptoms. Neuroimaging is necessary to demonstrate ventriculomegaly, identify or exclude obstruction to CSF flow within the ventricular system, and to assess other brain disorders that may be partially or entirely responsible for the patient's symptoms [56].

Gait Assessment

Gait disturbance is the most common and earliest symptom of iNPH, present in 94–100 of cases [44, 45]. The gait impairment of iNPH includes retropulsion and anteropulsion of stance, gait initiation failure, diminished foot clearance, and unsteadiness with turning [7]. Typically, the gait is wide based, slow, and shuffling [44]. Patients also have difficulty with transitional movements such as getting in or out of a chair. The absence of gait impairment is extremely uncommon in iNPH, and if gait impairment is not found, then other diagnoses should be evaluated before performing tests that are specific for iNPH. A gait assessment should be performed in all patients with suspected iNPH. The assessment serves as a benchmark for assessing either worsening or improvement in untreated patients, is needed to predict response to surgery when tests of CSF removal are performed, and is necessary for long-term follow-up and monitoring of surgical response [7, 57, 58]. Several tests that have been used to assess the gait of iNPH patients include the 10-meter walk test, timed up and go test, Tinetti assessment tool, and the Boon scale [59–62].

Cognitive Assessment

Cognitive difficulties are observed in 78–98% of iNPH patients. These tend to be gradual and progressive, and patients encounter the same difficulties as seen with other forms of dementia, such as difficulty managing medications, or banking, or appointments [7, 44, 63]. Over time, the cognitive dysfunction progresses to affect the ability to plan, problem solve, and to carry out daily self-care activities, which often preclude patients from safely living independently [7]. Depression, apathy, and sleep disturbance have also been associated with iNPH [7, 43, 44]. Delirium is not a feature of iNPH and its presence should raise the suspicion of a different or concomitant disease that requires treatment. Patients who have been admitted to the hospital with delirium or failure to thrive should not be assessed for iNPH until they have left the hospital and return to a stable baseline, because the delirium or underlying disorder can make it impossible to determine if a patient's response (or lack of response) to CSF removal is due to iNPH or the underlying disorder [7]. A number of screening tests have been used to assess cognitive impairment in iNPH, including the Montreal Cognitive Assessment, Beck Depression Inventory, and the Mini Mental Status Exam [64, 65]. While many cognitive domains may be affected, typically the deficits are primarily frontal-subcortical. The cognitive domains affected on neuropsychological testing include attention, concentration, executive function, working and recall memory, language, visuoconstructional skills, and conceptual thinking [66, 67]. The presence of an amnestic memory impairment (i.e., rapid forgetting that does not benefit from cueing) or significant impairment of language or naming should raise concern for a neurodegenerative dementia.

Urinary Incontinence Evaluation

Approximately, 76–83% of iNPH patients present with features of urinary frequency, urinary urgency, and incontinence. The characteristics of a patient's urinary dysfunction can be obtained through history taking. More importantly, other differential diagnoses such as neurogenic and urologic causes of urinary incontinence such as cervical or lumbar stenosis with myelopathy, spinal cord injury, prostatic hypertrophy, pelvic floor disorders, and overactive bladder should be ruled out [7, 37, 44, 68].

Diagnostic Criteria

Since 2004, two major guidelines to direct iNPH diagnosis and management have been published: the International guidelines [45, 69] and the Japanese guidelines [44, 58, 70]. In 2015, the American Academy of Neurology (AAN) published recommendations for iNPH management [71]. While there are subtle differences between the guidelines, they all emphasize clinical assessments to exclude the presence of other causes of the patient's symptoms before performing diagnostic testing. Neuroimaging is also emphasized. Ventricular enlargement is defined as an Evans ratio >0.3 [44, 63]. iNPH patients may be further categorized into three subgroups: "possible," "probable," and "definite" iNPH [44, 45, 58, 69, 70]. A patient ≥60-year-old with at least one symptom in the cognitive, gait, or urinary domains, plus having abnormal ventricular dilatation is classified as a "possible" iNPH. The criteria for "probable" iNPH is stricter and is diagnosed if a patient meets the possible iNPH criteria and has a confirmed CSF pressure ≤20 cmH_2O, plus either a Disproportionately Enlarged Subarachnoid Space Hydrocephalus (DESH) pattern of hydrocephalus on CT/MRI or a positive CSF tap or drainage test. A "definite" iNPH diagnosis is made after surgery, if a patient's symptoms improve after shunt surgery [44]. Table 12.1 compares the International and Japanese guidelines [7].

Neuroimaging

Evidence of abnormally enlarged ventricles on CT or MRI is necessary for the diagnosis of iNPH. High-resolution neuroimaging is also needed to look for obstruction to CSF flow, as 5–10% of patients with the iNPH syndrome have obstructive forms of hydrocephalus [72, 73]. Several measures have been described to determine whether the ventricles are enlarged, including the Evans Ratio, Frontal and Occipital Horn Ratio, and Callosal Angle [74, 75] (Fig. 12.1). The most widely used is the Evans Ratio, which is the ratio of the width of the frontal horns to the widest biparietal diameter. An Evans ratio >0.3 is considered abnormal [44, 45, 58, 69–71]. Even with evidence of enlarged ventricles, the confounder of hydrocephalus ex-vacuo (i.e., enlargement of the ventricles secondary to tissue loss) must be carefully assessed. As many as 21% of patients over the age of 70 who do not have iNPH have an Evans ratio of >0.3 [76]. In some iNPH patients, DESH, which is defined as the presence of hydrocephalus in the setting of relative effacement of the subarachnoid space at the vertex (high and tight) and disproportionate enlargement of the Sylvian fissures has been described [77].

Table 12.1 Comparison between the International and Japanese guidelines for the diagnosis of iNPH [7]

Feature	International guidelines	Japanese guidelines
Essential symptoms	Findings of gait/balance disturbance must be present, plus at least one other area of impairment in cognition, urinary symptoms, or both	More than one of the clinical triad: gait disturbance, cognitive impairment, and urinary incontinence
		Gait disturbance is the most prevalent feature, followed by cognitive impairment and urinary incontinence
Symptom onset	Insidious	Symptoms progress slowly
Symptom duration	Minimum duration of 3–6 months	
Age at onset	After age 40	After age 60
Etiology	No evidence of an antecedent event such as head trauma, intracerebral hemorrhage, meningitis, or other known causes of secondary hydrocephalus	Preceding diseases possibly causing ventricular dilation are not obvious, including subarachnoid hemorrhage, meningitis, head injury, congenital hydrocephalus, and aqueductal stenosis
Comorbid disorders	No other neurologic, psychiatric, or general medical conditions that are sufficient to explain the presenting symptoms	Clinical symptoms cannot be completely explained by other neurologic or non-neurologic diseases
		Other neurologic diseases, including Parkinson disease, Alzheimer disease, and cerebrovascular diseases, may coexist but should be mild
Gait impairment	At least two of the following should be present and not be entirely attributable to other conditions: Decreased step height Decreased step length Decreased cadence (speed of walking) Increased trunk sway during walking Widened standing base Toes turned outward on walking Retropulsion (spontaneous or provoked) En bloc turning (three or more steps for 180°) Impaired walking balance, as evidenced by two or more corrections out of eight steps on tandem gait testing	Small stride, shuffle, instability during walking, and increase of instability on turning

Table 12.1 (continued)

Feature	International guidelines	Japanese guidelines
Urinary urgency/ incontinence	One of the following should be present: Episodic or persistent urinary incontinence not attributable to primary urologic disorders Urinary and fecal incontinence Or any two of the following should be present: Urinary urgency (frequent perception of a pressing need to void) Urinary frequency (more than six voiding episodes in an average 12-h period) Nocturia (the need to urinate more than twice a night)	Overactive bladder, mainly manifesting as increased nocturnal urinary frequency, urgency, and urinary incontinence
Cognitive impairment	Documented impairment (adjusted for age and educational attainment) or decrease in performance on a cognitive screening instrument, or both	Cognitive impairment is detected on cognitive tests
	Or evidence of at least two of the following on examination that is not fully attributable to other conditions: Psychomotor slowing (increased response latency) Decreased fine motor speed Decreased fine motor accuracy Difficulty dividing or maintaining attention Impaired recall, especially for recent events Executive dysfunction Behavioral or personality changes	
Ventricular size	Ventricular enlargement not entirely attributable to cerebral size atrophy or congenital enlargement (Evans index 0.0.3 or comparable measure)	Ventricular dilation (Evans index 0.0.3)
Other neuroimaging features	No macroscopic obstruction to CSF flow	Sylvian fissures and basal cistern are usually enlarged
	At least one of the following supportive features: Enlargement of the temporal horns of the lateral ventricles not entirely attributable to hippocampus atrophy Callosal angle of 40° or more Evidence of altered brain water content, including periventricular signal changes on CT and MRI not attributable to microvascular ischemic changes or demyelination An aqueductal or fourth ventricular flow void on MRI	Periventricular changes are not essential Narrowing of the sulci and subarachnoid spaces over the high convexity/midline surface (DESH)

(continued)

Table 12.1 (continued)

Feature	International guidelines	Japanese guidelines
CSF pressure	CSF opening pressure in the range of 5–18 mm Hg (or 70–245 mm H2O), as determined by LP or a comparable procedure; appropriately measured pressures that are significantly higher or lower than this range are not consistent with a probable NPH diagnosis	CSF pressure of #200 mm H2O and normal CSF content

Reprinted with permission from Williams and Relkin [7]
Abbreviations: *DESH* disproportionately enlarged subarachnoid space hydrocephalus, *LP* lumbar puncture

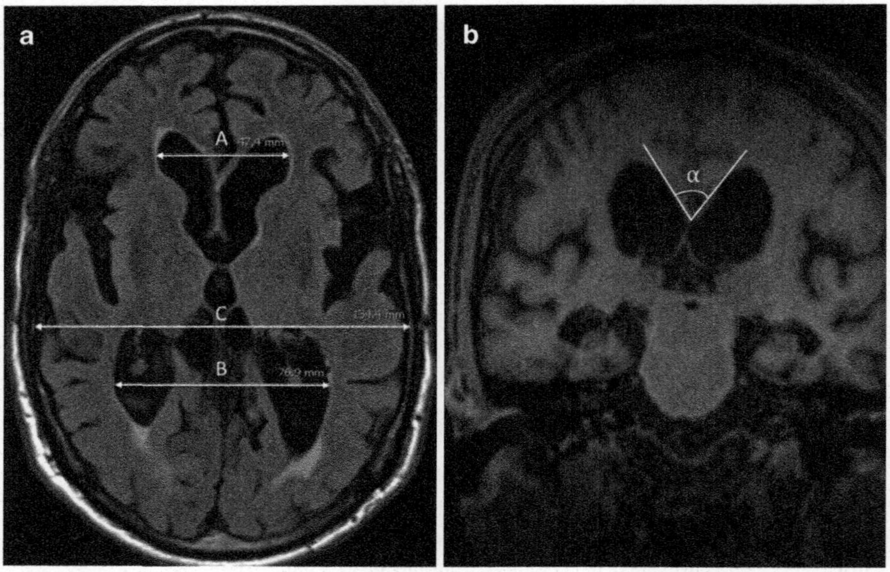

Fig. 12.1 MRI images of an 83-year-old male with iNPH. Image (**a**) is an axial T2-FLAIR image demonstrating enlarged ventricles with an Evan's ratio (*A*/*C*) of 0.35 and a frontal and occipital horn ratio (*A* + *B*)/2*C* of 0.46. Image (**b**) is a coronal T1-weighted image demonstrating a callosal angle, α of 70% at the level of the posterior commissure

DESH is believed to result from impaired CSF absorption, which leads to overaccumulation of CSF in the basal cisterns and a subsequent superoposterior displacement of the brain [78]. DESH has been described as a promising feature for shunt responsiveness in iNPH [50, 77, 78]. Kaziu et al. (2015) reported that of the 100 DESH-positive iNPH patients who underwent surgery, 80% demonstrated symptoms improvement irrespective of the results of their presurgical confirmatory test [50]. However, the negative predictive value (NPV) of DESH for shunt responsiveness in a retrospective cohort was found to be 25% [79], which suggests that going only by DESH criteria would miss a substantial proportion of potential iNPH shunt responders.

Table 12.2 Common diseases in the differential diagnosis of iNPH

	Gait	Dementia	Bladder
Stroke	x	x	x
Corticobasal syndrome	x	x	
Lewy body dementia	x	x	
Multiple system atrophy	x	x	
Parkinson's disease	x	x	
Progressive supranuclear palsy	x	x	
Cervical spondylotic myelopathy	x		
Hip and knee osteoarthritis	x		
Lumbar stenosis	x		x
Myopathy	x		
Polyneuropathy	x		
Alzheimer's disease		x	
Binzwanger disease		x	
Depression		x	
Psychosis		x	
Vascular dementia		x	x
Prostatic hyperplasia			x

Comorbidities and Differential Diagnosis

Because iNPH is seen in the older population, it is often associated with comorbidities such as osteoarthritis, heart disease, cerebral microvascular disease, Alzheimer dementia, diabetes, depression, falls, medication side effects, and impaired vision, all of which can exacerbate the iNPH symptoms or be entirely responsible for them in the absence of iNPH [15, 40, 41, 43, 64, 80–83]. Commonly, iNPH is overlooked or misdiagnosed as part of "normal aging" or as an early sign of neurodegeneration. Chronic conditions also have an impact on the outcomes of treatment for iNPH and should therefore be carefully examined or ruled out as the primary cause of the patient's presentation. Table 12.2 presents a list of comorbidities that may have clinical presentations similar to iNPH and may pose challenges to the accurate diagnosis of iNPH.

Presurgical CSF Dynamic Testing

Patients should undergo presurgical testing to predict their response prior to shunt surgery. The three most common confirmatory tests are large volume lumbar tap (tap test), extended lumbar drainage (ELD), and the CSF infusion test [57, 63].

Tap Test

The tap test involves removal of 30–50 cc of CSF via a standard lumbar puncture and testing the patient's gait and cognition before and after the procedure. It is recommended to wait 2–3 h before testing the patient's response. Patients may be tested again after 6–8 h if no improvement is noticed within the first 3 h, since some continue to show improvement even beyond the 24 h after a tap test [84]. The tap test has been shown to have a positive predictive value (PPV) of 73–100%, a negative predictive value (NPV) of 16–42% and an accuracy of 45–54% for shunting success in iNPH [85, 86].

External Lumbar Drainage

The external lumbar drainage (ELD) procedure involves inserting a spinal catheter through a Tuohy needle into the lumbar CSF cistern. The catheter is then connected to a sterile drainage system and drip chamber to drain 5–10 cc of CSF/hour over 24–72 h. While ELD may be used as first line, it is often performed as a second stage procedure for patients who do not show convincing improvement after a tap test. The ELD has been shown to be a more reliable method as it has a PPV of 80–100%, NPV of 36–100% and an accuracy of 58–100% when compared with the tap test [85]. However, the PPV of both the ELD and tap tests are reasonably high, which implies that when a patient shows improvement on either test, a positive response after shunting can be reliably predicted [85].

Infusion Test

The infusion test involves the insertion of two standard lumbar puncture needles to infuse artificial CSF into the subarachnoid space via one needle and to measure the pressure via the second needle to determine the CSF outflow resistance (Rout) [87, 88]. Different methods for performing infusion testing exist and the Rout values obtained are often method-dependent [87, 89–91]. Consequently, a universal cut off for Rout has not been established [86, 91], but values ranging from 8 to 18 mm Hg/ml/min have generally yielded positive predictive values ranging from 75% to 92% for good outcomes [59, 92, 93]. Nevertheless, a nonrandomized multicenter iNPH trial, in which all patients underwent both an infusion test and a tap test prior to shunting, found that neither Rout nor the results of a tap test correlates with patient outcome after 12 months post-shunting and should not be used to exclude patients from treatment [86].

Cerebrospinal Fluid Biomarkers

In the past decade, several studies have examined the CSF of iNPH patients to identify biomarkers to aid in the diagnosis and monitoring of treatment outcomes in iNPH [65, 94]. Specifically, biomarkers of neuronal injury and neurodegeneration such as amyloid precursor protein (APP) and its related isoforms, Amyloid-β (Aβ) and tau-protein, have been widely investigated [94–97], yet have yielded mixed results [94, 98, 99]. As such, CSF biomarkers have not been proven useful for the confirmation of the diagnosis and management of iNPH.

Treatment

iNPH is treated with surgical implantation of a shunt [94], which has three parts: a valve, proximal catheter, and a distal catheter. The proximal catheter may be inserted into the lateral ventricle (ventricular shunt) or in the lumbar subarachnoid space (lumbar shunt). The distal catheter may be placed in any body cavity that has good drainage and absorptive properties, commonly the peritoneal cavity. Ventriculoperitoneal (VP) and Lumboperitoneal (LP) shunting involves placement of the distal catheter in the peritoneal cavity and the proximal catheter within the cerebral ventricles or lumbar subarachnoid space, respectively. While VP shunts are the most widely used approach in Europe and North America, LP shunts predominates in Japan and other parts of Asia. Nevertheless, both have been shown to be effective for iNPH treatment [50, 77, 100]. An alternative to VP and LP shunts is a ventriculo-atrial (VA) shunt, which involves placement of the distal catheter at the superior vena cava-right atrial junction. While VA shunts may be utilized as first line, it is often reserved for patients whose medical history such as repeated peritoneal catheter obstruction, severe intra-abdominal adhesions, recurrent intra-abdominal infection, and abdominal wall issues increases their risk of perioperative complications for peritoneal catheter insertion [101–104].

While Endoscopic third ventriculostomy (ETV) has been pursued as an alternative to shunting in iNPH, the outcomes have not been favorable [105–107]. As such, ETV is not recommended for treatment of iNPH by any of the current guidelines [44, 45, 58, 69–71]. However, it may be considered in patients with iNPH symptoms who are found on neuroimaging to have obstructive hydrocephalus.

Outcomes

Delay in iNPH treatment has been shown to result in poorer outcomes [50, 51], and untreated iNPH has been associated with significant morbidity and mortality [52]. Approximately, 71–90% of patients who are treated have symptomatic relief in gait, bladder, and cognitive symptoms [77, 100, 108–112]. The 1-year improvement of iNPH symptoms following shunt surgery is 69–77% as measured by an improvement of ≥1 point(s) from baseline mRS score or ≥5 in iNPH grading score, respectively [77, 100, 113]. In an unblinded randomized controlled trial of iNPH patients who underwent immediate LP shunt versus delayed treatment, only 5% of the delayed group showed clinical improvement at 3 months compared with >65% of the treated group [50].

References

1. Rekate HL. A contemporary definition and classification of hydrocephalus. Semin Pediatr Neurol. 2009;16(1):9–15.
2. Larroche JC. Post-haemorrhagic hydrocephalus in infancy. Anatomical study. Biol Neonate. 1972;20(3):287–99.
3. Boop FA. Posthemorrhagic hydrocephalus of prematurity. In: Cinalli G, editor. Pediatric hydrocephalus. Milan: Springer-Verlag; 2005. p. 121–31.
4. Adams RD, Fisher CM, Hakim S, Ojemann RG, Sweet WH. Symptomatic occult hydrocephalus with "normal" cerebrospinal-fluid pressure. A treatable syndrome. N Engl J Med. 1965;273(3):117–26.
5. Hakim S. Algunas observaciones sobre la presion del L.C.R. Sindrome. Hidrocefalico en el Adulto con "Presion Normal" del L.C.R. (Presentacion de un Nuevo Sindrome). Bogota: School of Medicine, Javeriana University; 1964.
6. Hakim S, Adams RD. The special clinical problem of symptomatic hydrocephalus with normal cerebrospinal fluid pressure. Observations on cerebrospinal fluid hydrodynamics. J Neurol Sci. 1965;2(4):307–27.
7. Williams MA, Relkin NR. Diagnosis and management of idiopathic normal-pressure hydrocephalus. Neurol Clin Pract. 2013;3(5):375–85.
8. Malm J, Eklund A. Idiopathic normal pressure hydrocephalus. Pract Neurol. 2006;6(1):14–27.
9. Mori E. Idiopathic normal pressure hydrocephalus: the key to diagnosis. Jpn J Neurosurg. 2007;16(5):387–91.
10. Tarnaris A, Williams MA. Idiopathic normal pressure hydrocephalus: update and practical approach on diagnosis and management. Neurosurg Q. 2011;21(1):72–81.
11. Marmarou A, Black P, Bergsneider M, Klinge P, Relkin N, International NPHCG. Guidelines for management of idiopathic normal pressure hydrocephalus: progress to date. Acta Neurochir Suppl. 2005;95:237–40.
12. Kuriyama N, Miyajima M, Nakajima M, et al. Nationwide hospital-based survey of idiopathic normal pressure hydrocephalus in Japan: epidemiological and clinical characteristics. Brain Behav. 2017;7(3):e00635.
13. Jaraj D, Rabiei K, Marlow T, Jensen C, Skoog I, Wikkelso C. Prevalence of idiopathic normal-pressure hydrocephalus. Neurol. 2014;82(16):1449–54.
14. Vale FA, Miranda SJ. Clinical and demographic features of patients with dementia attended in a tertiary outpatient clinic. Arq Neuropsiquiatr. 2002;60(3-A):548–52.
15. Israelsson H, Carlberg B, Wikkelsö C, et al. Cardiovascular risk factors are associated with idiopathic normal pressure hydrocephalus. Fluids Barriers CNS. 2015;12(Suppl 1):O41.
16. Marmarou A, Young HF, Aygok GA. Estimated incidence of normal pressure hydrocephalus and shunt outcome in patients residing in assisted-living and extended-care facilities. Neurosurg Focus. 2007;22(4):E1.
17. Martin-Laez R, Caballero-Arzapalo H, Valle-San Roman N, Lopez-Menendez LA, Arango-Lasprilla JC, Vazquez-Barquero A. Incidence of idiopathic normal-pressure hydrocephalus in Northern Spain. World Neurosurg. 2016;87:298–310.
18. Martin-Laez R, Caballero-Arzapalo H, Lopez-Menendez LA, Arango-Lasprilla JC, Vazquez-Barquero A. Epidemiology of idiopathic normal pressure hydrocephalus: a systematic review of the literature. World Neurosurg. 2015;84(6):2002–9.
19. Graff-Radford NR, Godersky JC. Symptomatic congenital hydrocephalus in the elderly simulating normal pressure hydrocephalus. Neurol. 1989;39(12):1596–600.
20. Krefft TA, Graff-Radford NR, Lucas JA, Mortimer JA. Normal pressure hydrocephalus and large head size. Alzheimer Dis Assoc Disord. 2004;18(1):35–7.
21. Krauss JK, Regel JP, Vach W, Droste DW, Borremans JJ, Mergner T. Vascular risk factors and arteriosclerotic disease in idiopathic normal-pressure hydrocephalus of the elderly. Stroke. 1996;27(1):24–9.

22. Jaraj D, Agerskov S, Rabiei K, et al. Vascular factors in suspected normal pressure hydrocephalus: a population-based study. Neurol. 2016;86(7):592–9.
23. Bech RA, Waldemar G, Gjerris F, Klinken L, Juhler M. Shunting effects in patients with idiopathic normal pressure hydrocephalus; correlation with cerebral and leptomeningeal biopsy findings. Acta Neurochir. 1999;141(6):633–9.
24. Bech RA, Juhler M, Waldemar G, Klinken L, Gjerris F. Frontal brain and leptomeningeal biopsy specimens correlated with cerebrospinal fluid outflow resistance and B-wave activity in patients suspected of normal-pressure hydrocephalus. Neurosurgery. 1997;40(3):497–502.
25. Lee PH, Yong SW, Ahn YH, Huh K. Correlation of midbrain diameter and gait disturbance in patients with idiopathic normal pressure hydrocephalus. J Neurol. 2005;252(8):958–63.
26. Mocco J, Tomey MI, Komotar RJ, et al. Ventriculoperitoneal shunting of idiopathic normal pressure hydrocephalus increases midbrain size: a potential mechanism for gait improvement. Neurosurgery. 2006;59(4):847–50. discussion 850–41.
27. Pindrik J, Bastian A, Rigamonti D. Pathophysiology of gait dysfunction in normal pressure hydrocephalus. In: Rigamonti D, editor. Adult hydrocephalus. Cambridge: Cambridge University Press; 2014. p. 63–9.
28. Armand S, Allet L, Landis T, Beauchet O, Assal F, Allali G. Interest of dual-task-related gait changes in idiopathic normal pressure hydrocephalus. Eur J Neurol. 2011;18(8):1081–4.
29. Chistyakov AV, Hafner H, Sinai A, Kaplan B, Zaaroor M. Motor cortex disinhibition in normal-pressure hydrocephalus. J Neurosurg. 2012;116(2):453–9.
30. Blomsterwall E, Svantesson U, Carlsson U, Tullberg M, Wikkelso C. Postural disturbance in patients with normal pressure hydrocephalus. Acta Neurol Scand. 2000;102(5):284–91.
31. Del Bigio MR, Wilson MJ, Enno T. Chronic hydrocephalus in rats and humans: white matter loss and behavior changes. Ann Neurol. 2003;53(3):337–46.
32. Mataro M, Matarin M, Poca MA, et al. Functional and magnetic resonance imaging correlates of corpus callosum in normal pressure hydrocephalus before and after shunting. J Neurol Neurosurg Psychiatry. 2007;78(4):395–8.
33. Relkin N, Katzen H. The pathophysiologic basis of cognitive dysfunction in idiopathic normal pressure hydrocephalus. In: Rigamonti D, editor. Adult hydrocephalus. Cambridge: Cambridge University Press; 2014. p. 70–9.
34. Lenfeldt N, Larsson A, Nyberg L, et al. Idiopathic normal pressure hydrocephalus: increased supplementary motor activity accounts for improvement after CSF drainage. Brain. 2008;131(Pt 11):2904–12.
35. Klinge P, Berding G, Brinker T, Weckesser E, Knapp WH, Samii M. Regional cerebral blood flow profiles of shunt-responder in idiopathic chronic hydrocephalus--a 15-O-water PET-study. Acta Neurochir Suppl. 2002;81:47–9.
36. Klinge PM, Brooks DJ, Samii A, et al. Correlates of local cerebral blood flow (CBF) in normal pressure hydrocephalus patients before and after shunting–a retrospective analysis of [(15)O] H(2)O PET-CBF studies in 65 patients. Clin Neurol Neurosurg. 2008;110(4):369–75.
37. Sakakibara R, Kanda T, Sekido T, et al. Mechanism of bladder dysfunction in idiopathic normal pressure hydrocephalus. Neurourol Urodyn. 2008;27(6):507–10.
38. Klausner AP, Robinson SP. Incontinence and lower urinary tract symptoms in normal pressure hydrocephalus. In: Rigamonti D, editor. Adult hydrocephalus. Cambridge: Cambridge University Press; 2014. p. 80–90.
39. Gerstenberg TC, Gjerris F, Sorensen PS, Hald T. Detrusor hyperreflexia and detrusor sphincter incoordination and conductance to cerebrospinal-fluid outflow in normal pressure hydrocephalus. Acta Neurol Scand. 1982;65:296–7.
40. Malm J, Graff-Radford NR, Ishikawa M, et al. Influence of comorbidities in idiopathic normal pressure hydrocephalus - research and clinical care. A report of the ISHCSF task force on comorbidities in INPH. Fluids Barriers CNS. 2013;10(1):22.
41. Andren K, Wikkelso C, Sundstrom N, et al. Long-term effects of complications and vascular comorbidity in idiopathic normal pressure hydrocephalus: a quality registry study. J Neurol. 2018;265(1):178–86.

42. Pyykko OT, Nerg O, Niskasaari HM, et al. Incidence, comorbidities, and mortality in idiopathic normal pressure hydrocephalus. World Neurosurg. 2018;112:e624–31.
43. Israelsson H, Allard P, Eklund A, Malm J. Symptoms of depression are common in patients with idiopathic normal pressure hydrocephalus: The INPH-CRasH study. Neurosurgery. 2016;78(2):161–8.
44. Mori E, Ishikawa M, Kato T, et al. Guidelines for management of idiopathic normal pressure hydrocephalus: second edition. Neurol Med Chir (Tokyo). 2012;52(11):775–809.
45. Marmarou A, Bergsneider M, Relkin N, Klinge P, Black PM. Development of guidelines for idiopathic normal-pressure hydrocephalus: introduction. Neurosurgery. 2005;57(3 Suppl):S1–3. discussion ii-v.
46. Iseki C, Kawanami T, Nagasawa H, et al. Asymptomatic ventriculomegaly with features of idiopathic normal pressure hydrocephalus on MRI (AVIM) in the elderly: a prospective study in a Japanese population. J Neurol Sci. 2009;277(1–2):54–7.
47. Iseki C, Takahashi Y, Wada M, Kawanami T, Adachi M, Kato T. Incidence of idiopathic normal pressure hydrocephalus (iNPH): a 10-year follow-up study of a rural community in Japan. J Neurol Sci. 2014;339(1–2):108–12.
48. Razay G, Vreugdenhil A, Liddell J. A prospective study of ventriculo-peritoneal shunting for idiopathic normal pressure hydrocephalus. J Clin Neurosci. 2009;16(9):1180–3.
49. Scollato A, Tenenbaum R, Bahl G, Celerini M, Salani B, Di Lorenzo N. Changes in aqueductal CSF stroke volume and progression of symptoms in patients with unshunted idiopathic normal pressure hydrocephalus. AJNR Am J Neuroradiol. 2008;29(1):192–7.
50. Kazui H, Miyajima M, Mori E, Ishikawa M. Investigators S-. Lumboperitoneal shunt surgery for idiopathic normal pressure hydrocephalus (SINPHONI-2): an open-label randomised trial. Lancet Neurol. 2015;14(6):585–94.
51. Andren K, Wikkelso C, Tisell M, Hellstrom P. Natural course of idiopathic normal pressure hydrocephalus. J Neurol Neurosurg Psychiatry. 2014;85(7):806–10.
52. Jaraj D, Wikkelso C, Rabiei K, et al. Mortality and risk of dementia in normal-pressure hydrocephalus: a population study. Alzheimers Dement. 2017;13(8):850–7.
53. Mirzayan MJ, Luetjens G, Borremans JJ, Regel JP, Krauss JK. Extended long-term (>5 years) outcome of cerebrospinal fluid shunting in idiopathic normal pressure hydrocephalus. Neurosurgery. 2010;67(2):295–301.
54. Raftopoulos C, Massager N, Baleriaux D, Deleval J, Clarysse S, Brotchi J. Prospective analysis by computed tomography and long-term outcome of 23 adult patients with chronic idiopathic hydrocephalus. Neurosurgery. 1996;38(1):51–9.
55. Spagnoli D, Innocenti L, Bello L, et al. Impact of cerebrovascular disease on the surgical treatment of idiopathic normal pressure hydrocephalus. Neurosurgery. 2006;59(3):545–52. discussion 545–52.
56. Williams MA, Malm J. Diagnosis and treatment of idiopathic normal pressure hydrocephalus. Continuum (Minneap Minn). 2016;22(2 Dementia):579–99.
57. Ishikawa M, Hashimoto M, Mori E, Kuwana N, Kazui H. The value of the cerebrospinal fluid tap test for predicting shunt effectiveness in idiopathic normal pressure hydrocephalus. Fluids Barriers CNS. 2012;9(1):1.
58. Ishikawa M, Hashimoto M, Kuwana N, Mori E, Miyake H, Wachi A, et al. Guidelines for management of idiopathic normal pressure hydrocephalus: guidelines from the Guidelines committee of idiopathic normal pressure hydrocephalus, the Japanese society of normal pressure hydrocephalus. Neurol Med Chir (Tokyo). 2008;48(SUPPL): S1–S23.
59. Boon AJ, Tans JT, Delwel EJ, et al. Dutch normal-pressure hydrocephalus study: prediction of outcome after shunting by resistance to outflow of cerebrospinal fluid. J Neurosurg. 1997;87(5):687–93.
60. Tinetti ME. Performance-oriented assessment of mobility problems in elderly patients. J Am Geriatr Soc. 1986;34(2):119–26.
61. Podsiadlo D, Richardson S. The timed "Up & Go": a test of basic functional mobility for frail elderly persons. J Am Geriatr Soc. 1991;39(2):142–8.

62. Graham JE, Ostir GV, Fisher SR, Ottenbacher KJ. Assessing walking speed in clinical research: a systematic review. J Eval Clin Pract. 2008;14(4):552–62.
63. Relkin N, Marmarou A, Klinge P, Bergsneider M, Black PM. Diagnosing idiopathic normal-pressure hydrocephalus. Neurosurgery. 2005;57(3 Suppl):S4–16. discussion ii-v.
64. Vaes B, Pasquet A, Wallemacq P, et al. The BELFRAIL (BFC80+) study: a population-based prospective cohort study of the very elderly in Belgium. BMC Geriatr. 2010;10:39.
65. Tarnaris A, Toma AK, Pullen E, et al. Cognitive, biochemical, and imaging profile of patients suffering from idiopathic normal pressure hydrocephalus. Alzheimers Dement. 2011;7(5):501–8.
66. Picascia M, Zangaglia R, Bernini S, Minafra B, Sinforiani E, Pacchetti C. A review of cognitive impairment and differential diagnosis in idiopathic normal pressure hydrocephalus. Funct Neurol. 2015;30(4):217–29.
67. Saito M, Nishio Y, Kanno S, et al. Cognitive profile of idiopathic normal pressure hydrocephalus. Dement Geriatr Cogn Dis Extra. 2011;1(1):202–11.
68. Klausner AP, Ellen EF, Collins CW, et al. Characterization of urinary incontinence in patients with normal pressure hydrocephalus (NPH). J Urol. 2008;179(4):353.
69. Relkin N, Marmarou A, Klinge P, Bergsneider M, Black PM. INPH guidelines, part II: diagnosing idio-pathic normal-pressure hydrocephalus. Neurosurgery. 2005;57(3 SUPPL):S2-4–S2-16.
70. Ishikawa M. Guideline committe for idiopathic normal pressure hydrocephalus JSoNPH. clinical guidelines for idiopathic normal pressure hydrocephalus. Neurol Med Chir (Tokyo). 2004;44(4):222–3.
71. Halperin JJ, Kurlan R, Schwalb JM, Cusimano MD, Gronseth G, Gloss D. Practice guideline: idiopathic normal pressure hydrocephalus: response to shunting and predictors of response: report of the guideline development, dissemination, and implementation Subcommittee of the American Academy of Neurology. Neurology. 2015;85(23):2063–71.
72. Meier U, Zeilinger FS, Schonherr B. Endoscopic ventriculostomy versus shunt operation in normal pressure hydrocephalus: diagnostics and indication. Minim Invasive Neurosurg. 2000;43(2):87–90.
73. Tisell M, Tullberg M, Hellstrom P, Blomsterwall E, Wikkelso C. Neurological symptoms and signs in adult aqueductal stenosis. Acta Neurol Scand. 2003;107(5):311–7.
74. Virhammar J, Laurell K, Cesarini KG, Larsson EM. The callosal angle measured on MRI as a predictor of outcome in idiopathic normal-pressure hydrocephalus. J Neurosurg. 2014;120(1):178–84.
75. Reinard K, Basheer A, Phillips S, et al. Simple and reproducible linear measurements to determine ventricular enlargement in adults. Surg Neurol Int. 2015;6:59.
76. Jaraj D, Rabiei K, Marlow T, Jensen C, Skoog I, Wikkelso C. Estimated ventricle size using Evans index: reference values from a population-based sample. Eur J Neurol. 2017;24(3):468–74.
77. Hashimoto M, Ishikawa M, Mori E, Kuwana N. Study of Ioni. Diagnosis of idiopathic normal pressure hydrocephalus is supported by MRI-based scheme: a prospective cohort study. Cerebrospinal Fluid Res. 2010;7(1):18.
78. Ishikawa M, Oowaki H, Takezawa M, et al. Disproportionately enlarged subarachnoid space hydrocephalus in idiopathic normal-pressure hydrocephalus and its implication in pathogenesis. Acta Neurochir Suppl. 2016;122:287–90.
79. Mostafa T, Craven C, Patel NA, et al. DESH negative normal pressure hydrocephalus: can patients still benefit from shunt insertion? Fluids Barriers CNS. 2015;12(Suppl 1):O52.
80. Graff-Radford NR, Godersky JC. Idiopathic normal pressure hydrocephalus and systemic hypertension. Neurol. 1987;37(5):868–71.
81. Casmiro M, D'Alessandro R, Cacciatore FM, Daidone R, Calbucci F, Lugaresi E. Risk factors for the syndrome of ventricular enlargement with gait apraxia (idiopathic normal pressure hydrocephalus): a case-control study. J Neurol Neurosurg Psychiatry. 1989;52(7):847–52.
82. Krauss JK, Droste DW, Vach W, et al. Cerebrospinal fluid shunting in idiopathic normal-pressure hydrocephalus of the elderly: effect of periventricular and deep white matter lesions. Neurosurgery. 1996;39(2):292–9. discussion 299–300.

83. Jacobs L. Diabetes mellitus in normal pressure hydrocephalus. J Neurol Neurosurg Psychiatry. 1977;40(4):331–5.
84. Virhammar J, Cesarini KG, Laurell K. The CSF tap test in normal pressure hydrocephalus: evaluation time, reliability and the influence of pain. Eur J Neurol. 2012;19(2):271–6.
85. Mahr CV, Dengl M, Nestler U, et al. Idiopathic normal pressure hydrocephalus: diagnostic and predictive value of clinical testing, lumbar drainage, and CSF dynamics. J Neurosurg. 2016;125(3):591–7.
86. Wikkelso C, Hellstrom P, Klinge PM, Tans JT. European i NPHMSG. The European iNPH multicentre study on the predictive values of resistance to CSF outflow and the CSF tap test in patients with idiopathic normal pressure hydrocephalus. J Neurol Neurosurg Psychiatry. 2013;84(5):562–8.
87. Kahlon B, Sundbarg G, Rehncrona S. Comparison between the lumbar infusion and CSF tap tests to predict outcome after shunt surgery in suspected normal pressure hydrocephalus. J Neurol Neurosurg Psychiatry. 2002;73(6):721–6.
88. Kahlon B, Sundbarg G, Rehncrona S. Lumbar infusion test in normal pressure hydrocephalus. Acta Neurol Scand. 2005;111(6):379–84.
89. Katzman R, Hussey F. A simple constant-infusion manometric test for measurement of CSF absorption I. Rationale and method. Neurology. 1970;20(6):534–44.
90. Hussey F, Schanzer B, Katzman R. A simple constant-infusion manometric test for measurement of CSF absorption II. Clinical studies. Neurology. 1970;20(7):665–80.
91. Eklund A, Smielewski P, Chambers I, et al. Assessment of cerebrospinal fluid outflow resistance. Med Biol Eng Comput. 2007;45(8):719–35.
92. Malm J, Kristensen B, Fagerlund M, Koskinen LO, Ekstedt J. Cerebrospinal fluid shunt dynamics in patients with idiopathic adult hydrocephalus syndrome. J Neurol Neurosurg Psychiatry. 1995;58(6):715–23.
93. Malm J, Kristensen B, Karlsson T, Fagerlund M, Elfverson J, Ekstedt J. The predictive value of cerebrospinal fluid dynamic tests in patients with th idiopathic adult hydrocephalus syndrome. Arch Neurol. 1995;52(8):783–9.
94. Santangelo R, Cecchetti G, Bernasconi MP, et al. Cerebrospinal fluid amyloid-beta 42, total tau and phosphorylated tau are low in patients with normal pressure hydrocephalus: analogies and differences with Alzheimer's disease. J Alzheimers Dis. 2017;60(1):183–200.
95. Tarnaris A, Toma AK, Chapman MD, Keir G, Kitchen ND, Watkins LD. Use of cerebrospinal fluid amyloid-beta and total tau protein to predict favorable surgical outcomes in patients with idiopathic normal pressure hydrocephalus. J Neurosurg. 2011;115(1):145–50.
96. Tarnaris A, Toma AK, Kitchen ND, Watkins LD. Ongoing search for diagnostic biomarkers in idiopathic normal pressure hydrocephalus. Biomark Med. 2009;3(6):787–805.
97. Chen Z, Liu C, Zhang J, Relkin N, Xing Y, Li Y. Cerebrospinal fluid Aβ42, t-tau, and p-tau levels in the differential diagnosis of idiopathic normal-pressure hydrocephalus: a systematic review and meta-analysis. Fluids Barriers CNS. 2017;14(1):13.
98. Miyajima M, Nakajima M, Ogino I, Miyata H, Motoi Y, Arai H. Soluble amyloid precursor protein alpha in the cerebrospinal fluid as a diagnostic and prognostic biomarker for idiopathic normal pressure hydrocephalus. Eur J Neurol. 2013;20(2):236–42.
99. Moriya M, Miyajima M, Nakajima M, Ogino I, Arai H. Impact of cerebrospinal fluid shunting for idiopathic normal pressure hydrocephalus on the amyloid cascade. PLoS One. 2015;10(3):e0119973.
100. Miyajima M, Kazui H, Mori E, Ishikawa M. Sinphoni-investigators obot. One-year outcome in patients with idiopathic normal-pressure hydrocephalus: comparison of lumboperitoneal shunt to ventriculoperitoneal shunt. J Neurosurg. 2016;125(6):1483–92.
101. McGovern RA, Kelly KM, Chan AK, Morrissey NJ, McKhann GM 2nd. Should ventriculoatrial shunting be the procedure of choice for normal-pressure hydrocephalus? J Neurosurg. 2014;120(6):1458–64.
102. Al-Schameri AR, Hamed J, Baltsavias G, et al. Ventriculoatrial shunts in adults, incidence of infection, and significant risk factors: a single-center experience. World Neurosurg. 2016;94:345–51.

103. Ellegaard L, Mogensen S, Juhler M. Ultrasound-guided percutaneous placement of ventriculoatrial shunts. Childs Nerv Syst. 2007;23(8):857–62.
104. Hammersen S, Pietila TA, Brock M. Accurate placement of the distal end of a ventriculoatrial shunt catheter using Alphacard: direct intraoperative comparison with fluoroscopy. Acta Neurochir. 2000;142(5):563–6.
105. Gangemi M, Maiuri F, Naddeo M, et al. Endoscopic third ventriculostomy in idiopathic normal pressure hydrocephalus: an Italian multicenter study. Neurosurgery. 2008;63(1):62–7. discussion 67–69.
106. Longatti PL, Fiorindi A, Martinuzzi A. Failure of endoscopic third ventriculostomy in the treatment of idiopathic normal pressure hydrocephalus. Minim Invasive Neurosurg. 2004;47(6):342–5.
107. Tudor KI, Tudor M, McCleery J, Car J. Endoscopic third ventriculostomy (ETV) for idiopathic normal pressure hydrocephalus (iNPH). Cochrane Database Syst Rev. 2015;7(7):CD010033.
108. Eide PK, Sorteberg W. Outcome of surgery for idiopathic normal pressure hydrocephalus: role of preoperative static and pulsatile intracranial pressure. World Neurosurg. 2016;86(C):186–93.
109. Golz L, Ruppert FH, Meier U, Lemcke J. Outcome of modern shunt therapy in patients with idiopathic normal pressure hydrocephalus 6 years postoperatively. J Neurosurg. 2014;121(4):771–5.
110. Kahlon B, Sjunnesson J, Rehncrona S. Long-term outcome in patients with suspected normal pressure hydrocephalus. Neurosurgery. 2007;60(2):327–32. discussion 332.
111. Klinge P, Marmarou A, Bergsneider M, Relkin N, Black PM. Outcome of shunting in idiopathic normal-pressure hydrocephalus and the value of outcome assessment in shunted patients. Neurosurgery. 2005;57(3 Suppl):S40–52. discussion ii–v.
112. Pujari S, Kharkar S, Metellus P, Shuck J, Williams MA, Rigamonti D. Normal pressure hydrocephalus: long-term outcome after shunt surgery. J Neurol Neurosurg Psychiatry. 2008;79(11):1282–6.
113. Klinge P, Hellstrom P, Tans J, Wikkelso C. European i NPHMSG. One-year outcome in the European multicentre study on iNPH. Acta Neurol Scand. 2012;126(3):145–53.

Hydrocephalus Following Aneurysmal Subarachnoid Hemorrhage

13

David L. Dornbos III, Luke G. F. Smith, Varun Shah, Nicholas Musgrave, Patrick P. Youssef, Ciarán J. Powers, and Shahid M. Nimjee

Introduction

Hydrocephalus occurs in nearly two-thirds of patients following aneurysmal subarachnoid hemorrhage (SAH), and is a common source of morbidity for this patient population [1, 2]. The presence of post-SAH hydrocephalus has been shown to be associated with worsened cognitive deficits, increased 3-month Glasgow Outcome Scale severity, and worsened overall prognosis [3–5]. Nonetheless, prompt and appropriate management of hydrocephalus in this setting can ameliorate these adverse outcomes to some degree. While the etiology underlying acute and delayed hydrocephalus in this context has not been definitively identified, numerous mechanisms have been proposed, including inflammation and fibrosis secondary to hematologic degradation products, ultimately obstructing cerebrospinal fluid (CSF) flow or absorption. Management of SAH-associated hydrocephalus acutely following rupture typically involves temporary CSF diversion with an external ventricular drain (EVD), although permanent shunting is required in around 20–50% of patients [6].

Typically occurring acutely, hydrocephalus requiring permanent CSF shunting can occur in a delayed fashion, even months after the initial SAH. Numerous variables predictive of permanent shunting have been identified, including increased

D. L. Dornbos III · L. G. F. Smith · P. P. Youssef · C. J. Powers · S. M. Nimjee (✉)
Department of Neurological Surgery, The Ohio State University Wexner Medical Center, Columbus, OH, USA
e-mail: shahid.nimjee@osumc.edu

V. Shah· N. Musgrave
The Ohio State University Medical Center, Columbus, OH, USA

D. D. Limbrick, J. R. Leonard (eds.), *Cerebrospinal Fluid Disorders*,
https://doi.org/10.1007/978-3-319-97928-1_13

Fisher grades at presentation, degree of intraventricular hemorrhage (IVH), underlying posterior circulation aneurysm rupture, and numerous others, which will be discussed in detail [7, 8]. Importantly, patients who develop shunt-dependent hydrocephalus following SAH have worse short-term and long-term outcomes and longer hospitalizations [9]. This fact underscores the importance of prompt diagnosis, recognition, and management of both acute and delayed hydrocephalus to minimize their associated morbidity.

Etiology

While hydrocephalus requiring permanent CSF diversion is seen frequently following SAH (20–50%), the underlying molecular mechanisms, particularly in the setting of communicating hydrocephalus, remain largely unknown [2, 10–12]. Development of hydrocephalus may occur in the acute (<3 days), subacute (3–14 days), or chronic phases (>14 days) following aneurysm rupture [11, 12]. Acute development of hydrocephalus is most often secondary to obstruction of the CSF pathways with IVH or cisternal SAH [13]. Numerous studies have demonstrated a correlation between the quantity of ventricular and cisternal hemorrhage and the presence of acute hydrocephalus [13–15]. Nonetheless, acute hydrocephalus is still frequently seen in individuals following SAH in the absence of intraventricular blood clots, indicating other mechanisms underlying hydrocephalus in this setting [15, 16].

Inflammation, secondary to the presence of cisternal and ventricular hemorrhage, is also thought to play a crucial role. In the early stage following SAH, microglial activation and initiation of inflammatory cascades have been shown to promote blood–brain barrier (BBB) disruption, contributing to acute hydrocephalus [15, 17]. In addition to providing a blockade against CSF flow, it has also been postulated that the presence of IVH triggers a degree of choroid plexus inflammation, leading to increased CSF production [14, 18]. While these factors promote acute and subacute hydrocephalus, numerous other mechanisms underscore the development of communicating hydrocephalus in a chronic manner.

Hematologic breakdown products and the subsequent inflammatory response are believed to play a substantial role in the abnormal CSF secretion and reabsorption observed in chronic communicating hydrocephalus following SAH. In addition to stimulating hypersecretion of CSF, intraventricular blood triggers fibrosis of the arachnoid granulations, impairing CSF absorption [14, 15, 18]. Hemosiderin deposits and pathologic thickening of the leptomeninges further impede CSF flow and have been a target for potential therapies in preclinical models [19, 20]. Furthermore, the presence of intraventricular hemoglobin has been shown to directly induce the expression of proinflammatory cytokines, such as tumor necrosis factor (TNF)-α, interleukin-1β, and Toll-like receptor-4, in both periventricular white matter and CSF [21–23]. Hemoglobin has also been shown to increase expression of numerous aquaporins, triggering an increase in CSF production and fluid filtration across the BBB [11, 23, 24]. BBB breakdown is exacerbated following SAH, partially due to increased matrix metalloproteinase-9 expression, which results from the initial inflammatory response [11, 14]. Finally, the presence of iron has been shown to generate ventricular expansion in preclinical models [23, 25], and elevated ferritin levels acutely following SAH has been shown to correlate with chronic hydrocephalus development and need for permanent CSF shunting [11, 26].

Diagnosis

Development of acute hydrocephalus typically occurs within 48 h, whereas chronic hydrocephalus tends to present weeks to months following the initial hemorrhage [27]. The clinical findings in the setting of acute hydrocephalus following SAH are readily described and well known, including severe headache, nausea, vomiting, impaired consciousness, stupor or coma. Patients presenting in a delayed chronic manner may exhibit some of these symptoms, although gait abnormalities and mild cognitive impairment may be seen as well.

Several radiographic diagnostic criteria have been proposed and may be used to assist in establishing a diagnosis. The most commonly utilized metric is the bicaudate index (BCI), defined as the width of the frontal horns at the level of the caudate nuclei divided by the diameter of the brain [6, 28]. Previous studies have found this to be a reliable indicator of hydrocephalus when the BCI exceeds the 95th percentile after correcting for age (Table 13.1) [28]. Volumetric analysis and the rate of ventricular dilation have also been used, which may control for differences in ventricle shape [15]. Finally, the width of the third ventricle tends to be a reliable indicator of hydrocephalus progression in patients with both intraventricular and subarachnoid hemorrhage, although no clear cutoff exists to establish a diagnosis [29]. While these radiographic measurements of hydrocephalus may be helpful at times, decisions regarding treatment ultimately hinge on the clinical symptomatology.

Table 13.1 Age adjusted BCI values indicative of hydrocephalus

Age (Years)	BCI
<30	0.16
50	0.18
60	0.19
80	0.21
100	0.25

BCI threshold to establish a diagnosis of hydrocephalus, set at the 95th percentile for age. *BCI* bicaudate index

Acute Management

Management of acute hydrocephalus following aneurysmal SAH largely depends on the clinical presentation and initial radiographic findings. Radiographic evidence of hydrocephalus in the absence of clinical symptoms can be managed expectantly. Neurologic decline, such as decreased consciousness, altered sensorium, stupor, or coma, in the setting of aneurysmal SAH typically requires CSF diversion. While lumbar drainage or serial lumbar punctures can be pursued in the setting of communicating hydrocephalus, CSF diversion with a ventriculostomy is most commonly utilized and is recommended in patients with hydrocephalus and decreased consciousness in recent AHA guidelines (Fig. 13.1) [30]. In addition to providing CSF diversion, the EVD is beneficial in measuring intracranial pressure (ICP). Compared to lumbar drainage, it also prevents induction of brain herniation in noncommunicating hydrocephalus.

The use of prophylactic antibiotics throughout the course of the ventriculostomy duration has been a source of some debate. Administration of antibiotics prior to and during ventriculostomy placement is broadly accepted, and early studies demonstrated evidence for continued use of ongoing prophylactic antibiotics following placement [31, 32]. Later evaluation demonstrated no significant benefit to this practice. On the contrary, there was an increase in the incidence of antibiotic-resistant pathogens with ventriculostomy-associated infections when systemic antibiotics were utilized for greater than 24 h [33, 34]. Despite these mixed results

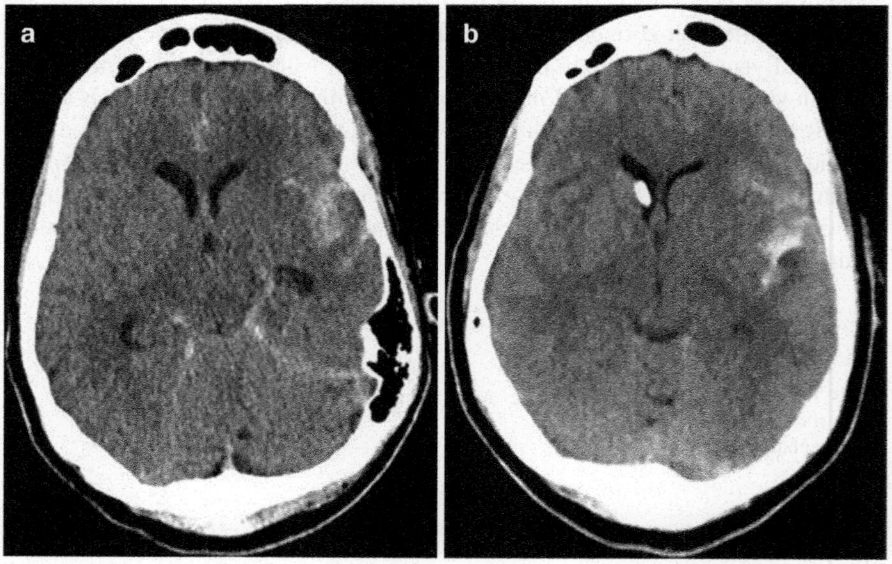

Fig. 13.1 Acute hydrocephalus following SAH. A 54-year-old male presenting with a Hunt and Hess grade 2, Fisher grade 3 SAH secondary to a ruptured left posterior communicating artery aneurysm with evidence of acute hydrocephalus on presentation (**a**). The patient was adequately treated with a temporary ventriculostomy (**b**). SAH = subarachnoid hemorrhage

utilizing prophylactic systemic antibiotics, the use of antibiotic-impregnated ventricular catheters has been shown to significantly decrease the rate of catheter-associated infections [35]. Given proper precautions, the risk of ventriculostomy-associated infections is quite low, although the number of drainage days is linearly correlated with an increased risk of infection. The overall infection rate has been previously found to be 6.3 infections per 1000 days of drainage [36], underscoring the need to promptly wean and remove ventricular catheters as soon as they are no longer needed.

In addition to ventriculostomy placement for the acute management of hydrocephalus, previous studies have shown that fenestration of the lamina terminalis and thorough irrigation of blood within the arachnoid cisterns may decrease shunt dependency [6]. A relatively simple maneuver during microsurgical clipping, this may help partially restore normal CSF dynamics but carries increased risk of CSF leakage, arterial injury, and hypothalamic damage [15]. Early studies demonstrated a 75–80% decrease in chronic shunt dependency in patients following lamina terminalis fenestration compared to their counterparts that did not undergo fenestration [6, 37, 38]. Nonetheless, more recent studies have not recapitulated this success [39], and while it may provide some benefit, it is not currently a standard of care practice.

Shunt Dependence Following SAH

Following SAH, the majority of patients do not require permanent or long-term CSF shunting. Numerous risk factors have been described, however, that do correlate with the need for ventriculoperitoneal (VP) shunt placement and can be helpful to assist in clinical decision-making and patient counseling. The initial Fisher grade on presentation strongly correlates with increased likelihood of shunt dependency [8, 40]. Patients presenting with Fischer grades 3 and 4 have an eightfold greater incidence of being shunt dependent than patients presenting with grades 1 or 2 [7]. This is likely due to increased occlusion and scarring of the arachnoid villi [41]. Similarly, the presence of IVH carries a fourfold increase in shunt dependency, with the highest risk resulting from when blood is present in the fourth ventricle [7, 8]. Similar to Fisher grade, patients who present with Hunt and Hess scores of 3–5 carry a threefold increase of shunt dependency compared to Hunt and Hess scores of 1–2 [7]. Patients presenting with a Hunt and Hess score of 3 or 4 demonstrate shunt dependency in 29.8% and 42.6% of cases, respectively [8]. Rupture of posterior circulation aneurysms may also confer some risk as one study found a 28.6% risk of shunt dependency with aneurysms in the posterior circulation compared to 18.4% in the anterior circulation [8]. Given their anatomic location, ruptured posterior circulation aneurysms may cause an obstructive pattern of hydrocephalus with blood impairing CSF flow at the level of the cerebral aqueduct or fourth ventricle. More recent studies have not observed a similar difference based on aneurysm location [7, 42].

The presence of acute hydrocephalus immediately following SAH portends a higher likelihood of long-term shunt dependency [43]. A recent meta-analysis found a sixfold increase in shunt dependency when patients present with acute hydrocephalus [7]. Using BCI as an objective measure of hydrocephalus, a BCI ≥ 0.2 was identified as an independent risk factor for shunt dependency [44]. Moreover, relative BCI (defined as patient BCI/upper limit BCI for age) exceeding 1.6 at any point has been shown to correlate with poor patient outcomes [15, 45]. Among patients initially presenting with acute hydrocephalus, CSF shunting was ultimately required in 20–50% [8, 46]. EVD placement within the first 24 h was also an independent predictor of the need for a permanent shunt [46], indicating that early, severe hydrocephalus is a stronger predictor for long-term CSF diversion than hydrocephalus of a more insidious onset. While studies have yielded mixed results [44, 47], a meta-analysis revealed a twofold increase in shunt dependency in patients experiencing a rehemorrhage following their initial hemorrhage [7], again signifying that a more severe SAH is more likely to require permanent CSF diversion.

Numerous complications and sequelae associated with the critical care of SAH patients are similarly associated with increased need for long-term CSF diversion. One of the most common sequelae following SAH, patients undergoing treatment for vasospasm were twice as likely to require permanent shunt placement [8]. Additionally, hyponatremia, ischemic stroke, nosocomial meningitis, and pneumonia correlated with increased risk of permanent shunt placement [4, 7, 46]. Altogether, these complications lead to a fivefold higher rate of shunt dependence [7].

Patient baseline demographics and history seem to play a role as well. Age greater than 60 years carries a twofold increased incidence in post-SAH shunt dependency [3, 7, 48], with a linear increase in shunt dependency with increasing age [8]. There does not appear to be any gender predilection for shunt dependence, despite a few early studies revealing a possible female predominance [7, 8]. Finally, the use of sympathomimetic drugs, notably cocaine, has been associated with not only increased vasospasm and mortality, but correlates with shunt dependence as well [7, 46, 49, 50]. While these various factors all demonstrate associations with increased shunt dependency, the diagnosis and treatment paradigm in the acute setting relies on the previously discussed clinical and radiographic findings.

Management of Posthemorrhagic Hydrocephalus

When needed, CSF diversion with an EVD is typically continued through the acute phase after SAH during the initial 7–14 days. Once the acute phase following SAH has passed and the patient has clinically and neurologically stabilized, attention can be turned toward determining the need for long-term CSF diversion. While acute hydrocephalus is a significant risk factor for the need for long-term CSF diversion, spontaneous neurologic improvement can be seen in up to 50% of patients [13, 28, 41]. Once neurologically stabilized, weaning of the EVD is performed through stepwise elevation of the EVD drip chamber and eventual clamping. When such maneuvers result in neurologic deterioration and/or increased ventricular size, permanent CSF diversion must be considered (Fig. 13.2). Although variable, additional indications for shunt placement include inability to

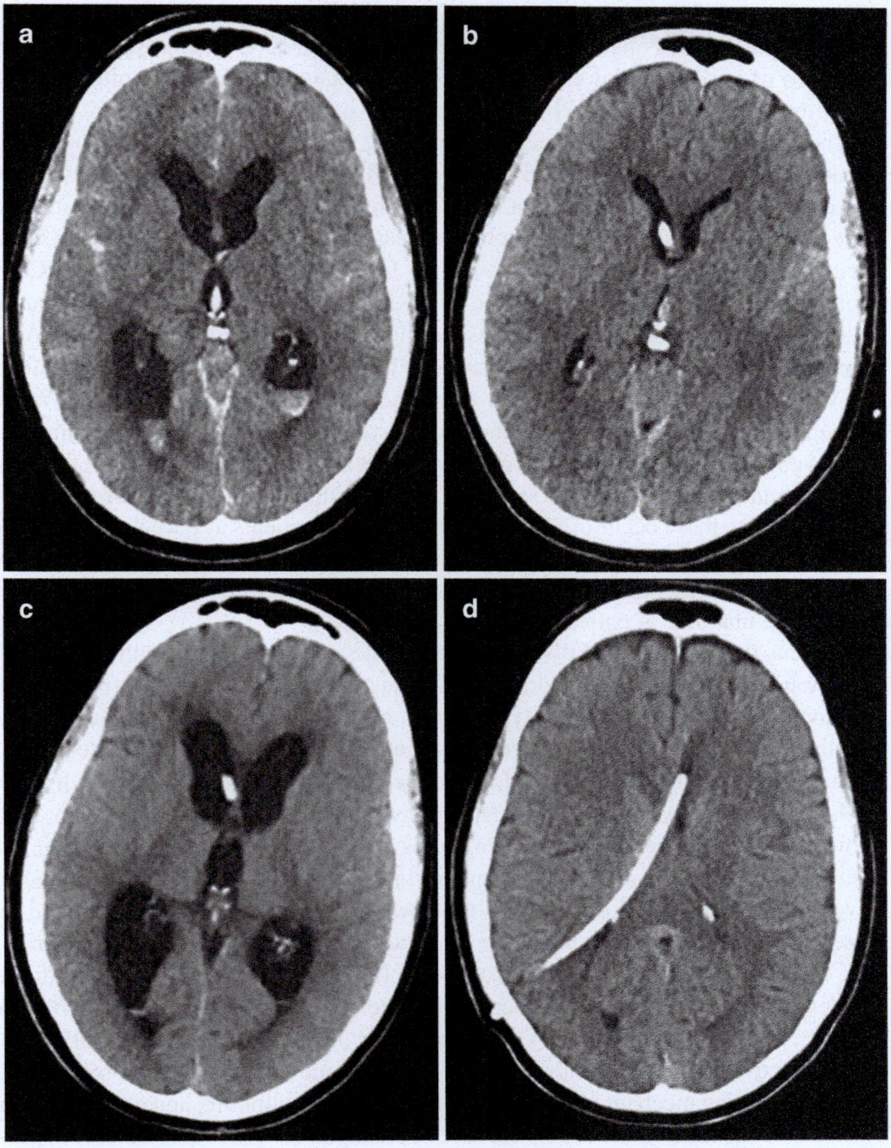

Fig. 13.2 Acute hydrocephalus requiring a ventriculoperitoneal shunt. A 49-year-old female presenting with a Hunt and Hess grade 3, Fisher grade 3 SAH secondary to a ruptured basilar apex aneurysm and acute hydrocephalus (**a**), managed with a ventriculostomy (**b**). Following 2 weeks of CSF drainage, the patient did not clinically or radiographically tolerate an EVD clamp trial (**c**), requiring placement of a VP shunt (**d**). *SAH* subarachnoid hemorrhage, *CSF* cerebrospinal fluid, *EVD* external ventricular drain, *VP* ventriculoperitoneal

tolerate ventriculostomy clamping, persistent high drainage volumes, persistent ICP elevations and consistently poor neurologic status. Overall, approximately one-third of patients require permanent CSF diversion during their initial hospitalization following SAH [51].

The timing of VP shunt placement regarding CSF content remains a source of debate. While allowing CSF red blood cell (RBC) counts and protein levels to decrease prior to implantation of a new shunt may be reasonable, previous studies have demonstrated that this may not be necessary [52]. An evaluation of 80 consecutive patients requiring conversion of an EVD to a VP shunt, with mean CSF protein levels of 124 mg/dl and median CSF RBC counts of 4600 RBCs/mm^3, found no significant association between these levels and shunt failure [52]. Furthermore, when placed in the acute setting, the same EVD site was shown to be a safe location for VP shunt placement, without an increased risk of failure or infection. While placement of a VP shunt for posthemorrhagic hydrocephalus is the most commonly employed treatment modality, it carries a significant 20–50% risk of complication and potential revision [15, 42, 53]. While nearly a third of patients require a subsequent revision, these occur in 50%, 90%, and 98% of patients at 2 weeks, 2 months, and 6 months, respectively [42]. Given that nearly all shunt failures occur within the first 6 months, it has been postulated that shunt dependency may be a transient issue in the large majority of patients.

Patients that are successfully weaned from the ventriculostomy without clinical or radiographic evidence of hydrocephalus must be closely monitored for delayed development of ventriculomegaly. Chronic hydrocephalus may arise weeks to months following the initial SAH, even without prior development of acute hydrocephalus. Symptoms often resemble those experienced in normal pressure hydrocephalus, commonly presenting with cognitive decline, urinary incontinence, gait difficulty, or headache [54]. These symptoms are typically accompanied by significant ventriculomegaly as well. The underlying etiology of delayed hydrocephalus development in this setting is largely unknown, although it has been postulated to arise secondary to both scarring of the arachnoid villi and exhaustion of compensatory responses to increased CSF production [51]. Although rare overall with an incidence of 1.3%, delayed hydrocephalus is seen with greater frequency (5.7%) in patients who required temporary CSF diversion during the initial hospitalization [51]. Moreover, in patients with evidence of high-grade SAH and greater severity of illness, including mechanical ventilation, microsurgical clipping, and discharge to a skilled nursing facility, the risk of chronic hydrocephalus was even greater [51, 55]. Greater than 90% of patients with these risk factors presented with delayed hydrocephalus within the first year [51], highlighting the need for close observation during follow-up visits after discharge.

Conclusion

Hydrocephalus is a common complication of aneurysmal SAH. While numerous risk factors portend a worse prognosis and potential need for permanent CSF diversion, the clinical decision-making in the acute setting relies on basic clinical and radiographic findings. Patients that are discharged without CSF diversion following SAH should be closely monitored for at least 1 year to monitor for clinical signs of potential delayed hydrocephalus development. Proper surveillance and management of hydrocephalus following SAH can ameliorate further sequelae of this potential devastating disease process.

References

1. Brinker T, Seifert V, Stolke D. Acute changes in the dynamics of the cerebrospinal fluid system during experimental subarachnoid hemorrhage. Neurosurgery. 1990;27(3):369–72.
2. Heros RC. Acute hydrocephalus after subarachnoid hemorrhage. Stroke. 1989;20(6):715–7.
3. Graff-Radford NR, Torner J, Adams HP Jr, Kassell NF. Factors associated with hydrocephalus after subarachnoid hemorrhage. A report of the Cooperative Aneurysm Study. Arch Neurol. 1989;46(7):744–52.
4. Sheehan JP, Polin RS, Sheehan JM, Baskaya MK, Kassell NF. Factors associated with hydrocephalus after aneurysmal subarachnoid hemorrhage. Neurosurgery. 1999;45(5):1120–7; discussion 1127–1128
5. Hutter BO, Kreitschmann-Andermahr I, Gilsbach JM. Cognitive deficits in the acute stage after subarachnoid hemorrhage. Neurosurgery. 1998;43(5):1054–65.
6. Germanwala AV, Huang J, Tamargo RJ. Hydrocephalus after aneurysmal subarachnoid hemorrhage. Neurosurg Clin N Am. 2010;21(2):263–70.
7. Wilson CD, Safavi-Abbasi S, Sun H, et al. Meta-analysis and systematic review of risk factors for shunt dependency after aneurysmal subarachnoid hemorrhage. J Neurosurg. 2017;126(2):586–95.
8. Dorai Z, Hynan LS, Kopitnik TA, Samson D. Factors related to hydrocephalus after aneurysmal subarachnoid hemorrhage. Neurosurgery. 2003;52(4):763–9; discussion 769–771
9. Wang YM, Lin YJ, Chuang MJ, et al. Predictors and outcomes of shunt-dependent hydrocephalus in patients with aneurysmal sub-arachnoid hemorrhage. BMC Surg. 2012;12:12.
10. Yolas C, Ozdemir NG, Kanat A, et al. Uncovering a new cause of obstructive hydrocephalus following subarachnoid hemorrhage: choroidal artery vasospasm-related ependymal cell degeneration and aqueductal stenosis-first experimental study. World Neurosurg. 2016;90:484–91.
11. Hua C, Zhao G. Biomarkers in adult posthemorrhagic hydrocephalus. Int J Stroke. 2017;12(6):574–9.
12. Varelas P, Helms A, Sinson G, Spanaki M, Hacein-Bey L. Clipping or coiling of ruptured cerebral aneurysms and shunt-dependent hydrocephalus. Neurocrit Care. 2006;4(3):223–8.
13. Shah AH, Komotar RJ. Pathophysiology of acute hydrocephalus after subarachnoid hemorrhage. World Neurosurg. 2013;80(3–4):304–6.
14. Wilson TJ, Stetler WR Jr, Davis MC, et al. Intraventricular hemorrhage is associated with early hydrocephalus, symptomatic vasospasm, and poor outcome in aneurysmal subarachnoid hemorrhage. J Neurol Surg A Cent Eur Neurosurg. 2015;76(2):126–32.
15. Chen S, Luo J, Reis C, Manaenko A, Zhang J. Hydrocephalus after Subarachnoid Hemorrhage: pathophysiology, Diagnosis, and Treatment. Biomed Res Int. 2017;2017:8584753.
16. Saliou G, Paradot G, Gondry C, et al. A phase-contrast MRI study of acute and chronic hydrodynamic alterations after hydrocephalus induced by subarachnoid hemorrhage. J Neuroimaging. 2012;22(4):343–50.
17. Chen S, Yang Q, Chen G, Zhang JH. An update on inflammation in the acute phase of intracerebral hemorrhage. Transl Stroke Res. 2015;6(1):4–8.
18. Kanat A, Turkmenoglu O, Aydin MD, et al. Toward changing of the pathophysiologic basis of acute hydrocephalus after subarachnoid hemorrhage: a preliminary experimental study. World Neurosurg. 2013;80(3–4):390–5.
19. Tan Q, Chen Q, Feng Z, et al. Cannabinoid receptor 2 activation restricts fibrosis and alleviates hydrocephalus after intraventricular hemorrhage. Brain Res. 2017;1654(Pt A):24–33.

20. Yan H, Chen Y, Li L, et al. Decorin alleviated chronic hydrocephalus via inhibiting TGF-beta1/Smad/CTGF pathway after subarachnoid hemorrhage in rats. Brain Res. 2016;1630:241–53.
21. Gram M, Sveinsdottir S, Ruscher K, et al. Hemoglobin induces inflammation after preterm intraventricular hemorrhage by methemoglobin formation. J Neuroinflammation. 2013;10:100.
22. Gram M, Sveinsdottir S, Cinthio M, et al. Extracellular hemoglobin – mediator of inflammation and cell death in the choroid plexus following preterm intraventricular hemorrhage. J Neuroinflammation. 2014;11:200.
23. Garton T, Keep RF, Wilkinson DA, et al. Intraventricular Hemorrhage: the Role of Blood Components in Secondary Injury and Hydrocephalus. Transl Stroke Res. 2016;7(6):447–51.
24. Bloch O, Auguste KI, Manley GT, Verkman AS. Accelerated progression of kaolin-induced hydrocephalus in aquaporin-4-deficient mice. J Cereb Blood Flow Metab. 2006;26(12):1527–37.
25. Gao C, Du H, Hua Y, Keep RF, Strahle J, Xi G. Role of red blood cell lysis and iron in hydrocephalus after intraventricular hemorrhage. J Cereb Blood Flow Metab. 2014;34(6):1070–5.
26. Suzuki H, Muramatsu M, Tanaka K, Fujiwara H, Kojima T, Taki W. Cerebrospinal fluid ferritin in chronic hydrocephalus after aneurysmal subarachnoid hemorrhage. J Neurol. 2006;253(9):1170–6.
27. Daniere F, Gascou G, Menjot de Champfleur N, et al. Complications and follow up of subarachnoid hemorrhages. Diagn Interv Imaging. 2015;96(7–8):677–86.
28. van Gijn J, Hijdra A, Wijdicks EF, Vermeulen M, van Crevel H. Acute hydrocephalus after aneurysmal subarachnoid hemorrhage. J Neurosurg. 1985;63(3):355–62.
29. Knol DS, van Gijn J, Kruitwagen CL, Rinkel GJ. Size of third and fourth ventricle in obstructive and communicating acute hydrocephalus after aneurysmal subarachnoid hemorrhage. J Neurol. 2011;258(1):44–9.
30. Morgenstern LB, Hemphill JC 3rd, Anderson C, et al. Guidelines for the management of spontaneous intracerebral hemorrhage: a guideline for healthcare professionals from the American Heart Association/American Stroke Association. Stroke. 2010;41(9):2108–29.
31. Poon WS, Ng S, Wai S. CSF antibiotic prophylaxis for neurosurgical patients with ventriculostomy: a randomised study. Acta Neurochir Suppl. 1998;71:146–8.
32. Blomstedt GC. Results of trimethoprim-sulfamethoxazole prophylaxis in ventriculostomy and shunting procedures. A double-blind randomized trial. J Neurosurg. 1985;62(5):694–7.
33. Alleyne CH Jr, Hassan M, Zabramski JM. The efficacy and cost of prophylactic and periprocedural antibiotics in patients with external ventricular drains. Neurosurgery. 2000;47(5):1124–7; discussion 1127–1129
34. Sonabend AM, Korenfeld Y, Crisman C, Badjatia N, Mayer SA, Connolly ES Jr. Prevention of ventriculostomy-related infections with prophylactic antibiotics and antibiotic-coated external ventricular drains: a systematic review. Neurosurgery. 2011;68(4):996–1005.
35. Kubilay Z, Amini S, Fauerbach LL, Archibald L, Friedman WA, Layon AJ. Decreasing ventricular infections through the use of a ventriculostomy placement bundle: experience at a single institution. J Neurosurg. 2013;118(3):514–20.
36. Scheithauer S, Burgel U, Ryang YM, et al. Prospective surveillance of drain associated meningitis/ventriculitis in a neurosurgery and neurological intensive care unit. J Neurol Neurosurg Psychiatry. 2009;80(12):1381–5.
37. Komotar RJ, Olivi A, Rigamonti D, Tamargo RJ. Microsurgical fenestration of the lamina terminalis reduces the incidence of shunt-dependent hydrocephalus after aneurysmal subarachnoid hemorrhage. Neurosurgery. 2002;51(6):1403–12; discussion 1412–1403
38. Tomasello F, d'Avella D, de Divitiis O. Does lamina terminalis fenestration reduce the incidence of chronic hydrocephalus after subarachnoid hemorrhage? Neurosurgery. 1999;45(4):827–31; discussion 831–822
39. Komotar RJ, Hahn DK, Kim GH, et al. Efficacy of lamina terminalis fenestration in reducing shunt-dependent hydrocephalus following aneurysmal subarachnoid hemorrhage: a systematic review. Clinical article. J Neurosurg. 2009;111(1):147–54.
40. Vale FL, Bradley EL, Fisher WS 3rd. The relationship of subarachnoid hemorrhage and the need for postoperative shunting. J Neurosurg. 1997;86(3):462–6.

41. Vermeij FH, Hasan D, Vermeulen M, Tanghe HL, van Gijn J. Predictive factors for deterioration from hydrocephalus after subarachnoid hemorrhage. Neurology. 1994;44(10):1851–5.
42. O'Kelly CJ, Kulkarni AV, Austin PC, Urbach D, Wallace MC. Shunt-dependent hydrocephalus after aneurysmal subarachnoid hemorrhage: incidence, predictors, and revision rates. Clinical article. J Neurosurg. 2009;111(5):1029–35.
43. Erixon HO, Sorteberg A, Sorteberg W, Eide PK. Predictors of shunt dependency after aneurysmal subarachnoid hemorrhage: results of a single-center clinical trial. Acta Neurochir. 2014;156(11):2059–69.
44. Rincon F, Gordon E, Starke RM, et al. Predictors of long-term shunt-dependent hydrocephalus after aneurysmal subarachnoid hemorrhage. Clinical article. J Neurosurg. 2010;113(4):774–80.
45. Dupont S, Rabinstein AA. Extent of acute hydrocephalus after subarachnoid hemorrhage as a risk factor for poor functional outcome. Neurol Res. 2013;35(2):107–10.
46. Motiei-Langroudi R, Adeeb N, Foreman PM, et al. Predictors of Shunt Insertion in Aneurysmal Subarachnoid Hemorrhage. World Neurosurg. 2017;98:421–6.
47. Gruber A, Reinprecht A, Bavinzski G, Czech T, Richling B. Chronic shunt-dependent hydrocephalus after early surgical and early endovascular treatment of ruptured intracranial aneurysms. Neurosurgery. 1999;44(3):503–9; discussion 509–512
48. Kwon JH, Sung SK, Song YJ, Choi HJ, Huh JT, Kim HD. Predisposing factors related to shunt-dependent chronic hydrocephalus after aneurysmal subarachnoid hemorrhage. J Korean Neurosurg Soc. 2008;43(4):177–81.
49. Howington JU, Kutz SC, Wilding GE, Awasthi D. Cocaine use as a predictor of outcome in aneurysmal subarachnoid hemorrhage. J Neurosurg. 2003;99(2):271–5.
50. Chang TR, Kowalski RG, Carhuapoma JR, Tamargo RJ, Naval NS. Cocaine use as an independent predictor of seizures after aneurysmal subarachnoid hemorrhage. J Neurosurg. 2016;124(3):730–5.
51. Walcott BP, Iorgulescu JB, Stapleton CJ, Kamel H. Incidence, timing, and predictors of delayed shunting for hydrocephalus after aneurysmal subarachnoid hemorrhage. Neurocrit Care. 2015;23(1):54–8.
52. Rammos S, Klopfenstein J, Augspurger L, et al. Conversion of external ventricular drains to ventriculoperitoneal shunts after aneurysmal subarachnoid hemorrhage: effects of site and protein/red blood cell counts on shunt infection and malfunction. J Neurosurg. 2008;109(6):1001–4.
53. Reddy GK. Ventriculoperitoneal shunt surgery and the incidence of shunt revision in adult patients with hemorrhage-related hydrocephalus. Clin Neurol Neurosurg. 2012;114(9):1211–6.
54. Yoshioka H, Inagawa T, Tokuda Y, Inokuchi F. Chronic hydrocephalus in elderly patients following subarachnoid hemorrhage. Surg Neurol. 2000;53(2):119–24; discussion 124–115
55. Spetzler RF, McDougall CG, Albuquerque FC, et al. The Barrow Ruptured Aneurysm Trial: 3-year results. J Neurosurg. 2013;119(1):146–57.

14 Posttraumatic Hydrocephalus

Jason Milton and Jeffrey R. Leonard

Overview

Traumatic brain injury (TBI) may result in posttraumatic hydrocephalus in 4% of patients experiencing a severe traumatic brain injury [23]. Posttraumatic hydrocephalus affects morbidity and mortality of severe traumatic brain injury patients, but the degree of its impact is difficult to assess due to an absence of clearly defined diagnostic criteria for hydrocephalus [10]. More often than not, posttraumatic hydrocephalus is nonobstructive and may arise due to a variety of physiologic factors.

Understanding the pathophysiology and diagnostic evaluation of posttraumatic hydrocephalus allows providers, who do not routinely manage chronic hydrocephalus, to effectively manage this condition as a rare but expected sequelae of a traumatic brain injury. Failure to recognize and appropriately manage this disease state can affect significantly morbidity and mortality in TBI patients.

Epidemiology

Posttraumatic hydrocephalus does not appear to have a predilection for either sex nor does race appear to play a role in the incidence. Age appears to affect the incidence and severity as older patients are more likely to develop posttraumatic hydrocephalus and older age is linked to a greater severity of hydrocephalus [19].

J. Milton
Department of Neurosurgery, OhioHealth, Columbus, OH, USA

J. R. Leonard (✉)
Nationwide Children's Hospital, Department of Neurosurgery, The Ohio State University College of Medicine, Columbus, OH, USA
e-mail: Jeffrey.Leonard@nationwidechildrens.org

D. D. Limbrick, J. R. Leonard (eds.), *Cerebrospinal Fluid Disorders*,
https://doi.org/10.1007/978-3-319-97928-1_14

The incidence of posttraumatic hydrocephalus ranges from 0.7% to 50% due to variations in study design, under diagnosis, and the variable presenting symptoms that can differ from a typical hydrocephalus patient. It is difficult to directly correlate the incidence of hydrocephalus with the initial lesion type, size, and location when evaluated on computed tomography. However, subarachnoid and intraventricular hemorrhage have an established relationship with the development of early ventricular enlargement as does diffuse axonal injury and hypoxic-ischemic insult with late ventricular enlargement. Moreover, there is a link between the development of hydrocephalus with operative head injuries, which likely corresponds to more severe brain injuries. Lastly, a correlation exists between the duration of a patient's coma and the development of hydrocephalus [21].

Pathophysiology

The pathophysiology of hydrocephalus in trauma is similar to that of patients without a history of trauma. It is caused by a variety of physiologic factors, including overproduction of CSF, insufficient reabsorption, or obstruction of CSF flow between communicating CSF spaces. Little research supports the theory of upregulation of CSF production in posttraumatic hydrocephalus during any phase of the disease state. It is believed that the two most common causes are abnormal or insufficient absorption of CSF via the arachnoid granulations or ineffective transit through fourth ventricular outlets [14].

The arachnoid villi of the granulations are thought to undergo a fibrotic transformation due to inflammation secondary to iron deposition from blood products related to the primary insult of the brain. The deposition of iron leads to oxidative injury similar to that of other organs where natural metals may accumulate [5]. Research efforts are focusing on this mechanism in hopes of arresting this process [25]. Outflow obstruction of the fourth ventricular outlets occurs via a similar mechanism related to inflammation because of the expected presence of blood products noted with intraventricular hemorrhage seen after traumatic brain injury.

There has been controversy whether posttraumatic hydrocephalus or ventriculomegaly is related to an active process related to CSF dynamics or if it is secondary to atrophy as a result of changing vascular dynamics related to secondary brain injury. Evaluation of CSF dynamics plays an important role in these patients, especially those without elevations in intracranial pressure and observed ventriculomegaly [7]. Evaluation of outflow resistance and intracranial elastance index serves to not only provide information in the diagnosis of this condition but also in predicting shunt responsiveness [8]. Elastance represents the reciprocal value of intracranial compliance, as it is the pressure/volume response at given levels of intracranial pressure [1]. Patients with ex vacuo changes typically do not exhibit flow dynamics with as great irregularity as those with posttraumatic ventriculomegaly. The variation in flow dynamics is represented in the waveform of intracranial pressure.

Hydrocephalus ex vacuo does not exhibit temporal horn enlargement as what may be seen in posttraumatic or normal pressure hydrocephalus [17]. Ex vacuo dilatation of the ventricular system results from atrophy due to ischemic injury, and intracranial pressure typically remains normal. Patients with ex vacuo dilatation typically do not exhibit the abnormal CSF dynamics noted in the typical posttraumatic hydrocephalus patient [10].

Some have linked the size of a patient's craniectomy defect to the development of posttraumatic hydrocephalus [9]. In addition, there is increasing data to support that early cranioplasty is associated with a decreased incidence in the development of posttraumatic hydrocephalus, even in the presence of subdural hygromas [24]. Epidural fluid collections after cranioplasty has not been linked to posttraumatic hydrocephalus. These collections have been associated with larger craniectomy defects and CSF leakage during cranioplasty [12]. These data sets, however, are small in size, and wide support of the practice of early cranioplasty has not been generally accepted.

Presentation

Posttraumatic hydrocephalus may present within 2 weeks of a traumatic brain injury, but may be seen years later. Up to 50% of patients may develop clinically evident hydrocephalus within the post-acute phase of a traumatic injury [19]. Hydrocephalus after TBI often presents in an atypical fashion when compared to other causes of hydrocephalus. Its presentation is often indolent and allows for the diagnosis to be easily missed. Conditions that affect the level of consciousness such as diffuse axonal injury or excessive administration of sedative chemicals may make it difficult to appreciate an improvement in condition with a subsequent decline in neurologic status.

TBI patients that present in the chronic phase experience a gradual decline in functional status or a progressive slowing in the rate of improvement. Others may present with progressive neurologic deficits, increased hypertonia, or increased tension at the surgical incision. The classic triad of symptoms (gait instability, bladder dysfunction, and mental status changes) found in normal pressure hydrocephalus may also be seen in patients with posttraumatic hydrocephalus [31]. Although treated the same, posttraumatic hydrocephalus patients will have most notable improvements in mental status.

Some patients may also present with asymptomatic posttraumatic hydrocephalus, which is easily confused with ex vacuo atrophic evolution of the primary and secondary insults to the brain. The following clinical vignette details the presentation of a patient that presented with an apparent asymptomatic course with progressively enlarging ventricles.

A 56-year-old male presented as a severe traumatic brain injury with an acute subdural hematoma and underwent decompressive craniectomy (Fig. 14.1a). His initial exam revealed a Glasgow Coma Score of 3T which improved to 7T in the immediate postoperative period with adequate resuscitation. The patient was managed expectantly with serial imaging and plans for a delayed

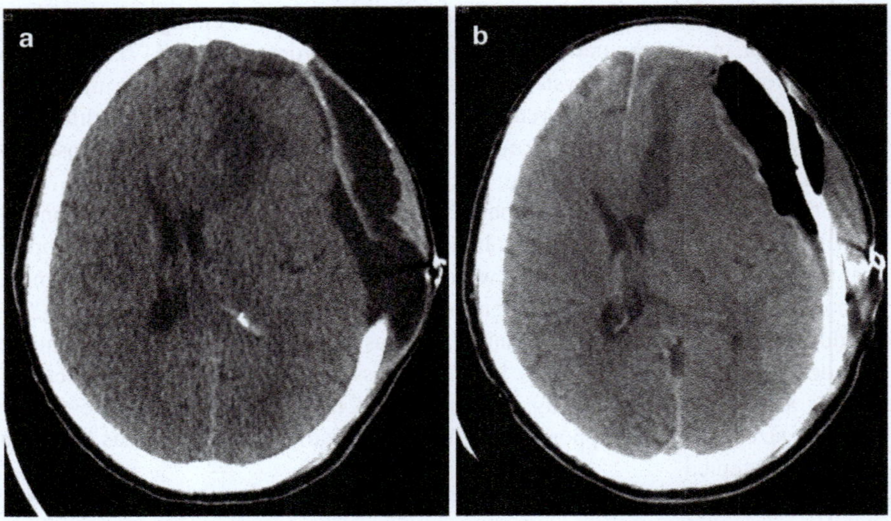

Fig. 14.1 Noncontrast CT head of a severe traumatic brain injury patient before (**a**) and after (**b**) cranioplasty using an autologous graft 3 weeks after a small decompressive craniectomy

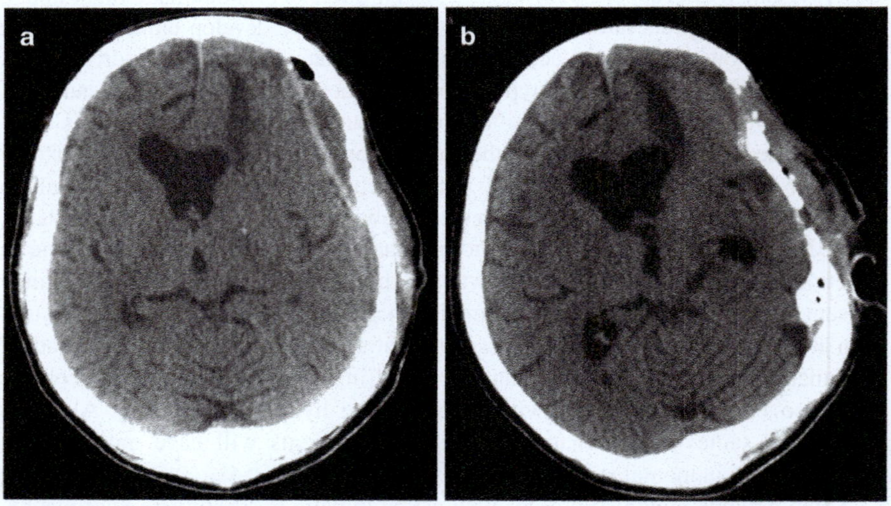

Fig. 14.2 Noncontrast CT head 4 (**a**) and 5 (**b**) weeks after cranioplasty revealing progressive ventriculomegaly

cranioplasty. The patient remained clinically stable and underwent cranioplasty 3 weeks after the decompressive craniectomy. Postoperatively, the patient developed a subdural fluid collection that eventually resolved. As the subdural fluid resolved, serial imaging showed progressive increases in ventricular size over 4 weeks (Fig. 14.2). The patient's exam remained stable throughout this course without any signs of neurologic dysfunction. An external ventricular

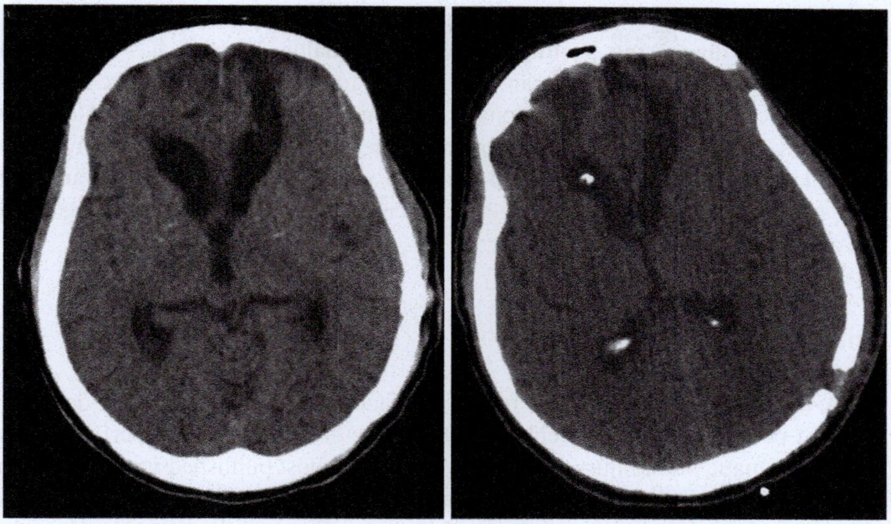

Fig. 14.3 Noncontrast CT head after placement of a right frontal external ventricular drain reveals decreased size of the lateral ventricles

drain was placed with an opening pressure of 5 mmHg. The ICP waveform was appropriate and was drained to achieve ventricular decompression with hopes of neurologic improvement. Over the course of 5 days, the patient intermittently improved to GCS 8T. The neurologic improvement noted after ventricular decompression supported the diagnosis of posttraumatic hydrocephalus despite the asymptomatic presentation following cranioplasty (Fig. 14.3). Wen et al. report that many patients in the subgroup of normal pressure posttraumatic hydrocephalus find benefit in shunt implantation [31].

The concept of an arrested phase in posttraumatic hydrocephalus is difficult to determine given the degree of parenchymal atrophy that tends to occur for these patients. This atrophy may often be progressive and continue at an accelerated rate compared to the noninjured patient. If hydrocephalus is suspected, it is best to obtain serial imaging as well as follow the patient clinically.

Diagnosis

Evaluation

A thorough medical evaluation to include imaging should be conducted prior to the diagnosis of posttraumatic hydrocephalus. Assessment of toxic, metabolic, and infectious etiologies should be ruled out. Progressive ventricular enlargement is one of the most definitive sign of posttraumatic hydrocephalus. Computed tomography is the standard, but magnetic resonance imaging may be beneficial to evaluate findings of the posterior fossa, including tonsillar herniation and stenosis of the aqueduct of Sylvius. Cisternography has previously been reported to be of assistance in diagnosing posttraumatic hydrocephalus, but this has since been refuted [28]. Lumbar puncture can also be used for evaluation, but there is only a slight association with mild functional improvement with the removal of 50 mL or more of CSF [16]. Clinical improvement suggests that permanent CSF diversion may likely be of benefit. Multiple failures to wean an external ventricular drain also serves as an indicator for the development of posttraumatic hydrocephalus in the acute phase [18].

Imaging

There are reports of radiographic prognostic factors that are linked to the development of posttraumatic hydrocephalus. Decompressive craniectomy, performed on severe traumatic brain injury patients, is one of the most published variables in the study of posttraumatic hydrocephalus. Kaen et al. reported that 80% of patients with interhemispheric hygromas after decompressive craniectomy developed hydrocephalus within 50 days of surgical intervention [13]. Furthermore, Vendantam et al. replicated this result with the addition of younger age at the time of decompressive craniectomy as an independent prognostic indicator [29]. However, the incidence of hygroma formation is reported to be less with duraplasty [22].

A greater degree of cortical atrophy in the post-acute phase is also thought to be related to developing hydrocephalus. In the presence of cortical atrophy, SPECT has been used to determine areas of hypoperfusion in posttraumatic hydrocephalus with the most common regions being the temporal and frontal lobes [19]. This study does not currently play a role in the diagnosis or the management of posttraumatic hydrocephalus.

Classification

Posttraumatic hydrocephalus is typically classified as obstructive (non-communicating) or nonobstructive (communicating) as defined by Dandy and Blackfan [6]. Traumatic brain injury lends to another classification system which should be noted in the evaluation and assessment. The phase of rehabilitation of a traumatic brain injury patient is important in regard to their clinical status and ability to recover. These phases are classified as acute, post-acute, and chronic. Posttraumatic hydrocephalus is typically elucidated in the post-acute phase of rehabilitation.

Medical Management

Despite inconsistent literature and limited benefits with the use of carbonic anhydrase inhibitors in children, the use of acetazolamide in adults has been shown to produce transient reductions in intracranial pressure [3]. This has been reported to serve as a good predictive response to shunting [3]. However, these patients have an impaired cerebrovascular response as the expected normal increase in cerebral flow is blunted in the presence of posttraumatic hydrocephalus [4]. Acetazolamide remains an adequate medication to use over a short period of time, but should not be a consideration of pharmacologic treatment in lieu of CSF diversion procedures.

In experimental models of TBI, deferoxamine has been used in rats to attenuate posttraumatic hydrocephalus caused by fluid percussion by affecting heme oxygenase-1 upregulation [33]. This chemical has yet to be tried in humans, and its utility is likely in the acute phase of posttraumatic hydrocephalus given the proposed mechanism of preventing fibrosis of the arachnoid villi. Its use may be limited given that posttraumatic hydrocephalus is most commonly diagnosed in the post-acute phase.

Surgical Intervention

Shunting of posttraumatic hydrocephalus improves level of consciousness, behavior, memory, and gait in patients with the most notable functional decline [19]. Ventriculoperitoneal shunting is the preferred procedure, but issues related to previous wound healing, history of a seizure disorder, or concerns regarding further iatrogenic brain penetration may dictate lumboperitoneal shunt placement. In addition, lumboperitoneal shunts are associated with their own unique set of complications, including, most notably, catheter migration. Programmable valves have enhanced the surgical treatment of posttraumatic hydrocephalus by allowing for greater variability in the adjustment of CSF diversion [2]. These adjustable valves allow providers to account for evolving CSF dynamics as cortical atrophy progresses. These valves are integral in the management of those patients in the normal pressure subgroup.

Literature purports that early CSF diversion results in improved outcomes while participating in inpatient rehabilitation programs [30]. There is always a question of timing with regard to appropriateness of shunt placement in patients with clearly evident posttraumatic hydrocephalus after decompressive craniectomy. One theory proposes simultaneous CSF diversion with cranioplasty to decrease operative time and anesthesia encounters for TBI patients with neurological deficits. A staged ventriculoperitoneal shunting following cranioplasty has been reported to have a decreased rate of infection and postoperative complications. Schuss et al. report a complication rate of 12% in staged procedures that is compared to 47% in simultaneous ventriculoperitoneal shunt placement with cranioplasty [27]. The rate of complication is increased proportionately to the amount of brain tissue herniating through the craniectomy defect [11]. The rate of cranioplasty infection does not change with regard to the timing of shunt placement. However, the rate of shunt infection is dramatically increased [20]. These results have been replicated with a reoperation rate of 20% for patients undergoing simultaneous procedures compared to 3% for those undergoing staged procedures [32].

Controversy surrounds whether or not endoscopic third ventriculostomy (ETV) is effective. A review by De Bonis et al. suggests that endoscopic third ventriculostomy should be considered as a viable option in patients with communicating posttraumatic hydrocephalus [8]. Performance of an ETV allows patients to remain shunt independent and may allow many patients to avoid the complications associated with lifetime shunt dependency. Proper evaluation of these patients is key, but the nuances of selection have yet to be elucidated given a paucity of research.

Complications

Complications of shunting in posttraumatic hydrocephalus are similar to those of patients with chronic hydrocephalus with some notable exceptions that are unique to patients with brain injuries. Overdrainage of CSF is an important complication to monitor as TBI patients often have evolving and progressing atrophic changes putting them at increased risk of developing subdural hematomas. For this reason, adjustable valves may be the most appropriate for posttraumatic hydrocephalus [15]. Subdural hygromas are often found prior to shunt implantation and may, in fact, be a harbinger of posttraumatic hydrocephalus. Although the incidence of shunt infection is elevated in relation to the timing of cranioplasty, there is no increased rate of infection of shunted patients without cranioplasty when compared to patients with chronic hydrocephalus [26]. As the body of information for these patients evolve, the rate of infection and timing considerations are likely to change.

Posttraumatic hydrocephalus patients exhibit a decreased rate of malfunction with need for revision when compared to patients with chronic hydrocephalus [26]. Shunt malfunction occurs in up to 32% of patients requiring revision during the lifetime of their shunt. The incidence does increase during the life of the shunt, but the rate of failure progressively slows [26].

Outcomes

The outcomes after shunt implantation in posttraumatic hydrocephalus show that greater than 50% of patients will have a clear benefit after CSF diversion. The best predictive parameter after implantation is the patient's preoperative clinical status. There is no direct correlation with outcome and age in reference to complications experienced with shunt devices for posttraumatic hydrocephalus [28]. However, it should be noted that older patients are more likely to develop posttraumatic hydrocephalus after a TBI. The most effective method of monitoring outcomes in posttraumatic hydrocephalus is by way of following neurologic status much like that of other patients with devices in place for CSF diversion.

Conclusion

Posttraumatic hydrocephalus is an underrecognized condition in TBI patients. It is a clinically distinct entity for which understanding the diagnosis and evaluation is paramount for proper treatment. Awareness of risk factors and prognostic indicators serve to guide evaluation and assessment of patients suspected to have posttraumatic hydrocephalus. Treatment of posttraumatic hydrocephalus is similar to that of chronic hydrocephalus and literature supports the use CSF diversion in these patients. Complications of shunt placement and shunt malfunction are similar to those of chronic hydrocephalus, but occur at a lesser rate. Staging of ventriculoperitoneal shunting with cranioplasty may decrease the rate of postoperative complications.

References

1. Anile C, De Bonis P, Mangiola A, Mannino S, Santini P. A new method of estimating intracranial elastance. Interdis Neuros. 2014;1:26–30.
2. Bergsneider M. Management of hydrocephalus with programmable valves after traumatic brain injury and subarachnoid hemorrhage. Curr Opin Neurol. 2000;13(6):661–4.
3. Chang CC, Asada H, Mimura T, Suzuki S. A prospective study of cerebral blood flow and cerebrovascular reactivity to acetazolamide in 162 patients with idiopathic normal-pressure hydrocephalus. J Neurosurg. 2009;111(3):610–7.
4. Chang CC, Kuwana N, Ito S, Ikegami T. Impairment of cerebrovascular reactivity to acetazolamide in patients with normal pressure hydrocephalus. Nucl Med Commun. 2000;21(2):139–41.
5. Chen Z, Gao C, Hua Y, Keep RF, Muraszko K, Xi G. Role of iron in brain injury after intraventricular hemorrhage. Stroke. 2011;42(2):465–70.
6. Dandy WE, Blackfan KD. Internal hydrocephalus: an experimental, clinical, and pathological study. Am J Dis Child. 1914;8:406.
7. De Bonis P, Mangiola A, Pompucci A, Formisano R, Mattogno P, Anile C. CSF dynamics analysis in patients with post-traumatic ventriculomegaly. Clin Neurol Neurosurg. 2013;115(1):49–53.
8. De Bonis P, Tamburrini G, Mangiola A, Pompucci A, Mattogno PP, Porso M, Anile C. Post-traumatic hydrocephalus is a contraindication for endoscopic third-ventriculostomy: isn't it? Clin Neurol Neurosurg. 2013;115(1):9–12.
9. Fotakopoulos G, Tsianaka E, Siasios G, Vagkopoulos K, Fountas K. Posttraumatic hydrocephalus after decompressive craniectomy in 126 patients with severe traumatic brain injury. J Neurol Surg A Cent Eur Neurosurg. 2016;77(2):88–92.
10. Guyot LL, Michael DB. Post-traumatic hydrocephalus. Neurol Res. 2000;22(1):25–8.
11. Heo J, Park SQ, Cho SJ, Chang JC, Park HK. Evaluation of simultaneous cranioplasty and ventriculoperitoneal shunt procedures. J Neurosurg. 2014;121(2):313–8.
12. Jeong SH, Wang US, Kim SW, Ha SW, Kim JK. Symptomatic epidural fluid collection following cranioplasty after decompressive craniectomy for traumatic brain injury. Korean J Neurotrauma. 2016;12(1):6–10.
13. Kaen A, Jimenez-Roldan L, Alday R, Gomez PA, Lagares A, Alén JF, Lobato RD. Interhemispheric hygroma after decompressive craniectomy: does it predict posttraumatic hydrocephalus? J Neurosurg. 2010;113(6):1287–93.
14. Katz RT, Brander V, Sahgal V. Updates on the diagnosis and management of posttraumatic hydrocephalus. Am J Phys Med Rehabil. 1989;68(2):91–6.
15. Kim KH, Yeo IS, Yi JS, Lee HJ, Yang JH, Lee IW. A pressure adjustment protocol for programmable valves. J Korean Neurosurg Soc. 2009;46(4):370–7.
16. Kim SW, Lee SM, Shin H. Clinical analysis of post-traumatic hydrocephalus. J Korean Neurosurg Soc. 2005;38:211–4.
17. Leborgne JM, Sheldon JJ, Goldstein MS, Smoak WM 3rd, Serafini AN. Differential diagnosis between normal pressure hydrocephalus and cerebral atrophy on computed tomography. Rev Interam Radiol. 1979;4(2):75–8.
18. Lewis A, Taylor KW. Prediction of ventriculoperitoneal shunt placement based on type of failure during external ventricular drain wean. Clin Neurol Neurosurg. 2014;125:109–13.

19. Mazzini L, Campini R, Angelino E, et al. Posttraumatic hydrocephalus: a clinical, neuroradiologic, and neuropsychologic assessment of long-term outcome. Arch Phys Med Rehabil. 2003;84(11):1637–41.
20. Meyer RM, Morton RP, Abecassis IJ, Barber JK, Emerson SN, Nerva JD, et al. Risk of complication with simultaneous cranioplasty and placement of ventriculoperitoneal shunt. World Neurosurg. 2017;107:830–3.
21. Meyers C, Levin H, Eisenberg H. Early versus late ventricular enlargement following closed head injury. J Neurol Neurosurg Psychiatry. 1983;46:1092–7.
22. Moon JW, Hyun DK. Decompressive craniectomy in traumatic brain injury: a review article. Korean J Neurotrauma. 2017;13(1):1–8.
23. Narayan RJ, Gokaslan ZL, Bontke CF. Neurologic sequelae of head injury. In: Rosenthal M, editor. Rehabilitation of the adult and child with traumatic brain injury. 2nd ed. Philadelphia: Davis; 1990. p. 94–106.
24. Rahme R, Weil AG, Sabbagh M, Moumdjian R, Bouthillier A, Bojanowski MW. Decompressive craniectomy is not an independent risk factor for communicating hydrocephalus in patients with increased intracranial pressure. Neurosurgery. 2010;67(3):675.
25. Raz E, Jensen JH, Ge Y, Babb JS, Miles L, Reaume J, et al. Brain iron quantification in mild traumatic brain injury: a magnetic field correlation study. AJNR Am J Neuroradiol. 2011;32(10):1851–6.
26. Reddy GK, Bollam P, Shi R, Guthikonda B, Nanda A. Management of adult hydrocephalus with ventriculoperitoneal shunts: long-term single-institution experience. Neurosurgery. 2011;69(4):774–80. discussion 780–1.
27. Schuss P, Borger V, Güresir Á, Vatter H, Güresir E. Cranioplasty and ventriculoperitoneal shunt placement after decompressive craniectomy: staged surgery is associated with fewer postoperative complications. World Neurosurg. 2015;84(4):1051–4.
28. Tribl G, Oder W. Outcome after shunt implantation in severe head injury with post-traumatic hydrocephalus. Brain Inj. 2000;14(4):345–54.
29. Vedantam A, Yamal JM, Hwang H, Robertson CS, Gopinath SP. Factors associated with shunt-dependent hydrocephalus after decompressive craniectomy for traumatic brain injury. J Neurosurg. 2017;16:1–6.
30. Weintraub AH, Gerber DJ, Kowalski RG. Posttraumatic hydrocephalus as a confounding influence on brain injury rehabilitation: incidence, clinical characteristics, and outcomes. Arch Phys Med Rehabil. 2017;98(2):312–9.
31. Wen L, Wan S, Zhan RY, Li G, Gong JB, Liu WG, et al. Shunt implantation in a special subgroup of post-traumatic hydrocephalus--patients have normal intracranial pressure without clinical representations of hydrocephalus. Brain Inj. 2009;23(1):61–4.
32. Yang XF, Wang H, Wen L, Huang X, Li G, Gong JB. The safety of simultaneous cranioplasty and shunt implantation. Brain Inj. 2017;12:1–5.
33. Zhao J, Chen Z, Xi G, Keep RF, Hua Y. Deferoxamine attenuates acute hydrocephalus after traumatic brain injury in rats. Transl Stroke Res. 2014;5(5):586–94.

Management of Intracranial Hypotension and Cerebrospinal Fluid Leaks

15

David L. Dornbos III, Nathaniel Toop, Ammar Shaikhouni, H. Wayne Slone, and John M. McGregor

Introduction

Intracranial hypotension and cerebrospinal fluid (CSF) leaks may occur secondary to numerous pathologies, including trauma, iatrogenic injury, or even in a spontaneous manner. A diagnostic hallmark of intracranial hypotension is the presence of low CSF volume rather than low CSF pressure. As such, intracranial hypotension may occur in the setting of low, normal, or elevated intracranial pressure. The diagnostic evaluation of this pathology, in addition to localization of a potential leak, can be challenging, requiring numerous noninvasive and invasive imaging modalities, including computed tomography (CT), magnetic resonance imaging (MRI), lumbar puncture, myelography, or cisternography. While medical management can provide symptomatic relief, definitive treatment of the source of the pathology depends on the etiology of the CSF leak. Depending on the source and localization of the CSF leak, less invasive means of CSF diversion may be sufficient, or patients may require definitive repair of the CSF fistula. Ultimately, proper evaluation and correct diagnosis of the pathology driving the CSF leak frame the paradigm for treatment of intracranial hypotension.

D. L. Dornbos III · N. Toop · A. Shaikhouni · J. M. McGregor (✉)
Department of Neurological Surgery, The Ohio State University Wexner Medical Center, Columbus, OH, USA
e-mail: john.mcgregor@osumc.edu

H. W. Slone
Department of Radiology, The Ohio State University Wexner Medical Center, Columbus, OH, USA

D. D. Limbrick, J. R. Leonard (eds.), *Cerebrospinal Fluid Disorders*,
https://doi.org/10.1007/978-3-319-97928-1_15

Etiology

Intracranial hypotension typically occurs secondary to trauma, iatrogenic injury or in a spontaneous manner nearly always resulting from a CSF leak. Traumatic injury to the skull base is the most frequent cause of intracranial hypotension, manifesting as rhinorrhea or otorrhea [1]. Following trauma, CSF leaks can be observed in approximately 3% of all closed head injury and 30% of all skull base fractures [2]. As an underlying source in 80% of all CSF leaks, those occurring secondary to traumatic etiology are often associated with significant morbidity [3]. Meningitis is a significant concern in this patient population, being cited in up to 32% of patients with persistent rhinorrhea [4]. For this reason, reparative measures are initiated early in the presence of a continuous leak. Uncommonly, prior traumatic brachial plexus avulsion injury can manifest in a delayed fashion as a spontaneous CSF leak as well [5].

Iatrogenic causes of intracranial hypotension can occur following endoscopic endonasal surgery [2, 6, 7]. While past studies have shown the risk of CSF leak following endonasal surgery to be as high as 10% [8], improvements in closure technique to mitigate potential CSF leaks have limited the rate of a persistent postoperative leak to approximately 1% [2]. Importantly, patients undergoing cranial skull base surgery carry a significant risk of developing hydrocephalus in the immediate postoperative setting, substantially increasing their risk of postoperative CSF leak [2]. Potential development of hydrocephalus must be monitored closely, allowing timely management of elevated intracranial pressure to preserve wound closure.

More commonly, iatrogenic intracranial hypotension can be seen following spinal surgery secondary to incidental durotomies. The incidence of durotomies sustained during spinal surgery varies between 1% and 17%, with higher rates associated with thoracic and lumbar location or in the setting of revision surgery [9–18]. These leaks are well known to cause positional headaches, photophobia, nausea/vomiting, and poor wound healing [19, 20]. More significant complications have also been noted, including subdural hematomas and meningitis [21–23]. The majority of CSF leaks following spinal surgery involve dural-cutaneous fistulas, although the possibility of a dural-pleural fistula following thoracic surgery is an important complication of which to be aware. In addition to the aforementioned complications, these rare leaks can also cause respiratory complications and persistent pleural effusions [24].

Intracranial hypotension secondary to spontaneous CSF leaks is rare, although most commonly arise from the spinal dural sac, with spontaneous skull base leaks being exceedingly rare [25]. One study found that symptoms and headaches consistent with intracranial hypotension are solely attributable to spine pathology [26]. While spontaneous CSF leaks remain diagnostically idiopathic, it has been postulated that an underlying weakness in the dura may allow for a relatively minor trauma, such as lifting, coughing, or physical exertion, to generate a CSF leak. While the underlying etiology in spontaneous CSF leaks often remains idiopathic, numerous mechanisms have been proposed, often related to a pre-existing weakness in the dura. Often seen in association with meningeal diverticula, spontaneous leaks are seen with increased frequency in patients with heritable connective tissue disorders [27, 28]. Notably, patients with Marfan syndrome have been previously shown to have an increased risk of meningeal diverticula, dural ectasia, and spontaneous CSF leaks [29–32]. Dural weaknesses may also arise secondary to degenerative disease, including osteophytic bone spurs and herniated discs [33, 34].

Regarding intracranial sources of spontaneous CSF leaks, CSF rhinorrhea may occur secondary to an erosive skull base tumor. However, up to one-third of patients presenting with spontaneous CSF rhinorrhea may have underlying idiopathic intracranial hypertension (IIH) [2]. These patients often display classic findings of intracranial hypotension on imaging, although typically without symptoms of intracranial hypotension despite recurrent CSF rhinorrhea. Diagnosis of IIH before surgical repair can be challenging as the leakage of CSF typically decreases intracranial pressure to normal physiologic levels, although this diagnosis must be addressed shortly after surgical repair as IIH treatment is paramount to preserving surgical closure of the associated CSF fistula.

Clinical Manifestation

Clinical Presentation

Patients with intracranial hypotension typically present with a classic orthostatic headache, although numerous variants have been described. Alternatively, patients may describe chronic lingering nonorthostatic headaches, neck pain, exertional headaches, acute thunderclap onset of orthostatic headaches, or even paradoxical headaches, in which severity is greater when in a recumbent position [35]. Numerous nonheadache symptoms have also been described, most commonly including nausea, visual complaints, radicular upper extremity pain, or cognitive difficulties [36]. With worsened CSF hypovolemia, cranial nerve deficits, such as cochleovestibular symptoms, diplopia secondary to sixth nerve palsies, or facial numbness, may arise [25]. Severe cases may even manifest with encephalopathy, stupor, and coma [37, 38].

Complications of Intracranial Hypotension

Severe or prolonged intracranial hypotension may manifest with a number of secondary complications. Meningitis is the most frequent complication arising from a persistent CSF leak, typically occurring with a persistent cutaneous CSF fistula. This is most often observed in the setting of CSF rhinorrhea, whether spontaneous, traumatic, or iatrogenic in nature. Spontaneous subdural hematomas may also arise, often following the development of subdural hygromas. While subdural hematomas are often small and asymptomatic, continued progression to the point that they become symptomatic or display increasing compression may require surgical intervention [39, 40].

Less commonly, cerebral venous sinus thrombosis may occur in the setting of intracranial hypotension, usually manifesting as a sudden worsening in the severity of headache [41], requiring subsequent treatment with anticoagulation. While exceedingly rare, bibrachial amyotrophy has been described as another sequelae to intracranial hypotension, manifesting as painless asymmetric bilateral weakness of the upper extremities [42]. Finally, rebound intracranial hypertension may follow successful CSF leak repair, presenting with severe headache and even papilledema [43]. While this is self-limiting, acetazolamide can be used for symptomatic relief.

Diagnosis

Evaluation of patients with symptoms suggestive of intracranial hypotension should largely be guided by history and physical examination. Following likely iatrogenic injury, such as a recent lumbar puncture, spinal surgery, or shunt placement, patients require minimal diagnostic workup and one can skip directly to treatment of the presumed source of the problem. Similarly, patients presenting with rhinorrhea or otorrhea following head trauma or skull base surgery should undergo targeted imaging of the skull base to localize the site of the potential CSF leak as outlined below. On the other hand, the diagnostic evaluation of patients presenting with classic symptoms of intracranial hypotension without a history of head trauma or surgery is substantially more challenging and may require the use of multiple imaging modalities to establish an etiology.

Diagnostic Criteria

The International Classification of Headache Disorders (ICHD-3) [44] defines headaches as being attributable to spontaneous intracranial hypotension if all the following diagnostic criteria are met:

1. Low CSF pressure (<60 mm CSF) and/or evidence of CSF leakage on imaging
2. Headache has developed in temporal relation to low CSF pressure or CSF leakage, or has led to its discovery
3. Headaches are not better accounted by another ICHD-3 diagnosis.

Lumbar Puncture

The use of lumbar puncture is seldom necessary to diagnose spontaneous intracranial hypotension, especially with MRI being widely available and with adequate sensitivity to establish the diagnosis. Nevertheless, in situations where MRI results are equivocal or when MRI is not feasible or available, then the use of lumbar puncture can help establish the diagnosis. An opening pressure of <6 cm of H_2O, measured in the lateral position, is diagnostic of spontaneous intracranial hypotension.

Up to 60% of patients, however, will be found to have an opening pressure in the normal range (between 6 and 20 cm of H_2O) [45, 46]. This phenomenon occurs secondary to the fact that intracranial hypotension is a condition of low CSF volume rather than one of low CSF pressure [47]. In certain patients, brain and spine compliance may be altered by body habitus or the disease course, allowing for CSF hypovolemia to coexist with normal CSF pressure. Normal opening pressure in spontaneous intracranial hypotension is more commonly encountered in patients with larger abdominal circumference and longer duration of symptoms [45]. The most common CSF profile in this patient population includes an increase in CSF protein and a mild lymphocytic pleocytosis, presumably due to an inflammatory reaction to the chronic CSF leak [25].

Imaging Modalities

Cranial Computed Tomography

There is limited use for CT in the diagnosis of spontaneous intracranial hypotension, although it can provide important clues as to potential etiologies, including areas of bony dehiscence or postoperative defects. Upon initial presentation when the diagnosis is unclear, it is often the first test ordered, typically to rule out more sinister diagnoses such as subarachnoid hemorrhage that can have a similar clinical presentation. When MRI is less available, a CT scan can prove to be useful [48]. The most commonly reported radiographic findings on CT in cases of intracranial hypotension include subdural hygromas, dural venous sinus distension, cerebellar ectopia, and pneumocephalus. While patients presenting with cranial CSF leaks rarely present with signs of intracranial hypotension, CT remains a useful tool to investigate the potential location of CSF leaks in cases of rhinorrhea or otorrhea [26] (Fig. 15.1). High-resolution CT of the skull base can show an area of dehiscence or bone defect and should be part of the investigation of cranial CSF leaks. In the setting of IIH, evidence of elevated intracranial pressure is often present, including thinning of the skull base, the presence of arachnoid pits, and multiple skull base defects, also providing clues for potential surgical repair of the underlying defect [49, 50] (Fig. 15.2).

Brain MRI

A brain MRI is the best initial diagnostic test in the evaluation of a patient with suspected intracranial hypotension. This should be done with and without contrast and can potentially confirm the diagnosis and rule out other etiologies. The most common diagnostic qualitative sign is pachymeningeal enhancement [25]. This can be differentiated from leptomeningeal enhancement in that pachymeningeal enhancement is constrained to the dural surfaces and spares the deep cortical sulci and brainstem arachnoid [51]. This pathophysiology is postulated to occur secondary to enlargement of the vascular compartment due to the shrinking CSF volume, resulting in meningeal enhancement when contrast is administered. This is more commonly seen in the acute phase of the disease, rather than in the chronic state [45].

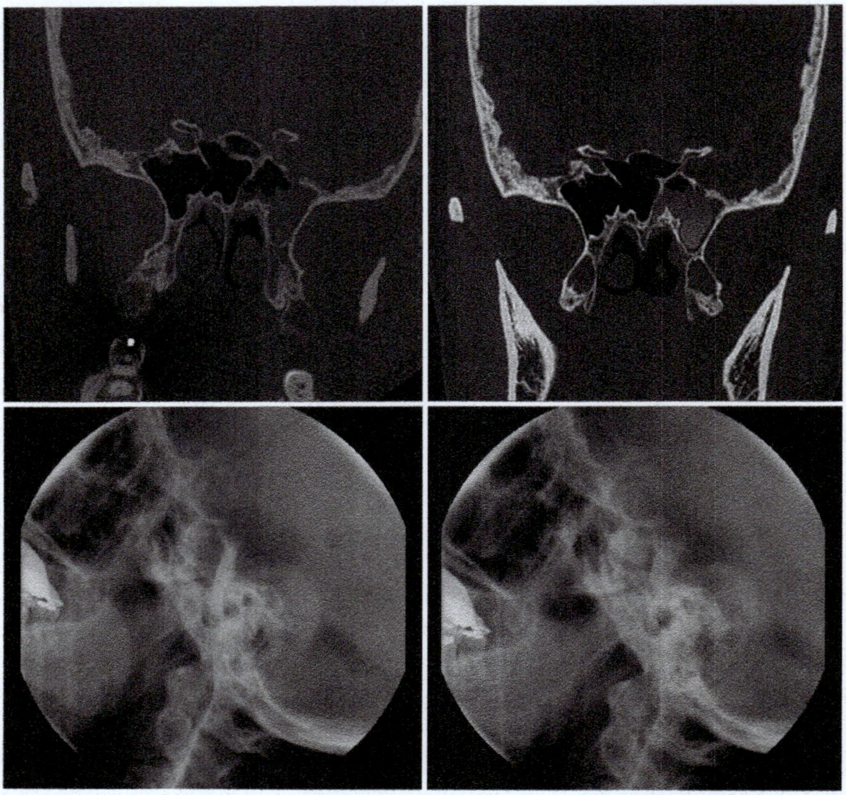

Fig. 15.1 High-resolution computed tomography (CT) of the skull base shows dehiscence at the foramen rotundum and fluid in the involved sphenoid sinus. The addition of intrathecal contrast shows contrast entering the sphenoid sinus on CT and plain films, confirming the communication with the subarachnoid space

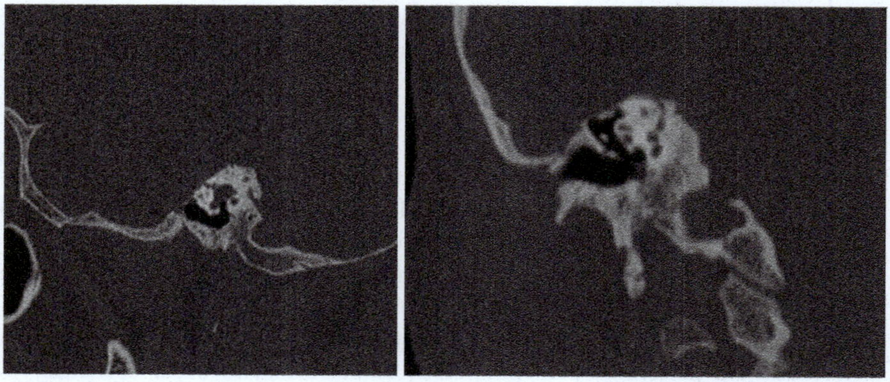

Fig. 15.2 High-resolution computed tomography scans in coronal and sagittal views show superior semicircular canal dehiscence in a 45-year-old patient with tinnitus and vertigo who developed cerebrospinal fluid leak following repair. The patient also had an elevated intracranial pressure of 35 cm H_2O consistent with idiopathic intracranial hypertension

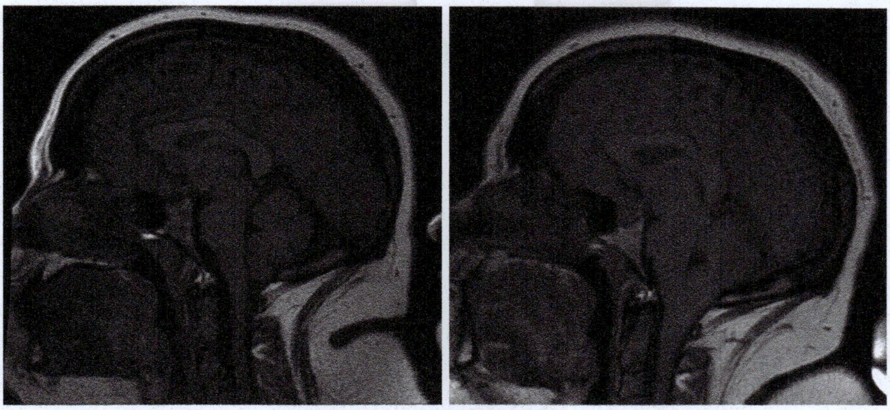

Fig. 15.3 Patient developed low cerebrospinal fluid (CSF) tension symptoms 9 years after placement of a lumboperitoneal shunt for treatment of idiopathic intracranial hypertension. Comparison of magnetic resonance imaging scans from prior to shunt placement to onset of positional headache symptoms identifies changes of CSF hypotension including pituitary enlargement, optic chiasm flattening, tonsillar herniation, decreased mamillopontine distance, and a decreased pontomesencephalic angle

Other common qualitative signs that have been described include subdural fluid collections (hygromas in the acute phase and hematomas in chronic situations), engorgement of the venous sinuses [52], pituitary enlargement and hyperemia [53], optic chiasm flattening [35], decreased ventricular size, and tonsillar herniation [54]. Infrequently, deep brain swelling may be observed due to venous engorgement, as severe brain sagging obstructs flow through the deep venous system [55]. A few quantitative signs of CSF hypotension have been described as well, including a decreased mamillopontine distance (shortest distance between the center of the mammillary bodies and top of the pons) below 5.5 mm and a decreased pontomesencephalic angle (the angle between a line drawn along the anterior margin of midbrain and another along the anterior superior margin of the pons) below 50° [56] (Fig. 15.3).

The presence of an encephalocele during MRI evaluation of a spontaneous CSF leak is often associated with an underlying diagnosis of IIH. Signs of long-standing elevated intracranial pressure, such as an encephalocele or an empty sella, can be seen in up to 50–90% of spontaneous CSF leaks [57–59]. Furthermore, past studies have shown reversal of an empty sella following improved control of elevated pressure whether through medical or surgical means [60]. While less common, dilated tortuous optic nerves and dilation of Meckel's cave have also been observed on MRI in patients with spontaneous CSF leaks, also indicative of underlying IIH [57, 61].

Spine MRI

In cases where a brain MRI reveals signs of intracranial hypotension, a spine MRI can localize the location of a potential CSF leak and help to confirm the diagnosis. Even in situations when the brain MRI is equivocal and there is a high suspicion for a spinal CSF leak, spinal MRI can be useful. To increase sensitivity, the MRI should include a T2 fat-suppression sequence and a T1 contrast-enhanced sequence [62].

The most common finding on spinal MRI is an epidural fluid collection with intensity similar to CSF, seen in 65–100% of patients [62]. These collections can be focal or can extend across multiple levels, forming due to an accumulation of CSF from a dural defect. Alternatively, they may form by transduction through an engorged epidural venous plexus. These epidural fluid collections are best visualized on T2 fat-suppressed sequences, allowing differentiation from epidural fat, which will also appear bright on T2 imaging. The location of the epidural collection identified on MRI does not always localize the leak. In particular, CSF pooling behind the dura between the C1-2 spinous processes can be seen in cases of spontaneous intracranial hypotension but does not necessarily indicate CSF leak location [62–65]. The sensitivity of MRI in identifying spinal CSF leaks is higher in cases of high-flow leaks, although MRI can often reveal low-flow leaks, especially when the leak is near a bony spur where CSF can pool locally [66].

In cases of spontaneous intracranial hypotension, spine MRI may reveal enlargement of epidural veins or the epidural venous plexus. This can also lead to dural enhancement with contrast administration via a similar mechanism as seen with brain MRI. Less commonly, MRI can reveal structural abnormalities such as meningeal diverticula, neural cysts, intradural disc herniations, or a pseudomeningocele that can shed light on the underlying cause of the CSF leak [62].

Conventional spine MRI with and without contrast with fat suppression sequences has a sensitivity above 90% in detecting CSF leaks when compared to CT myelography (CTM) [67]. Newer techniques can increase the achievable contrast by using heavy T2-weighted sequences coupled with three-dimensional image processing, a technique known as MR myelography, with a resultant improvement in sensitivity to diagnose and localize CSF leaks [68, 69]. These technological improvements have made conventional MRI of the spine a viable noninvasive method to diagnose and localize CSF leaks when compared to CTM.

Myelography Techniques

Myelography techniques are helpful in situations where MRI fails to detect the presence or location of a CSF leak. While conventional MRI can detect the presence of CSF leaks with high sensitivity, the localization accuracy is significantly lower. In low-flow leaks, conventional MRI can often localize the leak because the CSF spread is usually spatially confined. In high-flow leaks, CSF can spread for long distances along the spine, compromising the spatial accuracy. As a dynamic imaging technique, myelography can overcome the static nature of conventional MRI, and image acquisition can be tailored based on the type of leak [66] (Fig. 15.4).

CT Myelogram

In CTM, an iodinated contrast agent is injected intrathecally and followed by a spinal CT scan. This is the most widely used and recommended technique to diagnose and localize spinal CSF leaks [70]. CTM has a number of advantages compared to MRI, including better contrast between CSF and local tissue, allows the measurement of an opening pressure, and provides an opportunity to immediately target the

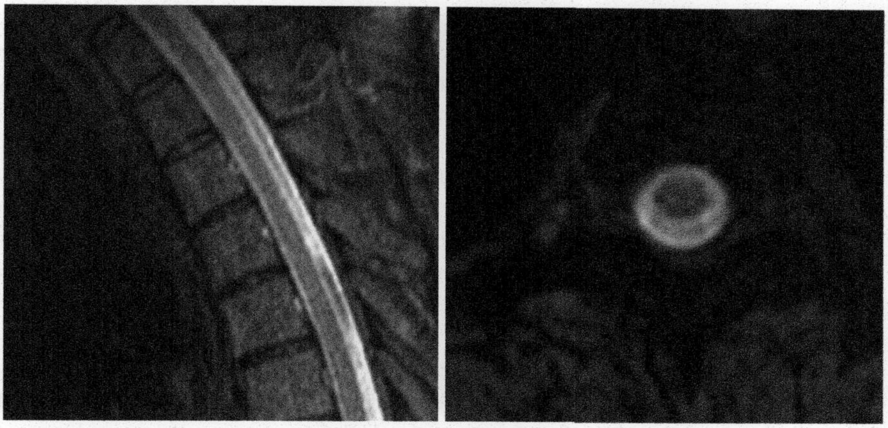

Fig. 15.4 Patient developed acute back pain after a lifting episode followed by a positional headache consistent with low cerebrospinal fluid (CSF) tension. Magnetic resonance imaging findings demonstrate longitudinal CSF collection in subdural space of the thoracic spine

leak with an epidural blood patch [71]. Furthermore, CTM has better temporal resolution as the study can be performed multiple times over a short time period, making it uniquely suitable for investigation of a high-flow leak that can be hard to localize with conventional spinal MRI [66]. The development of dynamic and ultrafast-dynamic CTM techniques allows the CT scan to be obtained at the same time as the intrathecal contrast injection. This provides extremely high spatial and temporal resolution and has been successfully used to detect high-flow CSF leaks in situations where other techniques have failed [72, 73]. Despite these advantages, the increased radiation exposure and invasive nature of the study are significant drawbacks that must be considered.

Digital Subtraction Myelography

For cases of very high-flow CSF leak that cannot be localized on CTM, digital subtraction myelography (DSM) is a newer technique that appears promising. In DSM, the patient is placed on a tilting fluoroscopy table and intrathecal contrast is injected while the patient is tilted so contrast remains in the dependent portion of the thecal sac. The patient is then tilted to allow contrast to flow cranially while fluoroscopic images are obtained in the region of interest, which can be repeated in a serial fashion. Subtraction of normal static tissue anatomy enhances the spatial resolution. This technique has been shown to detect high-flow leaks that were not detected using CTM [74, 75]. The high temporal resolution of this technique has also allowed the diagnosis of CSF-venous fistulas that were not identified with other modalities [76]. DSM is most useful in select cases of highly suspicious CSF leaks that cannot be detected or localized using other methods. Disadvantages of this technique include radiation exposure and either a very cooperative or anesthetized patient [66].

Nuclear Cisternography

Nuclear cisternography is a myelographic technique involving the intrathecal injection of the radioisotope in diethylene triamine pentaacetic acid (Indium-111 DTPA), followed by imaging at multiple time points, up to 48 h after injection. The radioisotope is injected in the lumbar cistern and ascends cephalad, reaching the basilar cisterns in 1–2 h, the sylvian and interhemispheric fissures by 3–4 h, and the cerebral convexity by 24 h. This method provides both direct and indirect evidence of a CSF leak [77]. A CSF leak can be directly observed as paradural extravasation of the isotope, although this is seen in a minority of cases [77]. Indirect evidence of a leak is more commonly observed and includes early detection of tracer in the bladder, delayed or incomplete appearance of the radioisotope over the cerebral convexity, and rapid washout of activity in the lumbar cisterns [77, 78]. Potential pitfalls with nuclear cisternography include leakage of the radioisotope into the epidural space during injection. This is often mistakenly interpreted as direct evidence of CSF leakage [77]. Similarly, leakage into the epidural space during injection can lead to early activity in the bladder, which may be misinterpreted as an indirect evidence of CSF leak [66]. While this technique has such disadvantages as low spatial resolution, need for intrathecal injections, and the use of specialized equipment [66, 77, 79], nuclear cisternography is uniquely able to detect intermittent and slow leaks as imaging takes place over a prolonged period of time.

MR Myelography

MR myelography with intrathecal gadolinium injection is a newer technique that is becoming more widely used. Studies have shown that this technique can detect CSF leaks not detected with CTM or standard spine MRI [80, 81]. This technique is especially useful in situations where other methods have failed in revealing the presence or location of the leak [66]. While the above studies demonstrate the safety of intrathecal gadolinium, it is still not FDA approved, and there have been multiple reports of encephalopathy and neurotoxicity due to overdosage of intrathecal gadolinium [82, 83]. Due to these reports, this technique is only currently recommended in rare situations where other methods do not yield significant results [66].

Management

Medical Management

Numerous conservative measures can often be employed prior to or in conjunction with potential surgical repair. Patients will often obtain significant symptomatic relief from bed rest and naturally tend to remain in a recumbent position given the severe orthostatic nature of the headache. Caffeine and theophylline may provide substantial relief [35], whereas classic analgesics have limited efficacy, and significant hydration can provide relief as well. While these maneuvers have been well demonstrated to provide symptomatic relief, their efficacy is limited in durability without obliteration of the CSF fistula, as they do not address the underlying pathology.

Traumatic CSF Leak

Management strategies of intracranial hypotension can vary significantly depending on the underlying etiology. In the setting of a traumatic CSF leak, a trial of conservative management is often initiated, resulting in resolution within 7–10 days in most cases [84–86]. Purely conservative measures include intracranial pressure mitigating maneuvers, such as strict bed rest, head of bed elevation, sneeze precautions, and stool softeners. These methods have been shown to be successful in up to 85% of patients, with higher success rates experienced with longer trials of conservative management [87–89]. The use of prophylactic antibiotics in the setting of traumatic CSF leak has been previously assessed, although current guidelines and recent randomized controlled trials do not support their use in this context [90]. Following failure of noninvasive conservative treatment, CSF diversion with a lumbar drain is often pursued, allowing time for the traumatic defect to heal. Lumbar drainage for 5–10 days successfully resolves persistent CSF leaks in those patients who fail initial conservative measures in 40–90% of patients [87–89]. Lumbar drain success rates are higher in cases in which they are placed earlier following the initial trauma [88, 89]. Nonetheless, randomized clinical studies have demonstrated that early lumbar drain placement and prolonged bed rest have similar rates of CSF leak resolution following traumatic injury; however, patients treated early with a lumbar drain had a significantly shorter duration of CSF leak [91]. Patients need to be closely monitored throughout a trial of conservative treatment as persistent CSF leaks carry a higher risk of meningitis [92, 93], and surgical correction should be considered in cases with persistent leaks. Surgical interventions for traumatic skull base CSF leaks are largely endoscopic in approach and have good outcomes, with efficacy nearing 100% [94]. Ultimately, surgical approach, when necessary, is dictated by the location of the skull base fracture.

Iatrogenic CSF Leak

Intracranial hypotension following endoscopic endonasal surgery is most commonly treated with revision surgery [86, 95]. Recent surgical advances have revolutionized reconstruction of skull base defects with a positive influence on the rate of CSF leaks. Historically, endoscopic closures were reinforced with synthetic, vascularized, or free grafts borrowed from the abdomen or temporoparietal fascia, requiring an additional incision and potential morbidity [96]. More recent use of pedicled nasal septal flaps supplied by the nasoseptal artery has significantly decreased the rate of postoperative CSF leaks [96–99].

The vast majority of durotomies during spinal surgery are recognized intraoperatively and are predominately treated with primary dural closure of the defect. This closure may at times be augmented with fibrin glue, autologous grafts, and other reinforcements. Intraoperative repair is able to prevent the development of a postoperative CSF leak in the majority of cases [10, 11, 17, 18]. Among patients without an observed intraoperative durotomy with evidence of CSF leak or intracranial hypotension in the postoperative period, conservative treatment with bed rest, fluid resuscitation, caffeine, with or without CSF diversion is a reasonable initial option [11, 18, 100, 101]. While conservative management without a lumbar drain has been successfully described, the addition of CSF diversion is highly correlated with successful treatment [10, 12, 14, 17, 20, 100, 101]. With persistent CSF leak despite these initial maneuvers, patients must typically return for definitive operative closure [11, 18, 101, 102]. Only 0.83% of unidentified CSF leaks present in a delayed fashion [20]. While some authors have proposed bed rest and lumbar drainage in these patients, nearly all require definitive surgical repair [20].

Spontaneous CSF Leak

Evidence of spontaneous intracranial hypotension is most often secondary to underlying spine pathology. For patients failing conservative management, an epidural blood patch is the initial invasive treatment of choice with the success rate of each patch being approximately 30% [103]. Epidural blood patches provide relief through two mechanisms. First, volume replacement secondary to dural tamponade typically provides immediate symptomatic relief. After this has occurred, a secondary, delayed effect occurs as the patch scars and seals the CSF leak to prevent recurrence. While epidural blood patches are most efficacious for headaches following lumbar puncture or when an exact level of CSF leak is known, they may provide relief even in the setting of an occult leak with symptoms of intracranial hypotension (Fig. 15.5).

Spontaneous cranial CSF leaks associated with intracranial hypertension have a high rate of recurrence following surgical repair of the leak (25–87%) [59], thought to be partially due to poor postoperative control of underlying IIH. When a spontaneous CSF leak can be localized, direct endoscopic repair is typically undertaken to obliterate the fistulous connection. Intrathecal injection of contrast or radioactive tracers can be used to assist in identifying the exact location of the leak [2]. Otherwise, intrathecal fluorescein can be used in the operating room to assist in endoscopic visualization of the leak. With this test, 5 mL of fluorescein (<5% concentration) is diluted in 10 mL of CSF and intrathecally injected via lumbar puncture [2]. The exact leak can then be seen under endoscopic visualization with the use of a Wood lamp, if necessary [104–106]. Fluorescein is neurotoxic, so limiting the volume and concentration is imperative. For repair, the choice of a graft or nasoseptal flap can vary significantly and depends on the location, defect size, and the availability of blood supply for a nasoseptal flap [59].

When IIH is strongly suspected in the setting of a spontaneous CSF leak, CSF diversion is often employed following primary repair. Lumbar or external ventricular drains can be used to provide temporary CSF diversion, allowing the surgical repair to appropriately heal [59]. While this may be successful in the short term, temporary CSF diversion is associated with late repair failure as intracranial hypertension resumes following treatment cessation [61]. Furthermore, studies have shown little impact on recurrence rates, with significantly longer hospital stays in

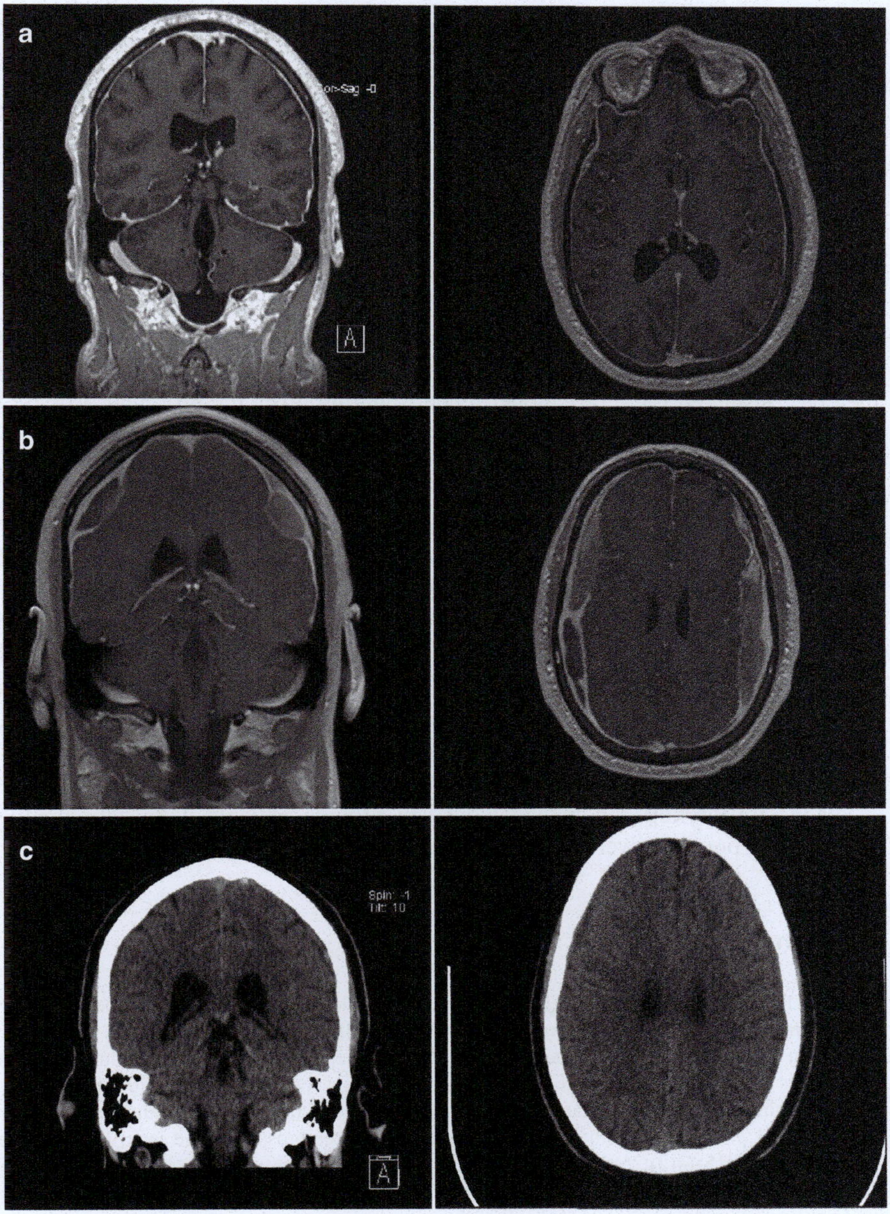

Fig. 15.5 Radiologic studies in a patient with spontaneous positional headache secondary to an occult cerebrospinal fluid leak. (**a**). Initial contrast enhanced magnetic resonance imaging (MRI) is consistent with intracranial hypotension with pachymeningeal enhancement constrained to the dural surfaces and sparing the deep cortical sulci. Symptoms were relieved following spinal epidural blood patch ×2. (**b**). Progressive intermittent headache and hemisensory symptoms developed at 12 weeks. MRI now shows bilateral mixed subdural hematomas treated successfully with burr hole evacuation (**c**)

patients treated with a lumbar drain [107]. Long term, approximately half of the patients treated for a spontaneous CSF leak require medical treatment with acetazolamide or surgical treatment with permanent CSF diversion via ventriculoperitoneal or lumboperitoneal shunting [59]. Active control of intracranial pressure following primary repair of spontaneous CSF rhinorrhea is associated with a significantly higher rate of successful repair. A recent study found that patients undergoing appropriate control of IIH following repair of spontaneous CSF rhinorrhea experienced a 93% success rate, whereas repair was only successful in 82% of patients without intracranial pressure management postoperatively [61]. In patients undergoing repair for a spontaneous CSF leak in the setting of suspected IIH, it is recommended that patients undergo a lumbar puncture to evaluate for an opening pressure 3–5 days following surgery [2]. Patients with elevated intracranial pressure should then be considered for ventriculoperitoneal shunting given the profound increased success in CSF leak repair with CSF diversion.

Conclusion

Arising from numerous etiologies, intracranial hypotension can range in severity from mild headaches to significant sequelae, including subdural hematomas and meningitis. Diagnostic workup can be challenging, but the advent of newer imaging techniques has improved accuracy and localization of potential CSF leaks. Aside from medical symptomatic management, treatment of intracranial hypotension largely depends on the underlying pathology. Traumatic CSF leaks can often be treated with conservative measures or temporary CSF diversion, iatrogenic causes typically require surgical repair, and the treatment of spontaneous CSF leaks depends on whether the leak is spinal or cranial in origin. Proper diagnostic workup and management can provide patients with symptomatic relief and prevent adverse sequelae.

References

1. Loew F, Pertuiset B, Chaumier EE, Jaksche H. Traumatic, spontaneous and postoperative CSF rhinorrhea. Adv Tech Stand Neurosurg. 1984;11:169–207.
2. Carrau RL, Snyderman CH, Kassam AB. The management of cerebrospinal fluid leaks in patients at risk for high-pressure hydrocephalus. Laryngoscope. 2005;115(2):205–12.
3. Hasheminia D, Kalantar Motamedi MR, Hashemzehi H, Nazeri R, Movahedian B. A 7-year study of 1,278 patients with maxillofacial trauma and cerebrospinal fluid leak. J Maxillofac Oral Surg. 2015;14(2):258–62.
4. Daudia A, Biswas D, Jones NS. Risk of meningitis with cerebrospinal fluid rhinorrhea. Ann Otol Rhinol Laryngol. 2007;116(12):902–5.
5. Hebert-Blouin MN, Mokri B, Shin AY, Bishop AT, Spinner RJ. Cerebrospinal fluid volume-depletion headaches in patients with traumatic brachial plexus injury. J Neurosurg. 2013;118(1):149–54.
6. Hegazy HM, Carrau RL, Snyderman CH, Kassam A, Zweig J. Transnasal endoscopic repair of cerebrospinal fluid rhinorrhea: a meta-analysis. Laryngoscope. 2000;110(7):1166–72.
7. Martin-Martin C, Martinez-Capoccioni G, Serramito-Garcia R, Espinosa-Restrepo F. Surgical challenge: endoscopic repair of cerebrospinal fluid leak. BMC Res Notes. 2012;5:459.

8. Janecka IP, Sen C, Sekhar LN, et al. Cranial base surgery: results in 183 patients. Otolaryngol Head Neck Surg. 1994;110(6):539–46.
9. Cammisa FP Jr, Girardi FP, Sangani PK, Parvataneni HK, Cadag S, Sandhu HS. Incidental durotomy in spine surgery. Spine (Phila Pa 1976). 2000;25(20):2663–7.
10. Enders F, Ackemann A, Muller S, Kiening K, Orakcioglu B. Risk factors and management of incidental durotomy in lumbar interbody fusion surgery. Clin Spine Surg. 2018;31(3):127–31.
11. Guerin P, El Fegoun AB, Obeid I, et al. Incidental durotomy during spine surgery: incidence, management and complications. A retrospective review. Injury. 2012;43(4):397–401.
12. Hannallah D, Lee J, Khan M, Donaldson WF, Kang JD. Cerebrospinal fluid leaks following cervical spine surgery. J Bone Joint Surg Am. 2008;90(5):1101–5.
13. Kotilainen E, Valtonen S, Carlson CA. Microsurgical treatment of lumbar disc herniation: follow-up of 237 patients. Acta Neurochir. 1993;120(3–4):143–9.
14. Rampersaud YR, Moro ER, Neary MA, et al. Intraoperative adverse events and related postoperative complications in spine surgery: implications for enhancing patient safety founded on evidence-based protocols. Spine (Phila Pa 1976). 2006;31(13):1503–10.
15. Saxler G, Kramer J, Barden B, Kurt A, Pfortner J, Bernsmann K. The long-term clinical sequelae of incidental durotomy in lumbar disc surgery. Spine (Phila Pa 1976). 2005;30(20):2298–302.
16. Stolke D, Sollmann WP, Seifert V. Intra- and postoperative complications in lumbar disc surgery. Spine (Phila Pa 1976). 1989;14(1):56–9.
17. Syre P, Bohman LE, Baltuch G, Le Roux P, Welch WC. Cerebrospinal fluid leaks and their management after anterior cervical discectomy and fusion: a report of 13 cases and a review of the literature. Spine (Phila Pa 1976). 2014;39(16):E936–43.
18. Wang JC, Bohlman HH, Riew KD. Dural tears secondary to operations on the lumbar spine. Management and results after a two-year-minimum follow-up of eighty-eight patients. J Bone Joint Surg Am. 1998;80(12):1728–32.
19. Gaucher DJ Jr, Perez JA Jr. Subdural hematoma following lumbar puncture. Arch Intern Med. 2002;162(16):1904–5.
20. Khazim R, Dannawi Z, Spacey K, et al. Incidence and treatment of delayed symptoms of CSF leak following lumbar spinal surgery. Eur Spine J. 2015;24(9):2069–76.
21. Lu CH, Ho ST, Kong SS, Cherng CH, Wong CS. Intracranial subdural hematoma after unintended durotomy during spine surgery. Can J Anaesth. 2002;49(1):100–2.
22. Pham MH, Tuchman A, Platt A, Hsieh PC. Intracranial complications associated with spinal surgery. Eur Spine J. 2016;25(3):888–94.
23. Sciubba DM, Kretzer RM, Wang PP. Acute intracranial subdural hematoma following a lumbar CSF leak caused by spine surgery. Spine (Phila Pa 1976). 2005;30(24):E730–2.
24. Deseyne S, Vanhouteghem K, Hallaert G, Delanghe J, Malfait T. Subarachnoidal-pleural fistula (SAPF) as an unusual cause of persistent pleural effusion. Beta-trace protein as a marker for SAPF. Case report and review of the literature. Acta Clin Belg. 2015;70(1):53–7.
25. Mokri B, Piepgras DG, Miller GM. Syndrome of orthostatic headaches and diffuse pachymeningeal gadolinium enhancement. Mayo Clin Proc. 1997;72(5):400–13.
26. Schievink WI, Schwartz MS, Maya MM, Moser FG, Rozen TD. Lack of causal association between spontaneous intracranial hypotension and cranial cerebrospinal fluid leaks. J Neurosurg. 2012;116(4):749–54.
27. Cilluffo JM, Gomez MR, Reese DF, Onofrio BM, Miller RH. Idiopathic ("ongenital") spinal arachnoid diverticula. Clinical diagnosis and surgical results. Mayo Clin Proc. 1981;56(2):93–101.
28. Schievink WI, Torres VE. Spinal meningeal diverticula in autosomal dominant polycystic kidney disease. Lancet. 1997;349(9060):1223–4.
29. Davenport RJ, Chataway SJ, Warlow CP. Spontaneous intracranial hypotension from a CSF leak in a patient with Marfan's syndrome. J Neurol Neurosurg Psychiatry. 1995;59(5):516–9.
30. Fukutake T, Sakakibara R, Mori M, Araki M, Hattori T. Chronic intractable headache in a patient with Marfan's syndrome. Headache. 1997;37(5):291–5.

31. Schrijver I, Schievink WI, Godfrey M, Meyer FB, Francke U. Spontaneous spinal cerebrospinal fluid leaks and minor skeletal features of Marfan syndrome: a microfibrillopathy. J Neurosurg. 2002;96(3):483–9.
32. Fattori R, Nienaber CA, Descovich B, et al. Importance of dural ectasia in phenotypic assessment of Marfan's syndrome. Lancet. 1999;354(9182):910–3.
33. Vishteh AG, Schievink WI, Baskin JJ, Sonntag VK. Cervical bone spur presenting with spontaneous intracranial hypotension. Case report. *J Neurosurg*. 1998;89(3):483–4.
34. Winter SC, Maartens NF, Anslow P, Teddy PJ. Spontaneous intracranial hypotension due to thoracic disc herniation. Case report. *J Neurosurg*. 2002;96(3 Suppl):343–5.
35. Mokri B. Spontaneous CSF leaks: low CSF volume syndromes. Neurol Clin. 2014;32(2):397–422.
36. Horton JC, Fishman RA. Neurovisual findings in the syndrome of spontaneous intracranial hypotension from dural cerebrospinal fluid leak. Ophthalmology. 1994;101(2):244–51.
37. Evan RW, Mokri B. Spontaneous intracranial hypotension resulting in coma. Headache. 2002;42(2):159–60.
38. Beck CE, Rizk NW, Kiger LT, Spencer D, Hill L, Adler JR. Intracranial hypotension presenting with severe encephalopathy. Case report. *J Neurosurg*. 1998;89(3):470–3.
39. de Noronha RJ, Sharrack B, Hadjivassiliou M, Romanowski CA. Subdural haematoma: a potentially serious consequence of spontaneous intracranial hypotension. J Neurol Neurosurg Psychiatry. 2003;74(6):752–5.
40. Mizuno J, Mummaneni PV, Rodts GE, Barrow DL. Recurrent subdural hematoma caused by cerebrospinal fluid leakage. Case report. *J Neurosurg Spine*. 2006;4(2):183–5.
41. Berroir S, Grabli D, Heran F, Bakouche P, Bousser MG. Cerebral sinus venous thrombosis in two patients with spontaneous intracranial hypotension. Cerebrovasc Dis. 2004;17(1):9–12.
42. Deluca GC, Boes CJ, Krueger BR, Mokri B, Kumar N. Ventral intraspinal fluid-filled collection secondary to CSF leak presenting as bibrachial amyotrophy. Neurology. 2011;76(16):1439–40.
43. Mokri B. Intracranial hypertension after treatment of spontaneous cerebrospinal fluid leaks. Mayo Clin Proc. 2002;77(11):1241–6.
44. Headache Classification Committee of the International Headache Society. The international classification of headache disorders, 3rd edition (beta version). Cephalalgia. 2013;33(9):629–808.
45. Kranz PG, Tanpitukpongse TP, Choudhury KR, Amrhein TJ, Gray L. How common is normal cerebrospinal fluid pressure in spontaneous intracranial hypotension? Cephalalgia. 2016;36(13):1209–17.
46. Mokri B, Hunter SF, Atkinson JL, Piepgras DG. Orthostatic headaches caused by CSF leak but with normal CSF pressures. Neurology. 1998;51(3):786–90.
47. Miyazawa K, Shiga Y, Hasegawa T, et al. CSF hypovolemia vs intracranial hypotension in "spontaneous intracranial hypotension syndrome". Neurology. 2003;60(6):941–7.
48. Yaffe D, Gordon CR. Noncontrast brain computed tomography findings of spontaneous intracranial hypotension in the emergency department setting. J Emerg Med. 2016;50(4):588–93.
49. Shetty PG, Shroff MM, Fatterpekar GM, Sahani DV, Kirtane MV. A retrospective analysis of spontaneous sphenoid sinus fistula: MR and CT findings. AJNR Am J Neuroradiol. 2000;21(2):337–42.
50. Schlosser RJ, Bolger WE. Nasal cerebrospinal fluid leaks: critical review and surgical considerations. Laryngoscope. 2004;114(2):255–65.
51. Smirniotopoulos JG, Murphy FM, Rushing EJ, Rees JH, Schroeder JW. Patterns of contrast enhancement in the brain and meninges. Radiographics. 2007;27(2):525–51.
52. Farb RI, Forghani R, Lee SK, Mikulis DJ, Agid R. The venous distension sign: a diagnostic sign of intracranial hypotension at MR imaging of the brain. AJNR Am J Neuroradiol. 2007;28(8):1489–93.
53. Alvarez-Linera J, Escribano J, Benito-Leon J, Porta-Etessam J, Rovira A. Pituitary enlargement in patients with intracranial hypotension syndrome. Neurology. 2000;55(12):1895–7.

54. Atkinson JL, Weinshenker BG, Miller GM, Piepgras DG, Mokri B. Acquired Chiari I malformation secondary to spontaneous spinal cerebrospinal fluid leakage and chronic intracranial hypotension syndrome in seven cases. J Neurosurg. 1998;88(2):237–42.
55. Savoiardo M, Minati L, Farina L, et al. Spontaneous intracranial hypotension with deep brain swelling. Brain. 2007;130(Pt 7):1884–93.
56. Shah LM, McLean LA, Heilbrun ME, Salzman KL. Intracranial hypotension: improved MRI detection with diagnostic intracranial angles. AJR Am J Roentgenol. 2013;200(2):400–7.
57. Silver RI, Moonis G, Schlosser RJ, Bolger WE, Loevner LA. Radiographic signs of elevated intracranial pressure in idiopathic cerebrospinal fluid leaks: a possible presentation of idiopathic intracranial hypertension. Am J Rhinol. 2007;21(3):257–61.
58. Schlosser RJ, Bolger WE. Spontaneous nasal cerebrospinal fluid leaks and empty sella syndrome: a clinical association. Am J Rhinol. 2003;17(2):91–6.
59. Chaaban MR, Illing E, Riley KO, Woodworth BA. Spontaneous cerebrospinal fluid leak repair: a five-year prospective evaluation. Laryngoscope. 2014;124(1):70–5.
60. Zagardo MT, Cail WS, Kelman SE, Rothman MI. Reversible empty sella in idiopathic intracranial hypertension: an indicator of successful therapy? AJNR Am J Neuroradiol. 1996;17(10):1953–6.
61. Teachey W, Grayson J, Cho DY, Riley KO, Woodworth BA. Intervention for elevated intracranial pressure improves success rate after repair of spontaneous cerebrospinal fluid leaks. Laryngoscope. 2017;127(9):2011–6.
62. Medina JH, Abrams K, Falcone S, Bhatia RG. Spinal imaging findings in spontaneous intracranial hypotension. AJR Am J Roentgenol. 2010;195(2):459–64.
63. Morgan JT, Scumpia AJ, Johnson AA, Schneider SJ. Case report: spontaneous intracranial hypotension in association with the presence of a false localizing C1-C2 cerebrospinal fluid leak. Surg Neurol. 2008;70(5):539–43; discussion 543–4
64. Schievink WI, Maya MM, Tourje J. False localizing sign of C1-2 cerebrospinal fluid leak in spontaneous intracranial hypotension. J Neurosurg. 2004;100(4):639–44.
65. Yousry I, Forderreuther S, Moriggl B, et al. Cervical MR imaging in postural headache: MR signs and pathophysiological implications. AJNR Am J Neuroradiol. 2001;22(7):1239–50.
66. Kranz PG, Luetmer PH, Diehn FE, Amrhein TJ, Tanpitukpongse TP, Gray L. Myelographic techniques for the detection of spinal CSF leaks in spontaneous intracranial hypotension. AJR Am J Roentgenol. 2016;206(1):8–19.
67. Starling A, Hernandez F, Hoxworth JM, et al. Sensitivity of MRI of the spine compared with CT myelography in orthostatic headache with CSF leak. Neurology. 2013;81(20):1789–92.
68. Tsai PH, Fuh JL, Lirng JF, Wang SJ. Heavily T2-weighted MR myelography in patients with spontaneous intracranial hypotension: a case-control study. Cephalalgia. 2007;27(8):929–34.
69. Wang YF, Lirng JF, Fuh JL, Hseu SS, Wang SJ. Heavily T2-weighted MR myelography vs CT myelography in spontaneous intracranial hypotension. Neurology. 2009;73(22):1892–8.
70. Mokri B. Spontaneous intracranial hypotension. *Continuum (Minneap Minn)*. 2015;21(4 Headache):1086–108.
71. Wendl CM, Schambach F, Zimmer C, Forschler A. CT myelography for the planning and guidance of targeted epidural blood patches in patients with persistent spinal CSF leakage. AJNR Am J Neuroradiol. 2012;33(3):541–4.
72. Luetmer PH, Mokri B. Dynamic CT myelography: a technique for localizing high-flow spinal cerebrospinal fluid leaks. AJNR Am J Neuroradiol. 2003;24(8):1711–4.
73. Thielen KR, Sillery JC, Morris JM, et al. Ultrafast dynamic computed tomography myelography for the precise identification of high-flow cerebrospinal fluid leaks caused by spiculated spinal osteophytes. J Neurosurg Spine. 2015;22(3):324–31.
74. Hoxworth JM, Patel AC, Bosch EP, Nelson KD. Localization of a rapid CSF leak with digital subtraction myelography. AJNR Am J Neuroradiol. 2009;30(3):516–9.
75. Hoxworth JM, Trentman TL, Kotsenas AL, Thielen KR, Nelson KD, Dodick DW. The role of digital subtraction myelography in the diagnosis and localization of spontaneous spinal CSF leaks. AJR Am J Roentgenol. 2012;199(3):649–53.

76. Schievink WI, Moser FG, Maya MM, Prasad RS. Digital subtraction myelography for the identification of spontaneous spinal CSF-venous fistulas. J Neurosurg Spine. 2016;24(6):960–4.
77. Mokri B. Radioisotope cisternography in spontaneous CSF leaks: interpretations and misinterpretations. Headache. 2014;54(8):1358–68.
78. Molins A, Alvarez J, Sumalla J, Titus F, Codina A. Cisternographic pattern of spontaneous liquoral hypotension. Cephalalgia. 1990;10(2):59–65.
79. Monteith TS, Kralik SF, Dillon WP, Hawkins RA, Goadsby PJ. The utility of radioisotope cisternography in low CSF/volume syndromes compared to myelography. Cephalalgia. 2016;36(13):1291–5.
80. Akbar JJ, Luetmer PH, Schwartz KM, Hunt CH, Diehn FE, Eckel LJ. The role of MR myelography with intrathecal gadolinium in localization of spinal CSF leaks in patients with spontaneous intracranial hypotension. AJNR Am J Neuroradiol. 2012;33(3):535–40.
81. Albayram S, Kilic F, Ozer H, Baghaki S, Kocer N, Islak C. Gadolinium-enhanced MR cisternography to evaluate dural leaks in intracranial hypotension syndrome. AJNR Am J Neuroradiol. 2008;29(1):116–21.
82. Arlt S, Cepek L, Rustenbeck HH, Prange H, Reimers CD. Gadolinium encephalopathy due to accidental intrathecal administration of gadopentetate dimeglumine. J Neurol. 2007;254(6):810–2.
83. Li L, Gao FQ, Zhang B, Luo BN, Yang ZY, Zhao J. Overdosage of intrathecal gadolinium and neurological response. Clin Radiol. 2008;63(9):1063–8.
84. Kerr JT, Chu FW, Bayles SW. Cerebrospinal fluid rhinorrhea: diagnosis and management. Otolaryngol Clin N Am. 2005;38(4):597–611.
85. Friedman JA, Ebersold MJ, Quast LM. Persistent posttraumatic cerebrospinal fluid leakage. Neurosurg Focus. 2000;9(1):e1.
86. Savva A, Taylor MJ, Beatty CW. Management of cerebrospinal fluid leaks involving the temporal bone: report on 92 patients. Laryngoscope. 2003;113(1):50–6.
87. Bell RB, Dierks EJ, Homer L, Potter BE. Management of cerebrospinal fluid leak associated with craniomaxillofacial trauma. J Oral Maxillofac Surg. 2004;62(6):676–84.
88. Yeo NK, Cho GS, Kim CJ, et al. The effectiveness of lumbar drainage in the conservative and surgical treatment of traumatic cerebrospinal fluid rhinorrhea. Acta Otolaryngol. 2013;133(1):82–90.
89. Yilmazlar S, Arslan E, Kocaeli H, et al. Cerebrospinal fluid leakage complicating skull base fractures: analysis of 81 cases. Neurosurg Rev. 2006;29(1):64–71.
90. Ratilal BO, Costa J, Pappamikail L, Sampaio C. Antibiotic prophylaxis for preventing meningitis in patients with basilar skull fractures. Cochrane Database Syst Rev. 2015;(4):CD004884.
91. Albu S, Emanuelli E, Trombitas V, Florian IS. Effectiveness of lumbar drains on recurrence rates in endoscopic surgery of cerebrospinal fluid leaks. Am J Rhinol Allergy. 2013;27(6):e190–4.
92. Brodie HA, Thompson TC. Management of complications from 820 temporal bone fractures. Am J Otol. 1997;18(2):188–97.
93. Schoentgen C, Henaux PL, Godey B, Jegoux F. Management of post-traumatic cerebrospinal fluid (CSF) leak of anterior skull base: 10 years experience. Acta Otolaryngol. 2013;133(9):944–50.
94. Virk JS, Elmiyeh B, Saleh HA. Endoscopic management of cerebrospinal fluid rhinorrhea: the charing cross experience. J Neurol Surg B Skull Base. 2013;74(2):61–7.
95. Stankiewicz JA. Complications of endoscopic intranasal ethmoidectomy. Laryngoscope. 1987;97(11):1270–3.
96. Kassam AB, Thomas A, Carrau RL, et al. Endoscopic reconstruction of the cranial base using a pedicled nasoseptal flap. *Neurosurgery*. 2008;63(1 Suppl 1):ONS44–52; discussion ONS52–43
97. Fraser S, Gardner PA, Koutourousiou M, et al. Risk factors associated with postoperative cerebrospinal fluid leak after endoscopic endonasal skull base surgery. J Neurosurg. 2018;128(4):1066–71.

98. Hadad G, Bassagasteguy L, Carrau RL, et al. A novel reconstructive technique after endoscopic expanded endonasal approaches: vascular pedicle nasoseptal flap. Laryngoscope. 2006;116(10):1882–6.
99. Paluzzi A, Fernandez-Miranda JC, Tonya Stefko S, Challinor S, Snyderman CH, Gardner PA. Endoscopic endonasal approach for pituitary adenomas: a series of 555 patients. Pituitary. 2014;17(4):307–19.
100. Tosun B, Ilbay K, Kim MS, Selek O. Management of persistent cerebrospinal fluid leakage following thoraco-lumbar surgery. Asian Spine J. 2012;6(3):157–62.
101. Kitchel SH, Eismont FJ, Green BA. Closed subarachnoid drainage for management of cerebrospinal fluid leakage after an operation on the spine. J Bone Joint Surg Am. 1989;71(7):984–7.
102. Eismont FJ, Wiesel SW, Rothman RH. Treatment of dural tears associated with spinal surgery. J Bone Joint Surg Am. 1981;63(7):1132–6.
103. Mokri B, Maher CO, Sencakova D. Spontaneous CSF leaks: underlying disorder of connective tissue. Neurology. 2002;58(5):814–6.
104. Oberascher G, Arrer E. Efficiency of various methods of identifying cerebrospinal fluid in oto- and rhinorrhea. ORL J Otorhinolaryngol Relat Spec. 1986;48(6):320–5.
105. Fransen P, Sindic CJ, Thauvoy C, Laterre C, Stroobandt G. Highly sensitive detection of beta-2 transferrin in rhinorrhea and otorrhea as a marker for cerebrospinal fluid (C.S.F.) leakage. *Acta Neurochir (Wien)*. 1991;109(3–4):98–101.
106. Skedros DG, Cass SP, Hirsch BE, Kelly RH. Sources of error in use of beta-2 transferrin analysis for diagnosing perilymphatic and cerebral spinal fluid leaks. Otolaryngol Head Neck Surg. 1993;109(5):861–4.
107. Adams AS, Russell PT, Duncavage JA, Chandra RK, Turner JH. Outcomes of endoscopic repair of cerebrospinal fluid rhinorrhea without lumbar drains. Am J Rhinol Allergy. 2016;30(6):424–9.

Part III

Treatment of CSF Disorders

Cerebrospinal Fluid Shunting

16

William E. Whitehead

History

Mainstream Treatments Prior to Shunting

In the first half of the twentieth century, the surgical treatment of hydrocephalus varied and the outcomes were dismal. Intermittent tapping of the lateral ventricles or the lumbar cistern was well described and a common practice [1–4]. This treatment strategy, performed under sterile conditions, provided temporary relief to patients but frequently led to death in time due to meningitis, bleeding, or herniation [5].

Another surgical treatment strategy was internalized drainage of cerebrospinal fluid (CSF) to lower pressure, body cavities with or without an implant. Most of these systems did not have a valve; however, if a valve was used, it was done by incorporating segments of autologous veins or bovine veins with intact venous flap valves. A variety of implant materials were tried to divert CSF including glass, metal, gold, silver, copper, and catgut [1, 6–8]. Passage ways for CSF flow into the dural sinuses, subarachnoid spaces, subdural space, subgaleal space, peritoneal cavity, bladder, and pleural cavity were all attempted with limited success [9–11]. Not surprising, most failures were due to infection, obstruction, or intraoperative death [12].

Third ventriculostomy was also introduced in the early twentieth century. In 1922, Dandy described a temporal craniotomy with sacrifice of the ipsilateral optic nerve to open the floor of the third ventricle into the subarachnoid space [13]. The first description of an endoscopic third ventriculostomy was by Mixter in 1923 [14]. A craniotomy for subfrontal approach to the lamina terminalis was described by

W. E. Whitehead
Texas Children's Hospital, Department of Neurosurgery, Houston, TX, USA
e-mail: wewhiteh@texaschildrens.org

D. D. Limbrick, J. R. Leonard (eds.), *Cerebrospinal Fluid Disorders*,
https://doi.org/10.1007/978-3-319-97928-1_16

Scarff and Stookey in 1936; the lamina terminalis was fenestrated and the floor of the third ventricle opened. Outcomes were poor even with endoscopy. Surgeons were limited by inadequate illumination, visualization, and instrumentation [15].

Controlling hydrocephalus by destruction of the choroid plexus either by removing it or cauterizing it was another treatment option. Both open and endoscopic techniques were described, but again success was limited and mortality rates were greater than 50% [16, 17].

The Early Implantable Valved Shunts and The Introduction of Silastic

The necessity of a valve to prevent backflow of CSF and the early obstruction of a shunt by blood clots, led to the manufacturing of one-way valves for CSF shunt systems. The earliest report of this treatment strategy was by Nulsen and Spitz [18]. Nulsen designed and created a one-way valve, which was implanted by Spitz in a patient with hydrocephalus in 1949 at the Children's Hospital of Philadelphia. This valve contained two ball valve units with platinum springs and an interposed pumping chamber. It was difficult to make, expensive, and was ultimately only used successfully in one patient [19, 20]. Improvements in valve design came over the next several years.

The second major breakthrough that led to the widespread use of CSF shunts in the treatment of hydrocephalus was the introduction of silastic tubing. Silastic was a byproduct of research being carried out during World War II to improve airplane construction. Silastic was found to be an outstanding biocompatible implant and very resistant to the mechanical stress of daily movement and the pulsations of the circulatory system [1]. This material was first used in a shunt in 1956 by Holter and Pudenz and thus began the current era of implantable valved shunts for the treatment of hydrocephalus [20, 21].

How Shunts Work

Mechanical Principles

CSF shunts are simple devices conceptually. Shunts carry fluid (CSF) from one container within the body (usually the ventricle) to another (usually the abdominal cavity) with a one-way valve to prevent backflow. Flow is driven by differences in pressure between the two compartments and is slowed by resistance across the valve or any other components spliced into the system.

Many factors can affect the pressure within the two cavities. Patients change positions. Changes in body position from flat to upright affect the differential pressure between the two body cavities and this will affect CSF flow. Other forces that intermittently affect pressure within the containers are pulse pressure, respirations, and brain compliance. Ultimately, flow through a CSF shunt is intermittent and subject to a variety of changing forces once implanted.

Shunts are also subject to the effects of siphoning when patients go from flat to upright. Siphoning is the use of gravity to move fluid from a higher to a lower location [22]. When siphoning from a closed container, like the ventricle, flow will continue until the pressure between the two chambers is equal (see Fig. 16.1). The pressure created from siphoning is proportional to the height of the column of fluid between the two chambers as shown in the diagram. For a ventriculoperitoneal shunt, this can be 60 cm or more depending on the patient's height.

It is clear that CSF shunt hydrodynamics is a significant variation from the normal physiology of CSF flow in a patient. It is unknown if this has any effect on the growth and development of the brain.

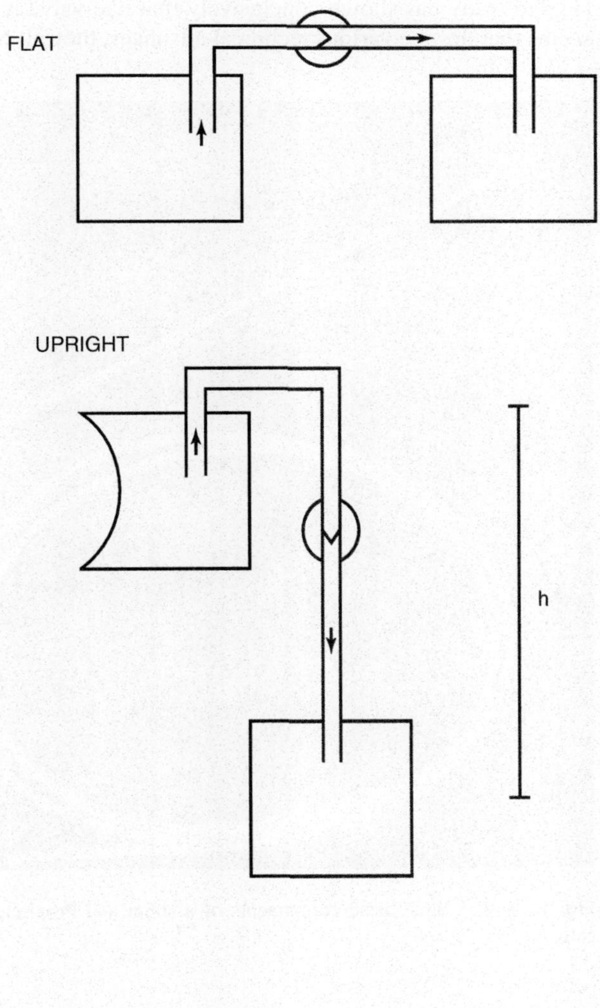

Fig. 16.1 The siphoning effect. In the flat position, the pressure between the two containers is the same minus the opening pressure of the valve. In the upright position, the pressure in the closed top container (ventricle) is proportional to the height of the column of fluid in the tubing (*h*)

Shunt Components

In its most common and basic form, CSF shunts consist of a proximal catheter, a valve, and a distal catheter (see Fig. 16.2). Additional components can be built in or added, such as a tapping reservoir, a pumping chamber, or an antisiphon device, but the utility of these devices is questionable.

Ventricular Catheters: The ventricular catheter carries CSF from the ventricle to the valve. It is inserted through the brain from the shunt entry site. The most proximal portion of the catheter contains multiple holes to allow for CSF flow. Configurations vary, but commonly there are three rows of eight holes within 2 cm of the tip of the catheter. It is unknown if the size and location of the holes have any bearing on shunt function [23].

Valves: There are over a hundred different CSF valves available in the market today [1]. No study has shown conclusively that one valve is better than another [24]. It seems that despite various technical advances, they all have similar outcomes when

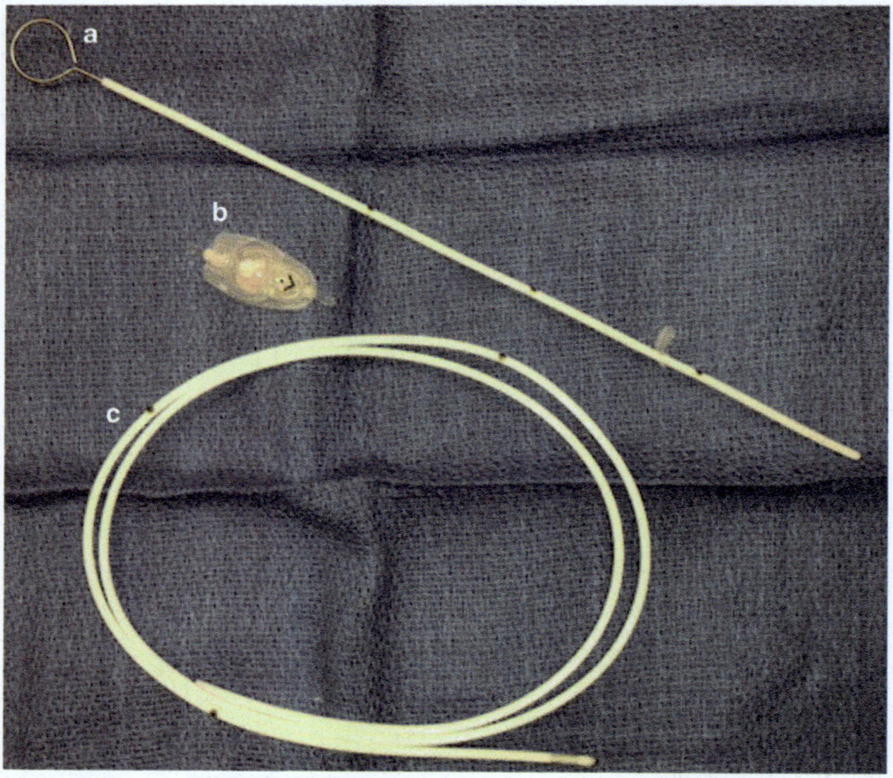

Fig. 16.2 The three basic components of a shunt. (**a**) Proximal catheter. (**b**) Valve. (**c**) Distal catheter

comparing large groups of patients. Valves can be classified based on their pressure-flow characteristics. Most valves are pressure-controlled with an opening pressure that once overcome allows flow and very little resistance (see Fig. 16.3a). The majority of these valves are made with a flexible diaphragm or a ball in cone design. Within this group, are valves with a set or fixed pressure (e.g., low, medium, or high) and valves that are adjustable after implantation. The opening pressure on an adjustable valve can be changed after it is implanted using an external magnet to unlock and then reset the opening pressure. The other less common valve type is a flow-controlled valve. Ideally, the pressure-flow curve for this type of valve system maintains a constant flow despite changes in differential pressure (see Fig. 16.3b). These valves are designed to change resistance to maintain constant flow.

Antisiphon Devices: These devices are designed to prevent the siphoning effect when patients change position from flat to upright. They are implanted to prevent symptoms from overdrainage and to keep the ventricles from becoming smaller than normal or slit-like. Surgeons implant them based on a theory that maintaining normal sized ventricles (or avoiding slit-like ventricle) will lead to a less contact of

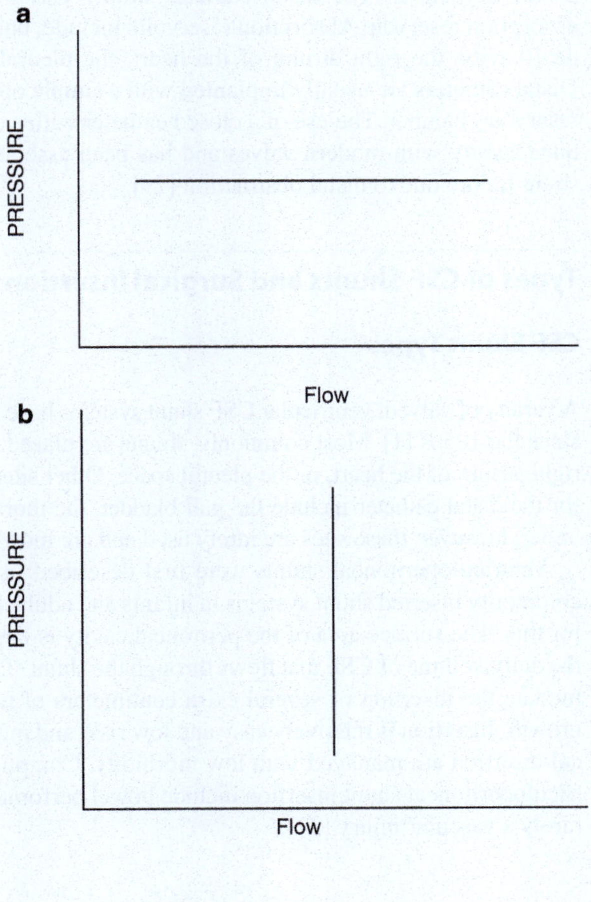

Fig. 16.3 Ideal pressure-flow curve for the two types of valve mechanics. (**a**) Pressure regulation. (**b**) Flow regulation

the ventricular catheter with the walls of the ventricle and choroid plexus, and the less contact will lead to fewer obstructions [25]. Although these devices clearly prevent siphoning during in-vitro bench testing, they have yet to show an ability to prevent ventricular collapse and they have yet to show an ability to prevent shunt failure [24, 26]. The technology, however, is promising and clearly clinical trials are necessary.

Reservoirs and Pumping Chambers: CSF shunt reservoirs are designed to allow tapping of the shunt to measure pressure and assess proximal flow. Some valves are manufactured with a built in reservoir; however, standalone reservoirs are made and can be spiced into the system. Reservoirs, ideally, are placed proximal to the valve so that intracranial pressure (ICP) can be directly measured if the proximal catheter is open (unobstructed). Many reservoirs are manufactured in a way to allow external pumping of the reservoir with the finger after implantation. The amount of pressure needed to depress the reservoir and the time it takes to refill can be used to determine shunt function. Although this is practiced widely, it has never been shown to be a sensitive or specific test in the evaluation of shunt function [27, 28].

Distal Catheters: The distal catheter simply caries CSF from the valve to the absorption reservoir. Absorption reservoirs include, but are not limited to the peritoneal cavity, the right atrium of the heart, the pleural space, and the gallbladder. Distal catheters are usually implanted with a simple open-ended tube going into the reservoir chamber. The use of a closed catheter with a distal slit valve or side slits is unnecessary with modern valves and has been associated with an increase rate of shunt failure due to distal obstruction [29].

Types of CSF Shunts and Surgical Insertion

CSF Shunt Types

A variety of valved, ventricular CSF shunt systems have been reported in the literature since the 1950s [1]. Most commonly, shunts are placed into the peritoneal cavity, the right atrium of the heart, or the pleural space. Other sites that can serve as a reservoir for the distal catheter include the gall bladder, the thoracic duct, fallopian tube, and ureter; however, these sites are rarely used and are mostly of historical interest only.

Ventriculoperitoneal shunts were first described in the 1950s and are the most commonly inserted shunt systems in infants and adults [30]. There are many reasons for this. The surface area of the peritoneal cavity is large and easily accommodates the daily volume of CSF that flows through the shunt. The abdomen can also accommodate the insertion of several extra centimeters of tubing that allows for patient growth. Insertion is relatively easy and low risk, and most complications from surgical insertion are managed with low morbidity. Complications associated with ventriculoperitoneal shunt insertion include bowel perforation, bladder perforation, and rarely a vascular injury [31].

Ventriculoatrial shunts are usually inserted when the peritoneal cavity is hostile or unsuitable for shunt insertion. Common clinical scenarios for this include necrotizing enterocolitis associated with prematurity, ruptured viscus, significant scarring within the peritoneal cavity from previous surgery, ascites, and previous distal catheter infection. The distal catheter is usually inserted into the external jugular, internal jugular, or subclavian vein and the passed intravascularly into the superior vena cava to the opening into the right atrium. Radiographic confirmation of catheter location in the operating room is routinely employed.

Ventriculopleural shunts are also a reasonable alternative to ventriculoperitoneal shunting. The distal catheter is inserted into the pleural space usually near the fifth intercostal space on the anterior axillary line and a variety of techniques have been described for insertion [32–34]. An excess of tubing can be inserted for growth. Distal complications due to failure of absorption or infection lead to pulmonary effusion and collapse of the lung. Patients usually present with dyspnea and require shunt externalization and rarely a chest tube.

Shunt Surgery

CSF shunt insertion or revision is a common surgical procedure for all neurosurgeons. It is a critical part of training and must be mastered. For the majority of pediatric neurosurgeons, it is still the most common indication for surgical intervention. Although it is not particularly complicated or high risk, it can easily result in significant morbidity or mortality is not performed well. The prevention of complications due to infection or poor surgical technique is important. The Hydrocephalus Clinical Research Network (HCRN), a collaborative group of pediatric specialist, has shown that the implementation of a surgical checklist to prevent infection lowers infection rates when there is high compliance with the protocol [35]. Surgical adjuncts such as endoscopy, ultrasound, and stereotaxy for proximal catheter insertion have been studied in prospective trial without significant effect on outcome [36–38]. Surprisingly, one large prospective cohort study found endoscopic placement of shunts for first-time shunt insertions to be harmful [39]. The impact these adjuncts have on revision surgeries, which often are technically more difficult, remains unclear, and requires further study.

Shunt insertion or revision surgery usually takes about an hour of surgical time and is done under general anesthesia. Prophylactic antibiotics are given within an hour of incision to prevent infection [40]. The patient is positioned so that the surgeon has access to the proximal catheter entry site on the head and the distal reservoir for CSF drainage (usually the peritoneal space). A meticulous surgical preparation of the skin is performed and any hair in the field is prepped or clipped to allow for surgical incisions.

The choice of entry site for the proximal catheter is determined by the surgeon and can be on the right or the left side of the skull. The two most common entry sites are anterior (1 cm anterior to the coronal suture on the mid-pupillary line), and posterior (6–8 cm above the external occipital protuberance on the mid-pupillary line)

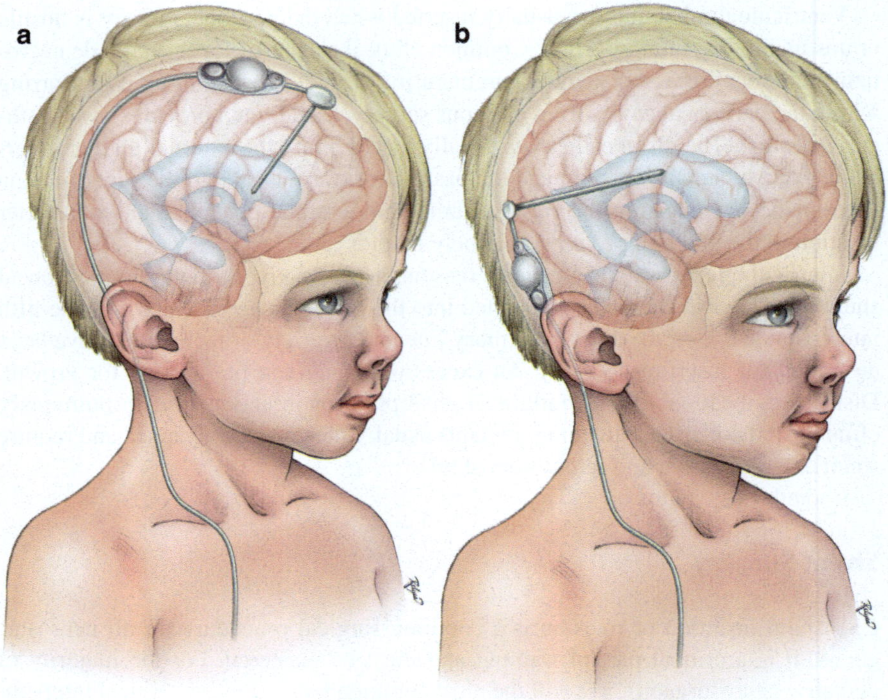

Fig. 16.4 Two commonly used cerebrospinal fluid shunt entry sites. (**a**) Anterior. (**b**) Posterior. (Image created by Katherine Relyea, MS, CMI and printed permission from Baylor College of Medicine)

(Fig. 16.4). These measurements are used in adults and must be modified in the pediatric patient based on head size and presence of fontanelles. They are well accepted and are not associated with any significant morbidity to the brain when the catheter is passed into the ventricle. It is unclear if one entry site is superior to the other; existing reports in the literature are conflicting [41–43]. Outcomes may be the same. A randomized trial is currently accruing subjects with results expected in 2020 [44].

The target for the tip of the ventricular catheter is generally accepted to be the frontal horn or the occipital horn of the lateral ventricle, away from the choroid plexus, and not touching the ventricular walls. It is believed that placement of the ventricular catheter tip into one of these sites will result in a lower risk of obstruction due to scar formation [26, 38]. A recent secondary analysis of a large cohort of first-time shunt insertions, however, was unable to confirm this theory [43]. That study concluded that any site within the ventricle was acceptable and no location within the ventricle improved shunt survival. Regardless, these sites are easily accessible from the above entry sites using standard anatomical landmarks [45].

Distal shunt placement requires the creation of a subcutaneous tunnel from the entry site to the distal reservoir insertion site. Shunt passers, long narrow steel rods, are used for this purpose [46]. Prior to insertion of the distal catheter flow of CSF through the shunt must be confirmed. If there is no flow through the system, the entire system is inspected to ensure that there are no disconnections, malfunctioning valves, or poorly placed proximal catheters.

Although CSF shunt surgery is considered by many to be one of the more mundane neurosurgical procedures, it requires a comprehensive knowledge of the patient's condition, careful planning and preparation, selection of implants, and attention to detail like all other surgical endeavors. Knowledge of the literature and clinical experience are invaluable. The surgeon's ability to influence shunt survival, achieve good outcomes, and avoid complications is a product of patient selection, planning, and surgical technique.

CSF Shunt Failures and Compilations

Although CSF shunts have significantly lowered mortality rates and improved outcomes for patients with hydrocephalus, they are not a cure. Shunts are associated with a very high failure rate and significant morbidities. In pediatric patients, it is hard to identify any other implantable device, which fails as frequently as a CSF shunt. Failures occur for a variety of reasons.

Shunt Obstruction

The most common reason for shunt failure is obstruction due to tissue or blood occluding the proximal catheter, but obstruction can also occur in the valve or distal catheter. Studies looking at the histopathology of tissue blocking the shunt catheter show a predominance of glial, choroid, and inflammatory cells [47]. When the proximal catheter comes into contact with the pulsating ventricular walls or choroid plexus, there is a mild inflammatory reaction with the proliferation of glial cells. The silastic tubing is encased in scar or walled off. Eventually the scar can block all of the ventricular catheters holes or occlude the lumen of the catheter [47]. An active area of research currently is the characterization of this reaction and the manufacturing of more biocompatible catheters [48–51].

Shunt Infection

Shunt failure due to infection has been a problem with CSF shunting since they were first introduced. Rates of infection vary between 3% and 27% depending on the definition used for infection and the patient population [52, 53]. Most shunt infections present with symptoms within the first 2–3 weeks of placement but may be longer in the setting of infection with less virulent organisms; over 90% of first infections present within 6 months of implantation. The vast majority of shunt infections are a consequence of microorganisms being introduced at the time of shunt insertion. Not surprisingly, one of the biggest risk factors for infections is number of shunt revisions [54, 55].

There is a predominance of Gram-positive organisms that cause these infections. Most series report a predominance of coagulase-negative staphylococci, typically *Staphylococcus epidermidis*, which as a group account for 32–53% of all shunt infections [52, 53, 56]. *Staphylococcus aureus* comprises the second most common cause of CSF shunt infection contributing to 23–38% of all infections, followed by Gram-negative rods accounting for 8–16% [57]. Shunts can also become secondarily infected from a ruptured viscus, such as the appendix, or an unrelated surgical procedure, such as placement of a percutaneous gastric tube.

When the diagnosis of shunt infection is made, it requires admission to the hospital, removal of the shunt, and placement of a drain in most cases, followed by days to weeks of antimicrobials to clear the infection, followed by reimplantation of the shunt. Hospitalization is long and multiple surgeries are required.

Shunt Fracture

Shunt fracture, or a break in the tubing, is a late complication. It is typically seen after the shunt has been in place for 10 years and most commonly occurs in the neck where there is the most movement. Calcification of scar around the tubing can contribute to a fracture. This complication is best diagnosed on plain X-ray films.

Shunt Disconnection

This is usually an early complication due to a poor connection between the shunt tubing and the valve. It can usually be prevented by good surgical technique carefully securing with a suture the tubing to the valve.

Shunt Migration

Shunts tubing is known to migrate from the initial placement over time. This occurs more commonly in infants than children. Catheters can migrate out of the ventricle into the subgaleal space, out of the subgaleal space and into the ventricle, out of the ventricle, and into the abdomen. A variety of complications from migration have been observed [58]. Anchoring the valve to the pericranium with a suture can reduce the incidence of this rare complication.

Overdrainage

Overdrainage is another less commonly seen CSF shunt complication occurring in less than 5% of cases, but it can result in significant morbidity for the patient [24]. Decompression of the ventricles from the placement of a shunt lowers intraventricular pressure. This can lead to collapse of the cortical mantle falling away from the subdural space. CSF will fill the subdural space creating what is known as a CSF hygroma. When this occurs, blood can also hemorrhage into this space when bridging veins are torn. Asymptomatic patients can be observed closely with serial exams, but symptomatic patients require additional surgery drain the subdural fluid. Adjustable valves may be useful in this condition because the opening pressure can be raised without additional surgery.

Underdrainage

Occasionally, the symptoms of hydrocephalus persist after shunt insertion and it is necessary to lower the resistance through the shunt system. This is done by changing the valve or adjusting it to a lower opening pressure.

Outcomes

Generally, the overall prognosis of patients with CSF shunts is determined by the underlying cause of hydrocephalus and not the presence of a shunt. CSF shunt failure, in its many forms, is associated with significant morbidity and mortality when treatment is delayed [59–61]. Additionally, from an economic perspective, there are significant costs to a healthcare system when it comes to maintaining CSF shunts.

Healthcare Costs

As described in this chapter, CSF shunt maintenance requires a significant commitment of time and resources from patients, families, healthcare providers, and hospital systems. The onset of headache, a common complaint associated with a multitude of ailments, can trigger the activation of a large healthcare team or system with access to neurosurgical expertise, cross-sectional imaging, and operating room resources. These resources must be available at all hours to prevent catastrophe. When the diagnosis is unclear, patients are admitted for observation, and when the shunt has failed, surgery is required. In the United States healthcare system from 1997 to 2003, it is estimated that pediatric hydrocephalus accounted for 40,000 admissions, 433,000 hospital days, and $2 billion in healthcare cost each year. Hydrocephalus in children accounted for 0.6% of all pediatric hospital admissions, 1.8% of all pediatric hospital days, and 3.1% of all hospital charges [62]. Economically, CSF shunts place a significant burden on healthcare systems.

Shunt Survival and the Associated Morbidity and Mortality

CSF shunts have a high failure rate when compared to other commonly used implants. After first-time shunt insertion approximately 30–40% of shunts will fail at least once in the first year [24, 38, 63]. This number increases to 50% by 2 years, and approximately 70–90% by 10 years [64]. Multiple studies have shown that young age is the most significant risk factor for shunt failure [39, 65–67]. The use of the endoscope and a coexisting cardiac comorbidity have also recently been shown to increase the risk of shunt failure [39]. No other significant, modifiable risk factors have been identified in the last 20 years despite significant effort.

The second most common cause of shunt failure is infection; roughly 20–30% of failures are due to infection. Recent advances aimed at reducing the risk of shunt infection have included the use of intrathecal injection of antibiotics at the time of shunt insertion and the use of antibiotic impregnated shunt catheters. The use of antibiotic impregnated catheters may play a role in lowering shunt infection rates. Multiple, moderate quality studies have shown an effect in lowering shunt infection rates [68–70]. However, the results of a randomized controlled trial in the United Kingdom comparing standard silicone catheter, to antibiotic impregnated, to silver impregnated are pending as the trial continues to enroll subjects (BASICS trial) [71].

Shunt infections can have a detrimental effect on patients. As described, they result in prolonged hospitalization and multiple surgeries, which have a significant impact on the quality of life of patients and families. There is also a well-established correlation between number of shunt infections and poor cognitive outcomes [72, 73].

Cognitive Outcomes and Quality of Life Measures

Evaluation of neuropsychological outcomes in the long term is becoming an increasingly important area in the field of hydrocephalus treatment. There is a real need for these types of assessments when comparing treatment options such as endoscopic third ventriculostomy alone, endoscopic third ventriculostomy with choroid plexus coagulation, and CSF shunting. Multiple tools are available and commonly used in the evaluation of pediatric shunt patients such as the Bayley Scales of Infant Development and the Capute Scales, but their use requires multidisciplinary evaluations, significant time, and additional costs.

Despite the fact that CSF shunts are not a cure for hydrocephalus, shunts continue to be the best treatment available for most patients. While the search for a cure should continue, it is paramount that research continue to improve shunt function until an alternative treatment is found.

References

1. Aschoff A, Kremer P, Hashemi B, Kunze S. The scientific history of hydrocephalus and its treatment. Neurosurg Rev. 1999;22:67–93; discussion 4–5
2. Wernicke C. Lehrbuch der Gehirnkrankheiten. Kassel: Fischer; 1881. p. 337–78.
3. Krause F. Chirurgie des Gehirns und des Ruckenmarks. Vienna: Urban and Schwarzenberg; 1911. p. 146–73.
4. Dandy WE. Ventriculography following the injection of air into ventricles. Ann Surg. 1918;68:5–11.

5. Fleischmann S. Die Ergebnisse der Lumbalpunktion. Dtsch Zeitschr Nervenheilk. 1896;10:342–67.
6. Henle A. Beitrag zur Pathologie und Therapie des Hydrocephalus. Mitt Grenzgeb Med Chir. 1896;1:264–302.
7. Payr E. Elfjähriger Dauererfolg einer Ventrikeldrainage bei Hydrocephalus. Med Klin. 1919;49:1247–51.
8. Ferguson AH. Intraperitoneal diversion of the cerebrospinal fluid in cases of hydrocephalus. N Y Med J. 1898;67:902–9.
9. Anton G, von Bramann FG. Balkenstich bei Hydrocephalien, Tumoren, end bei Epilepsie. Munch Med Wochenschr. 1908;11:1673–5.
10. Kanusch W. Die Behandlung des Hydrocephalus der kleinen Kinder. Arch Klin Chir. 1908;87:709–96.
11. Payr E. Drainage der Hirnventrikel mittels frei transplantierter Blutgefabe; Bemerkungen uber Hydrocephalus. Arch Klin Chir. 1908;87:801–85.
12. Fowler RS. The surgical treatment of internal hydrocephalus. Ann Surg. 1909;49(3):374–81.
13. Dandy WE. An operative procedure for hydrocephalus. Johns Hopkins Hosp Bull. 1922;33:189–96.
14. Mixter WJ. Ventriculoscopy and punture of the floor of the third ventricle. Boston Med Surg J. 1923;188:277–8.
15. Schmitt PJ, Jane JA Jr. A lesson in history: the evolution of endoscopic third ventriculostomy. Neurosurg Focus. 2012;33:E11.
16. Dandy WE. Extirpation of the choroid plexus of the lateral ventricles in communicating hydrocephalus. Ann Surg. 1918;37:569–79.
17. Grant JA. Victor Darwin Lespinasse: a biographical sketch. Neurosurgery. 1996;39:1232–3.
18. Nulsen FE, Spitz EB. Treatment of hydrocephalus by direct shunt from ventricle to jugular vein. Surg Forum. 1952;2:399–403.
19. Sandler AL, Sturrock D, Branfield J, et al. Marvelous medicine: the untold story of the Wade-Dahl-Till valve. J Neurosurg Pediatr. 2012;9:482–90.
20. Boockvar JA, Loudon W, Sutton LN. Development of the Spitz-Holter valve in Philadelphia. J Neurosurg. 2001;95:145–7.
21. Kalousdian S, Karlan MS, Williams MA. Silicone elastomer cerebrospinal fluid shunt systems. Council on Scientific Affairs, American Medical Association. Neurosurgery. 1998;42:887–92.
22. James JM, Sainte-Rose C. The shunt book. Cambridge, MA: Blackwell Science; 1995.
23. Harris CA, McAllister JP 2nd. Does drainage hole size influence adhesion on ventricular catheters? Child's Nerv Syst. 2011;27:1221–32.
24. Drake JM, Kestle JR, Milner R, et al. Randomized trial of cerebrospinal fluid shunt valve design in pediatric hydrocephalus. Neurosurgery. 1998;43:294–303; discussion 303–5
25. Gehlen M, Eklund A, Kurtcuoglu V, Malm J, Schmid Daners M. Comparison of anti-siphon devices-how do they affect CSF dynamics in supine and upright posture? Acta Neurochir. 2017;159:1389–97.
26. Tuli S, O'Hayon B, Drake J, Clarke M, Kestle J. Change in ventricular size and effect of ventricular catheter placement in pediatric patients with shunted hydrocephalus. Neurosurgery. 1999;45:1329–33; discussion 33–5
27. Piatt JH Jr. Pumping the shunt revisited. A longitudinal study. Pediatr Neurosurg. 1996;25:73–6; discussion 6–7
28. Nejat F, El-Khashab M. Why flushing the valve cannot be a reliable method to evaluate the ventriculoperitoneal shunt function? Iran J Pediatr. 2011;21:556.
29. Cozzens JW, Chandler JP. Increased risk of distal ventriculoperitoneal shunt obstruction associated with slit valves or distal slits in the peritoneal catheter. J Neurosurg. 1997;87:682–6.
30. Ames RH. Ventriculo-peritoneal shunts in the management of hydrocephalus. J Neurosurg. 1967;27:525–9.
31. Danan D, Winfree CJ, McKhann GM 2nd. Intra-abdominal vascular injury during trocar-assisted ventriculoperitoneal shunting: case report. Neurosurgery. 2008;63:E613; discussion E

32. Richardson MD, Handler MH. Minimally invasive technique for insertion of ventriculopleural shunt catheters. J Neurosurg Pediatr. 2013;12:501–4.
33. Kurschel S, Eder HG, Schleef J. Ventriculopleural shunt: thoracoscopic placement of the distal catheter. Surg Endosc. 2003;17:1850.
34. Nixon HH. Ventriculo-pleural drainage with a valve. Dev Med Child Neurol. 1962;4:301–2.
35. Kestle JR, Riva-Cambrin J, Wellons JC 3rd, et al. A standardized protocol to reduce cerebrospinal fluid shunt infection: the Hydrocephalus Clinical Research Network Quality Improvement Initiative. J Neurosurg Pediatr. 2011;8:22–9.
36. Whitehead WE, Riva-Cambrin J, Wellons JC 3rd, et al. No significant improvement in the rate of accurate ventricular catheter location using ultrasound-guided CSF shunt insertion: a prospective, controlled study by the Hydrocephalus Clinical Research Network. J Neurosurg Pediatr. 2013;12:565–74.
37. Nesvick CL, Khan NR, Mehta GU, Klimo P Jr. Image guidance in ventricular cerebrospinal fluid shunt catheter placement: a systematic review and meta-analysis. Neurosurgery. 2015;77:321–31; discussion 31
38. Kestle JR, Drake JM, Cochrane DD, et al. Lack of benefit of endoscopic ventriculoperitoneal shunt insertion: a multicenter randomized trial. J Neurosurg. 2003;98:284–90.
39. Riva-Cambrin J, Kestle JR, Holubkov R, et al. Risk factors for shunt malfunction in pediatric hydrocephalus: a multicenter prospective cohort study. J Neurosurg Pediatr. 2016;17:382–90.
40. Klimo P Jr, Van Poppel M, Thompson CJ, et al. Pediatric hydrocephalus: systematic literature review and evidence-based guidelines. Part 6: Preoperative antibiotics for shunt surgery in children with hydrocephalus: a systematic review and meta-analysis. J Neurosurg Pediatr. 2014;14(Suppl 1):44–52.
41. Albright AL, Haines SJ, Taylor FH. Function of parietal and frontal shunts in childhood hydrocephalus. J Neurosurg. 1988;69:883–6.
42. Bierbrauer KS, Storrs BB, McLone DG, Tomita T, Dauser R. A prospective, randomized study of shunt function and infections as a function of shunt placement. Pediatr Neurosurg. 1990;16:287–91.
43. Whitehead WE, Riva-Cambrin J, Kulkarni AV, et al. Ventricular catheter entry site and not catheter tip location predicts shunt survival: a secondary analysis of 3 large pediatric hydrocephalus studies. J Neurosurg Pediatr. 2017;19:157–67.
44. Whitehead WE. The CSF shunt entry site trial. NLM identifier: NCT02425761. http://www.clinicaltrials.gov/ct2/show/NCT00265317. Accessed 10 May 2018.
45. Lind CR, Tsai AM, Law AJ, Lau H, Muthiah K. Ventricular catheter trajectories from traditional shunt approaches: a morphometric study in adults with hydrocephalus. J Neurosurg. 2008;108:930–3.
46. Iantosca M, Drake J. Cerebrospinal fluid shunts. In: Albright A, Pollack IF, Adelson PD, editors. Operative techniques in pediatric neurosurgery. New York: Thieme; 2001. p. 3–14.
47. Sekhar LN, Moossy J, Guthkelch AN. Malfunctioning ventriculoperitoneal shunts. Clinical and pathological features. J Neurosurg. 1982;56:411–6.
48. Harris CA, Resau JH, Hudson EA, et al. Reduction of protein adsorption and macrophage and astrocyte adhesion on ventricular catheters by polyethylene glycol and N-acetyl-L-cysteine. J Biomed Mater Res A. 2011;98:425–33.
49. Harris CA, McAllister JP 2nd. What we should know about the cellular and tissue response causing catheter obstruction in the treatment of hydrocephalus. Neurosurgery. 2012;70:1589–601; discussion 601–2
50. Harris CA, Resau JH, Hudson EA, et al. Effects of surface wettability, flow, and protein concentration on macrophage and astrocyte adhesion in an in vitro model of central nervous system catheter obstruction. J Biomed Mater Res A. 2011;97:433–40.
51. Harris CA, Resau JH, Hudson EA, West RA, Moon C, McAllister JP 2nd. Mechanical contributions to astrocyte adhesion using a novel in vitro model of catheter obstruction. Exp Neurol. 2010;222:204–10.
52. McGirt MJ, Zaas A, Fuchs HE, George TM, Kaye K, Sexton DJ. Risk factors for pediatric ventriculoperitoneal shunt infection and predictors of infectious pathogens. Clin Infect Dis. 2003;36:858–62.

53. Lee JK, Seok JY, Lee JH, et al. Incidence and risk factors of ventriculoperitoneal shunt infections in children: a study of 333 consecutive shunts in 6 years. J Korean Med Sci. 2012;27:1563–8.
54. Simon TD, Butler J, Whitlock KB, et al. Risk factors for first cerebrospinal fluid shunt infection: findings from a multi-center prospective cohort study. J Pediatr. 2014;164:1462–8.e2.
55. McGirt MJ, Leveque JC, Wellons JC 3rd, et al. Cerebrospinal fluid shunt survival and etiology of failures: a seven-year institutional experience. Pediatr Neurosurg. 2002;36:248–55.
56. Odio C, McCracken GH Jr, Nelson JD. CSF shunt infections in pediatrics. A seven-year experience. Am J Dis Child. 1984;138:1103–8.
57. Davis SE, Levy ML, McComb JG, Masri-Lavine L. Does age or other factors influence the incidence of ventriculoperitoneal shunt infections? Pediatr Neurosurg. 1999;30:253–7.
58. Shahsavaran S, Kermani HR, Keikhosravi E, Nejat F, El Khashab M. Ventriculoperitoneal shunt migration and coiling: a report of two cases. J Pediatr Neurosci. 2012;7:114–6.
59. Iskandar BJ, Tubbs S, Mapstone TB, Grabb PA, Bartolucci AA, Oakes WJ. Death in shunted hydrocephalic children in the 1990s. Pediatr Neurosurg. 1998;28:173–6.
60. Sainte-Rose C, Piatt JH, Renier D, et al. Mechanical complications in shunts. Pediatr Neurosurg. 1991;17:2–9.
61. Tuli S, Tuli J, Drake J, Spears J. Predictors of death in pediatric patients requiring cerebrospinal fluid shunts. J Neurosurg. 2004;100:442–6.
62. Simon TD, Riva-Cambrin J, Srivastava R, et al. Hospital care for children with hydrocephalus in the United States: utilization, charges, comorbidities, and deaths. J Neurosurg Pediatr. 2008;1:131–7.
63. Kulkarni AV, Riva-Cambrin J, Butler J, et al. Outcomes of CSF shunting in children: comparison of Hydrocephalus Clinical Research Network cohort with historical controls: clinical article. J Neurosurg Pediatr. 2013;12:334–8.
64. Sainte-Rose C, Hoffman HJ, Hirsch JF. Shunt failure. Concepts Pediatr Neurosurg. 1989;9:7–20.
65. Tuli S, Drake J, Lawless J, Wigg M, Lamberti-Pasculli M. Risk factors for repeated cerebrospinal shunt failures in pediatric patients with hydrocephalus. J Neurosurg. 2000;92:31–8.
66. Simon TD, Whitlock KB, Riva-Cambrin J, et al. Association of intraventricular hemorrhage secondary to prematurity with cerebrospinal fluid shunt surgery in the first year following initial shunt placement. J Neurosurg Pediatr. 2012;9:54–63.
67. Piatt JH Jr, Carlson CV. A search for determinants of cerebrospinal fluid shunt survival: retrospective analysis of a 14-year institutional experience. Pediatr Neurosurg. 1993;19:233–41; discussion 42
68. Sciubba DM, Stuart RM, McGirt MJ, et al. Effect of antibiotic-impregnated shunt catheters in decreasing the incidence of shunt infection in the treatment of hydrocephalus. J Neurosurg. 2005;103:131–6.
69. Parker SL, McGirt MJ, Murphy JA, Megerian JT, Stout M, Engelhart L. Comparative effectiveness of antibiotic-impregnated shunt catheters in the treatment of adult and pediatric hydrocephalus: analysis of 12,589 consecutive cases from 287 US hospital systems. J Neurosurg. 2015;122:443–8.
70. Parker SL, McGirt MJ, Murphy JA, Megerian JT, Stout M, Engelhart L. Cost savings associated with antibiotic-impregnated shunt catheters in the treatment of adult and pediatric hydrocephalus. World Neurosurg. 2015;83:382–6.
71. Jenkinson MD, Gamble C, Hartley JC, et al. The British antibiotic and silver-impregnated catheters for ventriculoperitoneal shunts multi-centre randomised controlled trial (the BASICS trial): study protocol. Trials. 2014;15:4.
72. Vinchon M, Dhellemmes P. Cerebrospinal fluid shunt infection: risk factors and long-term follow-up. Child's Nerv Syst. 2006;22:692–7.
73. Schreffler RT, Schreffler AJ, Wittler RR. Treatment of cerebrospinal fluid shunt infections: a decision analysis. Pediatr Infect Dis J. 2002;21:632–6.

Shunts and Shunt Malfunction

17

Prashant Hariharan and Carolyn A. Harris

The Classic Versus Modern Shunt System

Perhaps one of the most intriguing events in neurosurgical history is the invention and use of the shunt system to treat hydrocephalus, despite the shunt's high failure rates. The shunt system, classically composed of a proximal catheter, valve, and distal catheter, was developed in the 1950s. The system was envisioned by tool-maker John Holter, whose son, Casey, had hydrocephalus. The concept, modeled after the nipple of a baby bottle, allowed for one-way flow through a pressure-regulated valve. The shunt system utilized surgical aseptic techniques (1860s), and followed historical predecessors: the external ventricular drain (1881), and ventricular-subdural shunts made of glass wool, gold tubes, bundled catgut (1890s), rubber (1903), glass, silver, and linen threads (1908–1926). Catheters from the ventricles to the cisterna magna and Nulsen-Spitz's ventriculo-jugular shunt were revolutionary precursors made of rubber or polyethylene (1940–1950) [1]. The Spitz–Holter valve is the result of these and Holter's efforts. The modern-day shunt remains similar now as when it was created (1955, implanted in 1957/58): slight modifications to the catheter, major iterations to the shunt valve, and the addition of compensators for gravity and siphoning are key improvements to treatment.

As is common practice, cerebrospinal fluid (CSF) in a patient with hydrocephalus typically travels from the central nervous system (CNS) outward through a shunt

P. Hariharan
Department of Chemical Engineering and Materials Science, Department of Biomedical Engineering, Wayne State University, Detroit, MI, USA

C. A. Harris (✉)
Department of Chemical Engineering and Materials Science Department of Biomedical Engineering, Department of Neurosurgery, Wayne State University Medical School, Detroit, MI, USA
e-mail: caharris@wayne.edu

D. D. Limbrick, J. R. Leonard (eds.), *Cerebrospinal Fluid Disorders*,
https://doi.org/10.1007/978-3-319-97928-1_17

system. Flow through shunt hardware moves from the cranial ventricles or atypically from the lumbar space, to the peritoneum, the heart's atrium, or the pleural cavity. The outward flow is intended to replicate an intricate balance between CSF production and absorption, but shunt failures and chronic headaches persist.

Since its inception, the shunt system has undoubtedly saved lives, but it also repetitively fails. Over the past decade, there has been an increase in the diagnosis of hydrocephalus and an increase in hydrocephalus prevalence in children and adults, necessitating the use of new clinical strategies and biomedical engineering approaches to inhibit failure. Still, 30% of shunts fail within the first year, 40% within the second year, and at least 85% within 10 years following implantation [2–4]. The question plaguing neurosurgical practice today, is, how and why do shunt systems fail, and equally important: what factors can be controlled for improved patient care?

Dependence on individual centers or surgeons brings about variations in failure; [5, 6] hydrocephalus etiology is a debatable factor, while age certainly plays a role [6–9]. There has been a great deal of recent research effort in manipulating the insertion path, showing that anterior entry has lower risk of shunt failure by one-third versus posterior entry [10, 11]. Although not discussed in detail in this chapter, manipulatable clinical aspects of shunt failure are important to revolutionizing patient care. Instead, we focus here on complications relevant to the shunt design and response to such, with more thorough clinical reports available [12, 13].

Whole System Shunt Failures and Complications

Ranging from infection, disconnection, overdrainage, and obstruction, the failure of a shunt system can occur days to decades after implantation.

Infection

Infections plague shunt insertion surgeries, with an infection rate of 3–20% [12]. The overall incidence of infection tapers, with 90% of infections within the first 6 months following shunt implantation; however, with each revision the cumulative risk of CSF infection rises per patient [14–17]. Multicenter studies have indicated significant quality improvement (decreased shunt infection) with standardized protocols across centers [18]. While infection seems to significantly vary institutions, other factors also play a role, including young age, female sex, African-American race, public insurance, etiology of intraventricular hemorrhage, respiratory complex chronic condition, subsequent revision procedures, hospital volume, and surgeon case volume [19]. Work is underway investigating the incidence of shunt infection, examined with new age technologies and with analyses of catheter biofilms.

The inception of antibiotic impregnated shunts (AIS) has led to a massive shift toward the incorporation of AIS in standard of care for the treatment of hydrocephalus. The release of impregnated antibiotics (namely, rifampicin and clindamycin, with gentamicin sulfate and diethanolamine fusidate and sodium fusidate tested [20]) will not likely influence pre-existing biofilms, but have been shown to prevent shunt catheter colonization in vitro [20, 21]. Still, data are controversial: some clinical reports indicate a significant reduction in infection rates, while others do not see as wide of an effect.

Antibacterial shunt systems impregnated with silver (silver-coated catheters, or SCCs), are the focus of many ongoing studies. There is no statistically significant difference between SCCs and AIS, but there is a decrease in CSF infection versus standard silicone catheters [22–25]. Hydrogel-coated ventricular catheters have shown a significant reduction in infection rates within 1 month of implantation, but correlate with an increase in general infection rate [26, 27]. High protein inhibits bacterial adhesion to catheter surfaces, but may also increase mammalian cell and tissue attachment [28, 29].

Disconnection, Fracture, and Migration

The inability to transfer CSF out of the CNS can be a direct result of disconnection, fracture, obstruction, or migration. The most recent statistics on disconnection date to 1991, which indicate a 15% failure, being second only to shunt obstruction [30]. Distal component tethering from foreign body reaction (FBR) elicits a pulling on the joints of the shunt system, causing misplacement of the ventricular catheter, disconnection, and in some cases migration. Suturing the proximal catheter or the valve to pericranium can help avoid some instances of migration; this paired with adding extra distal tubing reduces the risk of either catheter being misplaced.

Recently, snap-system ventricular catheters, with hydrophilic polyvinylpyrrolidone (PVP) coatings were recalled because of their increased incidence of disconnection. This is likely due to the lubricious nature of the PVP hydrogel. As indicated below, these coatings may inhibit the rate of protein adsorption and cell attachment [7, 30–34].

Nonphysiologic Outflow

Unfortunately, with the current standard of care, over- and underdrainage with persistent headache can develop. While the use of antisiphon devices significantly diminishes the progression of overdrainage, recent reports have observed dynamic fluctuations in intracranial pressure as a result of variable physiologic factors [35, 36]. Clinically, the use of lumbar-peritoneal shunt systems has been indicated in improving overdrainage-induced slit ventricle syndrome (SVS), with some potential to reduce shunt failure rate in this patient cohort [37].

As we continue to treat hydrocephalus with the shunt system, all future directions to prevent overdrainage must include improvement to valve testing and validation. The use of saline or water is standard practice, but neither represent physiologic conditions of proteinaceous CSF or pathologic CSF containing a variable degree of suspended cells. Certainly, increased CSF protein content leads to a reduction in CSF surface tension, which reduces the valve opening and closing pressures and creates a scenario in which the valve's operating pressure is likely lower in vivo than that which is specified by the manufacturer. The inclusion of detergent to manipulate surface tension, or the inclusion of proteins/cells in the valve test bed will likely mitigate this problem [38, 39].

Engineering improvements to overdrainage include the study and manipulation of the valve, [40] examination of flow through the shunt system with computational fluid dynamics, [41–45] and conversion from the shunt system to other treatment paradigms. Valve modifications to create more physiologic CSF outflow include membrane-control, flow-regulation, and gravity-assistance. There has also been a concerted effort to transition away from the shunt system in an effort to make outflow more physiologic: for instance, in the last decade there has been a resurgence of endoscopic third ventriculostomy paired with choroid plexus cauterization, [46–49] fabrication of artificial arachnoid granulations, [50–54] similar minimally invasive treatment, [55] and the use of intermittent tapping to delay or treat under-drainage [56, 57].

Obstructions Specific to the Shunt Valve

Modification to the modern shunt has primarily been focused on valve design. We will not hone in on fluctuations in failure rates between hardware. While variations in success have been reported across valve types, [58] surgeon-specific preference between valves, often dependent on the intricacies of each case, may be one driving factor of such differences. Complications with the shunt valve occur much less often than they do compared with complications with the shunt proximal or distal catheter, but nevertheless persist. It is often hypothesized that these differences have to do with highly proteinaceous or bloody CSF, although the viscosity of CSF itself is not directly correlated with valve failure [38]. Occlusion of the shunt valve is understudied. Revisions can be necessitated by either a failure of the mechanisms of the valve to function, or simply from an inability to detect if the shunt is functioning at full capacity.

Complications with the Shunt Catheter

Obstructions Specific to the Shunt Catheter

Modern-day shunt catheters are fabricated from polydimethylsiloxane (PDMS, silicone rubber), and come in varieties, which are impregnated with barium, infused with antibiotic, coated for lubricity, or processed to remove free silicone oligomers [59]. Systematic clinical, translational, and basic science reviews hone in on obstruction-centric shunt failure. Catheter obstruction remains the biggest source of shunt failure to date. Therefore, our focus here considers attempts to understand stepwise stages of obstruction, to deconvolute the mechanisms by which obstructions originate, and to ultimately develop a shunt catheter or insertion strategy that may elicit a more appropriate, biocompatible response.

Of importance to the research community now are the factors by which we can control and manipulate to reduce failure rates. PDMS was targeted in the 1940s and 50s for its elasticity, thermal stability, and bioinertness [2]. While PDMS works well in some environments, of course PDMS-shunt systems are not inert, and do not elicit a desirable response. Potentially obstructive cells and tissues can originate from single cells suspended in the CSF (from shedding periventricular white matter), from the catheter coming in contact with the ependymal wall or choroid plexus, or a response from the parenchyma due to a presence of a foreign body.

PDMS is not the only type of catheter that has been tested: polyethylene, poly-2-hydroxyethyl methacrylate, expanded polytetrafluoroethylene (e-PTFE), cellulose acetate, and polyurethane have been tested historically, among modifications to surface chemistry [2, 60]. Regardless of the material, however, biomaterials implanted into the body will evoke a FBR. This FBR needs to be understood and manipulated in order to improve device integration, and, in this case, maintain a patent shunt system for an extended time. From our perspective, this is the crucial mechanism for reducing shunt failure.

Stepwise Foreign Body Reaction

Biomaterials are typically designed to be nonimmunogenic, nontoxic, and physically and chemically stable. From cardiac pacemakers and hernia meshes to continuous glucose monitors and brain-stimulating or recording electrodes: biomaterials are susceptible to a host reaction. While emerging biomaterial device designs are moving toward manipulating these reactions, implanted devices are still destined for an end-stage response by which the body and the device persistently battle until homeostatic device encapsulation occurs. This response is called the FBR.

A survey of publications by Anderson [61] on FBR will help convey the fundamentals of this phenomenon. Following implantation, materials interact with the fluids in their environment, provoking further interaction with the immune cells, leading to matrix formation. In succession to this, acute and chronic inflammation occur in sequence. Acute inflammation, which resolves within a week (depending on the injury at the site of implantation), leads into chronic inflammation lasting for approximately 2 weeks. The chronic phase is usually confined to the interface of the biomaterial. After this stage, the emergence of granulation tissue is observed, which is classically identified by the presence of macrophages and infiltration of fibroblasts.

The following six events are fundamental to all FBRs to most biomaterials.

Protein Adsorption and Biofouling

FBR is initiated by the near-instantaneous adsorption of plasma proteins, namely albumin, fibrinogen, fibronectin, vitronectin, globulin, and others. In the case of the proximal (ventricular) catheter, the proteins that are found in the CSF will be the first to adsorb to the ventricular catheter. Our current understanding of adsorbed proteins tells us that it is a dynamic phenomenon where adsorption and desorption occur constantly (Vroman effect). As CSF proteins change because of hydrocephalus pathology, the adsorbed protein layer is also likely to change.

Proteomic analysis has shown that some constitutively expressed proteins adsorb to, and trigger the FBR by promoting the attachment of inflammatory cells [62]; this accentuates the notion that shunt catheter surface properties matter. The understanding of the relationships between surface properties and cell attachment has been used to design materials that allow less protein adsorption as a strategy to mitigate the FBR.

Inflammatory Cell Migration and Adhesion

Following protein adsorption to the material's surface, rapid extravasation and migration of neutrophils take place. These neutrophils then produce cytokines, chemokines, and reactive oxygen species (ROS). These products recruit undifferentiated monocytes and macrophages to the implant site over the next several days. Macrophages produce factors that recruit fibroblasts and may also fuse to form multinucleated foreign body giant cells (FBGCs). The presence of stimuli that encourage fusion is not sufficient to result in FBGCs; these signals must coincide with adsorption of a specific array of proteins to the surface of the biomaterial. In the case of the shunt system, this discussion must accommodate the immune cells of the brain: microglia and immunologically activated astrocytes. Participation of inflammatory cells from the blood does not typically drive the FBR in this space, but may in part, explain etiology-dependent variability with degrees of blood exposure [13].

Fusion and Frustrated Phagocytosis

Neutrophils and macrophages that have adhered to the biomaterial surface are challenged by shear stress caused by flow of bodily fluids. This may begin to disrupt their adhesion to the surface, which can then cause apoptosis ("anoikis"). To avoid death via anoikis, cells may fuse to form FBGCs. Fusion may also be induced by proinflammatory cytokines such as interleukin 4 or 13 (IL-4 or 13).

Encapsulation

The inability of the inflammatory cells to digest the intruding material invariably leads to the formation of a collagenous fibrotic capsule or a fibrin-predominant provisional matrix, which is usually the end stage of the FBR. This capsule can be up to several hundred micrometers thick, physically and physiologically separating the device from host tissue. The capsule usually lacks vasculature and is impermeable to metabolite transport. The provisional matrix becomes a zone with a high concentration of mitogens, chemoattractants, cytokines and growth factors, and other bioactive agents modulating macrophage proliferation and activation of other cell populations [63].

Mesure et al. [64] looked at the contributions of overexpressed genes using a GenMAPP analysis related to signaling and immune response in monocytes/macrophages isolated from FBRs and found that pathways related to cytokine release, innate immune response (IL-1a, IL-1b, IL-6, IL-10, and TNFa), cell adhesion (such as Icam-1, Vcam-1) and matrix remodeling (Mmp13) were the pathways that had the most overexpressed genes. This pattern of expression from inflammatory cell types will remain a common theme across FBRs in most organ systems. The same authors also noticed a progressive switch where macrophages go from the proinflammatory to an anti-inflammatory state. These two states have been canonically referred to as M1 (early, highly phagocytic response) and M2 (late stage, inflammatory resolution). The M1 and M2 paradigm fits macrophages better than it fits the immune cells of the CNS [65]. Results from transcriptomic profiling and ex vivo genome-wide expression profiling have discarded the idea that microglia may exist in states that lie on a spectrum between M1 and M2, or that they occupy either state separately. Consistent patterns of microglial responses emerging from genome-wide expression profiling are still under development.

Mechanisms Associated with Foreign Body Reaction Exclusive to the Central Nervous System

Stepping through the stage-wise response begs the question of how and why these reactions, which lead to obstruction and failure, occur around devices implanted in the CNS, and more specifically, to the shunt system ventricular catheter (Fig. 17.1).

Obstruction of the ventricular catheter dominates the discussion of pediatric shunt failure; as a result, there exists a focused effort to improve the interaction of this catheter with the CNS. The ventricular catheter's contact with CSF and neural tissue influences its patency. The CNS's response to the ventricular catheter is similar to other CNS implants, but it is also dependent on the specific location of insertion within the brain and mechanisms within that environment. Specifically, this means the response to the shunt system is dependent on contact with: CSF (entire shunt system but particularly ventricular catheter), parenchyma (ventricular catheter), subcutaneous space (valve), and the distal CSF absorption sites (peritoneum, atrium, pleural cavity, or subdural space).

CSF Contact

Since the ventricular catheter is partially bathed in CSF, hydrocephalus pathologies, and changes in fluid flow within that space, are crucial to the mechanisms by which protein adsorption and cell attachment occur (Fig. 17.1A). CSF contact yields dependencies with ependymal wall viability, CSF protein content, flow, and shear [42, 66]. A recent paradigm shift showed that flow and shear rates influence cell attachment in a similar conceptual framework to flow and shear on blood-contacting devices [67]. Using clinical shunt hardware, as flow and shear rates increase, astrocyte and microglia attachment increases [68, 69]. This occurs up to a defined threshold (shear stress approximately 0.1 N/m^2 but variable among devices), where cell attachment decreases for increasing flow [68]. It is hypothesized that increasing flow implements increased opportunity for cell integrins to bind to proteins already adsorbed to the shunt surface. But, as the flow and shear rates increase past the

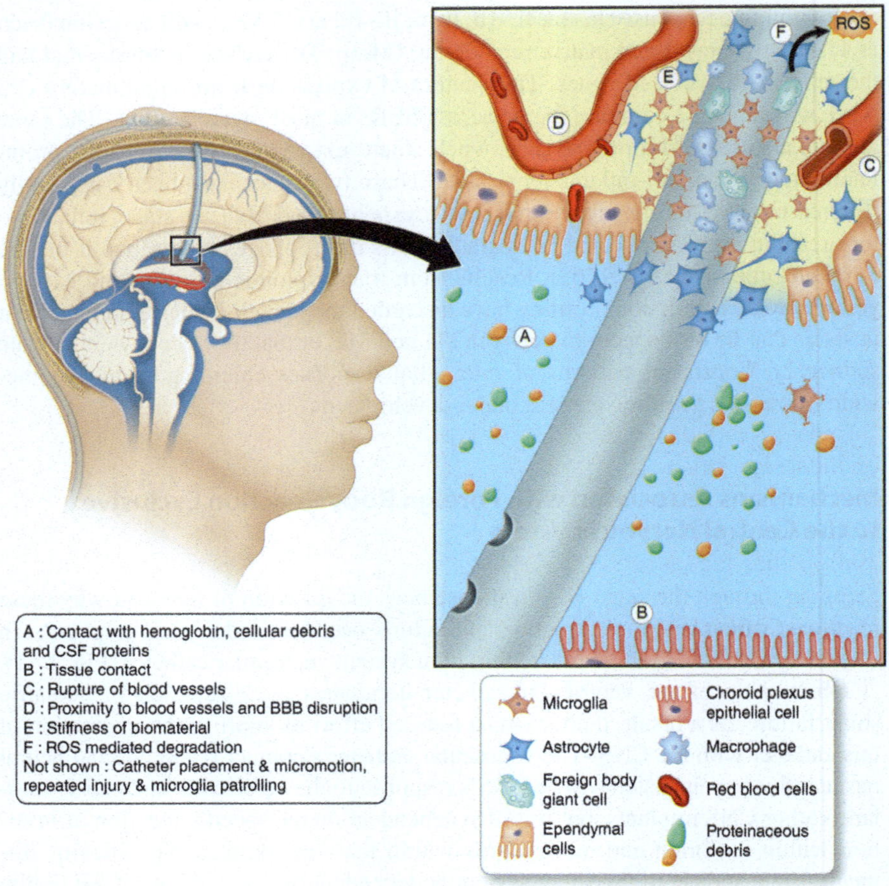

Fig. 17.1 Hypothesized mechanisms of ventricular catheter obstruction. Seen here is a sagittal view of a shunt ventricular catheter placed in the cerebral ventricles. The area around the catheter (inset) shows probable macro- and micro-triggers and responses following the ventricular catheter's placement, resulting in obstruction. For a detailed description of the scheme refer to section "Mechanisms Associated with Foreign Body Reaction Exclusive to the Central Nervous System" in this chapter. Image not to scale

aforementioned threshold, this increased propensity attach is overcome by high surface velocities that inhibit attachment [67]. These relationships are cell- and surface-dependent [39, 69].

Hemoglobin and Cellular Debris in the CSF

Metabolites of hemoglobin (Hb) may be suspended in CSF due to hydrocephalus etiology, secondary injury from hydrocephalus pathophysiology, or from injury during shunt placement (Fig. 17.1A). Mechanistically, Hb metabolites have been shown to cause inflammation of choroid plexus epithelium (CPE) and can subsequently result in hydrocephalus [70]. CPE faces damage caused by the extravasation of blood into intraventricular space; this can set off cytotoxic, oxidative and inflammatory pathways, and cause secondary tissue damage. Metabolites of extracellular Hb have been shown to activate endothelial cells through a NF-κB-mediated pathway and activate genes associated with downstream upregulation of chemotactic, proinflammatory molecules and cytokines [70]. Hemin, the oxidative form of heme, can participate in redox reactions, which release free radicals causing oxidative stress and caspase activation, injuring microglia, astrocytes and neurons [71].

Cellular debris from mechanical irritation and exfoliation may contribute to protein adsorption to ventricular catheters and surrounding inflammatory cascades; such failure is observed in intraocular lenses after the first months following implantation [72]. In a similar response, fibroblast-like cells and foreign-body giant cells adhere to the surface of intraocular lenses, degenerate, and leave an acellular proteinaceous membrane on the surface of the lens [73, 74]. The end result of this response is turbidity of the aqueous humor termed "aqueous flare", accompanied by cellular deposition. If this occurs in the CNS with ventricular catheters, it may manipulate CSF composition and influence shunt obstruction, especially when combined with shedding of the ventricular wall and a flux of CSF protein content surrounding the catheter.

Tissue Contact

Ventricular catheter-parenchymal tissue contact is thought to behave similarly to other CNS implants, which have direct tissue contact, like recording electrode probes and arrays, and deep brain stimulators. Although not directly shown on shunt systems, resident macrophages (microglia) become activated within 130 μm [75] of CNS implants immediately after implantation. Within the first 30 min, microglia begin to migrate toward the CNS implant surface where they extend their processes toward the implant and attempt to encapsulate it in their lamellipodia. With implants that are too big to be phagocytosed, microglia fail to encapsulate it and may at this stage begin to recruit more cells to the site of the implant. Within the first week of implantation, astrocytes become activated and proceed to form a compact sheet around the activated microglia over the next 2–3 weeks. This glial sheet forms a diffusion barrier with tight junctions around the CNS implant; this response is likely around the shunt system. This sheet formation is the body's attempt to reinstate homeostasis, but as a result there is secondary injury and neuronal cell death. The final stages of this process that happen over weeks to months are gliosis, scarring, and remodeling.

In the case of the shunt system specifically, astrocytes and microglia have been shown to be the dominant cell types bound directly to the catheter, they are the dominant cell types obstructing shunts, they are ubiquitous on all shunts, and their number and reactivity peak on failed shunts [76]. Astrocytes have been observed to dominate the response in catheters that had been implanted for an extended period (years), whereas microglia are dominant in the response to catheters that had been implanted for shorter periods (weeks–month) and a median between the two responses was observed in catheters implanted for an intermediate time span [2]. It has also been observed that in some cases the catheter comes in contact with and is obstructed by the choroid plexus (Fig. 17.1B).

Microglia and Patrolling

Two-photon microscopy has shown that microglia in the healthy CNS do not truly "rest," but engage in environmental surveillance by extending and retracting their processes. With this process motility, cells constantly sample their surroundings to maintain homeostasis and are able to become 'activated' if they encounter neuroprosthetics, like a shunt system [79, 80].

Size, Proximity to Blood Vessels, and Variability of Outcome

When accommodating the size of the implanted device, the brain sustains an insertion injury, which not only triggers biochemical pathways, but tears through extracellular matrix, and mechanically strains cells puncturing even distant cell membranes (Fig. 17.1C, D). The neurovascular architecture that gets damaged during the insertion of the shunt system dictates how quickly more immune cells get recruited to the injury site: damage to a major artery will have a different effect on the implant as compared to damage to many smaller capillaries. Avoiding visible blood vessels is standard of care, but should be considered when we tease apart mechanisms of failure and initial protein adsorption and cell attachment. In this light, correlations have been found between astroglial activation and proximity of the implant to the nearest major blood vessel. Shunt catheter size can also cause a local increase in pressure, pinching of the blood vessels, and subsequent ischemic and hypoxic cell death may result, caused by the reduced flow of oxygen and accumulation of waste [75, 81].

Blood–Brain Barrier Disruption

Blood–brain barrier (BBB) disruption as a consequence of hydrocephalus pathology, specific etiology (e.g., posthemorrhagic hydrocephalus), and shunt insertion can lead to an influx of plasma proteins like albumin, globulins, fibrin/fibrinogen, thrombin, plasmin, and red blood cells (Fig. 17.1D).

It is understood that the BBB disruption will lead to increased protein deposition onto CNS implant surfaces. Adsorption of CSF proteins does not occur in sufficient quantities to obstruct shunt catheters, [82] but likely contributes to cell activity in tissue and in CSF, ultimately playing a role in shunt obstruction. These plasma proteins do not increase CSF viscosity, [38, 83] but they likely play a role in cell activation and migration such that the degree of BBB disruption manipulates CSF protein content [84]. Albumin, for instance, has been shown to cause weakening of the BBB through the TGFβR (Transforming growth factor beta receptor)—MLCK (Myosin light-chain kinase) pathway [75]. Albumin has also been implicated in the activation of astrocytes through the MAPK pathway (Mitogen-activated protein kinases - a sequence of signaling proteins connecting receptors on the surface of cells to the DNA in the nucleus), upregulating the expression of IL-1β (Interleukin 1 beta), a cytokine and CX3CL1 (Fractalkine or Chemokine-(C-X3-C motif)-ligand 1), a chemokine which has been shown to induce adhesion and migration of cells. Fibrinogen and fibrin work through the TLR 4 (Toll-like receptor 4)—Mac1 (Macrophage-1 antigen) pathway, setting off phagocytic behavior in microglia [75]. The influx of plasma products can trigger the increase of ROS and reactive nitrogen species (RNS), which then act aggressively on cell lipids and proteins, increasing oxidation and exacerbating injury. This becomes a cascade when the ROS and RNS, downregulate tight junction proteins, and increases BBB permeability, allowing even more plasma proteins to enter the CNS. Proteins themselves can also participate in weakening the BBB. Some of these proteins can trigger downstream pathways that lead to increased production of ROS, which in turn can downregulate tight junction proteins [81]. This can compromise the integrity of the BBB and cause more leakage, leading to a damaging cascade in the microenvironment surrounding the device.

Stiffness

Astrocytic mechanosensitivity contributes significantly to the triggering of gliosis and FBR [77]. Around stiffer components of implants, significantly higher glial fibrillary acidic protein (GFAP) expression from reactive astrocytes and increased IL-1beta has been observed (Fig. 17.1E). Astrocytes take cues from the surface of implants to orient their filamentous structures, and under specific conditions, in response to specific features, can revert to a more primitive radial-glial phenotype [78]. Microglia are also influenced by surface features and surface chemistry, manifesting their response through a change in cytokine expression, which can intensify glial activation around the implant. In shunt ventricular catheters, astrocytes and microglia can take cues from the stiffness of the material to home themselves toward to surface, exacerbating the glial sheet formation [39].

Degradation Mediated by Reactive Oxygen Species and Enzymes

Some biomaterials rely on the degradation mediated by macrophages and the bioactive agents they release, to be cleared from the body [85]. Frustrated phagocytosis, the phenomenon where inflammatory cells are unable to successfully digest and remove the foreign body, leads to macrophages and FBGC releasing ROS and enzymes making the zone surrounding the biomaterial highly acidic [61, 86]. The high concentration of the ROS and enzymes trapped in the material's microenvironment by the fibrous capsule makes the material susceptible to degradation (Fig. 17.1F). An example of an application where this is used to our advantage is resorbable suture made of materials such as polylactic acid, polyglycolic acid, and polycaprolactone. If such ROS-mediated degradation occurs on the surface of the ventricular catheter, it could exacerbate the adsorption of CSF proteins and lead to more cellular adhesion to the catheter.

Catheter Placement and Micromotion

Although accurate catheter placement has been associated with prolonged shunt survival, [87] no conclusive guidelines have yet been defined. As was eluded earlier in the chapter, evidence seems to support the practice of surrounding the catheter tip with CSF to avoid contact with adjacent tissues; superior to the foramen of Monro and in the center of the lateral ventricle body has been identified as the ideal catheter tip position [88, 89]. Movement of the catheter and secondary collapse of ventricular walls can compound these findings. Correlations have been found between ventricular wall catheter contact and a presence of intraluminal glial tissue [90, 91]. Ultrasound-assisted ventricular catheter placements may improve catheter placement in the frontal horn [87].

Micromovement between implants and surrounding tissue has been shown to influence FBR in intracortical electrodes and other CNS implants and may play a similar role in exacerbating the FBR to a shunt system, particularly when it is secured to the skull [81]. Cells within 60 μm have been shown to incur damage from micromotion due to respiration, neck movement, and external vibrations [92, 93]. To this extent, the rate of insertion may also play some role in shunt catheter FBR.

Repeated Injury with Shunt Revisions

Markers in the CSF can be used to evaluate axonal damage, amyloid deposition, and synaptic loss in patients who have had repetitive mild traumatic brain injury (TBI) [94]. Neurodegenerative disorders, mainly Alzheimer's disease, have been linked to increased levels of CSF neurogranin, neurofilament light protein (a structural protein), GFAP, and other markers that reflect synaptic degeneration, glial activation, and injury to axons in the white matter. Considering these correlations, it is within reason to speculate that patients who have had multiple revisions will have markers in the CSF that could cause aggravated responses to their new catheter. An objective future assessment of these markers can help predict outcome of shunting.

A Response Beyond the Inflammatory FBR

While the initial influx and attachment of astrocytes and microglia in and around the shunt system is a crucial phase of shunt failure, [76, 91] choroid plexus and ependymal cells can subsequently attach and obstruct the catheter. Catheter contact with the ependymal wall causes ependymal denudation within 1 week of direct contact [95]. In animal and clinical models, tissue from the ventricular surface invaginates catheter holes [95, 96]. This is likely a result of direct tissue contact from catheter movement or misplacement, or conditions of overdrainage and SVS, and contain ependyma but largely vascularized astroglial pedicles.

For decades, choroid plexus infiltration has been indicated as one of the major mediators of shunt failure [14]. Recently, however, the role of the choroid plexus has been minimized. Especially considering its limited reactivity and drive to obstruct, choroid plexus in the catheter lumen is considered relatively rare (7%) [97]. Gross analyses of shunt catheters removed following failure is not an accurate measure of ingrowth and may have swayed our reliance on the hypothesis of choroid plexus being a major player for years.

Blood-derived immune cell types, namely lymphocytes, multinucleated giant cells, "connective tissue"/fibroblasts, and leptomeninges/mesothelial cells also attach [98]. The mechanism or role of these cells in overall obstruction is yet to be determined.

Distal Catheter Response

With a similar response to the basic FBR cascade, the distal (peritoneal) catheter can present with an initial host response and encapsulation. However, the peritoneal catheter does not fail at the rate of the proximal (ventricular) catheter, perhaps because of variability in organ system (environment), proximity to tissue, or degree of variability between intracranial and intra-abdominal pressure. Interestingly, there is recent speculation that peritoneal catheters fail more rapidly than ventricular catheter in adult cohorts.

Evolutionary Perspective: What Response Has the Brain Evolved to Produce to Brain Injury?

To fully understand the brain's response to an implanted material, and disentangle the mechanisms involved, it is worth asking if human brains have evolved a means to survive intrusion by a foreign object or a TBI. Weil et al. [99] note that individuals with such injuries should be evolutionarily selected. However, the very nature of these injuries makes survival (and therefore selection) highly implausible. It may be that the systems responsible for healthy brain function respond maladaptively under injury conditions. The response we see to biomaterials placed in the brain is likely a combination of (1) the brain's evolved responses to insults that guided evolution, and (2) the atypical, anomalous behavior of otherwise stable systems.

The classical role of inflammation is to protect against infection and to aid in repair through regeneration, and recent evidence after injury suggests that this may be true for the brain as well [100]. However, evidence has also shown that biomaterial adherent-macrophages/FBGCs have a cytokine profile that does not match either classically or alternatively activated macrophages [101]. In the future, a clearer understanding of cell–material interactions in the brain, especially their evolutionary underpinning, may help design therapies that can selectively modulate facets of the foreign body response.

Shunt Modifications

Since the inception of the shunt system, there have been significant modifications to the shunt valve, with manipulations ad nauseum to the functionality of the one-way pressure regulated valve. Because of the incredible renovation of the shunt valve, including the additions like antisiphon devices, patient care is dramatically improved. However, there have been limited modifications to the ventricular or peritoneal catheters: less than 40 significant modifications in the primary literature, even including those unsuccessful or suspended for funding issues. These modifications can be classified in multiple ways: based on the targeted stage of the FBR, [102] based on the nature of the approach (active or passive), or based on the nature of the modification (physical or chemical). Of course, not all modification strategies fall neatly into one category or the other.

An underlying commonality in the modification themes involving coatings or surface modification has been to improve the degree of wetting as a means to reduce protein adsorption. This strategy may, however, only show its benefits in the short term since the bulk of the catheter must still come in contact with the ventricular space and the cortex, where it will provoke a response due to bulk factors such as flow, BBB disruption, size, and stiffness [103]. To improve this long-term response, future modification strategies must hone in on inhibiting specific stages of the FBR, interrogate the glial bridge necessary for cells to bind, proliferate, and obstruct the shunt catheter, and take biointegration into consideration. Here we describe limited modifications that aid in our understanding of the molecular and bulk mechanisms governing cell–material interactions, which can be used to tackle specific steps of the inflammatory cascade to achieve long-term, sustainable outcomes.

Shunt modifications have taken advantage of a classic tier of biomaterial research in which polymer coatings are used to alter the interaction at the interface of the device and its environment. A few key examples of this strategy with shunt catheters include PVP (Bioglide by Medtronic); short- and long-chain monofunctional polyethylene glycol [29, 104]; *N*-acetyl-L-cysteine; [104] poly (3,4-ethylenedioxythiophene); e-PTFE, and poly (2-hydroxyethyl methacrylate) [2]. Trypsin, a proteolytic enzyme, has been immobilized onto the catheter surface to suppress the adhesive behavior of cells; [105] this is an example of an alternative to hydrogel coatings where a molecule is directly conjugated onto an implant's surface.

Some groups have worked on manipulating the architecture of the ventricular catheter based on physical surface properties, and how flow and shear stress affect cell attachment. Some examples of such architectural modifications are: adding flanges to catheters (Portnoy catheter), [2] using a floatation cell to keep the catheter tip away from tissue, manipulating hole size, [68] altering hole geometries such as rectangular bores with angled troughs to prevent direct exposure of the drainage holes, [43] and expandable membranes that filter CSF [106].

Attempts have also been made to produce "active" catheter designs that target obstruction while the cell and tissue attachment events are in progress, as opposed to previous techniques that are preventative. For example, these include, but are not limited to, a "self-cleaning" ventricular catheter with cantilever-based magnetic microactuators that physically disrupt obstructions [107].

Approaches such as cell-seeded biodegradable polymer coatings' [102, 108, 109] may hold promise because they address biointegration of the catheter. Future biomaterials could move adhering microglia toward a noninflammatory phenotype using surface chemistry [78]. Electrically conductive polymer coatings could be used to suppress microglia and astrocyte activation in the brain [110].

References

1. Weisenberg SH, TerMaath SC, Seaver CE, Killeffer JA. Ventricular catheter development: past, present, and future. J Neurosurg. 2016; Epub ahead:1–9.
2. Harris CA, McAllister JP. What we should know about the cellular and tissue response causing catheter obstruction in the treatment of hydrocephalus. Neurosurgery. 2012;70(6):1589–601.
3. Browd S. Bioengineering advancements to hydrocephalus treatment. In: Center for Integrative Brain Research Internal Review, Seattle Children's Research Institute. Seattle; 2012.
4. Enchev Y, Oi S. Historical trends of neuroendoscopic surgical techniques in the treatment of hydrocephalus. Neurosurg Rev. 2008;31(3):249–62.

5. Al-Tamimi YZ, Sinha P, Chumas PD, Crimmins D, Drake J, Kestle J, et al. Ventriculoperitoneal shunt 30-day failure rate: A retrospective international cohort study. Neurosurgery. 2014;74(1):29.
6. Riva-Cambrin J, Kestle JRW, Holubkov R, Butler J, Kulkarni AV, Drake J, et al. Risk factors for shunt malfunction in pediatric hydrocephalus: a multicenter prospective cohort study. J Neurosurg Pediatr. 2016;17(4):382.
7. Chen H, Riva-Cambrin J, Brockmeyer DL, Walker ML, Kestle JR. Shunt failure due to intracranial migration of BioGlide ventricular catheters. J Neurosurg Pediatr. 2011;7(4):408–12.
8. Khan F, Shamim MS, Rehman A, Bari ME. Analysis of factors affecting ventriculoperitoneal shunt survival in pediatric patients. Childs Nerv Syst. 2013;29(5):791.
9. Khan F, Rehman A, Shamim MS, Bari ME. Factors affecting ventriculoperitoneal shunt survival in adult patients. Surg Neurol Int. 2015;6:25.
10. Tuli S, O'Hayon B, Drake JM, Clarke M, Kestle J. Change in ventricular size and effect of ventricular catheter placement in pediatric patients with shunted hydrocephalus. Neurosurgery. 1999;45(6):1329–33.
11. Whitehead WE, Riva-Cambrin J, Kulkarni A, Wellons JC, Rozzelle CJ, Tamber M, et al. Ventricular catheter entry site and not catheter tip location predicts shunt survival: a secondary analysis of 3 large pediatric hydrocephalus studies. J neurosurg Pediatr [Internet]. 2017 [cited 2017 Oct 24];19(19):157–67. Available from: http://thejns.org/doi/pdf/10.3171/2016.8.PEDS16229.
12. Hanak BW, Bonow RH, Harris CA, Browd SR. Cerebrospinal fluid shunting complications in children. Pediatr Neurosurg [Internet]. 2017 [cited 2017 Oct 24];(0). Available from: http://www.ncbi.nlm.nih.gov/pubmed/28249297.
13. Drake JM, Kestle JR, Tuli S. CSF shunts 50 years on--past, present, and future. Childs Nerv Syst. 2000;16(10–11):800–4.
14. Molina ME, Lema A, Palacios MG, Somoza I, Tellado M, Pita S, et al. 25 years experience in cerebrospinal shunt. Are new systems better? Cir Pediatr. 2008;21(4):223–7.
15. McGirt MJ, Leveque J-C, Wellons JC, Villavicencio AT, Hopkins JS, Fuchs HE, et al. Cerebrospinal fluid shunt survival and etiology of failures: a seven-year institutional experience. Pediatr Neurosurg [Internet]. 2002 [cited 2017 Oct 24];36(5):248–55. Available from: http://www.ncbi.nlm.nih.gov/pubmed/12053043.
16. Choux M, Genitori L, Lang D, Lena G. Shunt implantation: reducing the incidence of shunt infection. J Neurosurg [Internet]. 1992 [cited 2017 Oct 13];77(6):875–80. Available from: http://thejns.org/doi/10.3171/jns.1992.77.6.0875.
17. Simon TD, Butler J, Whitlock KB, Browd SR, Holubkov R, Kestle JRW, et al. Risk factors for first cerebrospinal fluid shunt infection: findings from a multi-center prospective cohort study. J Pediatr [internet]. 2014 [cited 2017 Oct 24];164(6):1462–8.e2. Available from: http://www.ncbi.nlm.nih.gov/pubmed/24661340.
18. Kestle JR, Garton HJ, Whitehead WE, Drake JM, Kulkarni AV, Cochrane DD, et al. Management of shunt infections: a multicenter pilot study. J Neurosurg. 2006;105(3 Suppl):177–81.
19. Simon TD, Hall M, Riva-Cambrin J, Albert JE, Jeffries HE, Lafleur B, et al. Infection rates following initial cerebrospinal fluid shunt placement across pediatric hospitals in the United States. J Neurosurg Pediatr. 2009;4(2):156–65.
20. Bayston R, Milner RD. Antimicrobial activity of silicone rubber used in hydrocephalus shunts, after impregnation with antimicrobial substances. J Clin Pathol. 1981;34(9):1057–62.
21. Bayston R, Grove N, Siegel J, Lawellin D, Barsham S. Prevention of hydrocephalus shunt catheter colonisation in vitro by impregnation with antimicrobials. J Neurol Neurosurg Psychiatry. 1989;52(5):605–9.
22. Jenkinson MD, Gamble C, Hartley JC, Hickey H, Hughes D, Blundell M, et al. The British antibiotic and silver-impregnated catheters for ventriculoperitoneal shunts multi-Centre randomised controlled trial (the BASICS trial): study protocol. Trials. 2014 Jan;15(1):4.
23. Winkler KML, Woernle CM, Seule M, Held U, Bernays RL, Keller E. Antibiotic-impregnated versus silver-bearing external ventricular drainage catheters: preliminary results in a randomized controlled trial. Neurocrit Care. 2013 Apr;18(2):161–5.

24. Fichtner J, Güresir E, Seifert V, Raabe A. Efficacy of silver-bearing external ventricular drainage catheters: a retrospective analysis. J Neurosurg. 2010 Apr;112(4):840–6.
25. Xu H, Huang Y, Jiao W, Sun W, Li R, Li J, et al. Hydrogel-coated ventricular catheters for high-risk patients receiving ventricular peritoneum shunt. Medicine (Baltimore). 2016 Jul;95(29):e4252.
26. Ritz R, Roser F, Morgalla M, Dietz K, Tatagiba M, Will BE. Do antibiotic-impregnated shunts in hydrocephalus therapy reduce the risk of infection? An observational study in 258 patients. BMC Infect Dis. 2007 Dec;7(1):38.
27. Konstantelias AA, Vardakas KZ, Polyzos KA, Tansarli GS, Falagas ME. Antimicrobial-impregnated and -coated shunt catheters for prevention of infections in patients with hydrocephalus: a systematic review and meta-analysis. J Neurosurg. 2015 May;122(5):1096–112.
28. Brydon HL, Bayston R, Hayward R, Harkness W, Hayward R, Harkness W. Reduced bacterial adhesion to hydrocephalus shunt catheters mediated by cerebrospinal fluid proteins. J Neurol Neurosurg Psychiatry [Internet]. 1996 [cited 2017 Jul 28];60(6):671–5. Available from: http://www.ncbi.nlm.nih.gov/pubmed/8648336.
29. Berstrom K, Osterberg E, Holmberg K, Hoffman AS, Schuman TP, Kozlowski A, et al. Effects of branching and molecular weight of surface-bound poly(ethylene oxide) on protein rejection. J Biomater Sci Polym Ed. 1994;6(2):123–32.
30. Aldrich F, Harmann P. Disconnection as a cause of Ventriculoperitoneal shunt malfunction in multicomponent shunt systems. Pediatr Neurosurg. 1990;16(6):309–12.
31. Boelens JJ, Zaat SA, Meeldijk J, Dankert J. Subcutaneous abscess formation around catheters induced by viable and nonviable Staphylococcus epidermidis as well as by small amounts of bacterial cell wall components. J Biomed Mater Res. 2000;50(4):546–56.
32. Kaufmann AM, Lye T, Redekop G, Brevner A, Hamilton M, Kozey M, et al. Infection rates in standard vs. hydrogel coated ventricular catheters. Can J Neurol Sci. 2004;31(4):506–10.
33. Kestle JR, Riva-Cambrin J, Wellons JC, Kulkarni AV, Whitehead WE, Walker ML, et al. A standardized protocol to reduce cerebrospinal fluid shunt infection: the hydrocephalus clinical research network quality improvement initiative. J Neurosurg Pediatr. 2011;8(1):22–9.
34. Sainte-Rose C, Piatt JH, Renier D, Pierre-Kahn A, Hirsch JF, Hoffman HJ, et al. Mechanical complications in shunts. Pediatr Neurosurg. 1991–1992;17(1):2–9.
35. Venkataraman P, Browd SR, Lutz BR. A physical framework for implementing virtual models of intracranial pressure and cerebrospinal fluid dynamics in hydrocephalus shunt testing. J Neurosurg Pediatr [Internet]. 2016;18(3):296–305. Available from: http://www.ncbi.nlm.nih.gov/pubmed/27203135.
36. Lutz B, Venkataraman P, Browd S. New and improved ways to treat hydrocephalus: Pursuit of a smart shunt. Surg Neurol Int [Internet]. 2013 [cited 2017 Jun 30];4(2):38. Available from: http://surgicalneurologyint.com/surgicalint-articles/new-and-improved-ways-to-treat-hydrocephalus-pursuit-of-a-smart-shunt/.
37. Marupudi NI, Pavri T, Harris C, Haridas A, Ham S, Sood S. Lumbar-peritoneal shunting in hydrocephalus: preventing chiari malformations and decreasing shunt revisions. In: AANS 2016 annual scientific meeting [Internet]. Chicago: J Neurosurg; 2016 [cited 2017 Nov 1]. p. A1205–6. Available from: http://thejns.org/doi/pdf/10.3171/2016.4.JNS.AANS2016abstracts.
38. Brydon HL, Hayward R, Harkness W, Bayston R. Physical properties of cerebrospinal fluid of relevance to shunt function. 1: the effect of protein upon CSF viscosity. Br J Neurosurg. 1995;9(5):639–44.
39. Harris CA, Resau JH, Hudson EA, West RA, Moon C, McAllister JP. Mechanical contributions to astrocyte adhesion using a novel in vitro model of catheter obstruction. Exp Neurol. 2010;222(2):204–10.
40. Czosnyka Z, Czosnyka M, Richards H, Pickard JD. Hydrodynamic properties of hydrocephalus shunts. Acta Neurochir Suppl. 1998;71:334–9.
41. Weisenberg SH. Improving ventricular catheter design through computational fluid dynamics. [cited 2017 Nov 1]; Available from: http://trace.tennessee.edu/utk_gradthes/3817.

42. Thomale UW, Hosch H, Koch A, Schulz M, Stoltenburg G, Haberl EJ, et al. Performation holes in ventricular catheters -- is less more? Childs Nerv Syst. 2010;26(6):781–9.
43. Gimenez A, Galarza M, Pellicer O, Valero J, Amigo JM. Influence of the hole geometry on the flow distribution in ventricular catheters for hydrocephalus. Biomed Eng Online. 2016;15(Suppl 1):71.
44. Linford RG, Ryan NW. Pulsatile flow in rigid tubes. J Appl Physiol. 1965;20(5):1078–82.
45. Giménez Á, Galarza M, Thomale U, Schuhmann MU, Valero J, Amigó JM. Pulsatile flow in ventricular catheters for hydrocephalus. Philos Trans R Soc A Math Eng Sci [Internet]. 2017 [cited 2017 Nov 1];375(2096):20160294. Available from: http://www.ncbi.nlm.nih.gov/pubmed/28507239.
46. Warf BC. Endoscopic third ventriculostomy and choroid plexus cauterization for pediatric hydrocephalus. Clin Neurosurg. 2007;54:78–82.
47. Warf BC. Pediatric hydrocephalus in east Africa: prevalence, causes, treatments, and strategies for the future. World Neurosurg. 2010;73:296–300.
48. Warf BC, Dewan M, Mugamba J. Management of Dandy-Walker complex-associated infant hydrocephalus by combined endoscopic third ventriculostomy and choroid plexus cauterization. J Neurosurg Pediatr. 2011;8(4):377–83.
49. Warf BC. Hydrocephalus in Uganda: the predominance of infectious origin and primary management with endoscopic third ventriculostomy. J Neurosurg. 2005;102(1 Suppl):1–15.
50. Liu TL, Zahedi S, Garling RJ, Kralickk F, Harris CA, Cheng MMC. Prosthetic arachnoid granulations using 3D printing technology. In: Proceedings of the IEEE international conference on micro electro mechanical systems (MEMS). 2017. p. 542–5.
51. Kralick F, Oh J, Medina T, Noh HM. Micro-fabricated shunt to mimic arachnoid granulations for the treatment of communicating hydrocephalus. Acta Neurochir Suppl. 2012;114:239–42.
52. Oh J, Liu K, Medina T, Kralick F, Noh HM. A novel microneedle array for the treatment of hydrocephalus. Microsyst Technol. 2014;20(6):1169–79.
53. Schwerdt HN, Amjad U, Appel J, Elhadi AM, Lei T, Preul MC, et al. In vitro hydrodynamic, transient, and overtime performance of a miniaturized valve for hydrocephalus. Ann Biomed Eng. 2015;43(3):603–15.
54. Schwerdt HN, Bristol RE, Chae J. Miniaturized passive hydrogel check valve for hydrocephalus treatment. J Neurosurg [Internet] 2015;7(1):1205–18. Available from: https://doi.org/10.1016/j.mpaic.2015.01.003%5Cnhttp://www.annualreviews.org/doi/10.1146/annurev.bioeng.2.1.457%5Cnhttp://dx.doi.org/10.1016/j.joms.2016.02.004%5Cnhttp://dx.doi.org/10.1063/1.4905840%5Cnhttp://xlink.rsc.org/?DOI=C5LC00685F%5Cnhttp://dx.do.
55. CereVasc. Minimally invasive treatment of hydrocephalus | CereVasc [Internet]. [cited 2017 Nov 1]. Available from: http://cerevasc.com/treatment-of-hydrocephalus/.
56. Eskandari R, Packer M, Burdett EC, McAllister JP. Effect of delayed intermittent ventricular drainage on ventriculomegaly and neurological deficits in experimental neonatal hydrocephalus. Childs Nerv Syst. 2012;28(11):1849–61.
57. Lee J-B, Ahn H-Y, Lee H-J, Yang J-H, Yi J-S, Lee I-W. Cerebrospinal fluid lumbar tapping utilization for suspected ventriculoperitoneal shunt under-drainage malfunctions. J Korean Neurosurg Soc [Internet]. 2017 [cited 2017 Nov 1];60(1):1–7. Available from: https://doi.org/10.3340/jkns.2016.0404.002.
58. Drake JM, Kestle JR, Milner R, Cinalli G, Boop F, Piatt JJ, et al. Randomized trial of cerebrospinal fluid shunt valve design in pediatric hydrocephalus. Neurosurgery. 1998;43(2):294–5.
59. Millward CP, Perez da Rosa S, Williams D, Kokai G, Byrne A, Pettorini B. Foreign body granuloma secondary to ventriculo-peritoneal shunt: a rare scenario with a new insight. Pediatr Neurosurg [Internet]. 2013 [cited 2017 Oct 31];49(4):236–9. Available from: https://www.karger.com/Article/FullText/363330.
60. Harris CA, McAllister JP. Systems and methods for simulating flow of cerebrospinal fluid. Utah U of, editor. United States; 2010.
61. Anderson JM, Rodriguez A, Chang DT. Foreign body reaction to biomaterials. Semin Immunol. 2008;20:86.

62. Kim J-K, Scott EA, Elbert DL. Proteomic analysis of protein adsorption: serum amyloid P adsorbs to materials and promotes leukocyte adhesion. J Biomed Mater Res A. 2005 Oct;75(1):199–209.
63. Warburg O, Posener O, Negelein K, Hanahan E, Weinberg D, Hu RA. All charged up about implanted biomaterials. Nat Publ Gr. 2013;31(45):309–44.
64. Mesure L, De Visscher G, Vranken I, Lebacq A, Flameng W. Gene expression study of monocytes/macrophages during early foreign body reaction and identification of potential precursors of myofibroblasts. PLoS One. 2010;5(9):e12949.
65. Dondossola E, Holzapfel BM, Alexander S, Filippini S, Hutmacher DW, Friedl P. Examination of the foreign body response to biomaterials by nonlinear intravital microscopy. Nat Biomed Eng. 2016;1:0007. https://doi.org/10.1038/s41551-016-0007.
66. Ginsberg HJ, Sum A, Drake JM, Cobbold RS. Ventriculoperitoneal shunt flow dependency on the number of patent holes in a ventricular catheter. Pediatr Neurosurg. 2000;33(1):7–11.
67. Zhu C, Yago T, Lou J, Zarnitsyna VI, McEver RP. Mechanisms for flow-enhanced cell adhesion. Ann Biomed Eng. 2008;36(4):604–21.
68. Harris CA, McAllister JP. Does drainage hole size influence adhesion on ventricular catheters? Childs Nerv Syst. 2011;27(8):1221–32.
69. Harris CA, Resau JH, Hudson EA, West RA, Moon C, Black AD, et al. Effects of surface wettability, flow and protein concentration on macrohage and astrocyte adhesion in an in vitro model of central nervous system catheter obstruction. J Biomed Mater Res A. 2011;97(4):433–40.
70. Gram M, Sveinsdottir S, Cinthio M, Sveinsdottir K, Hansson SR, Mörgelin M, et al. Extracellular hemoglobin - mediator of inflammation and cell death in the choroid plexus following preterm intraventricular hemorrhage. J Neuroinflammation. 2014 Dec;11(1):200.
71. Karimy JK, Zhang J, Kurland DB, Theriault BC, Duran D, Stokum JA, et al. Inflammation-dependent cerebrospinal fluid hypersecretion by the choroid plexus epithelium in posthemorrhagic hydrocephalus. Nat Med [Internet]. 2017;advance on (July). Available from: https://doi.org/10.1038/nm.4361%0Ahttp://10.0.4.14/nm.4361%0Ahttp://www.nature.com/nm/journal/vaop/ncurrent/abs/nm.4361.html#supplementary-information.
72. Go KG, Ebels EJ, van Woerden H. Experiences with recurring ventricular catheter obstructions. Clin Neurol Neurosurg. 1981;83(2):47–56.
73. Özyol P, Özyol E, Karel F. Biocompatibility of intraocular lenses. Türk Oftalmol Derg. 2017;47(4):221–5.
74. Huang X-D, Yao K, Zhang Z, Zhang Y, Wang Y. Uveal and capsular biocompatibility of an intraocular lens with a hydrophilic anterior surface and a hydrophobic posterior surface. J Cataract Refract Surg. 2010 Feb;36(2):290–8.
75. Kozai TDY, Jaquins-Gerstl AS, Vazquez AL, Michael AC, Cui XT. Brain tissue responses to neural implants impact signal sensitivity and intervention strategies. ACS Chem Neurosci. 2015;6:48.
76. Hanak B, Ross EF, Harris CA, Browd S, Shain W. Toward a better understanding of the cellular basis for cerebrospinal fluid shunt obstruction: report on the construction of a bank of explanted hydrocephalus devices. J Neurosurg Pediatr. 2016:1–11. https://doi.org/10.3171/2016.2.PEDS15531.
77. Moshayedi P, Ng G, Kwok JCF, Yeo GSH, Bryant CE, Fawcett JW, et al. The relationship between glial cell mechanosensitivity and foreign body reactions in the central nervous system. Biomaterials. 2014;35(13):3919–25.
78. Pêgo AP, Pires LR, Rocha DN, Ambrosio L. The role of the surface on microglia function: implications for central nervous system tissue engineering.
79. Cherry JD, Olschowka JA, O'Banion M. Neuroinflammation and M2 microglia: the good, the bad, and the inflamed. J Neuroinflammation. 2014 Jun;11(1):98.
80. Ransohoff RM. A polarizing question: do M1 and M2 microglia exist? Nat Neurosci. 2016;19(8):987–91.
81. Saxena T, Karumbaiah L, Gaupp EA, Patkar R, Patil K, Betancur M, et al. The impact of chronic blood–brain barrier breach on intracortical electrode function. Biomaterials. 2013 Jul;34(20):4703–13.

82. Brydon HL, Keir G, Thompson EJ, Bayston R, Hayward R, Harkness W. Protein adsorption to hydrocephalus shunt catheters: CSF protein adsorption. J Neurol Neurosurg Psychiatry. 1998;64(5):643–7.
83. Bloomfield IG, Johnston IH, Bilston LE. Effects of proteins, blood cells and glucose on the viscosity of cerebrospinal fluid. Pediatr Neurosurg. 1998;28(5):246–51.
84. Jaeger CB, Winn SR, Tresco PA, Aebischer P. Repair of the blood-brain barrier following implantation of polymer capsules. Brain Res. 1991;551(1–2):163–70.
85. Sheikh Z, Brooks PJ, Barzilay O, Fine N, Glogauer M. Macrophages, foreign body giant cells and their response to implantable biomaterials. Materials. 2015;8:5671.
86. Love RJ, Jones KS. 2013. The recognition of biomaterials: Pattern recognition of medical polymers and their adsorbed biomolecules. J Biomed Mater Res Part A 2013:101A:2740–52.
87. Whitehead WE, Riva-Cambrin J, Wellons JC, Kulkarni AV, Browd S, Limbrick D, et al. Factors associated with ventricular catheter movement and inaccurate catheter location: post hoc analysis of the hydrocephalus clinical research network ultrasound-guided shunt placement study. J Neurosurg Pediatr J Neurosurg Pediatr. 2014;14(14):173–8.
88. Kemp J, Flannery A, DA Tamber M. Pediatric hydrocephalus: systematic literature review and evidence-based guidelines. Part 9: effect of ventricular catheter entry point and position. J Neurosurg Pediatr. 2014;14:72–6.
89. Yamada SM, Kitagawa R, Teramoto A. Relationship of the location of the ventricular catheter tip and function of the ventriculoperitoneal shunt. J Clin Neurosci. 2013 Jan;20(1):99–101.
90. Blegvad C, Skjolding AD, Broholm H, Laursen H, Juhler M. Pathophysiology of shunt dysfunction in shunt treated hydrocephalus. Acta Neurochir. 2013; epub ahead.
91. Del Bigio MR. Biological reactions to cerebrospinal fluid shunt devices: a review of the cellular pathology. Neurosurgery. 1998;42(2):319–25.
92. Sridharan A, Rajan SD, Muthuswamy J, Nguyen JK, Capadona JR, Stice P, et al. Brain micromotion around implants in the rodent. J Neural Eng. 2006;3:189–95.
93. Polanco M, Bawab S, Yoon H. Computational assessment of neural probe and brain tissue Interface under transient motion. Biosensors. 2016 Jun;6(2):27.
94. Shahim P, Tegner Y, Gustafsson B, Gren M, Ärlig J, Olsson M, et al. Neurochemical aftermath of repetitive mild traumatic brain injury. JAMA Neurol. 2016 Nov;73(11):1308.
95. Del Bigio MR, Bruni JE. Reaction of rabbit lateral periventricular tissue to shunt tubing implants. J Neurosurg. 1986;64(6):932–40.
96. Kraemer M, Iskandar BJ. Overdrainage-related ventricular tissue is a significant cause of proximal shunt obstruction. In: American Association of Neurological Surgeons. Chicago; 2016.
97. Sarkiss CA, Sarkar R, Yong W, Lazareff JA. Time dependent pattern of cellular characteristics causing ventriculoperitoneal shunt failure in children. Clin Neurol Neurosurg. 2014;127:30–2.
98. Sekhar LN, Moossy J, Norman GA. Malfunctioning ventriculoperitoneal shunts. J Neurosurg. 1982;56(3):411–6.
99. Weil ZM, Norman GJ, DeVries AC, Nelson RJ. The injured nervous system: a Darwinian perspective. Prog Neurobiol. 2008;86(1):48–59.
100. Jeong H-K, Ji K, Min K, Joe E-H. Brain inflammation and microglia: facts and misconceptions. Exp Neurobiol. 2013;22:59.
101. Jones JA, Chang DT, Meyerson H, Colton E, Kwon IK, Matsuda T, et al. Proteomic analysis and quantification of cytokines and chemokines from biomaterial surface-adherent macrophages and foreign body giant cells. J Biomed Mater Res A. 2007 Dec;83A(3):585–96.
102. Lotti F, Ranieri F, Vadalà G, Zollo L, DPino G. Invasive intraneural interfaces: Foreign body reaction issues. Front Neurosci. 2017;11:1–14.
103. Leung BK, Biran R, Underwood CJ, Tresco PA. Characterization of microglial attachment and cytokine release on biomaterials of differing surface chemistry. Biomaterials. 2008;29(23):3289–97.
104. Harris CA, Resau JH, Hudson EA, West RA, Moon C, Black AD, et al. Reduction of protein adsorption and macrophage and astrocyte adhesion on ventricular catheters by polyethylene glycol and N-acetyl- L -cysteine. J Biomed Mater Res A. 2011;98A(3):425–33.

105. Achyuta AKH, Stephens KD, Lewis HGP, Murthy SK. Mitigation of reactive human cell adhesion on poly(dimethylsiloxane) by immobilized trypsin. Langmuir. 2010 Mar;26(6):4160–7.
106. Medow J. The permeable proximal catheter project: a novel approach to preventing shunt obstruction. In: American Association of Neurological Surgeons Annual Meeting, Pediatric Section; 2005.
107. Yang Q, Nguyen T, Liu C, Miller J, Rhoads JF, Linnes J, et al. Polyimide-based magnetic microactuators for biofouling removal. 2016;1–14.
108. Damanik FFR, Rothuizen TC, van Blitterswijk C, Rotmans JI, Moroni L. Towards an in vitro model mimicking the foreign body response: tailoring the surface properties of biomaterials to modulate extracellular matrix. Sci Rep. 2015 May;4(1):6325.
109. Lee I, Vacanti JP, Taylor GA, Madsen JR. The living shunt: a tissue engineering approach in the treatment of hydrocephalus. Neurol Res. 2000;22(1):105–10.
110. Zhou K, Motamed S, Thouas GA, Bernard CC, Li D, Parkington HC, et al. Graphene functionalized scaffolds reduce the inflammatory response and supports endogenous neuroblast migration when implanted in the adult brain. Zhao F, editor. PLoS One. 2016;11(3):e0151589.

Endoscopic Third Ventriculostomy with Choroid Plexus Cauterization (ETV–CPC) Versus CSF Shunting

18

William B. Lo and Abhaya V. Kulkarni

Introduction

Cerebrospinal fluid (CSF) shunting remains the commonest surgical treatment for pediatric hydrocephalus of all etiologies since its invention in the 1950s. However, shunt complication rates, especially in infants, are high. Endoscopic treatment options have proved to be an effective alternative, with endoscopic third ventriculostomy (ETV), developed in the 1990s, being the commonest. However, ETV alone has a low success rate in infants, who are the largest age group for new onset hydrocephalus [1]. In the 2000s, Warf, at the CURE Children's Hospital of Uganda, showed that the addition of choroid plexus cauterization (CPC) to ETV was a safe and effective alternative, especially in infants [2, 3]. Warf's innovative development of the modern endoscopic CPC and robust scientific study in the unique setting brought a renaissance of choroid plexus obliteration to treat hydrocephalus. This chapter recounts the history of choroid plexus surgery, explains its biologic and pathophysiologic basis, describes the operative technique and outcome of ETV+CPC in the global setting, and compares it with other conventional treatments.

W. B. Lo · A. V. Kulkarni (✉)
Division of Neurosurgery, Hospital for Sick Children,
University of Toronto, Toronto, ON, Canada
e-mail: abhaya.kulkarni@sickkids.ca

D. D. Limbrick, J. R. Leonard (eds.), *Cerebrospinal Fluid Disorders*,
https://doi.org/10.1007/978-3-319-97928-1_18

Background

While CSF shunts, in particular ventriculoperitoneal (VP) shunts, have been the mainstay of treatment for hydrocephalus and saved many lives in the past 50 years, they are also associated with various time-dependent and shunt-specific complications. The risks are present for life and ongoing surveillance is required. Briefly, complications of shunting include infection (5–10%), obstruction (30–40% in the first 2 years), and overdrainage (10–15%) [4–6]. In addition to medical morbidity, any history of shunt infection, a history of 2 or more shunt revisions, and longer hospital stay for treatment of shunt complications are associated with worse long-term cognitive outcome and quality of life [7–10]. Furthermore, shunt insertion and complications place burden on the health care systems and carry an economic impact. In the United States, each year pediatric hydrocephalus accounts for over 38,000 admissions, 400,000 hospital days, and total hospital charges of $1.4–2.0 billion, equivalent to 3.1% of all pediatric hospital charges [11].

Since the early 1990s, with the improvement in endoscopy technology and surgical techniques, ETV has become the main alternative to shunting for hydrocephalus [12]. Because there is no implanted foreign shunt material, the main advantage of ETV is a lower infection rate [13]. As a result, in carefully selected patients, if an ETV remains complication-free at 6 months, the risk of developing any complication in the future is lower than compared to shunt (Fig. 18.1) [14–16]. Over the course of a lifetime, the better longevity translates to a significant improvement in recurrent clinical morbidities and, potentially, quality of life, although this has not been definitively shown.

Despite the promising medium-term results of ETV in some patient groups, ETV still carries a significant failure rate for many. The ETV Success Score (ETVSS), a predictive tool for probability of ETV success has identified age, etiology, and history of previous shunt as major contributing factors (Fig. 18.2) [1]. Infants have the highest associated failure rate, and thus ETV alone is rarely offered to this group of patients. Furthermore, the good ETV outcome reported by academic centers may not be reflective of all institutes in general. A recent retrospective analysis of for 5416 infants with hydrocephalus at 41 children's hospitals in the Pediatric Health Information Systems database showed that the 1-year failure rate was higher for ETV compared to shunt (65% vs 40%) [17]. Although this study included a heterogeneous population and contained a methodological limitation and an inherent selection bias, it potentially reveals "real-life" hydrocephalus treatment.

In the early 2000s, the addition of CPC to ETV was carefully investigated by Warf in Uganda, and has shown promising results in hydrocephalus of various etiologies, including postinfectious, non-postinfectious, posthemorrhagic, aqueductal stenosis, myelomeningocele, and Dandy–Walker complex [3]. In infants, the overall success rate of ETV–CPC was higher than ETV alone (66% vs 47%), with a surgical mortality of 1.3% and infection rate of less than 1%. Therefore, CPC+ETV seems to offer a novel safe and viable alternative for infants.

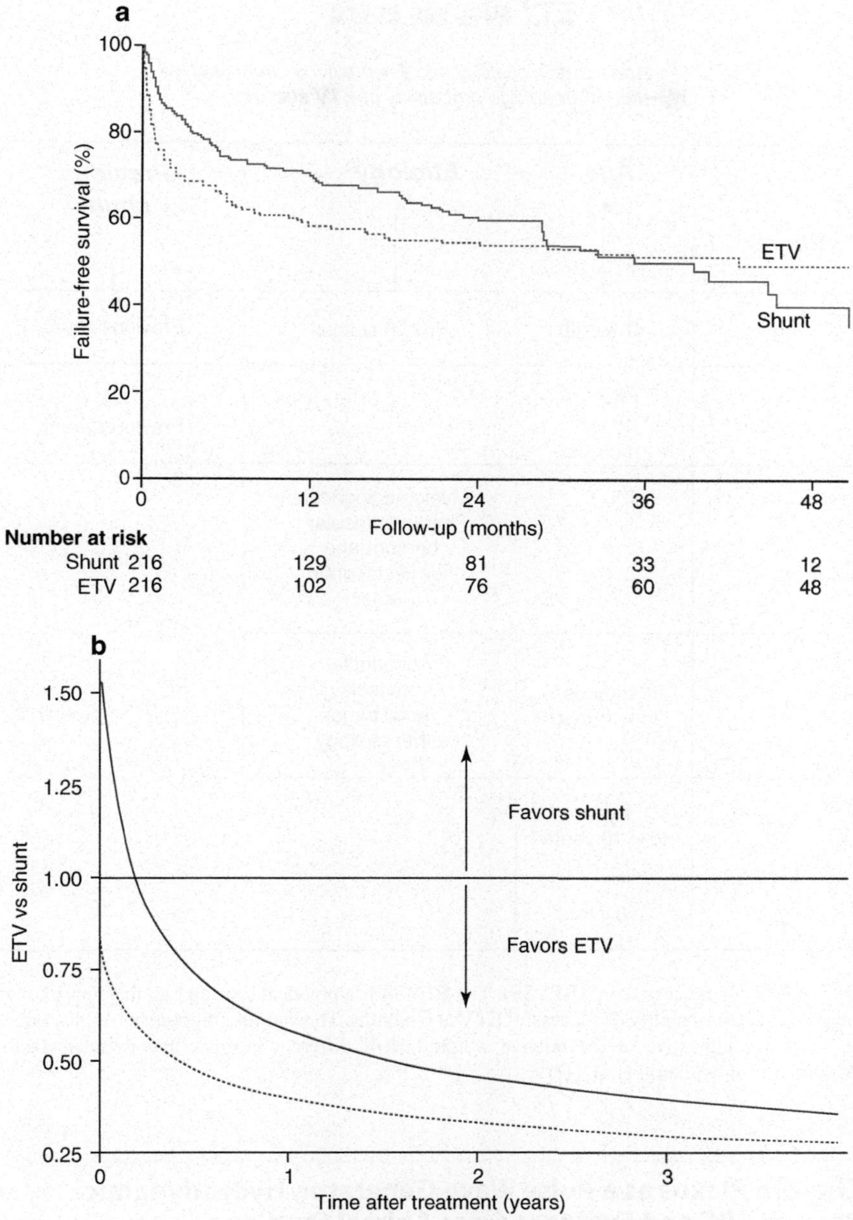

Fig. 18.1 Failure-free survival pattern for ETV and shunt. (**a**) Survival curve showing "failure-free treatment survival" for patients treated with ETV (dotted line) and shunt (solid line). For these curves, patient prognostic factors have been adjusted for with propensity score matching. (**b**) Graph showing the hazard ratios for ETV failure relative to shunt failure, modeled as a function of time. The dotted line represents an unadjusted model and the solid line represents the propensity score-matched model which balances prognostic factors. It can be seen that at 3 months, the hazard ratio crosses 1.00, indicating that the risk of treatment failure is less in ETV compared to shunt beyond 3 months. (Modified from Kahle et al. [16])

ETV success score

= Age score + etiology score + previous shunt score
≈ Percentage probability of ETV success

Score	Age +	Etiology +	Previous shunt
0	<1 Month	Post-infectious	Previous shunt
10	1 month to < 6 months		No Previous shunt
20		Myelomeningocele intra-ventricular hemorrhage non-tectal brain tumor	
30	6 months to < 1 year	Aqueductal stenosis tectal tumor other etiology	
40	1 year to < 10 years		
50	≥10 years		

Fig. 18.2 ETV success score (ETVSS). The ETVSS is a practical scoring tool that approximates the percentage probability of successful ETV at 6 months. The various components of the composite score are indicative of the relative weightings of different intrinsic and extrinsic factors. (Modified from Kulkarni et al. [1])

Choroid Plexus as a Pulse Wave Generator, Hydrodynamic Basis of CPC and Evidence from Animal Studies

A century ago, Dandy studied the experimental relationship between the choroid plexus and hydrocephalus using a dog model [18]. Occlusion of one foramen of Monro led to ipsilateral hydrocephalus. If both foramina of Monro were occluded, the lateral ventricle with choroid plexectomy collapsed while the contralateral ventricle with intact choroid plexus became enlarged. If the choroid plexus of both lateral ventricles was removed and the aqueduct of Sylvius was occluded with a piece of cotton, triventricular hydrocephalus still occurred, but at a reduced rate. The CSF production was attributed to the third ventricular choroid plexus. Collectively, these findings were indicative that the choroid plexus was a major CSF-producing structure and its removal delayed the development of hydrocephalus. At the time, it was believed that the reduction of CSF production was the only mechanism through which choroid plexus obliteration treated hydrocephalus. This bulk flow model would imply that if unilateral plexectomy was performed and the ipsilateral foramen of Monro was left open, the contralateral ventricle CSF production and back pressure proximal to an aqueduct occlusion would cause a symmetrical hydrocephalus. However, in 1962, Bering showed that this was not the case [19]. Instead, he proposed that the arterial pulsations in the choroid plexus created compression waves that transmitted through the ventricles and were normally dissipated by a patent CSF pathway, subarachnoid space, and intracranial venous compression. When the CSF pathway was impaired, these waves were absorbed by the local brain tissue instead, resulting in ventriculomegaly. This pulsatile mechanism of hydrocephalus formation was based on observations in a hydrocephalic dog model induced by intracisternal kaolin injection. When both foramina of Monro were left open, ventriculomegaly was seen only on the side with choroid plexus but not the side with plexectomy. Three additional observations supported this theory. First, focal areas of temporal horn enlargement were identified where plexectomy was not complete. Second, a subject with an absent septum pellucidum which underwent unilateral plexectomy developed symmetrical hydrocephalus. This occurred because there was no septum to act as a barrier to the pressure wave transmission. Third, intraventricular measurement showed larger pulse waves in the ventricle with choroid plexus. Wilson and Bertan also confirmed such notion in their experiments on hydrocephalic dogs [20]. Following the division of the right anterior choroidal artery, there was no difference in mean CSF pressure between the lateral ventricles. However, the right ventricular CSF pulse pressure decreased compared to the left. Also, the hydrocephalus was more severe on the left. Other nonsurgical methods of choroid plexus ablation have also been investigated. Weiss instilled intraventricular radioactive colloidal gold in kaolin-induced hydrocephalic dogs to cause selective radionecrosis of choroid plexus [21]. This resulted in a 78% reduction in CSF pressure, 32% reduction in CSF flow rate, and a reversal of ventriculomegaly. Selective choroid plexus radionecrosis and division of choroidal artery offered potential alternatives of hydrocephalus treatment, but were not further developed due to the associated morbidity and practicality.

In the late 1960s and early 1970s, Milhorat investigated the role of choroid plexus in CSF production in rhesus monkeys [22, 23]. Plexectomy was performed in both lateral ventricles and hydrocephalus was induced by inflation of a balloon in the fourth ventricle. Although the choroid plexus was not the only CSF-producing structure, its removal from the lateral ventricles resulted in a 33–40% reduction in CSF production as long as 9 months after the procedure.

Based on the above animal studies, choroid plexus does not only contribute to hydrocephalus by CSF production, that is, the bulk flow model, it also generates pulse pressure waves which is a main driver of ventriculomegaly. It is likely that in humans, while ETV works as a pulsation absorber, CPC functions as a pulsation reducer [24].

History of Open Plexectomy, Endoscopic Choroid Plexus Cauterization and Early Experience

The removal or cauterization of the choroid plexus as treatment for hydrocephalus is not a new concept, and was attempted as early as a century ago. As discussed above, Dandy demonstrated in dogs that choroid plexus was an organ of CSF production and its removal delayed the development of hydrocephalus [18]. Based on these findings, in 1918, he reported bilateral open extirpation of the choroid plexus for treatment of communicating hydrocephalus [25]. Although all 4 patients survived the operation, 3 died within 1 month, and the fourth one was alive after 10 months. Surgeries performed using a modified ventriculoscope with the addition of third ventriculostomy produced similar results [26, 27]. The poor outcome might have been, at least, partially due the open approach which required emptying of the bilateral ventricular CSF [28]. In 1934, Putnam described ventriculoscopic cauterization of choroid plexus for the first time [29]. The use of cautery allowed the CSF to be retained, thus avoiding the collapse of ventricles and severe shock, and the results were marginally better. In 1936, Scarff described a new ventriculoscope with the following features: (1) a "fore-oblique" lens system, which provided both "forward" and "oblique" vision with a wide angle (70°); (2) a maneuverable unipolar cauterizing electrode; (3) a lighting system; and (4) an irrigation system which had dual functions of clearing intraventricular blood from the operative field and replacing the fluid loss via the corticotomy. The results of CPC on 5 infants were 1 operative death, 1 failure, and 3 cases of arrested hydrocephalus. In 1956, Feld described a ventriculosope with an obliquely fixed mirror at the fore end of the lens system to provide a lateral view [30, 31]. Overall, in the early period of 1934–1957, a total of 95 cases were reported in 4 series by Putnam, Scarff, and Feld [32]. Collectively, the operative death rate was 14%, initial success rate 60%, and 5-year survival rate 30%.

The largest early experience with CPC was provided by Pople and Ettles [33]. Over 20 years (1973–1993), 116 patients underwent 156 operations. Of these, 104 patients were analyzed. The median age was 5 months and mean follow-up 10.5 years. Among those who had CPC as the first treatment, 80 (70%) were infants. Overall, 35% achieved long-term control without CSF shunts, although there was no significant reduction in ventricular size. Children with subacute communicating hydrocephalus had a better 64% shunt independent rate. Importantly, there was no mortality associated with the procedure and serious morbidity was low. Specifically, infection rate was 10% and, after vancomycin and gentamicin were added in the irrigation solution, it dropped to 0%. Patients who had CPC alone had significantly lower epilepsy rate than those who eventually required shunting (12% vs 48%). Other complications included 1 respiratory arrest in a premature infant, 1 low-pressure state, 8 ventricular drain displacement or blockage, 1 subdural effusion, and 2 abandonment of procedure due to intraoperative minor ventricular hemorrhage. Importantly, patients with successful CPC had better long-term educational outcome than those who required shunting.

Surgical Technique

The surgical technique has evolved significantly. The main modifications in the modern approach include putting the patient in supine position and using a unilateral frontal approach, made possible by the use of flexible neuroendoscope. The patient is supine with the head in the neutral position or turned to one side (in preparation for a possible shunt insertion, if ETV proves not to be feasible). A right-sided approach is preferred unless there is a significantly larger ventricle on the left or some other anatomical variant. The primary CSF diversion procedure of ETV is performed first with either a rigid or flexible neuroendoscope. At our institute, the preferred technique uses a linear dural opening, which will later be closed primarily, usually along a splayed coronal suture. If the suture is not splayed, then a small bone flap can be lifted and left partially attached by hinging it along the coronal suture. This is followed by introduction of a small rigid neuroendoscope (<4 mm diameter) via a peel-away sheath. The instruments of choice for creating the third ventricular floor stoma are a blunt stylette or Decq forceps [34]. Occasionally, a dilating balloon catheter, for example, Fogarty balloon catheter or NeuroBalloon (Integra LifeSciences) is used. The Lilliequest membrane is inspected and fenestrated. Following adequate ETV creation, the CPC begins in the body of the ipsilateral lateral ventricle with a monopolar cautery. The cautery should be set at the lowest current that is able to blanch the fronds of the plexus and coagulate the vascular pedicles. This process starts at the foramen of Monro and continues posteriorly to the glomus choroidea in the atrium. At this point, the flexible endoscope is used to enter the temporal horn and cauterize its choroid plexus. If the septum pellucidum is intact, a septostomy is performed. Through the septostomy, the CPC is performed in the contralateral body, atrium, and temporal horn. CPC is not performed in the third or fourth ventricles.

Recent Human Experience in Africa

In the early 2000s, Warf from CURE Children's Hospital of Uganda (CCHU) pioneered the combined ETV+CPC surgery in the sub-Saharan African setting [3]. The procedure was performed using a flexible endoscope and monopolar cautery, similar to the technique described above. In a prospective study of 550 children, 443 (81%) were infants. The ETV+CPC group had a superior outcome to ETV alone, with a success rate, that is, shunt avoidance, of 66% vs 47%. Subsequently, in studying the predictors for success for this patient group, CPC was identified as a major predicting factor, along with older age and myelomeningocele etiology (compared to postinfectious and others) [35]. Furthermore, the success rate is dependent on the extent of the CPC. Compared to no cauterization, partial unilateral and complete bilateral cauterization are associated with odds ratios of success of 2.0 and 4.8, respectively. Warf has since demonstrated in various specific subgroups the superior results by ETV+CPC compared to ETV alone, including congenital idiopathic communicating hydrocephalus (72% vs 20% success) and congenital aqueductal stenosis (82% vs 49%) [24, 36]. The ETV+CPC success rate in myelomeningocele was 76% compared to 35% with ETV alone [3, 37, 38]. This result was also superior to the 1-year shunt failure rate of 51% [39]. Beyond 1 year, ETV+CPC failure was rare, in contrast with the accumulative shunt failure risk of 31% in the second year and 12% per year in subsequent years [39]. Therefore, there was a clear advantage of ETV+CPC in the myelomeningocele subgroup. ETV+CPC also proved to be an effective and safe treatment in children with Dandy–Walker complex, offering a success rate of 75% [40].

Kulkarni et al. carried out a multicenter study comparing ETV+CPC in Africa to ETV alone performed in other countries [41]. Using risk-adjusted multivariable analysis, they showed that the superior success rate in the African patients could be explained entirely by known patient prognostic factors and the advantages by CPC. In terms of surgical morbidity, the overall operative mortality and infection rates for ETV+CPC are <1%, lower than shunting which were 4% and 9%, respectively [3, 42]. In terms of early development and neurocognitive function in a small group of children with myelomeningocele, there was no significant difference in Bayley Scales of Infant Development (BSID-III) scores between the ETV+CPC and VP shunt patients [43]. Warf et al. also showed that there was no difference in shunt survival or infection between those treated with a primary shunt compared to those who were shunted after failure of ETV+CPC [44].

Therefore, in brief, in the unique sub-Saharan African setting, ETV+CPC offers a higher success rate than ETV alone, with a more favorable long-term complication profile than shunting. A retrospective study found no survival advantage for non-shunt-treated children, that is, those receiving ETV+/–CPC, compared to shunt-treated children with a postinfectious hydrocephalus in Uganda (73% vs 68%) [45]. However, clinical equipoise still exists in terms of developmental and neurological outcome. This has fueled an ongoing National Institutes of Health-funded randomized trial to compare ETV+CPC and shunt with respect to safety, efficacy, developmental outcome, and brain/CSF volume metrics in infants with postinfectious hydrocephalus in Uganda [46–48].

Recent Human Experience Outside of Africa

Encouraged by the results in Uganda, ETV+CPC has been used increasingly in the rest of the world. Ogiwara et al. reported a 50% success rate in 18 patients treated with CPC, of whom 12 also had ETV [49]. Interestingly, in 3 patients who underwent repeat ETV, there was no regeneration of the choroid plexus, except for that in the proximity of the foramen of Monro, up to 38 months after CPC. Weil et al. reported the Miami experience in treating 85 children up to 24 months of age [50]. Intraventricular hemorrhage (IVH) of prematurity was the cause for just over half of the patients; other etiologies included myelomeningocele, congenital aqueductal stenosis, congenital communicating hydrocephalus, Dandy–Walker complex, postinfectious hydrocephalus, and other causes. The success rates were 42%, 38%, and 37% at 6, 12, and 24 months, which were higher than other series. However, it should be noted that a rigid endoscope was used, preventing complete CPC in the lateral ventricles. The median time to failure was 4.0 months. Prepontine scarring was associated with a higher treatment failure rate. Interestingly, both the ETVSS and CCHU ETV Success Score, which was developed for the sub-Saharan African population and accounted for the extent of CPC, were accurate in predicting treatment success in this North American cohort. There were 3 deaths, none related to the surgery. All 3 cases of infection had a background of IVH of prematurity with prior CSF reservoir. A different patient population might partly explain the lower success rate and mortality rate in this study. In a randomized trial, Malheiros et al. compared CPC (without ETV) to VP shunt for hydranencephaly and near-hydranencephaly [51]. They reported success in 80% of 10 patients who underwent CPC compared to 71% of 7 patients who had shunt placement, the difference of which was not significant. There was no perioperative complication. A recent meta-analysis of 10 studies by Zandian et al. reported a success rate of 67% for ETV+CPC (164 cases) compared to 55% for ETV alone (534 cases) in treating pediatric hydrocephalus [52]. The superiority of ETV+CPC was most marked in myelomeningocele (75% vs 49%).

The largest published North American experience to date comes from Warf himself. In an early report in 2011, 4 of 10 infants with posthemorrhagic hydrocephalus of prematurity were treated successfully by ETV+CPC. All cases of failed ETV+CPC had prepontine cistern scarring, in contrast to 1 in 4 for the successful cases. Following the initial report, Stone and Warf published the first North American prospective study, describing the Boston experience of 91 children undergoing primary ETV+CPC for hydrocephalus of various etiologies [53]. The success rate was 57% at 1 year, similar to African ETV+CPC (66%) and the North American primary shunt insertion outcome [3]. Including 3 successful redo ETVs, 65% of the patients remained shunt free to the limit of available follow-up (maximum approximately 4 years). Furthermore, in the patients with at least 6 months of follow-up, the ETV+CPC success at 6 months was 59%, higher than 45% that was predicted by the ETV Success Score. This suggested that CPC did add benefit to ETV alone in the North American setting, where there is a higher incidence of posthemorrhagic hydrocephalus related to prematurity, earlier presentation, and use of preoperative magnetic resonance imaging. This study also identified independent predictors of treatment failure: postinfectious etiology, age at treatment younger than 6 months, prepontine cistern scarring and prior CSF diversion. Finally, stratifying by age, 1-year success rates for infants younger and older than 6 months of age were roughly 60% and 80%, respectively. Because the success rate was just above 50%, the number of shunt placement could be halved by adopting a treatment strategy of primary

ETV+CPC. This could lead to a potential health care cost saving in the United States could amount to $1 billion annually [11].

The Hydrocephalus Clinical Research Network (HCRN) has also investigated the use of ETV+CPC in the North American population. A retrospective review included 36 children under 2 years of age from 7 HCRN centers, comparing them to a contemporaneous cohort of 758 children [2]. ETV+CPC was found to be safe and reasonably efficacious in the setting of HCRN. Specifically, there were no major perioperative morbidities or mortalities and the 1-year success rate was 52%. The lower success rate could be attributed to the disproportionately difficult cases in this retrospective series, and ETV+CPC was offered as a "salvage" procedure. Further retrospective analysis of 192 patients (unpublished data) showed a more frequent use of the procedure, performed on younger children and for a broader range of etiologies. Although the 1-year success rate was still lower compared to shunt (46% vs 67%), ETV+CPC had a very low incidence of intraoperative complications (0.5% severe hemorrhage and no major arterial injury) and postoperative complications (3.3% CSF leak, no infection, 1.7% postoperative hemorrhage, 1.7% postoperative seizure, 1.1% hyponatremia, and 0.6% new neurological deficit). Infants younger than 1 month of corrected age and IVH secondary to prematurity were identified as poor prognostic factors for success. In 2014, the HCRN started a prospective study of ETV+CPC in infants. As of the end of 2016, 179 infants had been recruited.

Future Directions

Regarding the optimal treatment option between ETV+CPC versus shunt, there remains a clinical equipoise. The decision-making for families and clinicians has to take into account several factors: (1) perioperative risks, which are slightly higher for ETV+CPC; (2) the inherent value families and patients might place on being "shunt free"; and (3) the relative neurocognitive outcomes for both, which is currently unknown. These uncertainties provide justification for a randomized trial in the North American setting, similar to the one ongoing in Uganda. Further avenues of study would also include the role of advanced neuroimaging and CSF biomarkers in terms of their prognostic values, use as outcome measures, and potential therapeutic roles. These topics are covered elsewhere.

Conclusion

Despite the incremental improvement in technology and technique, shunting and ETV appear to be approaching their maximal impact. The resurgence and refinement of ETV combined with CPC in a low-income country and subsequent popularization in high-income countries has produced promising results. This has the potential to be the third epic shift in hydrocephalus treatment, but will require further rigorous scientific validation in the form of prospective and, ideally, randomized studies.

References

1. Kulkarni AV, Drake JM, Mallucci CL, Sgouros S, Roth J, Constantini S. Endoscopic third ventriculostomy in the treatment of childhood hydrocephalus. J Pediatr. 2009;155(2):254–259.e1. https://doi.org/10.1016/j.jpeds.2009.02.048.
2. Kulkarni AV, Riva-Cambrin J, Browd SR, et al. Endoscopic third ventriculostomy and choroid plexus cauterization in infants with hydrocephalus: a retrospective hydrocephalus clinical research network study. J Neurosurg Pediatr. 2014;14(3):224–9. https://doi.org/10.3171/2014.6.PEDS13492.
3. Warf BC. Comparison of endoscopic third ventriculostomy alone and combined with choroid plexus cauterization in infants younger than 1 year of age: a prospective study in 550 African children. J Neurosurg. 2005;103(6 Suppl):475–81. https://doi.org/10.3171/ped.2005.103.6.0475.
4. Kulkarni AV, Riva-Cambrin J, Butler J, et al. Outcomes of CSF shunting in children: comparison of hydrocephalus clinical research network cohort with historical controls: clinical article. J Neurosurg Pediatr. 2013;12(4):334–8. https://doi.org/10.3171/2013.7.PEDS12637.
5. Drake JM, Kestle JRW, Miner R, et al. Randomized trial of CSF shunt valve design in pediatric hydrocephalus. Neurosurgery. 1998;43(August 1998):1–8.
6. Kestle JRW, Riva-Cambrin J, Wellons JC, et al. A standardized protocol to reduce cerebrospinal fluid shunt infection: the hydrocephalus clinical research network quality improvement initiative. J Neurosurg Pediatr. 2011;8(1):22–9. https://doi.org/10.3171/2011.4.PEDS10551.
7. Kulkarni AV, Drake JM, Rabin D, Dirks PB, Humphreys RP, Rutka JT. Measuring the health status of children with hydrocephalus by using a new outcome measure. J Neurosurg. 2004;101(2 Suppl):141–6. https://doi.org/10.3171/ped.2004.101.2.0141.
8. Hunt GM, Oakeshott P, Kerry S. Link between the CSF shunt and achievement in adults with spina bifida. J Neurol Neurosurg Psychiatry. 1999;67:591–5. https://doi.org/10.1136/jnnp.68.6.800.
9. Kulkarni AV, Shams I. Quality of life in children with hydrocephalus: results from the Hospital for Sick Children, Toronto. J Neurosurg. 2007;107(5 Suppl):358–64. https://doi.org/10.3171/PED-07/11/358.
10. Kulkarni AV, Cochrane DD, McNeely PD, Shams I. Medical, social, and economic factors associated with health-related quality of life in Canadian children with hydrocephalus. J Pediatr. 2008;153(5):689–95. https://doi.org/10.1016/j.jpeds.2008.04.068.
11. Simon TD, Riva-Cambrin J, Srivastava R, Bratton SL, Dean JM, Kestle JRW. Hospital care for children with hydrocephalus in the United States: utilization, charges, comorbidities, and deaths. J Neurosurg Pediatr. 2008;1(2):131–7. https://doi.org/10.3171/PED/2008/1/2/131.
12. Jones R, Stening W, Brydon M. Endoscopic third ventriculostomy. Neurosurgery. 1990;26(1):86–91. https://doi.org/10.1227/00006123-199001000-00012.
13. Drake JM. Endoscopic third Ventriculostomy in pediatric patients: the Canadian experience. Neurosurgery. 2007;60(5):881–6. https://doi.org/10.1227/01.NEU.0000255420.78431.E7.
14. Kulkarni AV, Drake JM, Kestle JR, Malluci CL, Sgouros S, Constantini S. Endoscopic third Ventriculostomy vs cerebrospinal fluid shunt in the treatment of hydrocephalus in children: a propensity score–adjusted analysis. Neurosurgery. 2010;67(3):588–93. https://doi.org/10.1227/01.NEU.0000373199.79462.21.
15. Kulkarni AV, Drake JM, Kestle JRW, Mallucci CL, Sgouros S, Constantini S. Predicting who will benefit from endoscopic third ventriculostomy compared with shunt insertion in childhood hydrocephalus using the ETV success score. J Neurosurg Pediatr. 2010;6(4):310–5. https://doi.org/10.3171/2010.8.PEDS103.
16. Kahle KT, Kulkarni A, Limbrick DD, Warf BC. Hydrocephalus in children. Lancet. 2016;136:788–199. https://doi.org/10.1016/B978-0-444-53486-6.00064-8.
17. Jernigan SC, Berry JG, Graham DA, Goumnerova L. The comparative effectiveness of ventricular shunt placement versus endoscopic third ventriculostomy for initial treatment of hydrocephalus in infants. J Neurosurg Pediatr. 2014;13(3):295–300. https://doi.org/10.3171/2013.11.PEDS13138.

18. Dandy WE. Experimental hydrocephalus. Ann Surg. 1919;70(2):129–42.
19. Bering EAJ. Circulation of the cerebrospinal fluid. Demonstration of the choroid plexuses as the generator of the force for flow of fluid and ventricular enlargement. J Neurosurg. 1962;19:405–13.
20. Wilson CB, Bertan V. Interruption of the anterior choroidal artery in experimental hydrocephalus. Arch Neurol. 1967;17(6):614–9. https://doi.org/10.1084/jem.19.1.106.
21. Weiss MH, Nulsen FE, Kaufman B. Selective radionecrosis of the choroid plexus for control of experimental hydrocephalus. J Neurosurg. 1972;36(3):270–5. https://doi.org/10.3171/jns.1972.36.3.0270.
22. Milhorat TH. Choroid plexus and cerebrospinal fluid production. Science (80-). 1969;166(3912):1514–6.
23. Milhorat TH, Hammock MK, Fenstermacher JD, Rall DP, Levin VA. Cerebrospinal fluid production by the choroid plexus and brain. Science (80-). 1971;173(3994):330–2.
24. Warf BC. Congenital idiopathic hydrocephalus of infancy: the results of treatment by endoscopic third ventriculostomy with or without choroid plexus cauterization and suggestions for how it works. Childs Nerv Syst. 2013;29(6):935–40. https://doi.org/10.1007/s00381-013-2072-1.
25. Dandy WE. Extirpation of the choroid plexuses of the lateral ventricle in communicating hydrocephalus. Ann Surg. 1918;68(6):569–79.
26. Dandy WE. The operative treatment of communicating hydrocephalus. Ann Surg. 1938;108:194–202.
27. Dandy WE. An operative procedure for hydrocephalus. Bull Johns Hopkins Hosp. 1922;33:189–90.
28. Scarff JE. Endoscopic treatment of hydrocephalus. Description of a ventriculoscope and preliminary report of cases. JAMA. 1936;451:853–61.
29. Putnam TJ. Treatment of hydrocephalus by endoscopic coagulation of the choroid plexus. Description of a new instrument and preliminary report of results. NEJM. 1934;210:1373–6.
30. Feld M. Ventriculoscope coagulant utilisé dans les hydrocephalies communicantes. Press médd. 1956;64:632.
31. Feld M. La coagulation des plexus choroides par ventriculoscopie directe dans l'hydrocephalie nonobstructive du nourrison. Neurochirurgie. 1957;3:70–9.
32. Scarff JE. Treatment of nonobstructive (communicating) hydrocephalus by cendoscopic cauterization of the choroid plexuses. Acta Psychiatr Scand. 1959;34(3):354–74. https://doi.org/10.1111/j.1600-0447.1959.tb07585.x.
33. Pople IK, Ettles D. The role of endoscopic choroid plexus coagulation in the management of hydrocephalus. Neurosurgery. 1995;36(4):698–701. https://doi.org/10.1227/00006123-199504000-00009.
34. Decq P, Le Guerinel C, Palfi S, Djindjian M, Kéravel Y, Nguyen J-P. A new device for endoscopic third ventriculostomy. J Neurosurg. 2000;93:509–12.
35. Warf BC, Mugamba J, Kulkarni AV. Endoscopic third ventriculostomy in the treatment of childhood hydrocephalus in Uganda: report of a scoring system that predicts success. J Neurosurg Pediatr. 2010;5(2):143–8. https://doi.org/10.3171/2009.9.PEDS09196.
36. Warf BC, Tracy S, Mugamba J. Long-term outcome for endoscopic third ventriculostomy alone or in combination with choroid plexus cauterization for congenital aqueductal stenosis in African infants. J Neurosurg Pediatr. 2012;10(2):108–11. https://doi.org/10.3171/2012.4.PEDS1253.
37. Warf BC. Hydrocephalus associated with neural tube defects: characteristics, management, and outcome in sub-Saharan Africa. Childs Nerv Syst. 2011;27(10):1589–94. https://doi.org/10.1007/s00381-011-1484-z.
38. Warf BC, Campbell JW. Combined endoscopic third ventriculostomy and choroid plexus cauterization as primary treatment of hydrocephalus for infants with myelomeningocele: long-term results of a prospective intent-to-treat study in 115 east African infants. J Neurosurg Pediatr. 2008;2(5):310–6. https://doi.org/10.3171/PED.2008.2.11.310.

39. Steinbok P, Irvine B, Douglas Cochrane D, Irwin BJ. Long-term outcome and complications of children born with meningomyelocele. Childs Nerv Syst. 1992;8(2):92–6. https://doi.org/10.1007/BF00298448.
40. Warf BC, Dewan M, Mugamba J. Management of Dandy-Walker complex-associated infant hydrocephalus by combined endoscopic third ventriculostomy and choroid plexus cauterization. J Neurosurg Pediatr. 2011;8(4):377–83. https://doi.org/10.3171/2011.7.PEDS1198.
41. Kulkarni AV, Warf BC, Drake JM, Mallucci CL, Sgouros S, Constantini S. Surgery for hydrocephalus in sub-Saharan Africa versus developed nations: a risk-adjusted comparison of outcome. Childs Nerv Syst. 2010;26(12):1711–7. https://doi.org/10.1007/s00381-010-1195-x.
42. Warf BC. Comparison of 1-year outcomes for the Chhabra and Codman-hakim micro precision shunt systems in Uganda: a prospective study in 195 children. J Neurosurg Pediatr. 2005;102(4 Suppl):358–62. https://doi.org/10.3171/ped.2005.102.4.0358.
43. Warf B, Ondoma S, Kulkarni A, et al. Neurocognitive outcome and ventricular volume in children with myelomeningocele treated for hydrocephalus in Uganda. J Neurosurg Pediatr. 2009;4(6):564–70. https://doi.org/10.3171/2009.7.PEDS09136.
44. Warf BC, Bhai S, Kulkarni AV, Mugamba J. Shunt survival after failed endoscopic treatment of hydrocephalus. J Neurosurg Pediatr. 2012;10(6):463–70. https://doi.org/10.3171/2012.9.PEDS1236.
45. Warf BC, Dagi AR, Kaaya BN, Schiff SJ. Five-year survival and outcome of treatment for postinfectious hydrocephalus in Ugandan infants. J Neurosurg Pediatr. 2011;8:502–8. https://doi.org/10.3171/2011.8.PEDS11221.
46. National Institutes of Health. Neurocognitive outcomes and changes in brain and CSF volume after treatment of post-infectious hydrocephalus in Ugandan infants by shunting or ETV/CPC: a randomized prospective trial (5R21TW009612–02). Res Portf Online Report Tools. 2012. https://projectreporter.nih.gov/project_info_description.cfm?projectnumber=5R21TW009612-02. Accessed 15 Aug 2017.
47. National Institutes of Health. Neurocogntive outcomes and changes in brain and CSF volume after treatment of post-infectious hydrocephalus in Ugandan infants by shunting or ETV/CPC: a randomized prospective trial (1R01HD085853–01). Res Portf Online Report Tools. 2015. https://projectreporter.nih.gov/project_info_description.cfm?projectnumber=1R01HD085853-01. Accessed 15 Aug 2017.
48. National Institutes of Health. Randomized Controlled Trial of Shunt vs ETV/CPC for PIH in Ugandan Infants (NCT01936272). US Natl Libr Med. 2013. https://clinicaltrials.gov/ct2/show/NCT01936272. Accessed 15 Aug 2017.
49. Ogiwara H, Uematsu K, Morota N. Obliteration of the choroid plexus after endoscopic coagulation. J Neurosurg Pediatr. 2014;14(3):230–3. https://doi.org/10.3171/2014.6.PEDS1438.
50. Weil AG, Fallah A, Chamiraju P, Ragheb J, Bhatia S. Endoscopic third ventriculostomy and choroid plexus cauterization with a rigid neuroendoscope in infants with hydrocephalus. J Neurosurg Pediatr. 2016;17:163–73. https://doi.org/10.3171/2015.5.PEDS14692.
51. Malheiros JA, Trivelato FP, Oliveira MM, Gusmão S, Cochrane DD, Steinbok P. Endoscopic choroid plexus cauterization versus ventriculoperitoneal shunt for hydranencephaly and near hydranencephaly: a prospective study. Neurosurgery. 2010;66:459. https://doi.org/10.1227/01.NEU.0000365264.99133.CA.
52. Zandian A, Haffner M, Johnson J, Rozzelle CJ, Tubbs RS, Loukas M. Endoscopic third ventriculostomy with/without choroid plexus cauterization for hydrocephalus due to hemorrhage, infection, Dandy-Walker malformation, and neural tube defect: a meta-analysis. Childs Nerv Syst. 2014;30(4):571–8. https://doi.org/10.1007/s00381-013-2344-9.
53. Stone SSD, Warf BC. Combined endoscopic third ventriculostomy and choroid plexus cauterization as primary treatment for infant hydrocephalus: a prospective north American series. J Neurosurg Pediatr. 2014;14(5):439–46. https://doi.org/10.3171/2014.7.PEDS14152.

Randomized Clinical Trials in Pediatric Hydrocephalus

19

Evan J. Joyce, Jay Riva-Cambrin, and John R. W. Kestle

Introduction

Among the options for research design for clinical investigators are case series (mostly retrospective), cohort studies (retrospective or prospective), case control studies, and randomized controlled trials. Analysis of data from prospective registries [1] using matching and/or propensity scores [2] has also gained popularity. Although nonexperimental design studies are frequently reported, randomized controlled trials have been considered the gold standard for the assessment of treatment efficacy, and the pros and cons have been extensively discussed in the literature [3, 4]. Randomized clinical trials of surgical procedures have some unique study design challenges and methods to address them. The most important attribute of randomized clinical trials, which is unique to that study design, is that randomization balances unknown confounders. Known confounders are also balanced, but this can be done with other research designs. Because it is not always possible to predict confounders in clinical research, randomization is the only method that has the ability to balance the unknown confounding factors.

Hydrocephalus is the most common condition treated by pediatric neurosurgeons. It is therefore the most common subject of clinical research in pediatric neurosurgery. Randomized controlled trials have been used to study a number of aspects of the care of pediatric hydrocephalus. This chapter will outline some of those trials, assess their methods, and discuss their findings (Table 19.1).

E. J. Joyce
University of Utah, Department of Neurological Surgery, Salt Lake City, UT, USA

J. Riva-Cambrin
Alberta Children's Hospital, Department of Clinical Neurosciences, Calgary, AB, Canada

J. R. W. Kestle (✉)
Primary Children's Hospital, University of Utah, Department of Neurosurgery, Salt Lake City, UT, USA
e-mail: John.kestle@hsc.utah.edu

D. D. Limbrick, J. R. Leonard (eds.), *Cerebrospinal Fluid Disorders*,
https://doi.org/10.1007/978-3-319-97928-1_19

Table 19.1 Randomized controlled trials in hydrocephalus research

Study	*n*	Sites	Dates	Entry criteria	Intervention	Primary outcome	Follow-up (mos.)	Blinded	Power (%)	Conclusion
Management of premature IVH										
Ventriculomegaly Trial Group (1990) [5]	157	15	1984–1987	Infants in NICU with IVH, ventricle width 97th percentile +4 mm	CSF removal based on ventricle size on US vs CSF removal based on head size/ symptoms	Survival, shunting, developmental assessment	12	Yes for developmental assessment, no for shunt	80	Early treatment had no benefit overall, perhaps helpful for nonmotor impairment in those with parenchymal lesions
Kennedy et al. (2001) [6]	177	55	1992–1996	Infants in NICU with IVH, ventricle width 97th percentile +4 mm	Standard rx ± acetazolamide and furosemide	Primary: death or shunt; Secondary: developmental assessment	12	Yes for developmental assessment, no for shunt	80	Acetazolamide and furosemide were of no benefit and were associated with increased neurologic morbidity
Whitelaw et al. (2010) [7]	77	4	February 2003–December 2006	<37 wks GA, IVH, ventricle width 97th percentile +4 mm, other ventricle size parameters	Drainage, irrigation and fibrinolytic therapy vs standard therapy	Severe cognitive or sensorimotor disability or death	24	Yes	Accrual stopped early due to secondary IVH	Despite secondary IVH, DRIFT reduced overall death and severe disability

de Vries et al. (2018) [8]	126	14	2006–2016	<34 wks GA, grade 3/4 IVH	Low threshold to begin CSF removal vs high threshold (both based on ventricle measurements)	Primary: shunt or death; Secondary: device failure/complications	Hospital discharge	Yes	80	No difference in shunt/death; low threshold group had more invasive procedures; follow-up for developmental outcome pending. Overall low rates of shunting.
Shunt valves										
Drake et al. (1998) [9]	344	10	October 1993–October 1995	First shunt insertion for hydrocephalus, <18 yrs. old, adjudication committee	Valves: Orbis-Sigma, Delta, differential pressure	Shunt failure, assessed by adjudication committee	36	Yes	80	No significant difference in the proportion of patients free of shunt failure
Pollack et al. (1999) [10]	377	13	June 1993–December 1995	Any age, shunt insertion or revision (including valve change)	Any commercially available shunt product vs Codman-Hakim programmable	Shunt survival	24	No	80	No significant difference in shunt survival
Surgical technique										
Bierbrauer et al. (1991) [11][a]	121	1	July 1988–October 1990	First shunt insertion	Frontal vs parieto-occipital entry site	Shunt survival	12	No	Not specified	Posterior shunts had significantly better survival

(continued)

Table 19.1 (continued)

Study	*n*	Sites	Dates	Entry criteria	Intervention	Primary outcome	Follow-up (mos.)	Blinded	Power (%)	Conclusion
Kestle et al. (2003) [12]	393	16	May 1996–November 1999	First shunt insertion for hydrocephalus, <18 yrs. old, adjudication committee	Ventricular catheter placement: endoscopic vs nonendoscopic	Shunt failure, assessed by adjudication committee	36	Yes	80	Endoscopic insertion of the initial VP shunt did not reduce shunt failure
Whitehead et al. (2017) [13]	448	14	Ongoing	First shunt insertion for hydrocephalus, <18 yrs. old, adjudication committee	Frontal vs parieto-occipital entry site	Shunt failure, assessed by adjudication committee	18	Yes	80	Study in progress
Endoscopy vs shunting										
Goyal et al. (2014) [14]	48	1	Not specified	Initial treatment of hydrocephalus in patients with definite, probable or possible tubercular meningitis	Shunt vs ETV	Success = improved clinical/radiographic profile	6	No	Not specified	No difference in % improved by 6 months

Kulkarni et al. (2016) [15]	158	27	2004–2013	First treatment of aqueduct stenosis	Shunt vs ETV	Procedure failure	60	No	Enrollment stopped due to low accrual in randomized arm	Higher rates of treatment failure with ETV. Health status outcome at 5 years pending
Kulkarni et al. (2017) [16]	100	1	May 2013–April 2015	Infants with postinfectious hydrocephalus	Shunt vs ETV/CPC	Cognitive score on BSID @ 12 mos	12	Yes	90	
Infection prevention										
Govender et al. (2003) [17]	153	1	Prior to 2003	Hydrocephalus patients (any age) having shunt insertion or revision	AIS[b] vs non-AIS	Shunt infection	≥6	No	80	Fewer infections in AIS group but a third of patients did not have endpoint assessed
Rozzelle et al. (2008) [18]	61 patients (84 procedures)	1	April 2005–December 2006	Hydrocephalus patients on pediatric neurosurgery service having shunt insertion or revision	AMS[c] vs non-AMS	Shunt infection	6	Yes	Not specified	Fewer infections in AMS group

NICU neonatal intensive care unit, *IVH* intraventricular hemorrhage, *CSF* cerebrospinal fluid, *US* ultrasound, *Rx* prescription, *GA* gestational age, *DRIFT* drainage, irrigation, and fibrinolytic therapy, *VP* ventriculoperitoneal

[a]Study was pseudorandomized

[b]*AIS* antibiotic-impregnated shunt catheters

[c]*AMS* antimicrobial suture

Management of Premature Intraventricular Hemorrhage

Babies who are born prematurely may experience bleeding into the ventricles. Several randomized trials have assessed the management of premature infants who have intraventricular hemorrhage (IVH). These studies have focused on interventions that would reduce the risk of shunt dependence, disability, or death in this fragile population.

Randomized Trial of Early Tapping in Neonatal Posthemorrhagic Ventricular Dilation

One of the first trials in this population of children compared an early aggressive approach to cerebrospinal fluid (CSF) removal with a more conservative regimen to evaluate whether aggressive action would improve neurodevelopmental assessment at a year of age [5]. Fifteen centers contributed patients from 1984 to 1987. These were premature children with IVH and ventricles that enlarged from the 97th percentile to the 97th percentile plus 4 mm on serial ventricular measurements on ultrasound. Early treatment was guided by ultrasound measurements. It began with lumbar punctures repeated as often as necessary if the ventricular width increased by 2 mm or more. If repeated taps were necessary for more than 4 weeks, permanent shunting "was discussed." The decision to insert a shunt also depended on the general condition of the infant, the infant's weight, and the protein concentration in the CSF.

The more conservative management plan did not depend on ultrasound measurements. Instead, CSF removal was performed by lumbar puncture when there was excessive head growth for at least 2 weeks or if there was symptomatic raised intracranial pressure (>12 mmHg). The criteria for inserting a shunt were the same as in the early treatment group. The shunting criteria in both groups did not seem very specific and were not independently adjudicated. The study was designed to have a power of 80% to detect a reduction in the proportion of children with severe impairments from 50% to 25%. A developmental pediatrician assessed the patients in follow-up. Neurodevelopmental outcome was known for 151 of the 157 patients in the trial. Overall, the results showed no difference in deaths or the need for ventriculoperitoneal (VP) shunt insertion. Fifty-eight patients (76%) in the early treatment group and 60 patients (80%) in the conservative management group died or were disabled. The results of a secondary analysis looked at patients with and without a parenchymal lesion. In patients without a parenchymal lesion, the aggressive treatment did not result in better outcomes. In patients with a parenchymal lesion, nearly all children had abnormal neuromotor signs, but those in the early treatment group had fewer impairments affecting other systems ($p = 0.05$; relative risk 0.67; 95% confidence interval [CI] 0.45–1.00). The authors concluded that there was no benefit to early treatment for children who did not have parenchymal lesions but that early treatment was associated with a significant reduction in other impairments among the children with parenchymal lesions. They state, and we agree, that these findings should be interpreted with caution.

Randomized Trial of Acetazolamide and Furosemide in Posthemorrhagic Ventricular Dilatation in Infancy

This trial [6] studied premature infants (median gestational age of 28 weeks) who were randomized to standard therapy or standard therapy plus drug therapy at a mean postnatal age of 3.6 weeks. Drug therapy consisted of acetazolamide plus furosemide. The primary outcome—death or shunt placement—occurred in more infants who received standard therapy plus drug therapy (56/88 vs 46/88). In addition, neurodevelopmental outcome of survivors at 1 year was better in the standard therapy group. Eighty-five percent of infants receiving drug therapy either died or were disabled at 1 year, compared with 70% of the standard therapy group.

The trial was well designed and executed. The entry criteria were largely based on imaging, and progressive dilation of the lateral ventricles to a ventricular index >4 mm above the 97th percentile was required. Dose route and administration of drug therapy were specified. Written guidelines were apparently provided for the standard therapy arm, but final clinical decisions regarding standard therapy were at the discretion of referring clinicians. Criteria for shunt insertion were specified, but the need for shunt insertion was not independently adjudicated. Developmental assessment was performed by a pediatrician in the child's community using Vineland Social Maturity Scales. "When possible," this individual was blind to the neonatal management. It is not clear how that was achieved or measured.

The study was designed to accrue 191 patients, giving a power of 80% to detect a reduction in shunting incidence from 60% to 40%. The trial was stopped early at 177 infants because it could not prove any advantage to the drug plus standard therapy arm. The primary outcome was known for all but 1 infant, and neurodevelopmental status was known for 98% of the survivors. The 177 infants were accrued from 55 centers worldwide. This means that some centers must have done very few patients, but the incorporation of patients from 55 centers worldwide enhances the generalizability of the results. The analysis also found that ventricular size at trial entry was the strongest predictor of shunt placement or death in the first year. This study highlighted the overall high risk of neurodevelopmental problems in these children and concluded that conservative management and explicit criteria for shunt insertion seemed to be the approach of least risk for these children.

Randomized Trial of Drainage, Irrigation, and Fibrinolytic Therapy (DRIFT) for Premature Infants with Posthemorrhagic Ventricular Dilatation

An aggressive treatment paradigm to reduce the cognitive and motor disability of premature infants with IVH was assessed in the DRIFT study. DRIFT therapy consisted of placement of two external ventricular drains (EVDs; right frontal and left occipital), followed by infusion of recombinant tissue plasminogen activator and artificial CSF. The artificial CSF was infused at 20 mL/kg/h into the right frontal catheter, and fluid was simultaneously drained from the left occipital catheter. The system had a transducer, and the drainage catheter height was adjusted to keep the intracranial pressure below 7 mmHg and to drain 60–100 mL/24 h more than the infused volume. The regimen continued until the drainage fluid became clear, and then the catheters were removed. Infusions were performed for a median of 3 days (range 2–7 days). This treatment was compared with standard therapy consisting of lumbar punctures and/or ventricular reservoir with tapping of 10–20 mL/kg/d to limit head growth below 2 mm/d. In the DRIFT group after completion of the DRIFT regimen, patients who met the same progressive head enlargement criteria were also treated with the same protocol of lumbar punctures and/or reservoir tapping. Criteria were defined for shunting in both groups when the patient reached 2500 g and the CSF protein fell below 1.5 g/L.

The early results, reported in 2007 [19], showed that DRIFT did not reduce the need for shunt placement surgery or death in the short term (up to 6 months post-treatment). In addition, there were some secondary IVHs in the intervention group. On the basis of these early findings, the researchers decided to stop accrual, but patient follow-up continued to assess the rates of death or severe developmental disability at 24 months corrected age [7]. All surviving infants were evaluated by a developmental assessor who was blind to the initial treatment allocation. The definition of severe disability (cognitive and sensory motor) was prespecified. Twenty-one (54%) patients in the DRIFT group were dead or disabled compared with 27 (71%) in the standard treatment group. The odds ratio adjusted for sex, birth weight, and IVH grade was 0.25 (95% CI 0.08–0.82).

This is one of the few interventions that has been demonstrated to benefit the survival and function of these children. Despite secondary hemorrhage in the treatment group, the neurodevelopmental outcome and survival was better with DRIFT. Recently, the 10-year data have been presented, and the benefit has persisted [20]. Among the 52 children assessed at 10 years, those in the DRIFT group had a 23.5-point cognitive quotient advantage and were 9 times more likely to be alive without severe cognitive disability than those in the control group.

Despite these encouraging results, the DRIFT approach has not been widely adopted. Perhaps the challenge of maintaining two external ventricular devices in a tiny, premature baby for several days has discouraged other centers. Since most of the patients were treated at 2 of the 4 study sites, the question of whether these techniques are generalizable to other centers has yet to be assessed. The trial has supported the notion that clot removal may be beneficial. Following that line of thinking, reports have started to emerge of clot evacuation at the time of reservoir insertion, but the experience is still very small [21, 22].

Treatment Thresholds for Intervention in Posthemorrhagic Ventricular Dilation: A Randomized Controlled Trial

A common question in the neonatal intensive care unit is when to intervene for children with IVH. Do we treat the patient when the ventricles enlarge, wait for the head size to cross percentiles, or wait for the condition to progress to a bulging fontanelle, split sutures, or bradycardia? This question was partially addressed by the

ELVIS (Early vs Late Ventricular Intervention Study) multicenter randomized trial [8]. The investigators randomized into two groups 126 premature infants born before 34 weeks of gestation with enlarged ventricles after Grades III and IV hemorrhage. The low-threshold (LT) group was treated when the ventricular index exceeded the 97th percentile and the anterior horn width (AHW) was >6 mm. The high-threshold (HT) group was treated when the ventricular index exceeded the 97th percentile plus 4 mm and the AHW was >10 mm. The primary outcome measure was the need for a VP shunt or death. The trial showed no significant difference between the two groups in primary outcome, although the LT group had more invasive procedures. Overall, this study showed a remarkably low rate of shunt insertion compared with previous studies.

This is another study that was carefully done in children from 13 neonatal intensive care units in Europe and 1 in the United States. Clear entry criteria included gestational age ≤34 weeks, Grade III or IV hemorrhage, age <28 days, and progressive enlargement of the ventricles, as described above. Serial ultrasounds were performed, and treatment began with lumbar punctures followed by reservoir placement if necessary, based on ventricular index criteria. Tapping of reservoirs was also adjusted according to the ultrasound measurements. Shunts were placed when children weighed 2000–2500 g, the CSF protein was below 1.5 g/l, and red blood cell count was <100/mm^2 if there was continued ventricular expansion and accelerated head growth. Two investigators blinded to treatment allocation reviewed ultrasounds and head size charts for infants from other centers to confirm that shunt criteria were met. In all cases, the reviewers agreed with the local decision to implant a shunt.

These children will continue to be followed for neurodevelopmental outcome at 2 years. Both treatment arms in this study were treated quite early. The very low shunting rate might therefore be due to tapping and reservoir placement in some children who might not have needed it, or those maneuvers might have been efficacious in avoiding the need for shunt placement. Despite the inclusion of 13 centers, it took 10 years to accrue 126 patients. Clearly, further work in this area will need multiple large centers in order to do trials in a timely fashion.

Shunt Valves

Numerous valves have been designed for the management of hydrocephalus. Many of them were intended to prevent overdrainage. Valves that can be adjusted to different settings via use of an external magnet began to appear in the late 1990s. Several randomized controlled trials have compared different shunt valve designs.

Randomized Trial of Cerebrospinal Fluid Shunt Valve Design in Pediatric Hydrocephalus

This trial assessed three of the most common valve designs on the market in the early 1990s [9, 23]. Claims that the new, more expensive valve designs reduced shunt malfunction compared with the conventional differential pressure valves led investigators to undertake this randomized comparison in pediatric hydrocephalus patients. In the study, 367 children at 12 North American or European pediatric centers were randomized to receive 1 of 3 valves: a differential pressure valve, a Delta valve, or an Orbis Sigma valve. The primary outcome was shunt failure, which was defined in detail in four categories: shunt obstruction, shunt overdrainage, loculated compartments in the ventricles, or infection. To minimize observer bias, clinical notes, case report forms, and imaging studies were blinded and then reviewed by an adjudication committee to determine whether the patient met shunt failure criteria. The study was designed to detect a 50% reduction in the 1-year shunt failure rate in any of the three groups. Follow-up assessments were done at 3 and 12 months and then annually for up to 3 years. In addition, patients were seen at any time there was a clinical concern for possible shunt malfunction.

Of the 367 patients randomized between October 1993 and October 1995, 23 were ruled ineligible by the blind adjudication committee, leaving 344 eligible randomized patients. The shunt survival rate was 61% at 1 year and 47% at 2 years. There was no difference among the three shunt valve groups overall or by individual pairwise comparisons. An adjusted Cox regression model also failed to show any significant differences among the valves. Follow-up was continued and reported in a separate paper extending the survival curves to 5 years [23]. The long-term follow-up did not alter the primary conclusions of the study, that none of the shunts was clearly better than the others.

Despite the large number of valves available, it is surprising that further randomized studies have not been performed or published. The frequency of shunt failure would suggest that valve trials are potentially important and in addition can be done with reasonable sample sizes. Further consideration should be given to studies in this area in the future.

A Randomized Controlled Study of a Programmable Shunt Valve Versus a Conventional Valve for Patients with Hydrocephalus

This multicenter randomized trial [10] compared the Codman Hakim programmable valve with a conventional valve of the surgeons' choice. Patients were included across the age spectrum (children and adults), and 235 underwent their first shunt implantation, whereas 142 had a shunt revision. Randomization was stratified by these two groups and by center. The median follow-up was 24 months, and the 2-year shunt survival was compared. For patients receiving their initial shunt insertion, there was no difference between the Codman Hakim adjustable shunt valve and the conventional valve systems (52% 2-year shunt survival vs 50%). In the group undergoing shunt revision, the results again showed no difference, with 43% of shunts surviving at 2 years in both groups.

The study did not specify indications for shunt revision, and neither the investigators nor the patients were blind to treatment group. The original valve settings in the experimental group were not specified, and the criteria for adjusting the valve in the experimental group were not provided. Two-thirds of patients in the experimental group had one or more valve pressure reprogrammings (mean 5 per patient). Most of the reprogrammings were performed in the first 6 months after valve insertion. In the control arm, any commercially available product could be used that the surgeons deemed appropriate, including a number of different commercial valves and/or antisiphon devices. Follow-up compliance was good, with more than 90% of patients completing the 3-, 12-, and 24-month evaluations. The ventricle size was also assessed, and again, there was no difference found between study groups. Survival curves comparing the time to failure of the original shunt systems in the experimental and control groups were virtually superimposed.

The authors concluded that patients with hydrocephalus can often be appropriately managed with fixed-valve pressure settings but that certain patients may require more precise selection of valve pressures. Although this may be true, the authors did not present data in this trial to support that statement. In fact, the trial seems to support the notion that adjustable valves are of no advantage since shunt failure rates and ventricle size were the same in experimental and control groups. The theoretical advantages of adjusting the shunt, while potentially valid, were not demonstrated in this trial. Many other reports of adjustable valves have been published, but none of them have been randomized in pediatric hydrocephalus.

Surgical Technique

The cranial entry site and the method of placing the ventricular catheter have been the subject of two previous randomized trials and a third study that is currently in progress.

A Prospective Randomized Study of Shunt Function and Infections as a Function of Shunt Placement

To determine whether shunt function was better after anterior or posterior placement, the investigators in this single-site study randomized 121 children between July 1988 and October 1990 [11]. Anterior shunts were placed anterior to the coronal suture and posterior shunts were placed in the parieto-occipital region. The location of the catheter tip within the ventricle was not specified. Overall, 59% of shunts in the anterior group and 70% of the shunts in the posterior group survived without revision or infection. The survival curves comparing these two groups were significantly different ($p < 0.05$).

Although presented as a randomized trial, the study was not actually randomized. The authors used a technique that is known as pseudorandomization, in which all shunts during even-numbered months were done via an anterior approach and shunts during odd-numbered months were done via a posterior approach. The problem with this type of "randomization" is that the study group is predictable before patients are entered. This is a significant disadvantage because it allows patients to be left out of the study if the predicted study group is not desirable to the surgeon or the family. In addition, it can lead to significant imbalances between the groups. For example, Surgeon B in this study entered 20 patients via a frontal approach and 8 patients via the posterior approach. True randomization would be extremely unlikely to result in such an imbalance.

The criteria for shunt malfunction are described in the chapter, but they are not very specific. In addition, there is no blinding or adjudication process to reduce observer bias. Despite these limitations, the study had reasonably well-balanced groups with regard to age and etiology, which are the important prognostic factors in pediatric hydrocephalus. The statistically significant difference in the survival of posterior shunts was interpreted cautiously. The authors concluded that there was no significant advantage to anterior shunts and that more patients needed to be studied for a longer period of time to determine whether there really is an advantage to posteriorly placed shunts. Because the study was performed at a single center, did not use true randomization, and had unblinded assessment of the outcomes, we think their cautious interpretation of the results is appropriate.

Hydrocephalus Clinical Research Network Entry Site Trial

Further research has continued since the Bierbrauer study [11] to determine whether anterior or posterior shunts have an advantage. On the basis of a secondary analysis of two previous randomized trials and another prospective observational study, Whitehead et al. [13] described evidence suggesting anterior shunts might have a survival advantage. Because of the opposing findings in the literature and common use of both anterior and posterior entry sites among pediatric neurosurgeons around the world, a large multicenter randomized trial has been organized by the Hydrocephalus Clinical Research Network (HCRN). Patients are randomized to anterior or posterior entry site with the goal of placing the catheter tip in the frontal horn or the occipital horn, away from the choroid plexus. The primary outcome is shunt failure, which is blindly adjudicated by an independent committee. The study is open to patients undergoing first-time shunt placement. Accrual of 448 patients is anticipated to be complete by the end of 2018, and analysis will begin after 18 months of follow-up.

Lack of Benefit of Endoscopic Ventriculoperitoneal Shunt Insertion: A Multicenter Randomized Trial

In the 1990s, uncontrolled evidence suggested that endoscopy could be used to assist with accurate placement of the ventricular catheter [24]. This led to promising reductions in the reported shunt failure rates. On the basis of these reports, a randomized trial was developed for infants undergoing their first treatment for hydrocephalus [12]. The infants were randomized to shunt placement with or without endoscopic assistance. The endoscope used in the trial was a small device that fit inside the lumen of the ventricular catheter so that the intraventricular anatomy could be assessed and the catheter could be placed away from the choroid plexus. Three hundred ninety-three children were randomized between May 1996 and November 1999. Children had a median age of 89 days, and the most common causes of hydrocephalus were myelomeningocele and IVH. As in the Shunt Design Trial [9, 23], shunt failure was clearly defined and blindly adjudicated by a committee. The study had a power of 80% to detect a reduction in the 1 year shunt failure rate from 0.5 to 0.35, from 0.4 to 0.25, from 0.3 to 0.2, or from 0.2 to 0.1.

The primary analysis showed there was no significant difference in time to shunt failure between the endoscopic and nonendoscopic groups. Shunts in 42% of endoscopic patients failed by 1 year and those in 34% of nonendoscopic patients failed in the same time window. The ventricular catheter position on the first postoperative scan was compared with the intraoperative observation and was found to be in the expected location about two-thirds of the time. This was similar in the endoscopic and nonendoscopic groups. A secondary analysis compared catheters that ended up away from the choroid plexus with catheters that ended up in the choroid plexus. The catheters away from the choroid plexus appeared to have a clear survival benefit. The authors concluded that catheter tip location is likely to be important in shunt survival, but endoscopic placement of the catheter did not improve catheter position or shunt survival.

Endoscopic Third Ventriculosotomy (ETV) (With or Without Choroid Plexus Coagulation [CPC]) Versus Shunting

The interest in endoscopic treatment of hydrocephalus has skyrocketed in the last couple of decades, and three trials have compared endoscopy with shunt insertion.

A Randomized Study of Ventriculoperitoneal Shunt Versus Endoscopic Third Ventriculostomy for Management of Tubercular Meningitis with Hydrocephalus

Although it is rare in the United States, tubercular meningitis (TBM) remains prevalent in many Asian countries, and hydrocephalus (TBMH) is the most common complication. Shunting is the standard treatment for TBMH, but CSF cell and protein content are often high, contributing to obstructive shunt failure. In these patients, ETV was considered a valid alternative to permanent shunt in order to avoid implanted hardware which is prone to failure.

In this study, the authors randomized 48 pediatric patients to compare the "radiographic and clinical" success of VP shunting versus ETV in the setting of TBMH [14]. They did not have a clearly stated primary outcome. They also recorded duration of illness, duration of antitubercular treatment, and preoperative clinical status via Modified Vellore grading (MVG; grading specific for TBMH) to determine whether these factors predicted shunt or ETV success. Patients were included if they had "definite, probable, or possible" TBM based on consensus definition as well as both clinical and radiographic evidence of hydrocephalus. The only exclusion criterion was previous CSF diversion. A randomization scheme based on random numbers was developed prior to study initiation, and CSF was sampled during the procedure for analysis and later comparisons. Follow-up was done at 1, 3, and 6 months to assess clinical and radiographic outcome (rated as improved or not improved/deteriorating) and determine complications related to each procedure.

Of the 48 patients (mean age ~4 years) enrolled, 26 had a VP shunt placed and 22 had an ETV. Of those who had shunts placed, 15 (54%) had "improvement in [their] clinical and radiological profile," 2 died, 4 required shunt repositioning, and 5 were lost to follow-up. In the ETV group, 10 (41%) had clinical and radiological improvement, 2 died (one because of meningitis from a postoperative CSF leak), and 10 patients had a shunt placed in the postoperative period because of ETV failure (although failure was not defined). The duration at which success was determined was not stated but was presumably 6 months. It is unclear whether the ETV group was analyzed as intention to treat, which is important given that 40% of patients crossed over to the shunt group. The authors reported that there was no statistically significant difference between the two groups in regard to treatment success ($p = 0.236$). The mean preoperative MVG was the same for both groups. While the shunted group did improve somewhat more at early follow-up, at 6 months the two groups were similar.

The most significant take-home message from this study is that ETV success was comparable to shunting at 6 months in TBMH, but the conclusions are limited by the lack of concise definitions for key endpoints and the lack of clarity in how the 10 crossover patients (ETV to shunt) were handled in the analysis.

International Infant Hydrocephalus Study: Initial Results of a Prospective Multicenter Comparison of Endoscopic Third Ventriculostomy and Shunt for Infant Hydrocephalus

The International Infant Hydrocephalus Study (IIHS) [15] was a partially randomized prospective cohort study. Children with triventricular hydrocephalus secondary to aqueduct stenosis who were less than 24 months of age were entered into the study. Families were asked whether they would agree to randomization and, if so, patients were randomized between shunt and third ventriculostomy. If they would not agree to randomization, patients were treated according to the parents' preference. The power calculation for the study required 182 randomized patients to detect a 0.10 difference in 5-year health status using the Health Utilities Index. Despite study recruitment beginning in 2004 and the eventual participation of 27 centers on 4 continents, recruitment was suspended in 2013, after the Data Safety Monitoring Committee determined that the effort to reach the targeted randomized sample size was futile. The analysis therefore combined the 52 randomized and 106 nonrandomized patients and compared overall results for 115 ETV patients and 43 shunt patients. When adjusted for important prognostic factors, the risk of procedure failure was significantly higher for ETV (Hazard ratio 3.17, $p = 0.004$). These are not the final results of this study. Follow-up is continuing until patients have the Health Utility Index completed 5 years after randomization.

The 5-year results will certainly be of interest, but there are some important findings from this early procedure-based analysis. It does appear that the failure rate of ETV is higher than that of shunt for infants with aqueduct stenosis. The broad distribution of 27 centers from around the world increases the generalizability of these results. On the other hand, it is surprising that a larger number of patients were not identified, and the chapter does not discuss eligible patients who were not entered. This chapter really highlights the challenge of performing a randomized trial comparing ETV and shunt. Surgeon and parental preferences can be very strong making randomization difficult. Of the 106 nonrandomized patients, 82 chose ETV. Another interesting observation is the temporal pattern of ETV failure. The ETV success rate between 1 and 3 months dropped from 82% to 68%, and then from 3 to 36 months, it stayed almost the same, decreasing to only 64%. In other words, after the first few months, the ETV success curve was almost flat. The third important observation was the effect of age. The survival curves for ETV and shunt were quite different for patients under 6 months of age (with ETV being worse). On the other hand, for patients over 6 months of age, the ETV and shunt survival curves were the same. The Health Utility outcomes at 5 years post-treatment are eagerly anticipated.

Endoscopic Treatment Versus Shunting for Infant Hydrocephalus in Uganda

This recently reported trial was conducted at CURE Children's Hospital of Uganda and included infants with postinfectious hydrocephalus who were less than 180 days of age [16]. Patients were randomly assigned to treatment with a Chhabra shunt or an ETV with choroid plexus coagulation (ETV/CPC). The primary outcome was the cognitive score on the Bayley Scales of Infant Development (BSID) at 12 months after surgery. This was assessed by a trained evaluator who was not aware of treatment assignment. Children wore hooded jackets to conceal the treatment assignment during the evaluation. The use of a developmental measure as the primary outcome is an important change in hydrocephalus clinical trials. Previously, studies focused on procedure failure, which was also recorded and analyzed in this study but was a secondary outcome.

One hundred children were enrolled between May 2013 and April 2015, and there was no significant difference between groups in the primary outcome at 12 months. In addition, there was no significant difference in failure-free shunt survival or language or motor scores from the BSID-3. Brain volume and CSF volume were measured in this study and, not surprisingly, CSF volume was lower in the shunt group, but brain volume did not differ between the groups. This raises the possibility that we should focus on brain volume rather than CSF volume, and perhaps brain volume will correlate better with functional outcome.

The authors expected the participating children to have a cognitive score of 6 ± 4 after treatment. In fact, the ETV/CPC group had a score of 4, and the shunt group had a score of 2. These scores are at the very low end of the range for the BSID and may reflect the postinfectious cause of hydrocephalus. Because these children were at the very low end of the cognitive scale, it is possible the children were too severely affected to benefit significantly from either treatment or to demonstrate differences between the two treatments.

The authors concluded that there was no significant difference between the two groups in cognitive outcome at 12 months. This is a very important finding in a very well done study. The continued follow-up of these children will be important. In addition, the assessment of these two procedures within other etiologies of hydrocephalus should be investigated.

Infection Prevention

CSF shunting devices have early infection rates of 5–15%. Treatment of shunt infection requires shunt removal, EVD insertion and antibiotic therapy until the infection is cleared, followed by shunt replacement. Because this subjects the patient to more invasive procedures, increases morbidity and mortality, and incurs significant direct/indirect costs, several randomized controlled trials have been undertaken to evaluate methods to prevent infection.

Evaluation of an Antibiotic-Impregnated Shunt System for the Treatment of Hydrocephalus

The use of antibiotic-impregnated shunts (AISs) to minimize the risk of infection has become common in the management of pediatric hydrocephalus. Surprisingly, only a single randomized trial has assessed these devices. In a study published in 2003 from a single center in South Africa, 153 patients requiring a VP shunt were randomized to an AIS or a non-AIS system [17]. A minimum sample size of 100 patients was calculated to identify whether AIS systems would reduce the existing infection rate of 11–4%, with an 80% power. The age distribution of patients in the trial is not described in detail but 64.5% of patients were <12 years old. Infection rates were compared in the 60 included patients with control shunts and the 50 with AISs. There were 10 infections (16.7%) in the control group and 3 infections (6%) in the AIS group ($p = 0.084$).

Unfortunately, the results are difficult to interpret. There were 153 patients initially enrolled, but 43 patients were excluded because of death prior to completion of follow-up, protocol violations, infected CSF at the time of shunt insertion, and loss to follow-up. With small event numbers and almost a third of enrolled patients without follow-up information, the internal validity of this study is questionable. Among the 13 infections, 9 occurred within 2 months of surgery, and 5.5% of patients in the study were human immunodeficiency virus (HIV) positive. All 10 control patients with shunt infections were found to have *Staphylococci*, whereas none of those with AIS infections had *Staphylococci* ($p = 0.038$). This trial appears to demonstrate that the devices had an effect on *Staphylococcus* infection rates, but conclusions are limited by the large number of patients whose outcome could not be determined, a percentage of children who were HIV positive, and a high baseline infection rate of 11%.

Antimicrobial Suture Wound Closure for Cerebrospinal Fluid Shunt Surgery: A Prospective, Double-Blinded, Randomized Controlled Trial

In 2008, a prospective, double-blinded, randomized controlled trial compared the use of triclosan-coated antimicrobial sutures (AMS; Vicryl Plus) versus placebo sutures (Vicryl) for fascia/galea closure to decrease shunt infections [18]. About 80% of participants were <21 years of age. The primary outcome was shunt infection within 6 months of surgery defined by positive CSF or hardware cultures. Eighty-four shunt placement procedures were performed in 61 patients during enrollment (40 new implants and 44 revisions), with the majority being VP shunts (81%). Patients were excluded if they had a ventricular access device (i.e., reservoirs or ventriculosubgaleal shunts), presented with active shunt infection, or were immunocompromised. Randomization to AMS or placebo was done with lettered cards and stratified by patient weight <4 kg, age <6 months, recent shunt infection (<1 month ago), and implant versus revision procedure. All participants were blinded except the scrub technician and operating room nurse. Patients who had a shunt failure or infection (treated) were randomized again. No patients were lost to follow-up. There were significantly fewer infections in the AMS group (2/46, 4.3%) than in the placebo group (8/38, 21%, $p = 0.038$).

This study assessed a simple intervention that is not expensive and is widely available, but the unusually high infection rate in the control group (21%) affects the generalizability of the results. In most centers currently, infection rates are much lower, so the impact of adding AMS sutures is not clear. A much larger trial would be needed to determine their efficacy.

Summary

Randomized trials are not suitable for answering all research questions. They require a large amount of work, careful planning and execution, and a large expensive infrastructure. Adequate sample sizes are necessary to achieve appropriate study power. Nevertheless, they are the best study design to answer important clinical questions for common conditions. Since hydrocephalus is the most common condition treated by pediatric neurosurgeons, it is likely that prospective randomized multicenter trials will continue to have a role. The papers outlined in this chapter cover a range of hydrocephalus topics and demonstrate that, under the right circumstances, rigorous trials are possible, bias can be minimized, and accurate information obtained.

References

1. Walicke P, Abosch A, Asher A, Barker FG, Ghogawala Z, Harbaugh R, et al. Launching effectiveness research to guide practice in neurosurgery: a National Institute Neurological Disorders and stroke workshop report. Neurosurgery. 2017;80:505–14.
2. Wang S, Stone S, Weil AG, Fallah A, Warf BC, Ragheb J, et al. Comparative effectiveness of flexible versus rigid neuroendoscopy for endoscopic third ventriculostomy and choroid plexus cauterization: a propensity score-matched cohort and survival analysis. J Neurosurg Pediatr. 2017;19:585–91.
3. Barker FG. Editorial: Randomized clinical trials and neurosurgery. J Neurosurg. 2016;124:552–6 discussion 556–557.
4. Mansouri A, Cooper B, Shin SM, Kondziolka D. Randomized controlled trials and neurosurgery: the ideal fit or should alternative methodologies be considered? J Neurosurg. 2016;124:558–68.
5. Randomised trial of early tapping in neonatal posthaemorrhagic ventricular dilatation. Ventriculomegaly Trial Group. Arch Dis Child. 1990;65:3–10.
6. Kennedy CR, Ayers S, Campbell MJ, Elbourne D, Hope P, Johnson A. Randomized, controlled trial of acetazolamide and furosemide in posthemorrhagic ventricular dilation in infancy: follow-up at 1 year. Pediatrics. 2001;108:597–607.
7. Whitelaw A, Jary S, Kmita G, Wroblewska J, Musialik-Swietlinska E, Mandera M, et al. Randomized trial of drainage, irrigation and fibrinolytic therapy for premature infants with posthemorrhagic ventricular dilatation: developmental outcome at 2 years. Pediatrics. 2010;125:e852–8.
8. de Vries LS, Groenendaal F, Liem KD, Heep A, Brouwer AJ, van' t Verlaat E, et al. Treatment thresholds for intervention in posthaemorrhagic ventricular dilation: a randomised controlled trial. Arch Dis Child Fetal Neonatal Ed. 2018.
9. Drake JM, Kestle JR, Milner R, Cinalli G, Boop F, Piatt J Jr, et al. Randomized trial of cerebrospinal fluid shunt valve design in pediatric hydrocephalus. Neurosurgery. 1998;43:294–303 discussion 303–305.
10. Pollack IF, Albright AL, Adelson PD. A randomized, controlled study of a programmable shunt valve versus a conventional valve for patients with hydrocephalus. Hakim-Medos Investigator Group. Neurosurgery. 1999;45:1399–408. discussion 1408–1411.
11. Bierbrauer KS, Storrs BB, McLone DG, Tomita T, Dauser R. A prospective, randomized study of shunt function and infections as a function of shunt placement. Pediatr Neurosurg. 1990;16:287–91.
12. Kestle JR, Drake JM, Cochrane DD, Milner R, Walker ML, Abbott R, et al. Lack of benefit of endoscopic ventriculoperitoneal shunt insertion: a multicenter randomized trial. J Neurosurg. 2003;98:284–90.
13. Whitehead WE, Riva-Cambrin J, Kulkarni AV, Wellons JC, Rozzelle CJ, Tamber MS, et al. Ventricular catheter entry site and not catheter tip location predicts shunt survival: a secondary analysis of 3 large pediatric hydrocephalus studies. J Neurosurg Pediatr. 2017;19:157–67.
14. Goyal P, Srivastava C, Ojha BK, Singh SK, Chandra A, Garg RK, et al. A randomized study of ventriculoperitoneal shunt versus endoscopic third ventriculostomy for the management of tubercular meningitis with hydrocephalus. Childs Nerv Syst. 2014;30:851–7.
15. Kulkarni AV, Sgouros S, Constantini S. International infant hydrocephalus study: initial results of a prospective, multicenter comparison of endoscopic third ventriculostomy (ETV) and shunt for infant hydrocephalus. Childs Nerv Syst. 2016;32:1039–48.
16. Kulkarni AV, Schiff SJ, Mbabazi-Kabachelor E, Mugamba J, Ssenyonga P, Donnelly R, et al. Endoscopic treatment versus shunting for infant hydrocephalus in Uganda. N Engl J Med. 2017;377:2456–64.
17. Govender ST, Nathoo N, van Dellen JR. Evaluation of an antibiotic-impregnated shunt system for the treatment of hydrocephalus. J Neurosurg. 2003;99:831–9.

18. Rozzelle CJ, Leonardo J, Li V. Antimicrobial suture wound closure for cerebrospinal fluid shunt surgery: a prospective, double-blinded, randomized controlled trial. J Neurosurg Pediatr. 2008;2:111–7.
19. Whitelaw A, Evans D, Carter M, Thoresen M, Wroblewska J, Mandera M, et al. Randomized clinical trial of prevention of hydrocephalus after intraventricular hemorrhage in preterm infants: brain-washing versus tapping fluid. Pediatrics. 2007;119:e1071–8.
20. Luyt K, Jary S, Lea C, Young G, Odd D, Miller H, et al. Drainage irrigation and fibrinolytic therapy (DRIFT) for post haemorrhagic ventricular dilatation: improved cognitive ability at school-age. Presented at Pediatric Academic Societies Meeting, San Francisco; 2017.
21. Etus V, Kahilogullari G, Karabagli H, Unlu A. Early endoscopic ventricular irrigation for the treatment of neonatal Posthemorrhagic hydrocephalus: a feasible treatment option or not? a multicenter study. Turk Neurosurg. 2018;28:137–41.
22. Schulz M, Buhrer C, Pohl-Schickinger A, Haberl H, Thomale UW. Neuroendoscopic lavage for the treatment of intraventricular hemorrhage and hydrocephalus in neonates. J Neurosurg Pediatr. 2014;13:626–35.
23. Kestle J, Drake J, Milner R, Sainte-Rose C, Cinalli G, Boop F, et al. Long-term follow-up data from the shunt design trial. Pediatr Neurosurg. 2000;33:230–6.
24. Taha J, Crone K. Endoscopically guided shunt placement. Techn Neurosurg. 1996;1:159–67.

Global Perspectives on the Treatment of Hydrocephalus

20

Johannes Marthinus Nicolaas Enslin
and Anthony Graham Fieggen

Hippocrates was among the first physicians to treat disorders of fluid in the brain by ventricular puncture in the fifth century BC, followed by legends of neuroanatomy such as Galen (200 AD) and later Vesalius (1560s), who made further contributions to the management of hydrocephalus [1]. However, successful management of this condition had to wait until the 1950s, when technological advances paved the way for shunts as a reliable intervention around the world—at least in areas where they could be afforded. Further advances in neuroendoscopy offered alternatives to shunting, given the high rate of failure due to obstruction, infection and disconnection [2]. Hydrocephalus has long challenged neurosurgeons, with modern neurosurgeons of our field such as Cushing and Dandy adding to our understanding and treatment of this condition, yet, as a paediatric neurosurgeon, one would be forgiven for feeling that we are little closer to managing, or understanding, this condition than our forefathers were, with shunt failure in the first 2 years after placement still in the region of 40–50% [3–5].

The Size of the Problem

Hydrocephalus is one of the most common birth defects, with an estimated 400,000 new cases of childhood hydrocephalus developing worldwide [6], and treating hydrocephalus is the most commonly performed neurosurgical operation in children. The incidence of hydrocephalus in the United States is 0.2–0.8/1000 live

J. M. N. Enslin (✉)
Red Cross Children's Hospital, Department of Neurosurgery, Cape Town, South Africa
e-mail: johannes.enslin@uct.ac.za

A. G. Fieggen
Division of Neurosurgery, University of Cape Town, Department of Surgery,
Cape Town, South Africa
e-mail: graham.fieggen@uct.ac.za

D. D. Limbrick, J. R. Leonard (eds.), *Cerebrospinal Fluid Disorders*,
https://doi.org/10.1007/978-3-319-97928-1_20

births [7], while in Japan the incidence in the first year of life is stated to be 0.58/1000 live births, equating to about 800 new cases of hydrocephalus per year [8]. Persson et al. [9] reported a prevalence in Sweden of 0.82/1000 live births. Hydrocephalus is a common concomitant of other conditions—approximately 1% of children who develop bacterial meningitis in their life, up to 4% of children who suffer traumatic brain injury will develop hydrocephalus [10, 11] and 12% of children with syndromic craniosynostosis may have hydrocephalus [11]. About 85% of patients with posterior fossa tumour present with hydrocephalus and up to 30% will have permanent hydrocephalus that will require surgical therapy [12], and subarachnoid haemorrhage is complicated by hydrocephalus in 20–30% of cases [13].

In Africa and India, the problem is even greater, with more than 6000 new cases of hydrocephalus estimated every year [14]. In Eastern Africa, hydrocephalus is the most common condition that requires neurosurgical management [14], and the problem is further complicated by the scarcity of neurosurgeons in Sub-Saharan Africa, with some countries having a ratio of 5–10 million people per neurosurgeon [14]. While this situation is rapidly improving, and countries like South Africa have one neurosurgeon for every 450,000 people, this discrepancy between the number of patients who need care and number of neurosurgeons to deliver care plays an important role in the global picture of hydrocephalus management. It is clear from a recent literature review done by Dewan et al. that the burden of hydrocephalus is highest in Africa, South-America and South-East Asia [6].

A Perspective on Hydrocephalus Globally

While it is used not to be a rare sight in some developing countries to have a child present with a head circumference of 100 cm or more, this has changed dramatically in the last 10 years, as there are more neurosurgeons being trained [15–17]. In some areas there is still stigma attached to children with hydrocephalus and other disabilities, so families, and even health care workers, may avoid seeking help for children with disabilities due to fear of being shunned by their communities. This makes caring for patients with hydrocephalus very difficult in some developing countries. The assumed poor prognosis that some clinicians ascribe to hydrocephalus is unfounded in general, as children with hydrocephalus seldom die early on, but survive and develop massive macrocrania, which leads to further social stigmatisation and caring difficulties. The mother may no longer be able to carry her child anymore due to the large head and weight [18], an absolutely avoidable situation if hydrocephalus is treated early on.

Financial issues are always at the forefront of health care worldwide. In some countries availability of a shunt depends on donors and philanthropic funders, and families may have to buy the shunt out of their own pocket in the absence of medical insurance [15]. Mission hospitals and other non-governmental institutions, where typically, patients are cared for by general surgeons or medical officers, have helped immensely to care for those who otherwise would not have had access to health care. This, unfortunately, also comes with the concern that while it may be straightforward to place a shunt, treating the complications that so often arise can challenge even the most experienced neurosurgeon, and these patients may then need referral to a neurosurgeon [15]. The cost associated with shunts has prompted various low income countries to develop their own valveless shunting systems like the "Harare shunt" and the "Malawi shunt" [19, 20]. The Chhabra shunt from India has for decades been the low-tech—but also low complication—shunt that many neurosurgeons have preferred [21, 22].

Aetiology of Hydrocephalus by Region

One of the most obvious facts is that there are clear regional differences in the aetiology of hydrocephalus in North America versus South America, Europe, Africa and India, as well as the East. These variations in aetiology have led to a distinct difference in the approach to hydrocephalus management as well. The effective implantable shunt that works very well and is the go-to option for the developed world, is the "expensive biofilm for the Staphylococci" in the developing country, that requires regular, unattainable follow-up visits to a far-off clinic or hospital.

Warf [14] found that congenital causes of hydrocephalus are much more common in developed countries, which is in stark contrast to the high incidence of acquired hydrocephalus in more underdeveloped countries in Africa [23, 24]. The incidence of post-infectious hydrocephalus is up to 60% in Uganda [25, 26]. Most infectious causes are bacterial, but non-bacterial infections also cause hydrocephalus: in Nepal and South America neurocysticercosis may cause obstructive hydrocephalus [27]. It is these post-infectious hydrocephalus cases that keep many paediatric neurosurgeons awake at night, as managing to create stomas between all the membranes and encysted ventricles is where you need as much help as one can get from neuronavigation and ultrasound guidance [28]. This is where the neuroendoscope comes into a realm of its own: either as a stand-alone procedure of septostomy with ventriculocisternostomy, or as an adjunct of septostomy followed by endoscopically guided shunt placement [28].

While the incidence of babies born with neural tube defects (NTDs) is on the decline in more developed countries, it is still a common problem in Africa and other developing nations. While antenatal diagnosis is usually available in developed countries, allowing parents the option of terminating a pregnancy, this is seldom available in developing countries, where families face the prospect not only of caring for a disabled child, but also managing the accompanying hydrocephalus in the majority of cases [29]. Hydrocephalus in this group of Chiari II-malformation patients is mostly treated by shunting in most areas around the world. Experience has been that the success of Endoscopic Third Ventriculosotomy (ETV) in this group is very low [30, 31], yet the experience of Warf in Uganda suggests that combining ETV with choroid plexus coagulation [14, 29] offers an alternative to shunt dependence in a population where aftercare of a shunted patient is incredibly difficult, and may be lacking altogether. Choroid plexus coagulation has also extended beyond the realm of Uganda to other centres around the globe which are now using the technique as an adjunct to ETV, or even in shunted patients with large cerebrospinal fluid (CSF) volumes [32, 33]. This is a great illustration of how the spread of technology can be a 2-way process, stimulated by the need to innovate in under-resourced settings.

Tuberculous meningitis (TBM) is a cause of hydrocephalus that almost exclusively occurs in the developing world [34]. While much progress has occurred in the treatment of TB, the optimal management of TBM, especially when complicated by hydrocephalus, remains an enigma [34–36]. Concerns about lifelong shunt dependence and the complications thereof have led physicians to explore medical options for temporising the hydrocephalus until medical management has taken full effect (in practice this may take up to as long as a month). Confirming communication in the CSF system and then performing regular lumbar CSF tapping may be effective in up to 50% of cases [35, 37–39].

Treatment Options for Hydrocephalus

Magnetic resonance imaging (MRI) as a standard modality in working up patients with hydrocephalus pre-operatively is not available in all countries—for example, none of the cases reported by Warf et al. [14, 25] and Kulkarni et al. [40] from the Ugandan subgroup, underwent MRI, while this is done routinely in the developed world prior to ETV [26]. Neuronavigation-assisted shunt placement, or navigation-guided endoscopy, which would be especially helpful for the daunting multiloculated hydrocephalus cases so commonly seen in Africa, are not widely available [28, 41]. Cranial ultrasound is very helpful [42], and widely available as most hospitals will have an ultrasound machine, but this only helps the neurosurgeon within the small window of opportunity presented by an open fontanelle. Other non-invasive techniques, such as ultrasound measurement of the optic nerve sheath diameter via orbital ultrasound for assessing raised intracranial pressure, hold great promise in under-resources settings [43].

As previously highlighted, necessity leads to invention and in certain countries, such as Uganda—ETV is the principal therapeutic option offered for hydrocephalus, shunting is only done for a failed ETV, in contrast to the selective approach to ETV in developed countries [26]. Since 2003 patients at CURE Children's Hospital of Uganda have also received choroid plexus coagulation as routine intervention during ETV [25, 44]. The benefit of the endoscopic techniques, apart from the range of management options, is that they offer the opportunity to treat hydrocephalus without implanting foreign material, nor creating a shunt-dependent patient with all the associated problems thereof [45]. These technically demanding cases of post-infectious hydrocephalus being treated with neuroendoscopy have challenged the skills of neuroendoscopists as "on the fly decisions" need to be made while endoscopically evaluating the cisterns and ventricular system to decide on best management option [40].

More expensive and better technology does not always equate to better care and function in the patient, though [46, 47]. This dictum is clearly demonstrated every day in practice caring for patients with hydrocephalus, as programmable valves and "fancy" shunts do not outlast or outperform simpler systems [5, 21, 48, 49]. As a community of health care providers, we need to look for ways to make health care accessible and equal for all [50–52].

Japanese neurosurgeons were the first to realise the value of having a flexible neuroendoscope that would allow the neurosurgeon to reach previously inaccessible areas, with the minimally invasive approach that endoscopy offers [53]. The relative poor image quality of flexible scopes has for many years been the drawback for many neurosurgeons, this was until the introduction of the videoscope which combines superior quality visualisation and optics with the manoeuvrability of the flexible endoscope [53].

Even caring for the wound after hydrocephalus management brings with it unique challenges in developing countries [54]. Facilities for basic hygiene may not be available in every household, which this makes caring for a delicate wound with high infection risk difficult. On the other hand, while developed countries fight a seemingly losing battle against antibiotic resistant bacteria, this is less of a problem in developing countries where antibiotics are less frequently used. Using absorbable sutures, which do not need the patient to come back to hospital for removal, as well as off-the-shelf products such as superglue® (the commercially available tissue glues are prohibitively expensive and therefore unavailable) to seal off the wound and prevent soiling, and the use of expensive dressings are all ways that a neurosurgeon in the developing world circumnavigates common problems.

Foetal surgery is no longer considered an experimental option, yet it is not yet performed widely [55]. Many centres in Europe, North American and Latin America have adopted foetal surgery as a management strategy in reducing the incidence of hydrocephalus in NTDs [56], but this is not practised in Africa and many other countries as yet. One of the concerns may be the higher risk of preterm labour and the difficulties that brings in an already resource scarce environment.

Who Manages Hydrocephalus?

While specialised neurosurgical care is readily available in most developed countries for managing hydrocephalus, many developing countries just have too large a ratio of neurosurgeons to patients (1:10,000,000) [14] to be able to offer this. In many other developing nations it is common for a general surgeon, or even a medical officer, to do all the surgical procedures in a community—shunts included [57]. While many of these doctors are highly skilled and are able to provide care not otherwise available, some have extended this concept to suggest that non-physicians may be trained to do basic neurosurgical procedures in developing countries [17, 58]. This certainly does stir up a hornet's nest in the age-old debate, where on the one hand we need to find ways to offer basic medical and surgical care for patients in developing countries which requires more people offering such services [59] while principles of equity demand that find innovative ways to bridge the gap between developed and developing countries [60]. We need to find ways of offering the same high quality service for people all around the globe and not be satisfied with second best for the developing world, while in the developed world, one would never let a non-neurosurgeon perform a neurosurgical operation [52].

Follow-up of Hydrocephalus

In developing countries, a decision on the effectiveness of an ETV or shunt procedure is based on control of the clinical signs of raised intracranial pressure (ICP), including head circumference, while in the developed world this decision is based on the same clinical signs in addition to routine follow-up imaging—often MRI [26]. Geographical barriers to follow-up are important considerations in Africa, South America as well as countries like Indonesia, where transport between clinics or hospitals are restrictive. Clinical follow-up remains the most commonly used method [61]. Ophthalmic examination is a key skill that all neurosurgeons and those caring for patients with hydrocephalus have to master [62].

In most developed countries imaging as part of follow-up is done via MRI. The renewed interest in limiting exposure to radiation has placed emphasis on measures to avoid routine computed tomography (CT) scanning for patients with hydrocephalus. In any paediatric neurosurgery service, it is not unknown to have children who undergo dozens of CT scans of their brain due to recurrent complications. MRI scanning does obviate the risks attached to radiation, but in a resource scarce environment, that firstly, may not even have access to MRI scanners, there are limited access during normal working hours only and in small children MRI scans mostly require anaesthetic support as well.

Paediatric neurosurgeons are also well aware that shunts do not respect office hours, and many patients present after hours when a decision about a shunt needs to be made on an emergency basis. Ultrasound offers a great alternative in small children and those in whom the anterior fontanel is still open. It is therefore a handy skill that every neurosurgeon should have to, at least, determine gross shunt malfunctions on ultrasound of the brain. There are even teams looking into options of using a smartphone to assist with placement guidance [63]. All of these are important factors to consider when evaluating a hydrocephalus service and all technological advancements to reduce the incidence of malposition of shunts, and procedure-related morbidity, are to be welcomed.

Neurocognitive evaluation in patients who undergo hydrocephalus management is also worthwhile, and this has seen renewed interest with the advent of choroid plexus coagulation in combination with other procedures [64]. This forms part of follow-up in developed countries like the United States and Europe, but is often simply not available in resource-limited areas [65, 66]. With greater collaboration of developed countries and developing countries, it may be possible to make more comprehensive follow-up possible [64]. This is very important as we are not merely managing fluid dynamics, but we should be primarily concerned with the cognition and function of the patient [67].

Great care therefore needs to be taken to ensure that every primary health care provider has experience in measuring head circumference and identifying the signs of raised intracranial pressure and shunt dysfunction. Every country should aim to develop infrastructure that can allow for referral of patients with hydrocephalus to centres where they can be managed adequately.

Outcomes of Hydrocephalus Treatment

Even though there is such a high incidence of post-infectious hydrocephalus in Africa (up to 60% of all cases of hydrocephalus in Uganda) [25], and generally accepted consensus is that the presence of post-infectious hydrocephalus is a poor prognostic factor in the overall success of an ETV [31], the group of Warf in Uganda reported a 70% success rate of ETV—if aqueduct stenosis is present, versus a 45% success rate in cases where the cerebral aqueduct was patent [25], although it should be noted that this study was not included in the review done by Kulkarni [31].

Guthara et al. [68] reviewed shunt outcomes in a rural hospital in Kenya and found 60% had poor outcome and 10% infection risk, which reflects the high percentage of post-infectious hydrocephalus (27.7%) and NTD-related hydrocephalus (49%). It is noteworthy that their outcomes with regard to congenital hydrocephalus are similar to those of developed countries. The studies of Warf and Kulkarni, as well as Constantini et al., all reflect the same outcomes [26, 69] and there is not much that differs if variables are accounted for in terms of hydrocephalus outcomes. The single most important factors seem to be aetiology and age, as well as head size at presentation [68].

Conclusion

Hydrocephalus is truly a global neurosurgical problem. The incidence of hydrocephalus varies greatly, as well as the main causes of the disease. Geographical, social, political and genetic factors all play a role in this. The playing field is definitely not level when it comes to managing hydrocephalus—with massive discrepancies in equipment, skilled personnel as well as well-developed long-term care plans. The important point, however, is that good care is not solely dependent on having access to the most expensive equipment and the best available shunts or endoscopes, many contributions to our knowledge of managing hydrocephalus have emanated from under-resourced areas. Our obligation as neurosurgeons is to embrace these differences between the developed and developing world, learn from each other and support each other. In the end it is all about giving each patient, independent of geographical location or socio-economic status, the best neurosurgical care possible. Hydrocephalus is one of the conditions in neurosurgery which lends itself to this collaborative effort (Table 20.1).

Table 20.1 Various options available to treat hydrocephalus

Hydrocephalus management options
Shunt placement
Endoscopic third ventriculostomy
ETV and choroid plexus coagulation
ETV and Omaya reservoir placement
Endoscopic ventricular lavage and subgaleal shunt placement
Endoscopic ventricular lavage only
Endoscopic ventricular lavage and Omaya reservoir placement with aspirations
Endoscopic aquaductoplasty
Endoscopic aquaductoplasty with stenting
Endoscopic septostomy and shunt placement
Endoscopic cystostomy and endoscopic assisted shunt placement
Programmable shunt use
Gravitation assisted shunt use
Flow controlled shunt use
Most basic shunt use (Chhabra/Harare)
Videoscope neuroendoscopy

References

1. Lifshutz JI, Johnson WD. History of hydrocephalus and its treatments. Neurosurg Focus. 2001;11(2):1–5.
2. Enchev Y, Oi S. Historical trends of neuroendoscopic surgical techniques in the treatment of hydrocephalus. Neurosurg Rev. 2008;31(3):249–62.
3. Kestle J, et al. Long-term follow-up data from the Shunt Design Trial. Pediatr Neurosurg. 2000;33(5):230–6.
4. Drake J, Kestle J, Tuli S. CSF shunts 50 years on–past, present and future. Childs Nerv Syst. 2000;16(10–11):800–4.
5. Drake JM, et al. Randomized trial of cerebrospinal fluid shunt valve design in pediatric hydrocephalus. Neurosurgery. 1998;43(2):294–303.
6. Dewan MC, et al. Global hydrocephalus epidemiology and incidence: systematic review and meta-analysis. J Neurosurg. 2018;27:1–15.
7. Chi JH, Fullerton HJ, Gupta N. Time trends and demographics of deaths from congenital hydrocephalus in children in the United States: National Center for Health Statistics data, 1979 to 1998. J Neurosurg Pediatr. 2005;103(2):113–8.
8. Tamakoshi A, et al. A nationwide survey of congenital hydrocephalus in Japan—estimated prevalence and incidence. Eur J Public Health. 1991;1(2):86–9.
9. Persson EK, Hagberg G, Uvebrant P. Hydrocephalus prevalence and outcome in a population-based cohort of children born in 1989–1998. Acta Paediatr. 2005;94(6):726–32.
10. Dodge PR, Swartz MN. Bacterial meningitis—a review of selected aspects: special neurologic problems, postmeningitic complications and clinicopathological correlations. N Engl J Med. 1965;272(18):954–60.
11. Guyot L, Michael D. Post-traumatic hydrocephalus. Neurol Res. 2000;22(1):25–8.
12. Riva-Cambrin J, et al. Predicting postresection hydrocephalus in pediatric patients with posterior fossa tumors. J Neurosurg Pediatr. 2009;3(5):378–85.

13. Chen S, et al. Hydrocephalus after subarachnoid hemorrhage: pathophysiology, diagnosis, and treatment. Biomed Res Int. 2017;2017:1–8.
14. Warf BC. Pediatric hydrocephalus in East Africa: prevalence, causes, treatments, and strategies for the future. World Neurosurg. 2010;73(4):296–300.
15. Jukonya L. Hydrocephalus management in Zimbabwe; 2018.
16. Adeloye A. The Rahima Dawood Memorial Guest Lecture–December 2006–Malawi. Pattern, practice and problems of neurological surgery in east and central Africa. East Cent Afr J Surg. 2006;12(2):4–16.
17. Attebery JE, et al. Initial audit of a basic and emergency neurosurgical training program in rural Tanzania. World Neurosurg. 2010;73(4):290–5.
18. Mangi DA. An exploration of social predicaments facing children with hydrocephalus: the case study of Muhimbili Orthopaedic Institute. The Open University of Tanzania; 2016.
19. Cotton M. The acute abdomen and HIV. Trop Dr. 2006;36(4):198–200.
20. Sibanda SE. Infection after Harare valve VP shunt operations: a review of 92 cases. Cent Afr J Med. 1991;37(12):397–403.
21. Warf BC. Comparison of 1-year outcomes for the Chhabra and Codman-Hakim Micro Precision shunt systems in Uganda: a prospective study in 195 children. J Neurosurg Pediatr. 2005;102(4):358–62.
22. Warf BC, et al. Costs and benefits of neurosurgical intervention for infant hydrocephalus in sub-Saharan Africa. J Neurosurg Pediatr. 2011;8(5):509–21.
23. Li L, et al. Association of bacteria with hydrocephalus in Ugandan infants. J Neurosurg Pediatr. 2011;7(1):73–87.
24. Laeke T, et al. Pediatric hydrocephalus in Ethiopia: treatment failures and infections: a hospital-based, retrospective study. World Neurosurg. 2017;100:30–7.
25. Warf BC. Hydrocephalus in Uganda: the predominance of infectious origin and primary management with endoscopic third ventriculostomy. J Neurosurg Pediatr. 2005;102(1):1–15.
26. Kulkarni AV, et al. Surgery for hydrocephalus in sub-Saharan Africa versus developed nations: a risk-adjusted comparison of outcome. Childs Nerv Syst. 2010;26(12):1711–7.
27. Agrawal J, et al. Kathmandu Univ Med J. 2012;9(2):1–2.
28. Spennato P, et al. Neuroendoscopic treatment of multiloculated hydrocephalus in children. J Neurosurg Pediatr. 2007;106(1):29–35.
29. Warf BC. Hydrocephalus associated with neural tube defects: characteristics, management, and outcome in sub-Saharan Africa. Childs Nerv Syst. 2011;27(10):1589.
30. Kulkarni AV, et al. Endoscopic third ventriculostomy in the treatment of childhood hydrocephalus. J Pediatr. 2009;155(2):254–259.e1.
31. Kulkarni AV, Riva-Cambrin J, Browd SR. Use of the ETV Success Score to explain the variation in reported endoscopic third ventriculostomy success rates among published case series of childhood hydrocephalus. J Neurosurg Pediatr. 2011;7(2):143–6.
32. Shitsama S, et al. Choroid plexus coagulation in infants with extreme hydrocephalus or hydranencephaly. J Neurosurg Pediatr. 2014;14(1):55–7.
33. Chamiraju P, et al. Endoscopic third ventriculostomy and choroid plexus cauterization in posthemorrhagic hydrocephalus of prematurity. J Neurosurg Pediatr. 2014;13(4):433–9.
34. Thwaites GE, van Toorn R, Schoeman J. Tuberculous meningitis: more questions, still too few answers. Lancet Neurol. 2013;12(10):999–1010.
35. Rajshekhar V. Management of hydrocephalus in patients with tuberculous meningitis. Neurol India. 2009;57(4):368.
36. Palur R, et al. Shunt surgery for hydrocephalus in tuberculous meningitis: a long-term follow-up study. J Neurosurg. 1991;74(1):64–9.
37. Figaji A, Fieggen A, Peter J. Endoscopic third ventriculostomy in tuberculous meningitis. Childs Nerv Syst. 2003;19(4):217–25.
38. Figaji A, Fieggen A, Peter J. Endoscopy for tuberculous hydrocephalus. Childs Nerv Syst. 2007;23(1):79–84.
39. Figaji AA, Fieggen AG. The neurosurgical and acute care management of tuberculous meningitis: evidence and current practice. Tuberculosis. 2010;90(6):393–400.

40. Warf BC, Kulkarni AV. Intraoperative assessment of cerebral aqueduct patency and cisternal scarring: impact on success of endoscopic third ventriculostomy in 403 African children. J Neurosurg Pediatr. 2010;5(2):204–9.
41. Kim S, et al. The use of frameless navigation during endoscopic interventions in children with multilocular hydrocephalus. Zh Vopr Neirokhir Im N N Burdenko. 2015;79(4):61–70.
42. Whitehead WE, et al. Accurate placement of cerebrospinal fluid shunt ventricular catheters with real-time ultrasound guidance in older children without patent fontanelles. J Neurosurg. 2007;107(5 Suppl):406–10.
43. Padayachy LC, et al. Change in optic nerve sheath diameter as a radiological marker of outcome from endoscopic third ventriculostomy in children. Childs Nerv Syst. 2015;31(5):721–8.
44. Warf BC, Campbell JW. Combined endoscopic third ventriculostomy and choroid plexus cauterization as primary treatment of hydrocephalus for infants with myelomeningocele: long-term results of a prospective intent-to-treat study in 115 East African infants. J Neurosurg Pediatr. 2008;2(5):310–6.
45. Stagno V, et al. Management of hydrocephalus around the world. World Neurosurg. 2013;79(2):S23.e17–20.
46. Oikonomou J, et al. New valves—new dangers? 22 valves (38 probes) designed in the 'nineties in ultralong-term tests (365 days). Eur J Pediatr Surg. 1999;9(S1):23–6.
47. Kamalo P. Point of view: exit ventriculoperitoneal shunt; enter endoscopic third ventriculostomy (ETV): contemporary views on hydrocephalus and their implications on management. Malawi Med J. 2013;25(3):78–82.
48. Ringel F, Schramm J, Meyer B. Comparison of programmable shunt valves vs standard valves for communicating hydrocephalus of adults: a retrospective analysis of 407 patients. Surg Neurol. 2005;63(1):36–41.
49. Pollack IF, Albright AL, Adelson PD. A randomized, controlled study of a programmable shunt valve versus a conventional valve for patients with hydrocephalus. Neurosurgery. 1999;45(6):1399–411.
50. Ravindra VM, et al. The need for cost-effective neurosurgical innovation—a global surgery initiative. World Neurosurg. 2015;84(5):1458–61.
51. Kalangu KK. Pediatric neurosurgery in Africa–present and future. Childs Nerv Syst. 2000;16(10–11):770–5.
52. Ibrahim GM, Bernstein M. Models of neurosurgery international aid and their potential ethical pitfalls. Virtual Mentor. 2015;17(1):49.
53. Oka K. Introduction of the videoscope in neurosurgery. Oper Neurosurg. 2008;62(suppl_5):ONS337–41.
54. Joseph RA, Killian MR, Brady EE. Nursing care of infants with a ventriculoperitoneal shunt. Adv Neonatal Care. 2017;17(6):430–9.
55. Clewell WH, et al. A surgical approach to the treatment of fetal hydrocephalus. N Engl J Med. 1982;306(22):1320–5.
56. Adzick NS, et al. A randomized trial of prenatal versus postnatal repair of myelomeningocele. N Engl J Med. 2011;364(11):993–1004.
57. Sader E, Yee P, Hodaie M. Barriers to neurosurgical training in sub-Saharan Africa: the need for a phased approach to global surgery efforts to improve neurosurgical care. World Neurosurg. 2017;98:397–402.
58. Kanyi JK, et al. Burr-hole craniostomy for chronic subdural hematomas by General Surgeons in Rural Kenya. World J Surg. 2018;42(1):40–5.
59. Dechambenoit G. Action Africa! World Neurosurg. 2010;73(4):251–3.
60. Warf BC. Educate one to save a few. Educate a few to save many. World Neurosurg. 2013;79(2):S15.e15–8.
61. Eriksen AA, et al. Implementing routine head circumference measurements in Addis Ababa, Ethiopia: means and challenges. World Neurosurg. 2016;91:592–596.e2.
62. Andersson S. Visual function and ocular morphology in children with surgically treated hydrocephalus. Göteborg: Institute of Neuroscience and Physiology. Department of Clinical Neuroscience and Rehabilitation; 2011.

63. Thomale U, et al. Smartphone-assisted guide for the placement of ventricular catheters. Childs Nerv Syst. 2013;29(1):131–9.
64. Warf B, et al. Neurocognitive outcome and ventricular volume in children with myelomeningocele treated for hydrocephalus in Uganda. J Neurosurg Pediatr. 2009;4(6):564–70.
65. Jacobs R, Northam E, Anderson V. Cognitive outcome in children with myelomeningocele and perinatal hydrocephalus: A longitudinal perspective. J Dev Phys Disabil. 2001;13(4):389–405.
66. Erickson K, Baron IS, Fantie BD. Neuropsychological functioning in early hydrocephalus: review from a developmental perspective. Child Neuropsychol. 2001;7(4):199–229.
67. Baron IS, Goldberger E. Neuropsychological disturbances of hydrocephalic children with implications for special education and rehabilitation. Neuropsychol Rehabil. 1993;3(4):389–410.
68. Gathura E, et al. Outcomes of ventriculoperitoneal shunt insertion in sub-Saharan Africa. J Neurosurg Pediatr. 2010;6(4):329–35.
69. Constantini S, Sgouros S, Kulkarni A. Neuroendoscopy in the youngest age group. World Neurosurg. 2013;79(2):S23.e1–S23.e11.

Technical Advances in the Treatment of Hydrocephalus: Current and Future State

21

Jason S. Hauptman, Barry R. Lutz, Brian W. Hanak, and Samuel R. Browd

In this chapter, we attempt to summarize the present and future state of technologies driven to diagnose and treat hydrocephalus. First, we focus on components of shunt devices, the most common surgical intervention employed to treat hydrocephalus. Second, we examine technologies used to diagnose shunt malfunction. While there has been considerable progress made over the last half-century, much work is left to be done.

Ventricular Catheters

Since the advent of the first modern internalized shunt systems in the early 1950s, which is generally credited to Frank Nulsen and Eugene Spitz, who reported on successful implantation of a ventriculojugular shunt employing a 12-Fr soft rubber catheter as the ventricular catheter in 1951 [1], the introduction of more inert silicone materials has been the greatest advance in the ventricular catheter technology [2, 3]. Robert Pudenz reported the successful implantation of a ventriculoatrial shunt made completely out of silicone rubber in 1957 [4], and the first silicone ventriculoperitoneal shunt was implanted a year later by Richard Ames [5]. To this day

J. S. Hauptman (✉)
Seattle Children's Hospital, University of Washington, Department of Neurosurgery, Seattle, WA, USA
e-mail: Jason.Hauptman@seattlechildrens.org

B. R. Lutz
Department of Bioengineering, University of Washington, Seattle, WA, USA

B. W. Hanak
University of Washington, Neurological Surgery, Seattle, WA, USA

S. R. Browd
Seattle Children's Hospital, University of Washington, Department of Neurological Surgery, Seattle, WA, USA

D. D. Limbrick, J. R. Leonard (eds.), *Cerebrospinal Fluid Disorders*,
https://doi.org/10.1007/978-3-319-97928-1_21

the vast majority of modern commercially available catheters are composed of polydimethylsiloxane (*PDMS*), although polyurethane catheters are also produced [6]. While the vast majority of catheters available to the practicing neurosurgeon are composed of the same base materials, the variety of catheter choices is largely a reflection of the numerous catheter embellishments—antibiotic impregnated, antimicrobial silver coated, hydrogel coated—in combination with the variety of catheter designs which can most readily be differentiated by their distinct cerebrospinal fluid (CSF) intake hole size, shape, and patterning. This section will review both the data on technology aimed at improving the accuracy of ventricular catheter operative implantation followed by a review of ventricular catheter technologies aimed at reducing shunt infection and forward-thinking strategies in pursuit of more obstruction-resistant ventricular catheters.

Ventricular Catheter Design

Most ventricular catheter innovations have been designed with an eye toward addressing one of the two most costly and morbid shunt complications: infection and failure secondary to obstruction. First, we will review data on antimicrobial catheter technologies in widespread commercial use. Next, we will briefly describe the mechanisms of noninfectious ventricular catheter obstruction and describe some forward-thinking catheter technology design strategies that may be able to combat this problem, which, alone, accounts for over 50% of failures in the pediatric population [7] and approximately 20% of failures in the adult population [8].

Antimicrobial Catheters

Catheters with antimicrobial properties, predominantly antibiotic-impregnated (rifampin with either clindamycin or minocycline) and silver-coated catheters (combination of metallic silver and an insoluble silver salt), have become widely adopted in North American clinical practice. Although the literature has been somewhat mixed regarding the efficacy of antibiotic-impregnated and silver-coated catheters with respect to successfully reducing shunt infection rates [9–11], two recent reviews have concluded that overall there is class III evidence supporting the notion that the use of antimicrobial modified-catheters modestly reduces postoperative infection rates [12, 13]. Several studies have advocated for the routine use of more costly antimicrobial catheters on the basis of overall cost-savings with even modest reductions in the shunt infection rate given the high cost of a hospitalization for shunt infection (approximately $50,000) [9, 14, 15]. Although one finding of concern from the Konstantelias et al. meta-analysis is that when infections do occur in patients with antibiotic-impregnated or silver-coated catheters, the organisms cultured tend to be more virulent/antibiotic-resistant, including methicillin-resistant *Staphylococcus aureus* and gram-negative bacilli. Certainly this observation warrants further study. Hopefully the multicenter randomized trial currently underway in the UK (BASICS; British Antibiotic and Silver-Impregnated Catheters for VP Shunts) will provide more high quality prospective data on shunt infection rates with the use of antimicrobial catheters as well as antibiotic resistance patterns for those infections that do occur [16].

In addition to antibiotic-impregnated and silver-coated catheters, one commercialized catheter with a polyvinylpyrrolidone hydrogel coating that demonstrated promising reductions in bacterial attachment in vitro is commercially available (BioGlide, Medtronic, Dublin, Ireland) [17]. Disappointingly, early clinical studies with polyvinylpyrrolidone coated external ventriculostomy drain catheters failed to demonstrate reduced infection rates [18], and largest study looking at their use in internalized shunt systems actually found that they were associated with increased infection rates in the pediatric population studied [19]. However, a more recent retrospective study from a Chinese group looking at high-infection-risk adult and pediatric patients demonstrated a decreased rate of shunt infection with the use of BioGlide catheters [20], raising the question of whether further prospective study in selected patient populations is warranted.

Noninfectious Ventricular Catheter Obstruction and the Pursuit of Obstruction-Resistant Catheters

In the historical literature, a wide variety of cell/tissue types, including choroid plexus, astrocytes, macrophages/microglia/foreign body giant cells/granulomatous reactions, eosinophils, lymphocytes, monocytes, brain parenchyma, ependyma, connective tissue and fibrin networks, leptomeninges, necrotic debris, hemorrhage, and calcification, have been implicated in ventricular catheter obstruction. Recent work has brought into focus the innate immune cells of the central nervous system, microglia, and astrocytes, as the likely pathophysiologic lynchpin in typical nonallergic, noninfectious, ventricular catheter obstruction. However, before proceeding with a discussion of the most common mechanism of ventricular catheter obstruction, the caveat of "non-allergic" in the prior statement warrants further explanation. In patients presenting with repeated short-interval catheter obstructions, one must always consider the possibility that they are mounting an allergic response to the implant, a diagnosis that can be made in the context of CSF eosinophilia and sterile cultures [21, 22]. Although the PDMS catheter material is the most commonly implicated allergen [2, 23], it has also been posited that the ethylene oxide used to sterilize many commercialized shunts may be the inciting agent [24]. Patients with shunt hardware allergy should have their standard PDMS catheter exchanged for a polyurethane or "extracted" PDMS catheter, which has been through a series of solvents to extract any unpolymerized silicone oil and polymerization catalysts, as this commonly alleviates the problem [23].

As evidenced by the panoply of cell/tissue times reported to cause ventricular catheter obstruction in the historical literature, it is clear that the field of neurosurgery has generally not had a unified grasp on the pathophysiology of the catheter obstruction. Historically, ingrowth of choroid plexus has been the most commonly stated hypothesis for the majority of obstructions, based largely on Hakim's 1969 report describing choroid plexus to be the obstructive material in 80% of "15 or more" catheters examined [25]. In spite of a growing body of literature which has been progressively shifting the focus away from choroid plexus over the last

35 years [26–29], the choroid plexus obstruction model has been reiterated in neurosurgery textbooks and remains entrenched in the minds of practicing neurosurgeons based on the observation that the majority of respondents (66%) in a recent survey of American Society of Pediatric Neurosurgeons members stated that choroid plexus is the tissue responsible for most proximal catheter obstructions [30], in spite of the disappointing results seen with the numerous ventricular catheters designed specifically to prevent choroid plexus attachment to the CSF-intake holes, such as the multiflanged Portnoy catheter [31–33]. Our group as studied the problem of ventricular obstruction extensively through analysis of explanted (obstructed) ventricular catheters from shunt dependent Seattle Children's Hospital utilizing comprehensive multichannel confocal microscopy [34]. With this approach, we found that microglia and astrocytes are the only cell types bound directly to the ventricular catheter surface in great numbers and that the microglia:astrocyte ratio on the catheter is time dependent. We observed that microglia are the first cells to attach to the CSF-intake holes in great numbers, based on the observation that failed catheters with a microglia dominant cellular response have generally been implanted for a shorter durations (mean: 24.7 days) than those demonstrating an astrocyte dominant cellular response (mean: 1183 days; $p = 0.027$). When choroid plexus was seen, it was always bound to the catheter secondarily via a sheet/bridge of astrocytes. Our finding that astrocytes don't appear on catheter CSF-intake holes in great numbers within the first 2 months of implantation helps to explain why only long-term indwelling catheter removals require use of Bugbee wire electrocautery to safely detach any affixed vascularized choroid plexus pedicles [35] and why choroid plexus attachment to external ventriculostomy drains implanted for less than 2 weeks is virtually unheard of. We suspect that microglia are the first cell type to arrive on the catheter surface in great numbers simply because they are exceptionally mobile in vivo following tissue injury [36, 37]. However, it is possible that co-stimulatory cytokine signaling between microglia and astrocytes may partially explain the later arrival of astrocytes on the catheter surface in this context [38]. On the basis of our microglia/astrocyte-centric model of ventricular catheter obstruction, our group is currently developing ventricular catheters with novel anti-inflammatory small-molecule surface modifications that are showing promise in early in vivo animal studies (unpublished data). While far more animal/safety testing will be required before first-in-human trials of any CNS implants designed to promote localized immune modulation, the authors are hopeful that further study of the innate immune response mounted to CNS implants will guide the logical development of more obstruction-resistant catheters.

Although numerous groups have attempted to improve ventricular catheter design through both structural [32, 39, 40] and chemical [41] modifications, no currently available ventricular catheter has demonstrated superiority with respect to noninfectious failure rates. One ventricular catheter design consideration that is intuitively very attractive is the notion of varying CSF-intake hole size so as to create greater flow uniformity throughout the intake holes along the length of the intraventricular portion of the catheter given the observation that 50–75% of CSF flow occurs via the two most proximal sets of intraventricular CSF-intake holes in traditional catheter designs with uniform CSF-intake hole sizes [42–44]. Introduced in 2007, the Rivulet catheter (Medtronic) is the first commercially available ventricular catheter designed to promote uniform CSF flow via variable CSF-intake hole sizes, with large holes near the catheter tip progressively decreasing in size in the more proximal portions of the ventricle [3]. However, while the principle behind the Rivulet catheter design is quite logical, more than a decade since its introduction, there have been no published reports demonstrating reductions in obstruction rates with the use of this catheter.

While catheters with unique structural designs are commercially available, the majority of modern ventricular catheters implanted remain *PDMS*-based blind-end tubes lined with roughly 500 μm-diameter CSF-intake holes with little science behind their design [32, 45]. The CSF-intake holes of these catheters are constructed by sharply "punching out" pieces of PDMS from preformed catheter tubing. This method for CSF-intake hole construction, while cost-effective, results in irregular, rough conduits that serve as an excellent substrate for attachment of astrocytes and microglia, the primary mediators of the central nervous system's foreign body immune response (Figs. 21.1 and 21.2) [47–49]. With this in mind our group is exploring various strategies to produce catheters possessing CSF-intake holes with smooth, irregularity-free features given the intuitive notion that making catheter CSF-intake holes as less favorable substrate for cell attachment will result in lower rates of hole occlusion (and therefore shunt failure). Given the importance of maintaining patency of ventricular catheter CSF-intake holes, other groups [50–52] have been exploring more hi-tech approaches to addressing this problem through the development of catheters with magnetic microactuators to clear cells/debris from CSF-intake holes. Still in the early stages of development, ventricular catheters with debris-clearing magnetic microactuators will require more testing before human trials. Notably, while magnetic microactuators are appealing because they can be controlled non-invasively using externally applied magnetic fields and therefore do not require an implanted power supply [53], it is this responsiveness to external magnetic fields that raises concerns regarding compatibility of these devices with magnetic resonance imaging (MRI) techniques [50, 54].

Ventricular Catheter Placement

Numerous technological innovations designed to improve the accuracy of ventricular catheter placement have been developed, although none of these technologies have demonstrated superiority over free-hand technique with respect to shunt failure rates when studied systematically [46]. The first device designed to specifically guide ventricular catheter placement, the simple Ghajar Guide (Neurodynamics, New York, NY), which is essentially a tripod with a central channel through which a ventricular catheter is placed, effectively ensuring a trajectory orthogonal to the skull surface, continues to endure [55]. As successful as any of the more hi-tech catheter placement aides to follow the Ghajar Guide has been shown to increase radiographically optimal catheter placement [56]. A Thomale Guide (Miethke,

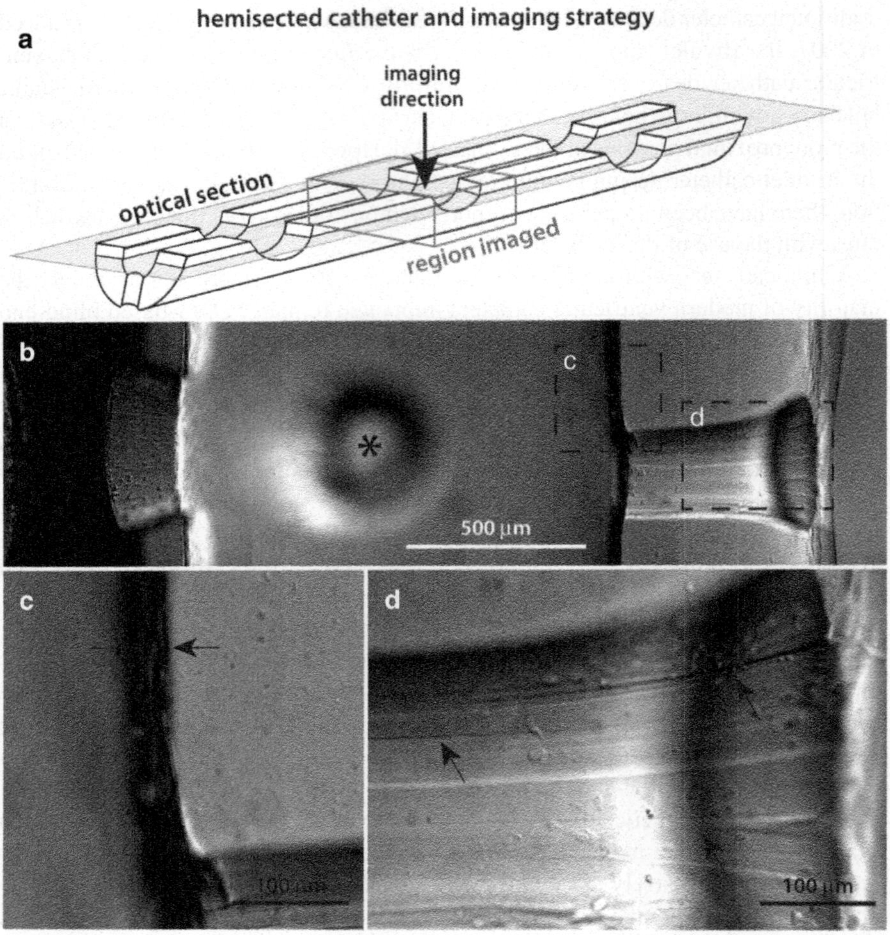

Fig. 21.1 Differential interference contrast imaging of explanted Codman® ACCU-FLO® ventricular catheter demonstrating surface irregularities. (**a**) A schematic demonstrating the method for imaging a longitudinally sectioned catheter. (**b**) 10× image of a single optical section (2.5 μm in depth) demonstrating irregularities of the catheter surface; note the out-of-focus CSF-intake hole which has an orthogonal orientation to the plane of imaging is denoted by (*). Enlarged views of the luminal (**c**) and CSF-intake hole (**d**) surfaces clearly demonstrate undulations and grooves (arrows), which serve as anchor points for cell attachment. (Reprinted with permission from Hanak et al. [46])

Potsdam, Germany) is similar to the Ghajar Guide in principle, although it allows for the angulation of the catheter trajectory to be adjusted in accordance with the patient's unique ventricular anatomy. Recently, a smartphone application has been developed that will compute frontal bur hole distance from midline, catheter length, and Thomale Guide angle based on a screenshot of a coronal plane image at the level of the anterior commissure [57]. Similar to the Ghajar Guide, the use of more hi-tech frameless stereotactic image guided systems for catheter placement results

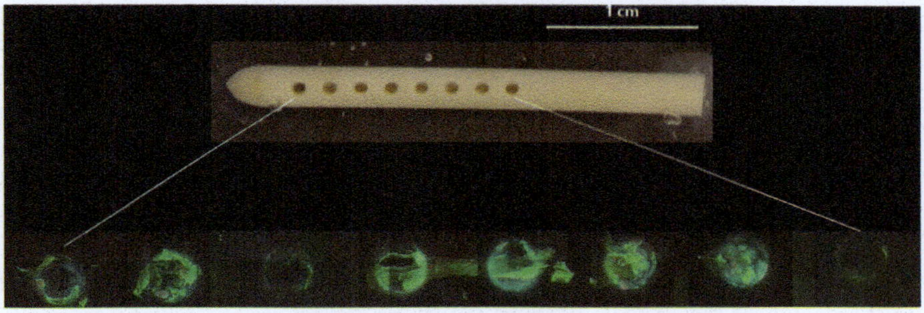

Fig. 21.2 Robust cellular attachment is seen at the CSF-intake holes of ventricular catheters explanted from patients. This gross photograph of an explanted Medtronic® Ares® antibiotic impregnated catheter alongside 3D confocal microscopy imaging of the same CSF-intake holes demonstrates extensive astrocyte attachment (GFAP labeled in green channel, nuclear stain in blue) to CSF-intake holes with a relative paucity of cell attachment to the comparatively smooth surfaces between the holes. (Reprinted with permission from Hanak et al. [34])

in higher rates of radiographically optimal catheter positions, although this has not translated to shunt failure rate reductions [58]. Endoscopic and ultrasound-guided catheter placement techniques have fared worse as they fail to improve catheter placement accuracy and the former technique may actually increase failure rates in pediatric patients [59, 60]. However, it bears mentioning, that although routine use of endoscopic techniques for shunt placement does not confer a benefit, the use of a rigid endoscope to assist with postinfectious intraventricular cyst fenestration in cases of multiloculated hydrocephalus is safe, if not safer, than performing cyst fenestration via open craniotomy [61].

In spite of considerable investment in the development of catheter placement technology, a firm consensus regarding the optimal surgical approach for ventricular catheter implantation has not been settled on, with some studies favoring the frontal/anterior and others the posterior parieto-occipital/posterior approach [62–65]. The largest and most recent study looking at the subject, a retrospective review of three large pediatric hydrocephalus studies (858 pediatric patients receiving a first time shunt), found the anterior approach to be superior to the posterior approach with approximately a one-third lower failure rate (HR 0.65; 95% CI 0.51–0.83) [66]. A randomized trial of anterior versus posterior ventricular catheter entry sites is currently enrolling across nine HCRN centers in the hope of providing a more definitive answer to this question [67].

Shunt Valves

In current state, there are a variety of readily available valves on the market from manufacturers such as Codman, Integra, Medtronic, Aesculap, and Sophysa. The main control mechanisms for these valves include differential pressure and flow regulation, with the possible addition of antisiphon components and the ability to magnetically change valves to several adjustable pressure settings [40]. While incremental changes have come onto the market regarding MRI compatibility and sizing options, little has changed in the fundamental design and function of the valves in many decades. All depend on the astute clinician to choose the right valve prior to surgery based on assumed or implied hydrocephalus physiology, and all have limits on functionality that must be weighed carefully prior to surgery. On occasions where the patient's needs exceed the scope of the valve, an additional surgery is required to change it. Furthermore, like ventricular catheters, valves are mechanical devices prone to occlusion or mechanical dysfunction [33].

As we have described in prior publications [45], many investigators are involved in the design of the so-called "smart valve" or "smart shunt," which essentially implies auto-adjusted CSF drainage according to feedback from measured physiologic conditions. These conditions can include intracranial pressure, the flow rate of CSF, or the position of the patient. We term this component of the smart shunt the *sensor*. One of the challenges with regard to sensors has been the extraordinary low flow rate of CSF, which has been an area of innovation within microsensor technology. Innovations have included using a thermistor and Wheatstone bridge to predict flow rate [68], looking at heat dissipation from a thermal source [69], impedance-based sensors [70], and pressure-sensitive capacitors [71]. These sensors must have low power needs (of which power sourcing is an additional challenge), they must be biocompatible and moisture-resistant, and they have controlled or resettable calibration while in vivo. Several groups have been actively working on sensors that can be added in line to existing valves and provide measurements at single time points [72, 73]. The ideal smart shunt system, however, will require continuous measurements to in turn allow for real-time feedback control. Of course, continuous sensing would require a substantial power draw. Another secondary point to consider is whether continuous sensing would occur with real-time monitoring/alerts vs wireless/Bluetooth data transmission to a computer source or cellular device, or whether the device would generate a historical record for the physician to review offline.

Pressure sensing has been a particular challenge to date due to the concerns over "drift," while many pressure sensors available today have drifts within an acceptable range over weeks or months the concerns remain about inaccuracies that can develop with a chronically implanted system that hopefully last for years if not decades. As an example, a highly accurate pressure sensor today may have a drift of ±1 mmHg/month. If the drift ends up being nonrandom, pressure readings upon which clinical decision are made could be inaccurate relative to atmospheric pressure by 12 mmHg or more, a significant and potentially misleading variance. Referencing or recalibrating to atmospheric pressure remains the objective but without the ability to sample pressures outside of the body, recalibration to the gold standard of atmospheric pressure remains an unsolved engineering dilemma. Our group and others have been working on solutions that leverage various forms of internal recalibration against known standards. This remains an area of active research in various laboratories and is fundamental to providing accurate representation of intracranial pressure if that ultimately the desired mechanism to control a "smart" shunt system.

In addition to sensors, smart shunts need to have mechanisms by which to control fluid motion (either using pumps or valves that are on/off or of variable resistance), an actuator which physically generates the flow of CSF [74], a power source (likely battery-dependent), a way to communicate with the device (Bluetooth, for example), and a housing unit that allows for CSF contact with the sensor and actuator but not the electrical components, and that allows for reference to atmospheric pressure [45]. These issues are formidable. Powering a smart shunt is a challenge especially if you are considering continuous monitoring of ICP. The minimally acceptable life span for a device is likely to be 5 years of continuous use before revision operation is undertaken similar to pacemakers and other devices such as baclofen pumps. Newer technologies such as inductive charging and energy scavenging may allow devices to "recharge" extending battery life and device function indefinitely. The housing in which devices reside is also a considerable challenge as the body normally attempts to "wall-off" and encapsulate foreign bodies with fibrous tissue. This is a particular challenge to ensure the device is waterproof and any "windows" that might be put on the device to act as sensors must be robust.

Assuming the technical challenges of building a smart shunt can be overcome, including the ability to regulate to pressure and/or flow, it remains unknown how best to manage these systems to best mimic normal human physiology. Many factors need to be taken into account as devices become smarter. Transients such as Valsalva maneuvers can increase the ICP to over 50 mmHg for short periods of time, children crying, coughing, bowel movements, periods of exercise, and exertion all can lead to marked but transient elevations in ICP. Smart systems will need to be able to recognize and manage transient events but similarly identify when a transient event becomes prolonged and represents a meaningful sign of shunt system failure. It is recognized that CSF flow can also be intermittent and variable. When does lack of flow represent a potential device failure versus normal physiology? Given the ability to record and analyze ICP waveforms, does this ultimately become the controlling modality? Significant complexities and variability are seen in ICP waveforms, and smart systems will need to be able to identify and distinguish between variances in wave form morphology due to the cardiac cycle, Valsalva events, and other complex physiologic events. It remains unclear whether a complex management system driven by multiple data points is necessary to achieve optimal control of a smart shunt, and others (Dr. Jack Walker-personal communication) suggest managing to flow may be perfectly satisfactory to achieve good results.

Diagnosis and Treatment of Shunt Malfunction

In current clinical practice, the diagnosis of a malfunctioning ventricular shunt can be challenging. Because there is no direct noninvasive physical method of observing the flow of fluid through the ventricular catheter, valve, and distal tubing, the functionality of a CSF shunt is inferred in a variety of ways. Clinical symptoms typical of shunt malfunction include headache, nausea, vomiting, an increase in baseline seizure frequency, lethargy, irritability, lability, or coma. Clinical signs can include pupillary changes, papilledema, alterations in level of consciousness, vital sign changes including bradycardia or hypertension, fluid around the shunt valve or leakage from shunt incisions, or changes in the fontanelle and cranial suture examination in infants. Radiographic examinations are typically employed, including X-rays, computed tomography (CT), MRI, and nuclear medicine studies. X-rays can demonstrate kinks, discontinuities, or malposition of shunt components. CT and MRI studies of the brain can demonstrate changes in ventricular caliber or configuration characteristic of shunt failure. Nuclear medicine studies may demonstrate lack of dispersion in the ventricular system or abdomen, or a significant delay in transit of the radiotracer through the shunt system. Invasive studies include shunt taps, which can determine proximal patency and allow for measurement of an intracranial pressure through direct manometry, or operative shunt exploration. All of our noninvasive tools have drawbacks, unfortunately. Shunted patients can exhibit a wide variability in their clinical signs and symptoms of shunt failure, and some children with neurological and psychiatric comorbidities may be quite difficult to examine. Some children may not change their ventricular caliber with shunt failure. CTs expose children to ionizing radiation [75], while MRIs may alter the programming of magnetic shunt valves (and even occasionally break them) [76–78]. Nuclear medicine shunt studies have demonstrated variable sensitivity and specificity even under stringent conditions [79].

Various technologies and concepts have been put forth to either diagnosis shunt malfunction or provide a mechanism to treat or prevent obstructions from occurring. Non-invasive ICP monitoring has been the holy grail sought for diagnosing a variety of neurosurgical maladies. In regard to hydrocephalus, many groups have been working on devices that can be placed in series with the shunt valve to provide on-demand ICP measurements that can guide clinical decision making. To date these devices have not reached clinical trials and remain challenging due to issues raised about sensor drift and recalibration. The ability to sense ICP and especially elevated ICP remains a desired clinical tool. CSF flow is also another potential diagnostic modality.

The use of telemetry has been used in cardiology for some time and devices exist that provide feedback to the patient and record physiologic variables that can be analyzed and shared with healthcare providers remotely. There is a desire from patients to have similar systems for hydrocephalus management whereby indicators of shunt patency or function can be assessed real time. For example, is a patient's headache due to shunt malfunction or simply something that should be treated with an analgesic? Knowing the functional status of the shunt system would be a highly sought-after feature and would reduce the anxiety of patients and families and reduce the cost of hydrocephalus care immensely. The caveat is these systems will need to be highly reliable with rare false negative readings or analysis.

Several devices have been described and are in various stages of commercial development that are aimed at clearing a shunt obstruction. Various techniques have been proposed including mechanical disruption of obstruction at the proximal catheter by accessing the shunt through a reservoir and mechanically removing the obstruction via use of electrocautery or other means of tissue removal such as rotatory blades similar to devices used in peripheral artery recanalization. Other systems include new devices that are either integrated into the valve or ride in series that allow for "back-flushing" of the device after obstruction occurs (Fig. 21.3). These types of devices have not been shown to work clinically after obstruction has already occurred. Other groups are making systems whereby "new" holes can be exposed in a proximal catheter after the "existing" holes become obstructed. Our group has been interested in developing systems that maintain patency from the time implantation essentially creating an electromechanical mechanism to provide repeated countermeasures aimed at preventing cell adhesion, migration, and ultimately obstruction at the proximal catheter inlets.

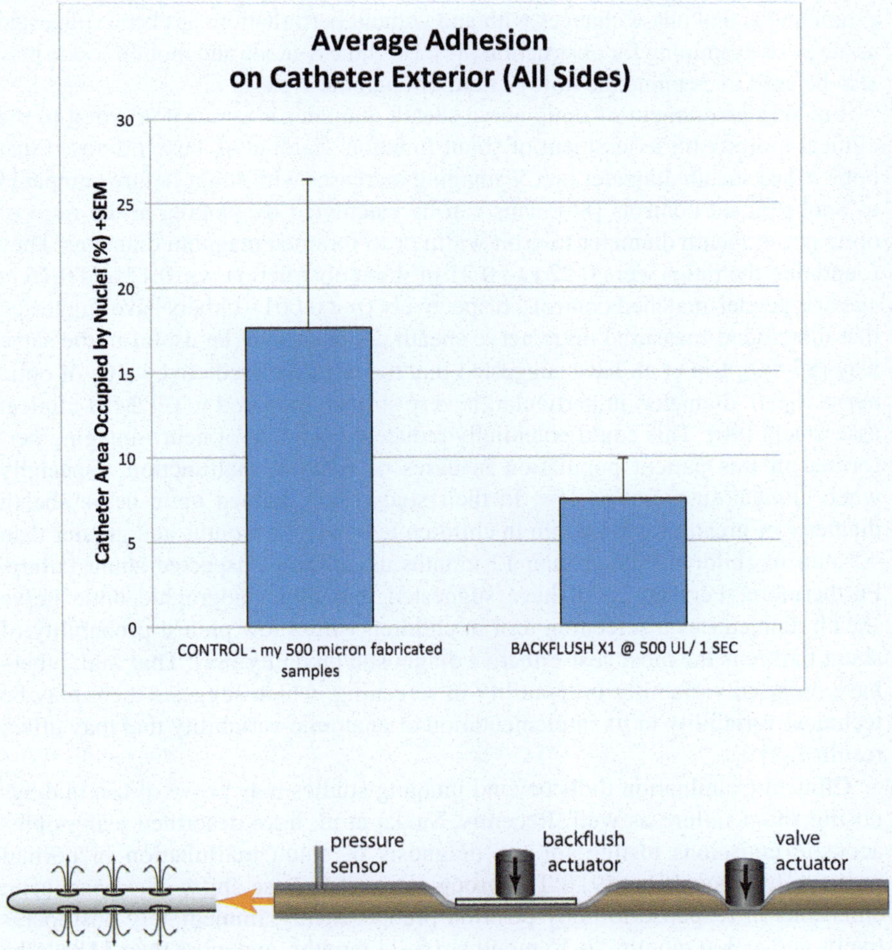

Fig. 21.3 Above: Backflushing reduces cellular debris (unpublished data). Below: A schematic of an in-line valve and backflush actuator to mitigate obstruction

Existing Clinically Relevant Imaging and Examination Modalities

Original attempts at noninvasively assessing shunt patency used MR imaging to quantify the flow of CSF through the tubing. Using a model shunt system and tubing designed for MR studies, Frank et al. were able to demonstrate the spin echo images could potentially differentiate between flow rates of 2.5–20 mL/h [80]. Two years later in a follow-up study, they were able to demonstrate sensitivity to 0.8 mL/h flow [81]. Unfortunately, attempts to translate this technique to clinical use were hamstrung by the fact that the position of the shunt valve and catheter significantly altered the measurement and flow, limiting its reliability and accuracy [82]. Another noninvasive imaging modality described to assess shunt patency is contrast enhanced ultrasound, which has been shown in vitro to differentiate between flow rates low enough to be relevant physiologically [83]. Even non-contrasted ultrasound, by examining signal phase changes with and without perturbation, has been suggested as a way of examining for obstruction [84]. Brightness-mode and motion-mode may also be used to examine the flow of fluid through the system.

Imaging assessment of optic nerve sheath diameter is a recent addition to the clinical toolbox for assessment of shunt function. Zaidi et al. have proposed that optic nerve sheath diameter on CT imaging increases with shunt failure compared to unobstructed controls [85]. This can by calculated by looking at the ratio of optic nerve sheath diameter to orbit width or to foramen magnum diameter. They found that the ratios were 0.22 and 0.21 in shunt obstruction, vs. 0.17 and 0.16 in age and gender-matched controls, respectively ($p < 0.001$). Others have suggested that ultrasound-measured optic nerve sheath diameter may be useful in the same way [85–90]. Lin et al. have suggested that the negative predictive value of optic nerve sheath diameter, in particular, is very strong compared to CT/MRI clinical assessment [90]. This could potentially reduce the amount of neuro-imaging performed in this patient population in cases of rule-out malfunction, especially when clinical suspicion is low. In their study, they defined optic nerve sheath diameter of greater than 4.0 mm in children less than 12 months and greater than 4.5 mm in children greater than 12 months as defining suspected shunt failure. Furthermore, Pershad et al. have suggested that ultrasonographic optic nerve sheath diameter as a screening tool in children with a low pretest probability of shunt failure is the most cost-effective diagnostic modality [89]. That said, others have reported variability in its utility in screening, which suggests there may be technical variability in its implementation or anatomic variability that may affect results [87].

Clinical examination tools beyond imaging studies may prove of use in diagnosing shunt failure as well. Recently, Sakka et al. have described using opto-acoustic emissions testing for the diagnosis of shunt malfunction in normal pressure hydrocephalus [91]. The group measured phase shifts of optoacoustic emissions in response to body position preoperatively, immediately postoperatively, and at 3–6 months, 7–15 months, 16–24 months, and more than 24 months postoperatively. They found that changes in phase shifts may predict the need for shunt revision and may change in relation to valve adjustments. Since this study was small and largely descriptive, it is not clear how this will translate into sensitivity and specificity for shunt failure in a larger and more diverse hydrocephalus population, particularly in etiologies other than normal pressure hydrocephalus.

Novel Biomedical Devices

The ShuntCheck device (NeuroDx, Yardley, PA), now in its third iteration, is a biomedical device that uses thermal dilution methods to detect flow through shunt tubing. Simply put, it transcutaneously transduces the temperature of CSF by placing an ice pack on proximal shunt tubing and the sensor over the clavicle, where tubing is usually apparent and fairly superficial. It detects whether the cooled fluid reaches the transducer to determine if there is flow through the tubing. Unfortunately, to date, the scientific rigor with which this device has been studied is limited and the results have been variable. In 2005, Neff demonstrated that flow in a functioning shunt could be demonstrated using this technique in nine out of ten attempts, with positive and negative predictive values at least as good as existing radiographic studies [92]. Madsen et al. used the device on 100 shunted patients, of which 48 were evaluated for shunt malfunction and 24 went onto surgical exploration [93]. They found that while the device was 80% sensitive and 100% specific for flow at surgery, it was unable to distinguish between those that when onto surgery and those that were discharged without it. Many patients were identified in clinical visits as not having flow but did not have suspected shunt malfunction—thus, surgical decision-making could not depend on the results. Marlin and Gaskill had a similar experience using the ShuntCheck device, showing that flow was demonstrated in only 51% of functioning shunts [94]. Likely more work will need to be done to understand how the ShuntCheck can be optimized for clinical use in evaluating the shunted patient.

Technology integrated within the shunt system will have a future role in diagnosis of shunt failure as well. Microelectromechanical systems (MEMS), for example, may detect in addition to mitigate shunt failure. MEMS has been described in approaches to designing better, non-obstructing ventricular catheters [50, 51] and "smarter" valves [95]. MEMS sensors can monitor CSF flow transcutaneously across a dynamic range of flow rates and pressures [96]. Song et al. have described a microfluidic pressure sensor essentially consisting of a PDMS film bonded over a reservoir to form a fluidic capacitor [97]. This allows for wireless monitoring of pressure and flow through shunt valves. Kim et al. have reported a parylene MEMS patency sensor that could potentially be integrated into shunt systems for wireless detection of performance [98]. In preliminary studies with external ventricular drains, promise has been shown for detecting obstruction. These sensors, which can perform across a wide range of flow rates and temperatures, may be the future of shunt systems.

Endovascular Devices to Manage Hydrocephalus

The use of endovascular techniques to address hydrocephalus is now appearing. There is a recent entrant, the CereVasc eShunt, (CereVasc, LLC, Auburndale, MA) that accesses the inferior petrosal sinus via an endovascular approach then deploys a tubing set through the dural into the cerebellopontine angle cistern. The idea is to treat communicating hydrocephalus via a direct shunt from CSF cistern to venous outflow portal. Our understanding at the time of this manuscript is that the group has performed this in animal models but has not reached human trials. It remains to be seen if this highly novel technique will be safe, effective or potentially reduce the risks of shunt malfunction inherent in current devices implanted today.

Conclusions

We tried to provide a general overview in the technical advances within hydrocephalus treatment, and provide a conceptual framework off which we can think about future developments. Hopefully we are entering an era where we can transition from incremental advances in the technological approaches to hydrocephalus to more substantive paradigm shifts. Ventricular catheter design will focus on avoidance of obstruction and infection. Valve design will focus on data collection/transmission and feedback mechanisms to alter flow rates. Advances in imaging and novel biomedical devices will facilitate the noninvasive detection of shunt obstruction. Several devices are currently on the market or coming to market that require rigorous study and physician-facilitated modification to enhance care delivery. It is clear that our engineering colleagues require surgeon engagement and feedback to optimize devices for meaningful clinical use.

References

1. Nulsen FE, Spitz EB. Treatment of hydrocephalus by direct shunt from ventricle to jugular vain. Surg Forum. 1951:399–403.
2. Tomei KL. The evolution of cerebrospinal fluid shunts: advances in technology and technique. Pediatr Neurosurg. 2017;52(6):369–80.
3. Weisenberg SH, et al. Ventricular catheter development: past, present, and future. J Neurosurg. 2016;125(6):1504–12.
4. Pudenz RH, et al. Ventriculo-auriculostomy; a technique for shunting cerebrospinal fluid into the right auricle; preliminary report. J Neurosurg. 1957;14(2):171–9.
5. Ames RH. Ventriculo-peritoneal shunts in the management of hydrocephalus. J Neurosurg. 1967;27(6):525–9.
6. Izci Y, et al. Initial experience with silver-impregnated polyurethane ventricular catheter for shunting of cerebrospinal fluid in patients with infected hydrocephalus. Neurol Res. 2009;31(3):234–7.
7. Kestle J, et al. Long-term follow-up data from the Shunt Design Trial. Pediatr Neurosurg. 2000;33(5):230–6.
8. Korinek AM, et al. Morbidity of ventricular cerebrospinal fluid shunt surgery in adults: an 8-year study. Neurosurgery. 2011;68(4):985–94; discussion 994–5
9. Attenello FJ, et al. Hospital costs associated with shunt infections in patients receiving antibiotic-impregnated shunt catheters versus standard shunt catheters. Neurosurgery. 2010;66(2):284–9; discussion 289

10. Ritz R, et al. Do antibiotic-impregnated shunts in hydrocephalus therapy reduce the risk of infection? An observational study in 258 patients. BMC Infect Dis. 2007;7:38.
11. Kestle JR, et al. A new Hydrocephalus Clinical Research Network protocol to reduce cerebrospinal fluid shunt infection. J Neurosurg Pediatr. 2016;17(4):391–6.
12. Konstantelias AA, et al. Antimicrobial-impregnated and -coated shunt catheters for prevention of infections in patients with hydrocephalus: a systematic review and meta-analysis. J Neurosurg. 2015;122(5):1096–112.
13. Klimo P Jr, et al. Pediatric hydrocephalus: systematic literature review and evidence-based guidelines. Part 7: Antibiotic-impregnated shunt systems versus conventional shunts in children: a systematic review and meta-analysis. J Neurosurg Pediatr. 2014;14(Suppl 1):53–9.
14. Parker SL, et al. Cost savings associated with antibiotic-impregnated shunt catheters in the treatment of adult and pediatric hydrocephalus. World Neurosurg. 2015;83(3):382–6.
15. Klimo P Jr, et al. Antibiotic-impregnated shunt systems versus standard shunt systems: a meta- and cost-savings analysis. J Neurosurg Pediatr. 2011;8(6):600–12.
16. Jenkinson MD, et al. The British antibiotic and silver-impregnated catheters for ventriculoperitoneal shunts multi-centre randomised controlled trial (the BASICS trial): study protocol. Trials. 2014;15:4.
17. Bridgett MJ, et al. In vitro assessment of bacterial adhesion to Hydromer-coated cerebrospinal fluid shunts. Biomaterials. 1993;14(3):184–8.
18. Kaufmann AM, et al. Infection rates in standard vs. hydrogel coated ventricular catheters. Can J Neurol Sci. 2004;31(4):506–10.
19. Kestle JR, et al. A standardized protocol to reduce cerebrospinal fluid shunt infection: the Hydrocephalus Clinical Research Network Quality Improvement Initiative. J Neurosurg Pediatr. 2011;8(1):22–9.
20. Xu H, et al. Hydrogel-coated ventricular catheters for high-risk patients receiving ventricular peritoneum shunt. Medicine (Baltimore). 2016;95(29):e4252.
21. Tung H, Raffel C, McComb JG. Ventricular cerebrospinal fluid eosinophilia in children with ventriculoperitoneal shunts. J Neurosurg. 1991;75(4):541–4.
22. Traynelis VC, et al. Cerebrospinal fluid eosinophilia and sterile shunt malfunction. Neurosurgery. 1988;23(5):645–9.
23. Ellis MJ, et al. Treatment of recurrent ventriculoperitoneal shunt failure associated with persistent cerebrospinal fluid eosinophilia and latex allergy by use of an "extracted" shunt. J Neurosurg Pediatr. 2008;1(3):237–9.
24. Pittman T, et al. The role of ethylene oxide allergy in sterile shunt malfunctions. Br J Neurosurg. 1994;8(1):41–5.
25. Hakim S. Observations on the physiopathology of the CSF pulse and prevention of ventricular catheter obstruction in valve shunts. Dev Med Child Neurol Suppl. 1969;20:42–8.
26. Sarkiss CA, et al. Time dependent pattern of cellular characteristics causing ventriculoperitoneal shunt failure in children. Clin Neurol Neurosurg. 2014;127:30–2.
27. Blegvad C, et al. Pathophysiology of shunt dysfunction in shunt treated hydrocephalus. Acta Neurochir. 2013;155(9):1763–72.
28. Del Bigio MR. Biological reactions to cerebrospinal fluid shunt devices: a review of the cellular pathology. Neurosurgery. 1998;42(2):319–25; discussion 325–6
29. Sekhar LN, Moossy J, Guthkelch AN. Malfunctioning ventriculoperitoneal shunts. Clinical and pathological features. J Neurosurg. 1982;56(3):411–6.
30. Kraemer MR, et al. Shunt-dependent hydrocephalus: management style among members of the American Society of Pediatric Neurosurgeons. J Neurosurg Pediatr. 2017;20(3):216–24.
31. Haase J, Weeth R. Multiflanged ventricular Portnoy catheter for hydrocephalus shunts. Acta Neurochir. 1976;33(3–4):213–8.
32. Harris CA, McAllister JP 2nd. What we should know about the cellular and tissue response causing catheter obstruction in the treatment of hydrocephalus. Neurosurgery. 2012;70(6):1589–601; discussion 1601–2
33. Browd SR, et al. Failure of cerebrospinal fluid shunts: part I: obstruction and mechanical failure. Pediatr Neurol. 2006;34(2):83–92.

34. Hanak BW, et al. Toward a better understanding of the cellular basis for cerebrospinal fluid shunt obstruction: report on the construction of a bank of explanted hydrocephalus devices. J Neurosurg Pediatr. 2016;18(2):213–23.
35. Chambi I, Hendrick EB. A technique for removal of an adherent ventricular catheter. Pediatr Neurosci. 1988;14(4):216–7.
36. Davalos D, et al. ATP mediates rapid microglial response to local brain injury in vivo. Nat Neurosci. 2005;8(6):752–8.
37. Kim JV, Dustin ML. Innate response to focal necrotic injury inside the blood-brain barrier. J Immunol. 2006;177(8):5269–77.
38. Morales I, et al. Neuroinflammation in the pathogenesis of Alzheimer's disease. A rational framework for the search of novel therapeutic approaches. Front Cell Neurosci. 2014;8:112.
39. Harris CA, McAllister JP 2nd. Does drainage hole size influence adhesion on ventricular catheters? Childs Nerv Syst. 2011;27(8):1221–32.
40. Drake JM, Sainte-Rose C. The shunt book. New York: Wiley; 1995.
41. Harris CA, et al. Effects of surface wettability, flow, and protein concentration on macrophage and astrocyte adhesion in an in vitro model of central nervous system catheter obstruction. J Biomed Mater Res A. 2011;97(4):433–40.
42. Harris CA, et al. Reduction of protein adsorption and macrophage and astrocyte adhesion on ventricular catheters by polyethylene glycol and N-acetyl-L-cysteine. J Biomed Mater Res A. 2011;98(3):425–33.
43. Lin J, et al. Computational and experimental study of proximal flow in ventricular catheters. Technical note. J Neurosurg. 2003;99(2):426–31.
44. Galarza M, et al. Computational fluid dynamics of ventricular catheters used for the treatment of hydrocephalus: a 3D analysis. Childs Nerv Syst. 2014;30(1):105–16.
45. Lutz BR, Venkataraman P, Browd SR. New and improved ways to treat hydrocephalus: pursuit of a smart shunt. Surg Neurol Int. 2013;4(Suppl 1):S38–50.
46. Hanak BW, et al. Cerebrospinal fluid shunting complications in children. Pediatr Neurosurg. 2017;52(6):381–400.
47. Craighead HG, et al. Chemical and topographical surface modification for control of central nervous system cell adhesion. Biomed Microdevices. 1998;1(1):49–64.
48. Minev IR, et al. Interaction of glia with a compliant, microstructured silicone surface. Acta Biomater. 2013;9(6):6936–42.
49. Turner AM, et al. Attachment of astroglial cells to microfabricated pillar arrays of different geometries. J Biomed Mater Res. 2000;51(3):430–41.
50. Lee H, et al. Mechanical evaluation of unobstructing magnetic microactuators for implantable ventricular catheters. J Microelectromech Syst. 2014;23(4):795–802.
51. Lee SA, et al. Magnetic microactuators for MEMS-enabled ventricular catheters for hydrocephalus. Conf Proc IEEE Eng Med Biol Soc. 2006;1:2494–7.
52. Yoon HJ, et al. Micro devices for a cerebrospinal fluid (CSF) shunt system. Sens Actuators A Phys. 2004;110(1–3):68–76.
53. Judy JW, Muller RS. Magnetic microactuation of torsional polysilicon structures. Sens Actuators A Phys. 1996;53(1–3):392–7.
54. Lee H, et al. Evaluation of magnetic resonance imaging issues for implantable microfabricated magnetic actuators. Biomed Microdevices. 2014;16(1):153–61.
55. Ghajar JB. A guide for ventricular catheter placement. Technical note. J Neurosurg. 1985;63(6):985–6.
56. O'Leary ST, et al. Efficacy of the Ghajar Guide revisited: a prospective study. J Neurosurg. 2000;92(5):801–3.
57. Ozerov S, et al. The use of a smartphone-assisted ventricle catheter guide for Ommaya reservoir placement-experience of a retrospective bi-center study. Childs Nerv Syst. 2018;34(5):853–9.
58. Levitt MR, et al. Image-guided cerebrospinal fluid shunting in children: catheter accuracy and shunt survival. J Neurosurg Pediatr. 2012;10(2):112–7.

59. Whitehead WE, et al. No significant improvement in the rate of accurate ventricular catheter location using ultrasound-guided CSF shunt insertion: a prospective, controlled study by the Hydrocephalus Clinical Research Network. J Neurosurg Pediatr. 2013;12(6):565–74.
60. Riva-Cambrin J, et al. Risk factors for shunt malfunction in pediatric hydrocephalus: a multicenter prospective cohort study. J Neurosurg Pediatr. 2016;17(4):382–90.
61. Akbari SH, et al. Surgical management of complex multiloculated hydrocephalus in infants and children. Childs Nerv Syst. 2015;31(2):243–9.
62. Sainte-Rose C. Shunt obstruction: a preventable complication? Pediatr Neurosurg. 1993;19(3):156–64.
63. Hoffman HJ, Smith MS. The use of shunting devices for cerebrospinal fluid in Canada. Can J Neurol Sci. 1986;13(2):81–7.
64. Buster BE, et al. Proximal ventricular shunt malfunctions in children: factors associated with failure. J Clin Neurosci. 2016;24:94–8.
65. Becker DP, Nulsen FE. Control of hydrocephalus by valve-regulated venous shunt: avoidance of complications in prolonged shunt maintenance. J Neurosurg. 1968;28(3):215–26.
66. Whitehead WE, et al. Ventricular catheter entry site and not catheter tip location predicts shunt survival: a secondary analysis of 3 large pediatric hydrocephalus studies. J Neurosurg Pediatr. 2017;19(2):157–67.
67. Whitehead WE. A randomized controlled trial of anterior versus posterior entry site for CSF shunt insertion. 2014. Available from: http://hcrn.org/research/entry-site/.
68. Qin C, Stamos B, Dasgupta PK. Inline shunt flow monitor for hydrocephalus. Anal Chem. 2017;89(15):8170–6.
69. Bork T, et al. Development and in-vitro characterization of an implantable flow sensing transducer for hydrocephalus. Biomed Microdevices. 2010;12(4):607–18.
70. Basati S, et al. Impedance changes indicate proximal ventriculoperitoneal shunt obstruction in vitro. IEEE Trans Biomed Eng. 2015;62(12):2787–93.
71. Raj R, et al. Demonstration that a new flow sensor can operate in the clinical range for cerebrospinal fluid flow. Sens Actuators A Phys. 2015;234:223–31.
72. Wakeland W, McNames J, Goldstein B. Calibrating an intracranial pressure dynamics model with clinical data—a progress report. Conf Proc IEEE Eng Med Biol Soc. 2004;1:746–9.
73. Wakeland W, Goldstein B. A review of physiological simulation models of intracranial pressure dynamics. Comput Biol Med. 2008;38(9):1024–41.
74. Szczesny S, Jetzki S, Leonhardt S. Review of current actuator suitability for use in medical implants. Conf Proc IEEE Eng Med Biol Soc. 2006;1:5956–9.
75. Antonucci MC, et al. The burden of ionizing radiation studies in children with ventricular shunts. J Pediatr. 2017;182:210–216.e1.
76. Watanabe A, Seguchi T, Hongo K. Overdrainage of cerebrospinal fluid caused by detachment of the pressure control cam in a programmable valve after 3-tesla magnetic resonance imaging. J Neurosurg. 2010;112(2):425–7.
77. Lavinio A, et al. Magnetic field interactions in adjustable hydrocephalus shunts. J Neurosurg Pediatr. 2008;2(3):222–8.
78. Bullivant KJ, Mitha AP, Hamilton MG. Management of a locked Strata valve. J Neurosurg Pediatr. 2009;3(4):340–3.
79. Thompson EM, et al. Using a 2-variable method in radionuclide shuntography to predict shunt patency. J Neurosurg. 2014;121(6):1504–7.
80. Frank E, Buonocore M, Hein L. The use of magnetic resonance imaging to assess slow fluid flow in a model cerebrospinal fluid shunt system. Br J Neurosurg. 1990;4(1):53–7.
81. Frank E, Buonocore M, Hein L. Magnetic resonance imaging analysis of extremely slow flow in a model shunt system. Childs Nerv Syst. 1992;8(2):73–5.
82. Frank E, Buonocore M, Hein L. The effect of position on magnetic resonance evaluation of cerebrospinal fluid shunt function. Neurol Res. 1994;16(3):168–70.
83. Hartman R, et al. Quantitative contrast-enhanced ultrasound measurement of cerebrospinal fluid flow for the diagnosis of ventricular shunt malfunction. J Neurosurg. 2015;123(6):1420–6.

84. Aralar AJ, et al. Ultrasound characterization of interface oscillation as a proxy for ventriculoperitoneal shunt function. Conf Proc IEEE Eng Med Biol Soc. 2016;2016:215–8.
85. Zaidi SJ, Yamamoto LG. Optic nerve sheath diameter measurements by CT scan in ventriculoperitoneal shunt obstruction. Hawaii J Med Public Health. 2014;73(8):251–5.
86. Newman WD, et al. Measurement of optic nerve sheath diameter by ultrasound: a means of detecting acute raised intracranial pressure in hydrocephalus. Br J Ophthalmol. 2002;86(10):1109–13.
87. Hall MK, et al. Bedside optic nerve sheath diameter ultrasound for the evaluation of suspected pediatric ventriculoperitoneal shunt failure in the emergency department. Childs Nerv Syst. 2013;29(12):2275–80.
88. Ertl M, et al. Measuring changes in the optic nerve sheath diameter in patients with idiopathic normal-pressure hydrocephalus: a useful diagnostic supplement to spinal tap tests. Eur J Neurol. 2017;24(3):461–7.
89. Pershad J, et al. Imaging strategies for suspected acute cranial shunt failure: a cost-effectiveness analysis. Pediatrics. 2017;140(2):pii: e20164263.
90. Lin SD, et al. The use of ultrasound-measured optic nerve sheath diameter to predict ventriculoperitoneal shunt failure in children. Pediatr Emerg Care. 2017; https://doi.org/10.1097/PEC.0000000000001034.
91. Sakka L, et al. Validation of a noninvasive test routinely used in otology for the diagnosis of cerebrospinal fluid shunt malfunction in patients with normal pressure hydrocephalus. J Neurosurg. 2016;124(2):342–9.
92. Neff S. Measurement of flow of cerebrospinal fluid in shunts by transcutaneous thermal convection. Technical note. J Neurosurg. 2005;103(4 Suppl):366–73.
93. Madsen JR, et al. Evaluation of the ShuntCheck noninvasive thermal technique for shunt flow detection in hydrocephalic patients. Neurosurgery. 2011;68(1):198–205; discussion 205
94. Marlin AE, Gaskill SJ. The use of transcutaneous thermal convection analysis to assess shunt function in the pediatric population. Neurosurgery. 2012;70(6):181–3.
95. Johansson SB, et al. A MEMS-based passive hydrocephalus shunt for body position controlled intracranial pressure regulation. Biomed Microdevices. 2014;16(4):529–36.
96. Apigo DJ, et al. An Angstrom-sensitive, differential MEMS capacitor for monitoring the milliliter dynamics of fluids. Sens Actuators A Phys. 2016;251:234–40.
97. Song SH, et al. Inductively coupled microfluidic pressure meter for in vivo monitoring of cerebrospinal fluid shunt function. J Med Eng Technol. 2012;36(3):156–62.
98. Kim BJ, et al. Parylene MEMS patency sensor for assessment of hydrocephalus shunt obstruction. Biomed Microdevices. 2016;18(5):87.

Index

D. D. Limbrick, J. R. Leonard (eds.), *Cerebrospinal Fluid Disorders*,
https://doi.org/10.1007/978-3-319-97928-1

The manufacturer's authorised representative in the EU is Springer Nature Customer Service Centre GmbH, Europaplatz 3, 69115 Heidelberg, Germany. If you have any concerns regarding our products, please contact ProductSafety@springernature.com

Printed and bound by CPI Group (UK) Ltd, Croydon, CR0 4YY
22/09/2026
02221065-0007